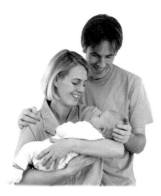

Encyclopedia of

FAMILY
HEALTH

& FIRST AID

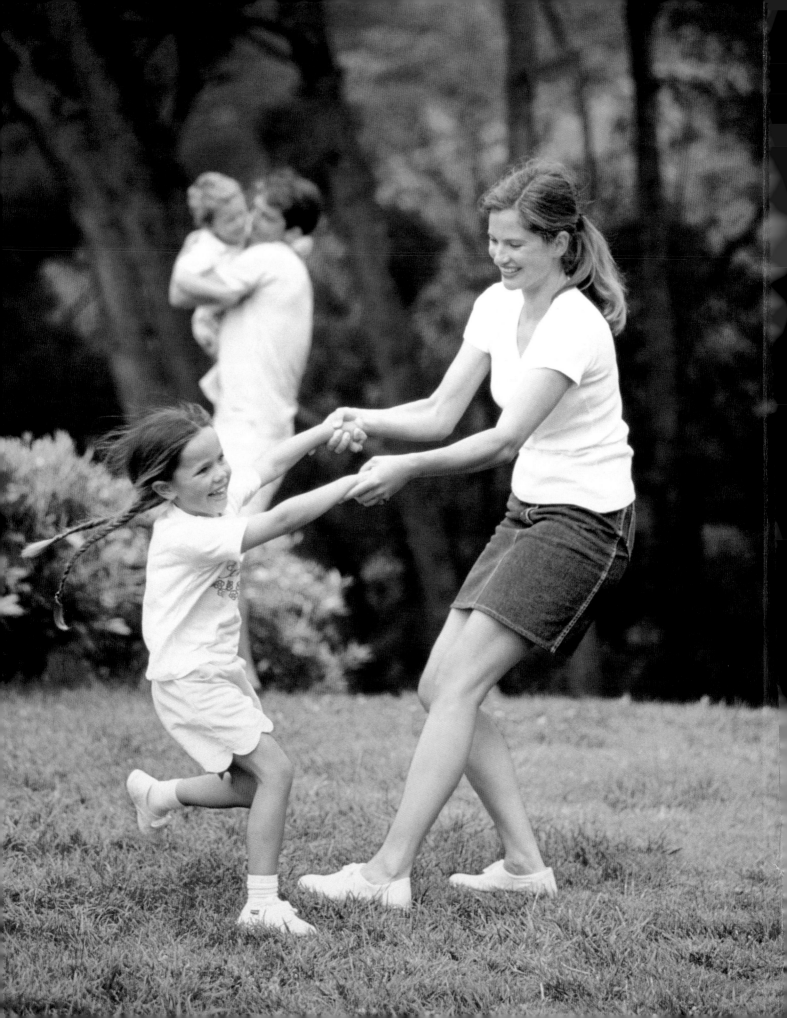

Encyclopedia of

FAMILY HEALTH

& FIRST AID

CONSULTANT EDITOR

Dr Susan Lipscombe

CONTRIBUTORS

Anita Kerwin – Nye

Dr Trevor Rees

Ellen Dupont

This is a Parragon Book

First published in 2003

Parragon
Queen Street House
4 Queen Street
Bath BA1 1HE, UK

Created and produced for Parragon by

THE BRIDGEWATER BOOK COMPANY LIMITED

CREATIVE DIRECTOR Terry Jeavons

ART DIRECTOR Michael Whitehead

EDITORIAL DIRECTOR Jason Hook

SENIOR PROJECT EDITOR Hazel Songhurst

PROJECT EDITOR Sara Harper

DESIGNER Alistair Plumb

PHOTOGRAPHER Mike Hemsley at Walter Gardiner

PICTURE RESEARCHER Lynda Marshall

ILLUSTRATIONS Michael Courtney, Coral Mula

FIRST AID CONSULTANT The Red Cross, Sussex Branch

PHOTO-SHOOT COORDINATORS Rebecca Gerlings and Claire Shanahan

INDEXER Ursula Caffrey

ISBN: 1-40541-539-8

Printed in China

CONTENTS

INTRODUCTION

In the developed world, medical advances over the past century have slashed the rate of deaths from infectious diseases and increased life expectancy by many years. However, many people are still becoming disabled by or dying prematurely from diseases that could often be prevented. Simple lifestyle changes, immunisation and screening, and awareness of the signs of illness, could mean the difference between life and death. The aim of Family Health and First Aid *is to provide people with the information they need in order to maintain a healthy and happy life.*

HOW THIS BOOK IS ORGANISED

This book is arranged into six main parts. The first and last cover first aid: PART ONE *is a detailed step-by-step guide,* PART SIX *is a ready-reference manual for use in an emergency. In between are four thematic sections that deal with aspects of well-being, health needs throughout life, illness and medical care. Each section has an introduction that provides an overview of the entire contents of the section, and contains a number of articles that deal with a specific subject, such as a certain disease, how to give rescue breaths, or another aspect of family health.*

WHAT EACH SECTION CONTAINS

PART ONE *is a step-by-step guide to first aid, the immediate help given to somebody who has been injured, or who suddenly becomes ill, before medical help is available. In-depth articles give information on how to practice first aid quickly, calmly and effectively. Reading this section gives you the underpinning knowledge to carry out first aid, and even if you are untrained, there are simple*

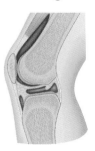

measures that
you can take
in an
emergency that
can save lives.

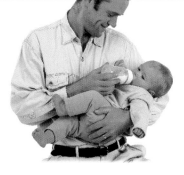

PART TWO: THE WELL BODY, *is divided
into two main sections. The first is a
guide to the human body, describing
all the different systems that work
together to sustain life. The second
section focuses on healthy living, with
detailed information on how to achieve
a healthy lifestyle, mainly through diet
and exercise, to reduce your risk of
developing certain diseases, make you
feel better and stay active for longer.*
PART THREE: FAMILY HEALTH, *takes
into account all aspects of health
throughout the various stages of life,
from conception to old age. Your
susceptibility to particular illnesses is
affected by your sex and changes as
you age.*
PART FOUR: ILLNESSES, *considers
the common illnesses we are
likely to encounter. This section
is not intended to be a
substitute for medical
treatment, but protecting*

*your health is often a matter of
understanding what causes disease so
you can take steps to avoid it.*
PART FIVE: MEDICAL CARE, TESTS,
TREATMENTS AND MEDICINES,
*describes the basics of medical care,
including various tests, methods of
treatment and medicines that are
routinely prescribed.*
PART SIX: FIRST AID IN ACTION,
*summarises a particular aspect of first
aid described in full in* PART ONE.

GOOD HEALTH IN YOUR HANDS
*Information on health abounds, from
government information campaigns, to
self-help groups, to the explosion of
internet sites. However, much advice is
confusing and contradictory, and*
Family Health and First Aid *aims to
provide a reliable, comprehensive, one-
stop guide to all aspects of
looking after yourself,
from the basics of
maintaining a healthy
lifestyle from infancy
to old age, to what
to do if a medical
emergency arises.*

PART ONE

PRACTICAL
FIRST AID

CONTENTS

INTRODUCTION

First aid is the immediate help given to somebody who has been injured, or who suddenly becomes ill, before medical help is available. First aid has three key aims: to keep the injured or ill person alive; to stop the condition worsening; and to promote the recovery of the patient. These aims can be met with simple skills that require little or no special equipment, but you must always put your own safety first. If you become a victim yourself, you will not be able to help the person and will make the situation worse.

The following pages give detailed information on how to practice first aid quickly, calmly and effectively. Reading this section gives you the underpinning knowledge to carry out first aid, but the term first aider is generally applied to somebody who has completed a set standard of training with an accredited training provider, such as the British Red Cross. Taking a practical course in first aid is the best preparation for dealing with an emergency. However, even if you are untrained there are simple measures that you can take at an emergency scene that can save lives.

This section aims to provide you with clear instructions to help you deal with common first aid situations, should they arise. Each spread in this chapter covers a particular aspect of first aid. Boxes describe signs and symptoms and give clear instructions on what and what not to do, and photographic step-by-step illustrations are used throughout to clarify the procedures. First aid for children and infants often requires different techniques, and these are clearly explained when they need to be done.

Articles describe how to assess a casualty so that appropriate treatment can be given while you wait for professional medical help to arrive. There are also practical discussions of emergency procedures, including checking for breathing and circulation, placing a person in the recovery position, and life-saving techniques such as giving rescue breaths (mouth-to-mouth resuscitation) if breathing has stopped, and chest compression if both breathing and circulation have ceased. Using these techniques will ensure that vital organs such as the brain receive enough oxygen to keep the person alive until medical help is at hand.

Further articles describe how to deal with other life-threatening situations or injuries, such as drowning, choking, shock, burns, poisoning and severe bleeding. Asthma, heart attack, epilepsy and allergic reactions may also require emergency treatment.

Specific injuries such as head and eye injuries, broken bones and spinal injuries are also covered in this section. Although these may not be immediately life-threatening, first aid may help someone recover more quickly and avoid permanent damage.

Most first aid situations will involve no more than minor cuts and bruises, but you should be equipped to deal with major accidents or emergencies, and you will need to understand and practice the techniques detailed in this section to give first aid effectively. You should also keep a well-stocked first aid box that is accessible in an emergency but kept out of the reach of children.

AT THE EMERGENCY SCENE

You will have to follow a set routine and establish your priorities when faced with an emergency. If possible, send someone to call for medical help while you deal with the situation. Make sure that you are in no danger and make the scene safe. Then check the victim's condition and carry out treatment as appropriate.

GETTING APPROPRIATE HELP

Life-threatening emergencies require professional medical assistance. If possible, ask a bystander to contact the emergency services by dialling 999 or 112 (112 is the single emergency number for all EU countries). Useful information to have to hand includes:

- *Details of what happened.*
- *Number of people injured.*
- *Type of illness or injuries.*
- *Whether a person is not breathing.*
- *The exact address with landmarks if possible.*
- *A contact phone number.*

Do not hang up until the operator tells you to. He or she may be able to guide you through first aid procedures if you are unsure what to do next.

MAKING THE SCENE SAFE

The cardinal rule of first aid is to ensure that you can give assistance without endangering yourself. Do not rush to the scene: walk slowly and steadily, looking around you for potential dangers and an overview of what has happened. Be prepared to take charge unless someone more qualified than you is present. Identify dangers and remove them if it is safe to do so, but if you cannot eliminate the danger, call for emergency help and advice and consider whether the danger poses a continuing risk to the injured person. If it does, assess whether you can safely move him or her. If in doubt, do not approach the scene. Keep everybody else back and call for emergency help.

BELOW *The best people to deal with first aid emergencies are qualified medical personnel. There are many sources of medical assistance available, from the ambulance crews who deal with road traffic accidents, to accident and emergency departments, doctor's surgeries and pharmacies. Keep a list of useful numbers by your telephone or stored in your mobile.*

Sources of medical help

- Ambulance
- Hospital Accident and Emergency Department
- Doctor's surgery
- Minor injuries clinics
- Pharmacists
- NHS Direct

There is a variety of sources of medical assistance throughout the country. Investigate what is available locally before an emergency happens, and keep a list of useful numbers by the phone or stored in your mobile.

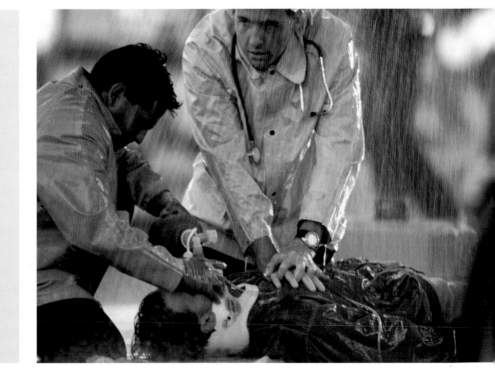

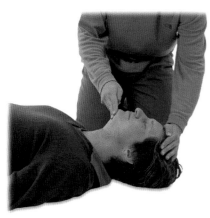

ABOVE *When a person is unconscious he is at risk of the airway becoming blocked by the tongue. To keep the airway open, place the victim on his back and open the airway by tilting the head and lifting the chin.*

RIGHT *To see if a person who has collapsed is still conscious, squeeze the shoulders gently (because the neck may be injured) and ask the person if he is all right. Speak loudly and clearly.*

Potential dangers include:

- *At the scene of an accident – other cars, broken glass or metal, and an unsteady crash vehicle.*
- *Chemicals, fire or electricity.*
- *Aggressive behaviour in those who may be ill, hysterical or as a result of drugs or alcohol.*
- *Sharp objects on the floor such as a knife or syringe.*

TREATING THE INJURED OR ILL

If you can give first aid safely, your priorities are to maintain an open airway and resuscitate if necessary, to treat serious bleeding and to treat for shock. If faced with several injured people, always approach the quietest first – a person who is shouting is at least able to maintain a clear airway.

Determining what may be wrong with an injured person is part of the treatment. To help you reach a provisional diagnosis you need to consider:

- *What actually happened (from what you or a bystander has observed).*
- *The signs (what you can see, hear, touch or smell on the casualty such as pale skin, swelling, noisy breathing, or alcohol on the breath.*
- *The symptoms (what the injured or ill person tells you – for example, he or she feels dizzy or is in pain).*

First aid by its very nature is often a highly emotional activity. It is important that you have the chance to discuss what happened with your family and friends, what you did and how you feel after helping at the scene of an accident.

BELOW *While waiting for help to arrive, place the victim in the recovery position. This keeps the airway open and allows fluid to flow out of the mouth if the victim vomits.*

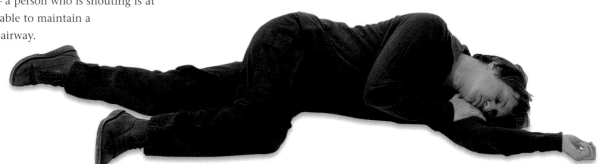

ACTION IN AN EMERGENCY

DANGER

Is anyone in danger?

✚ If yes, can the danger be easily managed?

✚ If it cannot, call for emergency help and protect the scene.

RESPONSE

Move to the quietest victim first

✚ Gently shake the shoulders and ask him or her a question.

✚ If there is a response, treat any life-threatening condition before checking the next person.

✚ If there is no response, check the airway.

ACT ON YOUR FINDINGS

If **not** breathing

✚ Give 2 rescue breaths by pinching the nose, sealing your mouth over his or her mouth and breathing into the person.

✚ If you are alone call for an ambulance as soon as you determine that the casualty is not breathing.

ACT ON YOUR FINDINGS

If breathing

✚ Check for and treat any life-threatening conditions and place in the recovery position.

AIRWAY

Open the airway

✚ *Lift the chin, check the mouth for any obstructions and remove, then tilt the head back gently.*

BREATHING

Check for breathing

✚ *Place your cheek to his or her mouth and listen and feel for breathing. Look to see if the chest is moving.*

NOT BREATHING

Look for signs of circulation

✚ *If victim is a child, or an adult who has suffered drowning or an accident, proceed direct to CPR (cardiopulmonary resuscitation).*

✚ *Otherwise look for signs of life such as movement and normal skin colour for 10 seconds.*

CIRCULATION PRESENT

Continue Rescue Breaths

✚ *Check for signs of circulation every minute.*

CIRCULATION NOT PRESENT

Start CPR (cardiopulmonary resuscitation)

✚ *Combine rescue breaths with chest compressions.*

ASSESSING A CASUALTY

Prompt action during an emergency could mean the difference between life and death. The following article describes how to assess a casualty's airway and breathing. For further information, see pages 18-19.

CHECK THE RESPONSE

If faced with a person who appears to be unresponsive, check the response by gently shaking the shoulders and asking loudly, 'Are you all right?' Speak loudly and clearly and shake gently because there may be a neck injury.

IF THERE IS NO RESPONSE

Shout for help. If possible, leave the casualty in the position in which you found him and open the airway. When it is not possible to carry out an assessment of the casualty in the position found, turn the person on to his back and open the airway.

OPEN THE AIRWAY

1 *Place one hand on the forehead and gently tilt the head back. Open the casualty's mouth and remove any obvious obstructions, including dislodged dentures, but leave well-fitting dentures in place.*

2 *Place the fingertips of the other hand under the point of the casualty's chin and lift the chin. If injury to the neck is suspected, handle the head very gently and try to avoid tilting the head.*

3 *Look, listen and feel for breathing for no more than 10 seconds.*

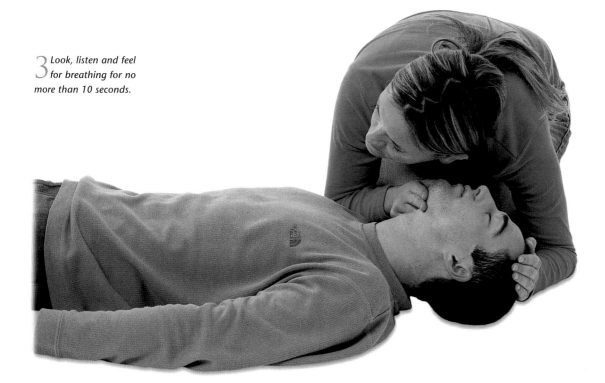

Apply the same techniques for a child as for an adult. For a baby, use only one finger under the chin and be very careful not to over-extend the neck when tilting the head back.

CHECK FOR BREATHING
Keep the airway open and look, listen and feel for breathing for no more than 10 seconds.

• Look for chest movement.
• Listen for sounds of breathing.
• Feel for breath on your cheek.

SIGNS AND SYMPTOMS OF A NON-BREATHING CASUALTY
• Unconsciousness, stillness.
• Pale skin with possible blue lips.
• No movement of the chest.
• No feeling or sound of breathing.

Assessing a baby or toddler
If the casualty is a toddler or a baby, it is important to handle them with care.
Roll the baby gently on to her back with one hand, making sure you cradle the head with the other. To open the airway, place only one finger under the chin and tilt the head back slowly. Do not tip the head back too far as this may cause damage to the neck. Once you are sure the airway is clear, check for breathing for no more than ten seconds.

Opening airway and checking breathing

DO
• *Check to see if the casualty is conscious.*
• *Open the airway gently by lifting the chin, checking in the mouth and tilting the head.*
• *Check for breathing for up to 10 seconds.*

DO NOT
• *Sweep blindly in the mouth for obstructions.*

WHAT IF
• *The person is unconscious? Treat any other injuries as necessary.*
• *The person is breathing? Turn into the recovery position (see pages 22-25).*
• *The person is not breathing? Give rescue breaths (see pages 26-29).*

MAINTAINING AIRWAY, BREATHING AND CIRCULATION

The most important principle of first aid is the ABC of resuscitation, which stands for Airway, Breathing and Circulation. This is a life-saving procedure that will enable you to decide whether a casualty who has collapsed needs rescue breaths or CPR (cardiopulmonary resuscitation). The airway must be open, breathing must be checked and circulation must be assessed. Always follow the ABC sequence before giving any other treatment if the casualty is unconscious.

RESUSCITATION

Resuscitation is the name given to the set of procedures that are applied when a person is not breathing, and their heart has possibly stopped. The full set of procedures is known as cardiopulmonary resuscitation (CPR). *Cardio* relates to the heart and *pulmonary* to the lungs.

The person whose heart has stopped (cardiac arrest), or who is not breathing (respiratory arrest), needs immediate treatment to improve the chances of survival. As speed is a key factor in survival, the treatment needs to be started before the arrival of the emergency ambulance and, as most cardiac arrests happen in the home or in the presence of a family member, friend or colleague, CPR skills are essential for everyone to know.

The best outcomes from cardiac or respiratory arrest are achieved when all the steps in the Chain of Survival (see panel) are in place.

Chain of survival

- *Early call for help*
- *Early CPR*
- *Early defibrillation (see below)*
- *Early medical care*

The first two of these steps are often in the hands of the first aider.

ABC of Resuscitation

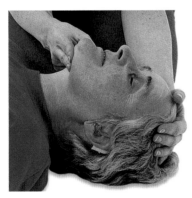

ABOVE Lay the victim on his back, tilt the head back and lift the chin to open the airway. Look at the casualty's chest for signs of breathing.

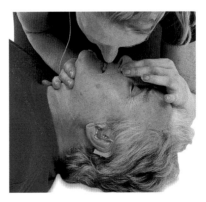

ABOVE If the person is not breathing, pinch the nose shut and keep the chin tilted. Seal your mouth over the casualty's and give 2 breaths.

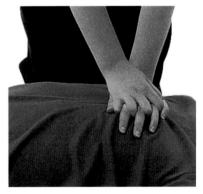

ABOVE Place interlocked hands on the casualty's breastbone, press down, then release. Alternate 15 chest compressions with 2 rescue breaths.

AN EARLY CALL FOR HELP

Ambulances today carry a range of equipment and treatments vital to the survival of seriously ill casualties. Calling for an ambulance early is an essential part of the Chain of Survival, particularly for a casualty whose heart has stopped.

EARLY CPR

CPR works by putting oxygen into the blood through breathing into the casualty's mouth or nose and by pushing the blood around the body by pressing on the chest and compressing the heart. The aim is to keep the person alive until emergency help arrives. Sometimes CPR alone will revive somebody whose heart has stopped but more often it is used to buy time until more advanced procedures are available.

EARLY DEFIBRILLATION

The most effective treatment for an adult whose heart has stopped pumping blood is defibrillation. In simple terms, this is an electric shock delivered in a very specific way to encourage the heart to begin beating effectively again. Defibrillators are carried in most ambulances but are also increasingly found in public places such as shopping malls, railway stations and airports, where local workers will have been trained in their use. Their early use is an essential factor in their effectiveness, highlighting again the need for an early call for help.

EARLY MEDICAL CARE

Medical treatments following cardiac and respiratory arrest are improving all the time. Early access to such treatments in the ambulance and in hospital play a major role in long-term survival rates.

THE PRINCIPAL STEPS OF RESUSCITATION

These are detailed on the following pages.

- *Check for danger to yourself and the casualty.*
- *Check for a response from the casualty.*

If there is no response
- *Open the airway.*

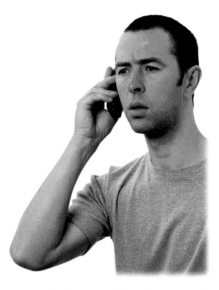

ABOVE *Call for an ambulance immediately if you are alone and the casualty has stopped breathing. The person is likely to have had a heart attack and will need early defibrillation from trained personnel.*

- *Check for breathing.*

If there is no breathing
- *Give 2 effective rescue breaths.*
- *Check for signs of circulation.*

If there are no signs of circulation
- *Start CPR.*

When to call an ambulance

1 If you are alone, breathing is absent and the casualty is an adult, call for an ambulance and/or for access to a defibrillator as soon as you realise the casualty is not breathing. The cause is most likely to be a heart attack leading to cardiac arrest, and the most effective treatment is CPR and very early access to defibrillation.

2 If you are alone and the casualty is an infant or a child under 8 years of age, provide 1 minute of rescue breaths or full CPR before calling for an ambulance. The cause is most likely to be a problem with breathing, such as choking or drowning etc., and the most effective treatment is to get oxygen into the lungs.

If you are not alone, send a bystander for the ambulance as soon as you have confirmed that the casualty is not breathing.

Calling for an ambulance

- *Dial 999 or 112 (the emergency number in all EU countries).*
- *Ask for the ambulance service.*
- *Listen to the operator – he will ask for your name, contact details and where you are.*
- *The operator will ask a series of questions about the casualty and what has happened – give as much information as you can.*
- *Often the operator will give you advice on what to do next.*
- *Do not put the phone down until you are told to do so.*

WHAT TO DO WHEN SOMEBODY HAS COLLAPSED

Facing a situation where somebody has collapsed is frightening, particularly if it is somebody you know. However, there are some very simple steps that you can take to help you decide the best course of action, which in an emergency could mean the difference between life and death.

CHECK THE SCENE

Is it safe for you to approach the person who has collapsed?

Do not become a victim yourself. Check for dangers such as chemicals, electricity or traffic. If you can safely remove the danger, do so. If not, consider if you can safely and easily move the person from the danger, or whether you need to call for additional help such as the fire service.

CHECK THE RESPONSE

Is the person who has collapsed conscious?
- *Gently squeeze the shoulders and ask loudly, 'Are you all right?'*
- *Speak loudly and clearly.*
- *Always assume there may be a neck injury and squeeze gently.*

For babies and young children, do not squeeze the shoulders – try to provoke a response by stroking the cheek or the sole of the foot and speaking loudly.

IF THERE IS NO RESPONSE

If there is no response, the immediate danger is that the casualty might be unconscious and may have a blocked airway or be in need of resuscitation.

- *Shout for help.*
- *If possible, leave the casualty in the position in which you found him and open the airway.*
- *When it is not possible to carry out an assessment of the casualty in the position found, turn him on to his back and open the airway.*

BELOW *The most important rule of first aid is never to put yourself in danger. Do not rush to the scene; look around you to assess potential dangers. If in doubt, stay back.*

What can block the airway?

The airway is made up of the nose, mouth and windpipe (trachea). These carry air, containing oxygen, to the lungs and remove the waste product carbon dioxide from the lungs. If the airway becomes blocked, the oxygen levels in the body drop and eventually the vital organs such as the brain and heart stop working. Death will follow unless action is taken.

A number of things can block the airway: blood, food and vomit are among the main culprits. In an unconscious person, however, the biggest risk is from the tongue. When a person loses consciousness the muscles relax. If the person is lying on his back the tongue will

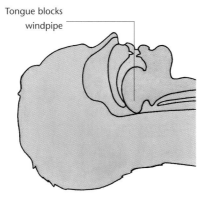
Tongue blocks windpipe

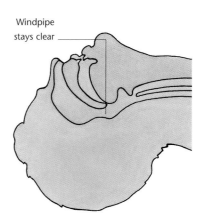
Windpipe stays clear

fall to the back of the mouth, blocking off the windpipe and stopping oxygen getting into the body.

Clearing the airway is the first step of the essential ABC of first aid. The

method of clearing an airway blocked by the tongue is very simple. By tilting the head back and lifting the chin, the tongue is prevented from falling to the back of the throat and the windpipe remains clear.

OPEN THE AIRWAY
- *Place one hand on the forehead and gently tilt the head back.*
- *Remove any obvious obstructions from the casualty's mouth, including dislodged dentures, but leave well-fitting dentures in place.*
- *Place the fingertips of two fingers under the point of the casualty's chin and lift the chin. If injury to the neck is suspected, handle the head very gently and try to avoid tilting the head too much.*

For a baby, use only one finger to lift the chin and take particular care not to overtilt the head.

CHECK FOR BREATHING
Once the airway is open, the next priority is to check whether or not the person is breathing. Keep the airway open with one hand on the forehead

and one hand lifting the chin. Put your cheek to the victim's face and look down the chest.

- *LOOK for the movement of the chest and stomach.*
- *LISTEN for breath sounds.*
- *FEEL for breathing on the side of your face.*

If the casualty is breathing, turn into the recovery position.

IF THE CASUALTY IS NOT BREATHING

- *Call for emergency help.*

If you have not already done so, make sure that an ambulance has been called.

- *Start resuscitation.*

ABC of resuscitation

AIRWAY Ensure a clear airway.

BREATHING Check breathing and give rescue breaths to the non-breathing person.

CIRCULATION Check that the person has a good circulation and help them if their circulation has stopped or is damaged.

THE RECOVERY POSITION FOR ADULTS

An unconscious person is always at risk of the airway becoming blocked by the tongue. There is also the possibility of choking on stomach contents as the valve holding food down often relaxes, allowing food to come back up into the mouth. If there is damage to the mouth or internal injuries, a person may also be at risk of choking on blood. To try to reduce these risks, most unconscious people are safest if placed in the recovery position while waiting for help to arrive. This is a secure position that keeps the airway open and allows liquids to drain from the mouth.

ASSESSING A CASUALTY

If somebody is unconscious (not responsive) but breathing, your priorities are: to ensure that he stays breathing by keeping the airway unblocked and regularly looking, listening and feeling for breaths; to treat any life-threatening injuries such as serious bleeding; and to call for emergency help. For an unconscious person who you know to be breathing, do a quick check for life-threatening injuries such as severe bleeding and treat if necessary, then turn the victim into the recovery position.

HOW TO TURN AN ADULT INTO THE RECOVERY POSITION

1 *Kneel beside the casualty. Remove spectacles and any bulky objects from the pockets. Ensure the airway is open by lifting the chin and tilting the head. Make sure both legs are straight, then place the arm nearest to you at right angles to the casualty's body, with the elbow bent and the palm facing upwards.*

ABC of first aid

AIRWAY Use the recovery position to help maintain an open airway.

BREATHING Continue to check breathing while the person is in the recovery position.

CIRCULATION Treat any life-threatening bleeding.

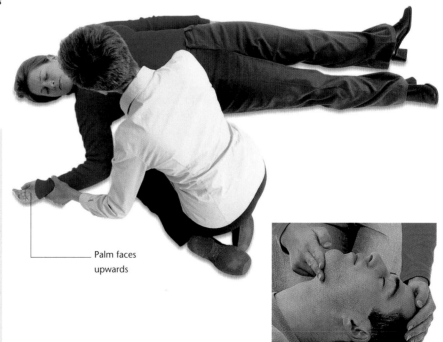

Palm faces upwards

Lift the chin to open the airway

2 *Bring the arm furthest away from you across the victim's chest and hold the back of the hand against the cheek nearest to you.*

3 *With your other hand, grasp the far leg just above the knee and pull it up, keeping the foot flat on the ground.*

4 *Keeping the casualty's hand pressed against his or her cheek, pull on the far leg and roll the casualty towards you and on to his or her side. Adjust the upper leg so that both the hip and knee are bent at right angles.*

Grasp leg above knee and pull up

Hold back of casualty's hand against cheek

Hip and knee at right angles

Spinal injury

If the casualty has been involved in an accident that involved a lot of force, such as a fall from a height or a car accident, the back or neck may be injured. The priority in an unconscious person will always be ABC. If you suspect a person may have a neck or back injury, or other broken bones, you may wish to adjust the recovery position to minimise movement. Gently move the head to a position where vomit or blood will drain out. If you are concerned about breathing then the person must be moved into a safer position. See also Spinal Injury, pages 92-93.

Warning: Never move someone if you suspect spinal injury unless breathing is hindered or the person needs to be removed from danger.

5 *Tilt the head back so that the airway remains open. If necessary, adjust the hand under the cheek to make sure the casualty's head remains tilted and the airway* stays open. *Call for emergency help if this has not already been done. Check the breathing regularly, and check the lower arm for any loss of colour or warmth. If it turns white or blue, or if it gets cold, gently move it until the colour or warmth returns.*

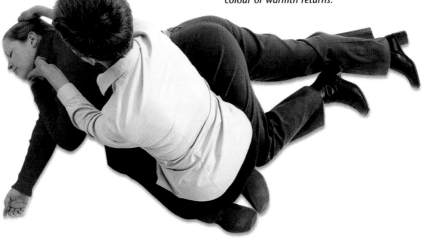

THE RECOVERY POSITION FOR CHILDREN AND BABIES

KEEPING THE AIRWAY CLEAR

The recovery position keeps the airway open and allows liquids to drain from the mouth. This is the safest position in which to place an unconscious child or baby until medical help arrives. It prevents the airway becoming blocked by the tongue, and reduces the risks of choking on blood or stomach contents.

The priorities for an unconscious child are the same as for an unconscious adult: to ensure that the child stays breathing by keeping the airway unblocked and regularly looking, listening and feeling for breaths; to treat any life-threatening injuries such as serious bleeding; and to call for emergency help. For an unconscious child who you know to be breathing, do a quick check for life-threatening injuries such as severe bleeding and treat if necessary, then turn the victim into the recovery position.

HOW TO TURN A CHILD INTO THE RECOVERY POSITION

1 *Kneel beside the child.*
Remove spectacles and any bulky objects from the pockets. Ensure the airway is open by lifting the chin and tilting the head. Make sure both legs are straight, then place the arm nearest to you at right angles to the child's body, with the elbow bent and the palm facing upwards.

ABC of first aid

AIRWAY Use the recovery position to keep the child's airway open.

BREATHING Continue to check breathing while the child is in the recovery position.

CIRCULATION Treat any life-threatening bleeding.

Spinal injury

If a child has been involved in an accident that involved a lot of force, such as a fall from a height, or a car accident, you need to consider carefully the possibility of an injury to the back or neck. The priority in an unconscious child or infant will always be ABC (check for an open airway, maintain breathing and ensure circulation). If you suspect that a child may have a neck or back injury, or other broken bones, then you may wish to adjust the recovery position to minimise movement. If the child is already lying on her side then just gently move the head to a position where vomit or blood will drain out. However, if at any time you are concerned about breathing, the child must be moved into a safer position. See Spinal Injury, pages 92-93.

Warning: Never move a child if you suspect spinal injury unless breathing is hindered or the child needs to be removed from danger.

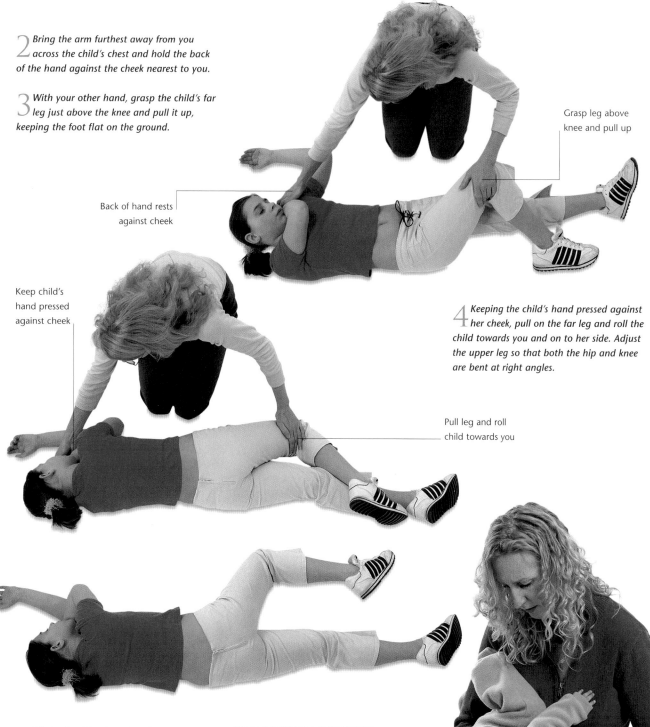

2 Bring the arm furthest away from you across the child's chest and hold the back of the hand against the cheek nearest to you.

3 With your other hand, grasp the child's far leg just above the knee and pull it up, keeping the foot flat on the ground.

Grasp leg above knee and pull up

Back of hand rests against cheek

Keep child's hand pressed against cheek

4 Keeping the child's hand pressed against her cheek, pull on the far leg and roll the child towards you and on to her side. Adjust the upper leg so that both the hip and knee are bent at right angles.

Pull leg and roll child towards you

5 Tilt the head back so that the airway remains open. If necessary, adjust the hand under the cheek to make sure the child's head remains tilted and the airway stays open. Call for emergency help if this has not already been done. Check the breathing regularly, and check the lower arm for any loss of colour or warmth. If it turns white or blue, or if it gets cold, gently move it until the colour or warmth returns.

RECOVERY POSITION FOR BABIES

For a baby or a very young child who is unconscious, the easiest way to maintain an open airway is to cradle the infant in your arms on its side, with a gentle movement to open the airway by lifting the chin and tilting the neck.

GIVING RESCUE BREATHS FOR ADULTS

When a person is not breathing the body suffers from shortage of oxygen, and if action is not taken this will eventually lead to death. The air that a healthy adult breathes out contains a valuable amount of oxygen, which can be blown into a person who is not breathing and help restore his or her oxygen levels. This process is often called mouth-to-mouth resuscitation or artificial respiration; the actual breaths are called rescue breaths.

GIVING RESCUE BREATHS

Rescue breaths are given to a person who is not breathing. When an adult is not breathing, the cause is very likely to be a problem with the heart. It is therefore essential that as soon as you realise that an adult is not breathing, you make sure that an ambulance has been called. If you have a face shield or mask and know how to use it, this can be valuable, but do not waste time looking for one.

In the case of face injury or if a person has been poisoned, give mouth-to-nose rescue breaths. Lift the chin, tilt the head, seal the mouth and breathe into the nose, removing your mouth to let air escape.

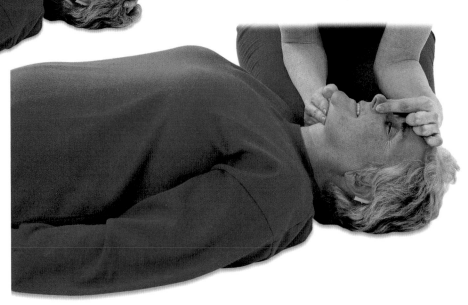

1 *Place the casualty on her back. Open the airway by tilting the head and lifting the chin with two fingers.*

2 *Pinch the soft part of the nose closed with the finger and thumb of the hand that was on the forehead. Open the mouth.*

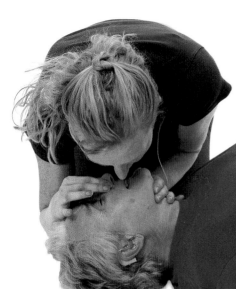

3 Take a deep breath to fill your lungs with air and place your lips around the casualty's mouth, making sure you have a good seal.

ABC of resuscitation

AIRWAY   Use head tilt and chin lift to keep an open airway while giving rescue breaths.

BREATHING   Give rescue breaths to somebody who is not breathing.

CIRCULATION   Check for signs of circulation.

4 Blow steadily into the mouth and watch the chest rise. Maintaining head tilt and chin lift, take your mouth away and watch the chest fall.

An effective breath is one where you see the chest rise and fall, and your aim is to give 2 effective breaths. Try up to 5 attempts to give 2 effective breaths.

What to do if the chest does not rise

• *Check for any obvious obstruction around the neck or on the chest which may be preventing the breath from going in.*
• *Re-open the airway. Tilt the head, look for and remove any obvious obstructions and lift the chin.*
• *Re-seal the nose and mouth and breath in again.*
• *Try up to 5 attempts to give 2 effective breaths.*

If the chest still does not rise, it is likely that the airway is blocked either by an object such as food or vomit or because the air passages have swollen up due to a condition such as anaphylaxis (see pages 46–47). In these circumstances, the best treatment is to move straight to CPR: checking for circulation and combining further attempts at rescue breaths with chest compressions.

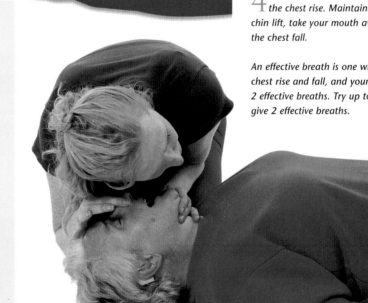

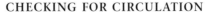

CHECKING FOR CIRCULATION

After giving 2 effective breaths, the next step in the ABC of first aid is to check that the oxygen is being circulated around the body. Look, listen and feel for breathing, coughing, movement, normal colour or any other sign of life for not more than 10 seconds. If there are clear signs of circulation, then continue to give rescue breaths at a rate of 1 every 6 seconds, until help arrives or the person begins to breathe for himself. Continue to check for signs of circulation throughout.

If there are no signs of circulation, you will need to move to giving the casualty full CPR — combining rescue breaths with chest compressions (see page 31).

GIVING RESCUE BREATHS FOR CHILDREN AND BABIES

If your child has lost consciousness and is not breathing, you will need to give rescue breaths in order to prevent brain damage and heart failure. When a child is not breathing, the cause is very likely to be a problem with the intake of oxygen, for example, through drowning, an accident or through choking. The priority, therefore, is to provide oxygen. If you are by yourself and an ambulance has not yet been called, do not leave to call an ambulance until you have given a minute's worth of rescue breaths (or if the circulation has also stopped, a minute's worth of CPR, where rescue breaths are combined with chest compressions).

GIVING RESCUE BREATHS FOR A CHILD

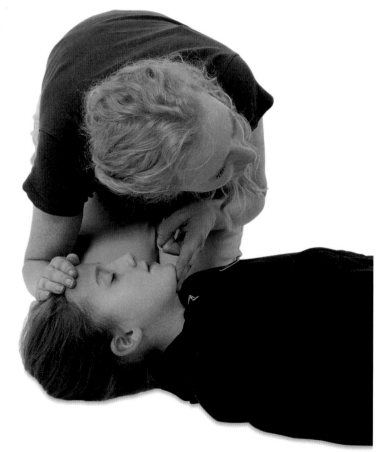

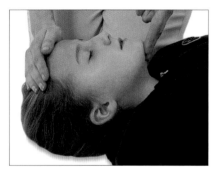

1 *Place the child on his back. Open the airway by tilting the head and lifting the chin up with your fingers.*

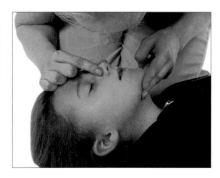

2 *Pinch the soft part of the nose closed with the finger and thumb of the hand that was on the forehead. Open the mouth.*

3 *Take a deep breath to fill your lungs with air and place your lips around the child's mouth, making sure you have a good seal.*

4 *Blow into the mouth and watch the chest rise. Maintaining head tilt and chin lift, remove your mouth and watch the chest fall.*

GIVING RESCUE BREATHS FOR A BABY

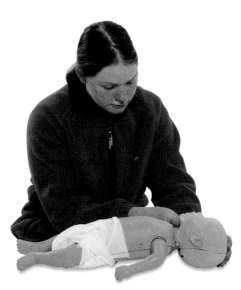

1 Open the airway by lifting the chin; use minimum head tilt.

2 You may find it easier to seal your mouth over the baby's mouth and nose rather than trying to pinch the nose separately. Open the infant's mouth. Empty your cheeks of air rather than blowing hard into the mouth. Watch the chest rise.

3 Keeping the baby's chin lifted, take your mouth away and watch the chest fall.

An effective breath is one where you see the chest rise and fall, and your aim is to give 2 effective breaths. Try up to 5 attempts to give 2 effective breaths.

CHECKING FOR CIRCULATION

After giving 2 effective breaths, the next step in the ABC of first aid is to check that oxygen is being circulated around the body. Look, listen and feel for breathing, coughing, movement, normal colour or any other sign of life for no more than 10 seconds. If there are clear signs of circulation, then continue to give rescue breaths at a rate of 1 every 6 seconds, until help arrives or the child begins to breathe for himself. Continue to check for signs of circulation throughout.

If there are no signs of circulation, move to giving full CPR – combining rescue breaths with chest compressions (see pages 30-33).

In the case of face injury or if a child has been poisoned, give mouth-to-nose rescue breaths. Lift the chin, tilt the head, seal the mouth and breathe into the child's nose, removing your mouth to let air escape.

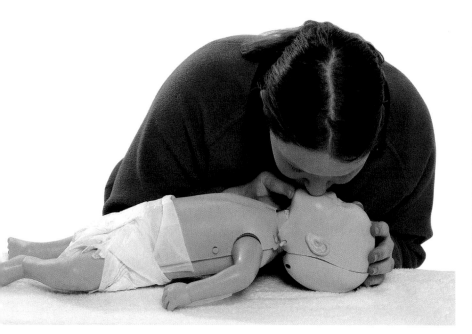

ABC of resuscitation

AIRWAY Use head tilt and chin lift to keep an open airway while giving rescue breaths.

BREATHING Give rescue breaths to somebody who is not breathing.

CIRCULATION Check for signs of circulation.

What to do if the chest does not rise

• Check for any obvious obstruction around the neck or on the chest which may be preventing the breath from going in.
• Re-open the airway. Tilt the head, look for and remove any obvious obstructions and lift the chin.
• Re-seal the nose and mouth and breathe in again.
• Try up to 5 attempts to give 2 effective breaths.

If the chest still does not rise, it is likely that the airway is blocked either by an object such as food or vomit or because the air passages have swollen up due to a condition such as anaphylaxis (see pages 46-47). In these circumstances, the best treatment is to move straight to CPR – combining further attempts at rescue breaths with chest compressions.

CPR FOR ADULTS

Cardiopulmonary resuscitation (CPR) combines rescue breaths with chest compressions to circulate oxygen around the body while waiting for further emergency help. CPR does not normally restart a person's heart but when it is combined with early emergency help, early defibrillation (whereby a brief electric shock is given to the heart) and early advanced hospital care, it has saved many lives. Ribs are often broken during CPR but this is preferable to dying.

GIVING CPR

After giving the initial rescue breaths (see pages 26-27), you need to check the circulation to see if the heart is effectively pumping blood, and therefore oxygen, around the body. Look, listen and feel for breathing, coughing, movement, normal colour or any other sign of life for not more than 10 seconds. If there are no signs of circulation, or you are at all unsure, start chest compressions. These must be given with the casualty lying on his back on a firm surface.

CHEST COMPRESSIONS

1 *With your lower hand, locate one of the bottom ribs. Slide the fingers of one hand along the rib to the point where the rib meets the breastbone. Place one finger at this point and the finger next to it above it on the breastbone. Place the heel of your other hand on the breastbone and slide it down until it reaches your index finger. This is the point at which you should apply pressure.*

ABC of resuscitation

AIRWAY Use head tilt and chin lift to keep the airway open while giving rescue breaths.

BREATHING Give rescue breaths to somebody who is not breathing.

CIRCULATION Check for signs of circulation and combine rescue breaths with chest compressions if you think the heart has stopped beating.

2 *Place the heel of your first hand on top of the other hand and interlock your fingers. Lean well over the casualty and, with your arms straight, press down vertically and depress the breastbone one-third of the depth of the chest, which on an adult is 4–5 cm.*

3 *Release the pressure without losing contact between your hands and the breastbone. Compress the chest 15 times, at a rate of 100 compressions per minute. Compression and release should take an equal amount of time.*

COMBINING CHEST COMPRESSIONS WITH RESCUE BREATHS

Chest compressions circulate blood to the vital organs such as the brain. To ensure that this blood contains oxygen, you need to combine chest compressions with rescue breaths.

After 15 compressions, tilt the head, lift the chin and give 2 effective breaths. Continue this cycle of 15 compressions to 2 effective breaths. Do not interrupt the CPR sequence unless the casualty makes a movement or takes a breath on his own. Continue this procedure until:

- *Emergency help arrives and takes over.*
- *The casualty shows signs of circulation.*
- *You become so exhausted you cannot*

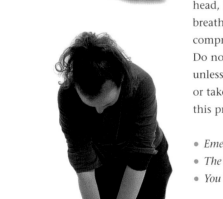

If the casualty vomits

The combination of being unconscious with no muscle tone to hold in the stomach contents, air possibly being blown into the stomach through rescue breaths, and compressing the chest may result in the casualty being sick. He or she will often have lost the reflex that causes gagging so the vomit may stay at the back of the throat or come into the mouth. If this happens it is important to clear this promptly:

- *Roll the victim towards you, supporting the head.*
- *Open the mouth and sweep out any vomit with two fingers.*
- *Turn the victim on to his back and start the ABC process again.*

You may wish to use a face shield when giving rescue breaths to somebody who has been sick, but not having one should not be a deterrent to performing CPR. You could give breaths through a handkerchief.

carry on (in which case, try to find someone else to take over this procedure until medical help arrives).

CPR FOR CHILDREN AND BABIES

If a child or infant has no pulse and is not breathing you will need to give CPR (cardiopulmonary respiration) to enable the body's vital organs to continue functioning. After giving the initial rescue breaths, check the circulation to see if the heart is effectively pumping blood, and therefore oxygen, around the body. Look, listen and feel for breathing, coughing, movement, normal colour or any other sign of life for no more than 10 seconds. If there are no signs of circulation, or if you are at all unsure, start chest compressions. This must be given with the child lying on her back on a firm surface.

CHEST COMPRESSIONS FOR CHILDREN

These techniques broadly apply for a child between 1 and 7 years old. However, you should take into account the size of the child when deciding whether to use the techniques for children or infants.

1 *Place the heel of one hand on the lower half of the breastbone. Lean well over the casualty and, with your arm straight, press vertically down and depress the breastbone one-third of the depth of the chest.*

2 *Release the pressure without losing contact between your hands and the breastbone. Compress the chest 5 times at a rate of 100 compressions per minute. Compression and release should take an equal amount of time.*

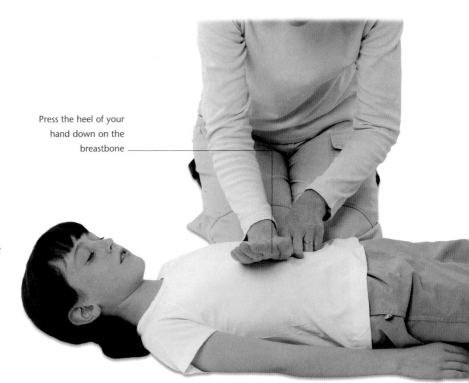

Press the heel of your hand down on the breastbone

COMBINING CHEST COMPRESSIONS WITH RESCUE BREATHS FOR CHILDREN

Chest compressions circulate blood to the vital organs such as the brain. To ensure that this blood contains oxygen, you need to combine chest compressions with rescue breaths.

The procedure is the same as CPR for an adult but the chest compressions are not as forceful and the rate of breaths

and compressions is different. After 5 compressions, tilt the head, lift the chin and give 1 effective breath. Continue this cycle of CPR. Do not interrupt the CPR sequence unless the child makes a movement or takes a breath on her own.

Continue until:
* *Emergency help arrives and takes over.*
* *The casualty shows signs of circulation.*
* *You become so exhausted you cannot carry on (in which case, try to find someone else to take over until medical help arrives).*

CHEST COMPRESSIONS FOR BABIES

These techniques broadly apply for a baby under one year. However, a large baby may require the techniques for a child and a small child may be better with the techniques for a baby.

1 *Place the two fingers of one hand on the lower half of the breastbone. Lean well over the baby and, with your arm straight, press vertically down and depress the breastbone one-third of the depth of the chest.*

2 *Release the pressure without losing contact between your hands and the breastbone. Compress the chest 5 times at a rate of 100 compressions per minute. Compression and release should take an equal amount of time.*

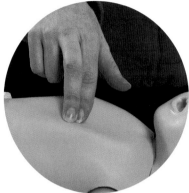

ABOVE *If the baby has no pulse and is not breathing you will have to give CPR. Lay her down on a firm surface and position two fingers in the middle of the chest.*

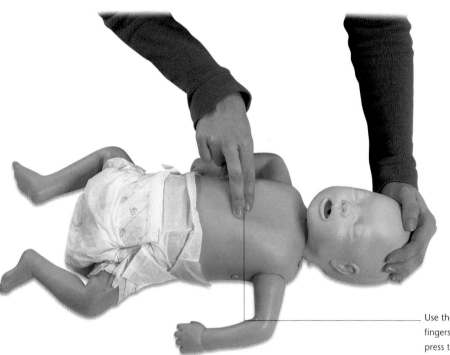

Use the tips of your fingers, taking care not to press too hard

COMBINING CHEST COMPRESSIONS WITH RESCUE BREATHS FOR BABIES

Chest compressions circulate blood to the vital organs, and to ensure that this blood contains oxygen, chest compressions need to be combined with rescue breaths.

After 5 compressions, lift the chin and give 1 effective breath. Continue this cycle of 5 compressions to 1 effective breath. Do not interrupt the CPR sequence unless the baby makes a movement or takes a breath on her own. Continue until emergency help arrives and takes over; the infant shows signs of circulation; or you become so exhausted that you cannot carry on.

WHEN TO CALL FOR HELP

With children and babies, the heart is most likely to stop because of problems with breathing. Therefore, if you are alone and have to call for an ambulance yourself, you should give one minute of CPR before leaving to make the call. This will ensure that oxygen has been circulated around the body, the most effective treatment for breathing problems. If the child is small enough, you may be able to carry her to the phone with you. Try not to leave the child unattended. If the infant recovers at any time, stop performing CPR but monitor the breathing and circulation rates until medical help arrives.

ABC of resuscitation

AIRWAY Use head tilt and chin lift to keep airway open while giving rescue breaths.

BREATHING Give rescue breaths to somebody who is not breathing.

CIRCULATION Check for signs of a circulation and combine rescue breaths with chest compressions if you think the heart has stopped beating.

CHOKING IN ADULTS

Choking is a blockage in the windpipe that makes it difficult or impossible for a person to breathe as air cannot pass into the lungs. Somebody who is choking will often do so quietly, initially turning red as he or she struggles to take air in, grasping at the neck and mouth and eventually losing colour, with a blue tinge to the lips. Without treatment, a person will become unconscious and will die. Choking in adults is often as a result of eating a meal too quickly or of eating on the move.

TREATMENT FOR AN ADULT WHO IS CHOKING

Check the mouth to see if anything can be easily removed. Do not sweep in the mouth blindly, and take great care not to push into the throat. Encourage the casualty to continue coughing if he or she is able. If the person shows signs of becoming weak or stops breathing or coughing, do 5 back slaps. If back slaps fail, do 5 abdominal thrusts.

GIVING BACK SLAPS

Bend the casualty over as far as you can, providing support as needed. Using the palm of your hand, hit him or her up to 5 times between the shoulder blades. Check the mouth to see if the object has been dislodged.

Use the palm of your hand to slap between the shoulder blades

Bend the victim forwards and give support

RIGHT **When someone is choking, prompt, calm action can save their life.**

GIVING ABDOMINAL THRUSTS

If the casualty continues to cough without dislodging the object, stand or kneel behind him and put both arms around the upper abdomen. Make sure the casualty is bending well forwards. Clench your fist and place it between the belly button and the bottom of the breastbone. Grasp it with your other hand. Pull sharply inwards and upwards 5 times. The purpose is to relieve the obstruction with each abdominal thrust.

If the obstruction is still not relieved, recheck the mouth for any object that can be reached with a finger and remove it if possible. If not, continue with alternating 5 back slaps and 5 abdominal thrusts. Repeat the cycle 3 times then call for emergency help.

WHAT IF THE PERSON BECOMES UNCONSCIOUS?

Open the airway by tilting the head, checking the mouth and lifting the chin. If the casualty is breathing, falling unconscious might have freed the object sufficiently to allow air through. Turn the person into the recovery position (see pages 22-23), maintaining a careful check on breathing. If the casualty is not breathing, give rescue breaths (see pages 26-27) and move on to the normal CPR procedures (see pages 30-31).

If you know that the person has choked and the chest does not rise when rescue breaths are attempted, move straight to chest compressions without assessment of circulation. Check the mouth after every set of compressions. The chest compressions act as an artificial cough and may help expel the object from the windpipe. Make sure that an ambulance is called as early as possible.

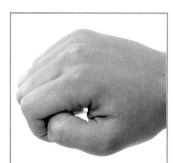

ABOVE *Make a fist and then position it thumb first in the middle of the casualty's abdomen, just below the breastbone.*

Place your hand over your fist and pull inwards and upwards

Use interlocking fingers to thrust down on chest

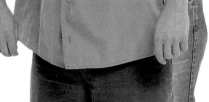

CHOKING IN CHILDREN AND BABIES

Children often put small objects into their mouths which may cause choking. This is an obstruction in the windpipe that makes it difficult or impossible to breathe as air cannot pass into the lungs. A child who is choking will often do so quietly, initially turning red as he or she struggles to take air in, grasping at the neck and mouth and eventually losing colour, with a blue tinge to the lips. Without treatment, a child will become unconscious and will die.

CHOKING IN CHILDREN

Choking is a major cause of death in young children and should be considered whenever a child has breathing difficulties. Look for small beads or coins that the child may have been playing with, or ask playmates to identify clues that choking may be the cause of unconsciousness in the child.

TREATMENT

Check a child's mouth for obstruction but do not feel blindly in the mouth as you may push the object further into the windpipe. Look to see if there is anything that can be easily removed. If the child is breathing, encourage her to continue coughing because this may dislodge the obstruction. If the child weakens, stops breathing or coughing, do 5 back slaps. If back slaps fail, perform 5 chest thrusts. If the chest thrusts fail, give 5 abdominal thrusts.

GIVING BACK SLAPS

Bend the child over or, if small enough, put the child over your legs with the head down. With the palm of your hand, give up to 5 blows between the shoulder blades. Check the mouth to see whether the object has been dislodged.

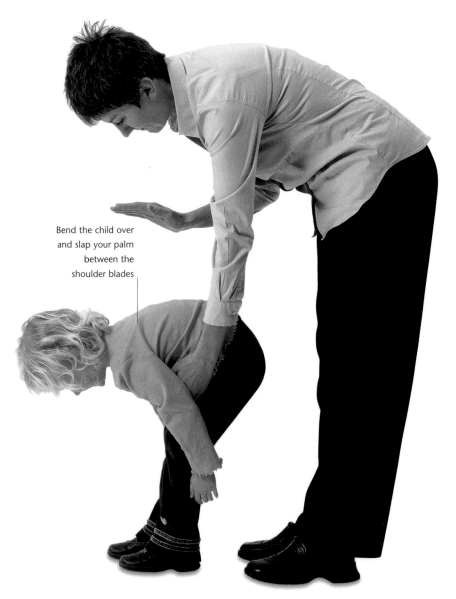

Bend the child over and slap your palm between the shoulder blades

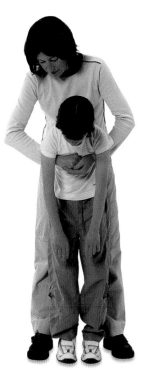

Giving chest thrusts to a child

GIVING CHEST THRUSTS

Chest thrusts work by producing an artificial cough. Stand or kneel behind the child. Make a fist and place it against the lower half of the breastbone. Grasp the fist with your other hand. Pull sharply inwards and upwards. Perform 5 chest thrusts at a rate of 1 every 3 seconds. The aim is to relieve the obstruction with each chest thrust rather than necessarily doing all 5.

GIVING ABDOMINAL THRUSTS

If chest thrusts fail and the windpipe is still blocked, stand or kneel behind the child and put both arms around the upper abdomen. Make sure the child is bending well forwards. Clench your fist and place it between the belly button and the bottom of the breastbone. Grasp it with your other hand. Pull sharply inwards and upwards 5 times. The aim is to relieve the obstruction with each abdominal thrust.

If the obstruction is still not relieved, recheck the mouth for any object that

can be reached with a finger and remove it if possible. If not, continue alternating 5 back slaps, 5 chest thrusts and 5 abdominal thrusts. Repeat the cycle 3 times before calling for emergency help.

CHOKING IN BABIES

Babies under one year are most likely to choke on their vomit. Look in the mouth. If you can easily remove the cause of the problem, then do so, but take great care not to touch the back of the throat or to push the object further in.

1 *As with a child, move the baby so that the head is downwards. Apply back slaps as for a child but with slightly less force, and check the mouth carefully for the object.*

2 *If back slaps do not work, then apply chest thrusts as for a child but using only two fingers.*

Do not perform abdominal thrusts on a baby. If the obstruction is still not relieved, recheck the mouth for any object that can be reached with a finger and remove it if possible. If not, continue alternating 5 back slaps and 5 chest thrusts. Repeat the cycle 3 times then call for emergency help.

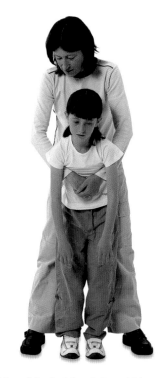

Giving abdominal thrusts to a child

WHAT IF THE CHILD OR BABY BECOMES UNCONSCIOUS?

Begin CPR (see pages 32-33). If the infant is not breathing and the chest does not rise when rescue breaths are attempted, move straight to chest compressions without assessment of circulation. Check the mouth after every set of compressions.

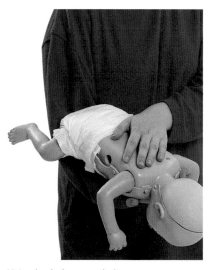

Giving back slaps to a baby

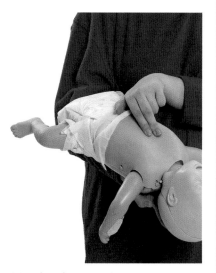

Giving chest thrusts to a baby

DROWNING

When a person is drowning, the air passages close up to prevent water going into the lungs. This also prevents air entering the lungs, depriving the victim of oxygen and eventually leading to unconsciousness and death. Usually, only if the victim has been unconscious in the water for some time do the lungs fill up with water. More commonly, the water goes into the stomach. A secondary risk for the rescued person is that he or she may choke on vomit as water in the stomach forces the stomach contents upwards. A near-drowning victim also faces the risk of hypothermia. Children and young adults are at the greatest risk of drowning.

RESCUING A DROWNING PERSON

As in all first aid, the key rule is to protect yourself. A person who is drowning will hit out and pull down even the most competent swimmer; dirty water can hide dangers such as metal rubbish with sharp edges; and cold water can cause the muscles to seize up very quickly.

Where possible, reach to the person from the safety of solid ground using a pole, rope or buoyancy aid to enable him to help himself out of the water. If in doubt about your ability to rescue the person safely, call for emergency help.

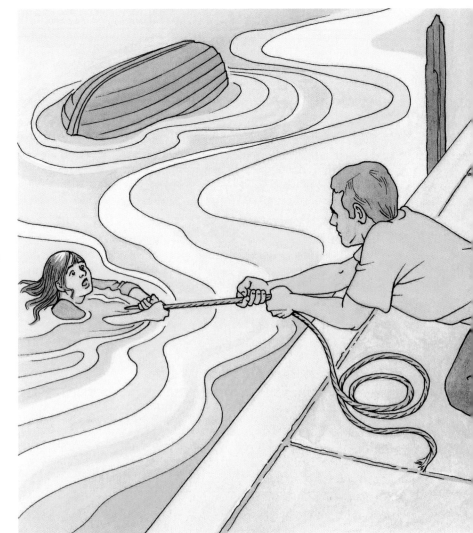

RIGHT *Make sure you are safe before attempting to rescue a drowning person; if in doubt call for emergency help. If possible, reach out to the person using a pole, a piece of rope or buoyancy aid from the safety of solid ground.*

TREATMENT OF A NEAR-DROWNING VICTIM

Your priority is to ensure an open airway and that the person is breathing.

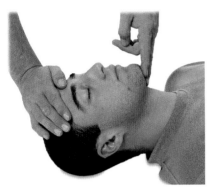

1 Open the airway by tilting the head, checking the mouth and lifting the chin. Check for breathing for up to 10 seconds.

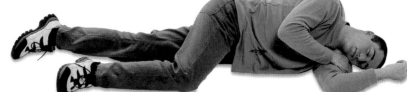

2 If the victim is breathing, place into the recovery position (see pages 22-25).

3 If the victim is not breathing, give rescue breaths (see pages 26-29) before moving on to an assessment of circulation and full CPR (see pages 30-33) as necessary.

BEING SICK

A person who has nearly drowned is very likely to be sick. Maintain a close watch for this. If the victim is sick while you are resuscitating him, turn him towards you, and clear out the mouth before turning him on to the back and resuming rescue breaths. If the victim is sick while in the recovery position, clear out the mouth and keep a close check on breathing to ensure that it has not stopped. If the victim is conscious and sick, encourage him to lean forward and give support while he is vomiting.

Do not make any effort to remove water from the lungs by applying chest compressions or abdominal thrusts. The risk of water in the lungs is minimal, while compressing the chest or stomach will increase the risk of the victim choking on his own vomit.

HYPOTHERMIA

Hypothermia is a lowering of the body's core temperature and is a very common secondary problem of near-drowning. If untreated, hypothermia

leads to the breathing and heart rate slowing down and eventually stopping.

To reduce the risks of hypothermia in a victim of near-drowning, place him on a blanket or layer of coats to insulate him from the ground. Remove wet clothing if you are able to replace it quickly with warm and dry clothing; if not, then cover the wet clothing with blankets and coats. Cover the head, as much heat is lost from here. Warm the external environment where possible.

Even in a conscious person, hypothermia can be a risk. Seek medical help as soon as possible.

For further information on hypothermia, see pages 112-113.

Cover with a warm blanket to reduce the risk of hypothermia

BREATHING DIFFICULTIES

In a first aid situation you are likely to encounter a casualty who has breathing difficulties. Psychological stress may trigger breathing problems that affect the blood's chemical composition, causing a range of symptoms that make the victim feel unwell. Accidents that include a heavy impact to the chest can cause injuries that result in severe breathing difficulties.

HYPERVENTILATION

This is a breathing difficulty that may be triggered by the stress of an accident or some other form of emotional shock. The person over-breathes, causing the level of carbon dioxide in the blood to drop. This leads to a combination of the signs and symptoms listed below:

- *Fast, shallow breathing*
- *Feeling of pins and needles in the limbs*
- *Dizziness*
- *Cramps*
- *Panic attacks*

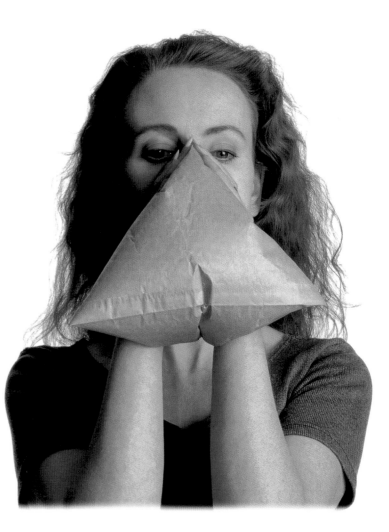

Reduced carbon dioxide levels in the blood can be restored to normal by slowly breathing into and out of a paper bag about 10 times and then breathing normally for 15 seconds until the rapid breathing ceases.

TREATMENT

1 If the casualty is otherwise uninjured, remove her from the scene of the accident to a quiet place where there is no audience. People who are hyperventilating often subconsciously react to onlookers, making themselves worse.

2 Reassure the casualty but remain calm and speak firmly. Encourage the casualty to regain control of her breathing.

3 If the situation persists, and you are certain that there is no other underlying condition such as asthma or chest injury, let the casualty inhale her own breathed-out air from a paper

bag. This air contains more carbon dioxide and this will help restore the balance of oxygen and carbon dioxide in the blood.

4 Call a doctor or ambulance if symptoms do not disappear. Do not slap the casualty – she may become violent and attack you, and you run the risk of being charged with assault.

SIGNS AND SYMPTOMS OF COLLAPSED LUNG AND OTHER CHEST INJURIES

- *History of chest impact or recent illness affecting breathing*
- *Chest rises as the person breathes out (paradoxical breathing)*
- *Swelling or indentation along the line of the ribs*
- *Open fractures*
- *Difficulty in breathing*
- *Pain on breathing*
- *Shock, as there is likely to be some degree of internal bleeding (see pages 68-69)*
- *Bright red, frothy blood coming from the mouth and/or nose. (This is an indication of a punctured lung as oxygenated blood is escaping from the respiratory system. There may or may not be an associated sucking wound to the chest.)*
- *Sucking wound to the chest*

TREATMENT

Ensure that an early call for emergency medical help has been made. If the casualty is conscious, she will often find it easier to breathe if sitting up. Help the casualty into a sitting-up position if possible and provide support to remain in this position comfortably. If you can determine the side of the injury, lean the casualty to the injured side. This helps relieve pressure on the good lung, allowing the casualty to breathe a little easier.

If there is an open sucking wound to the chest, cover this up as soon as possible. The best cover comes from using plastic sealed on three sides over the wound area. Help the casualty remove blood from her mouth. If the person becomes unconscious, place into the recovery position (see pages 22-25) on the injured side and monitor breathing carefully. Treat any open wound (see pages 60-65) once the person is in the recovery position. Treat any broken ribs (see pages 90-91).

CHEST INJURIES

Serious injuries following an accident, or the aftermath of any illnesses causing problems with breathing, can lead to the lung collapsing. Air enters the space between the lung and the chest wall, making breathing very difficult. In severe cases, the pressure affects the uninjured lung and the heart, causing a tension pneumothorax, a condition requiring urgent medical attention if the casualty is to survive.

Chest injuries with more than one broken rib will often result in the casualty having difficulty in breathing as the chest wall is unable to move effectively. There may also be an open break on the chest wall where ribs have sprung out. Remember that the ribs extend around the back and there may be injuries here as well as on the front. See also *Fractures of the Rib Cage*, pages 90-91.

Chest injuries may be accompanied by a sucking wound to the chest (see page 64). Here there is a direct passage between the outside and the lungs, often caused by a puncture injury from a sharp object pushing through the chest wall.

ASTHMA

Asthma attacks cause the muscles of the air passages to go into spasm, making it very difficult for the sufferer to breathe, particularly to exhale. Attacks may be triggered by an allergy or by stress, for example being involved in an accident. Sometimes the cause of the attacks for a particular sufferer is never identified. There is evidence to suggest that asthma appears to be increasing in frequency, or at least in diagnosis. For more information on asthma, see pages 366-67.

Signs and symptoms

• *History of the condition (although some people may not realise that they are asthmatic and the first attack may be a very severe one)*
• *Difficulty in breathing, particularly breathing out*
• *Wheezing or otherwise noisy breathing*
• *Inability to speak*
• *Pale skin and potential blueness, particularly around the lips, caused by lack of oxygen*
• *Distress, dizziness and confusion as it becomes harder to get oxygen into the body*
• *Unconsciousness and then breathing stopping*

TREATMENT

An asthma attack should not be underestimated. While the preventive treatments are very effective, and the drugs to relieve attacks usually work very well, left untreated, a serious attack can be fatal. The strain of a serious asthma attack can cause the breathing to stop or the heart to cease beating (see resuscitation, pages 26-29). You should be prepared to give CPR (see pages 30-33) if necessary.

1 *Reassure the casualty as this will have a positive effect on his breathing.*

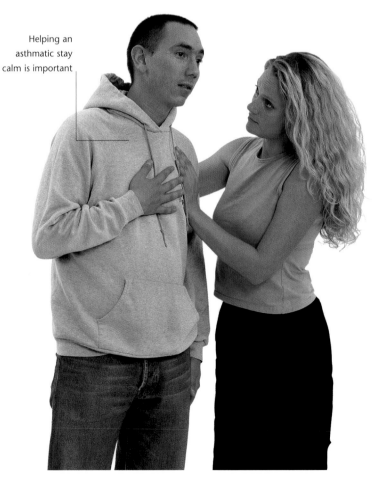

Helping an asthmatic stay calm is important

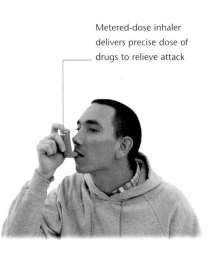

Metered-dose inhaler delivers precise dose of drugs to relieve attack

3 *If the casualty has medication, enable him to use it. Inhalers are the main form of treatment and are generally blue.*

If this is the first attack, the medication does not work within 5 minutes or the casualty is in severe distress, then call an ambulance. Help the casualty to take medication every 5 to 10 minutes.

If the attack eases and the casualty finds it easier to breathe, he will not need immediate medical attention but should advise a doctor of the attack. A person will often be very tired following an attack so it is best to ensure that he is accompanied home to rest.

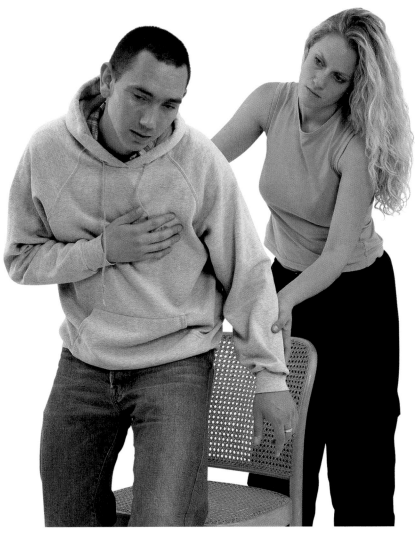

2 *Help the casualty into a sitting position, leaning slightly forwards, as most people with asthma find this an easier position for breathing.*

Using an inhaler

Known asthmatics are usually prescribed an inhaler, a device that administers a measured dose of drugs inhaled directly into the lungs, where it will have a near-instant effect. Inhalers for prevention are generally brown and inhalers for the relief of attacks are usually blue.

Young children may find it hard to use an ordinary aerosol inhaler and will need a spacer instead. Medication is put into the end of the spacer and the child breathes normally to take this in.

Children under the age of four will usually require a face mask to use with the spacer as they cannot coordinate their breathing to inhale the drugs.

If a member of your family is an asthmatic, make sure that everyone understands the importance of knowing where the inhaler is and that there is always enough medication in the house.

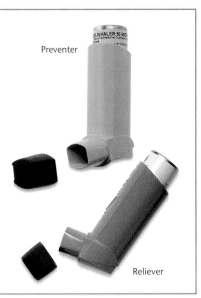

Preventer

Reliever

SHOCK

The word shock can be used in a range of ways, but when used in a first aid context it describes a physical condition that results from a loss of circulating body fluid. It should not be confused with emotional shock that might occur, say, when a person has received bad news (although the external signs are very similar).

WHAT HAPPENS IN CASES OF SHOCK

A severe loss of body fluid will lead to a drop in blood pressure. Eventually the blood's circulation around the body will deteriorate and the remaining blood flow will be directed to the vital organs such as the brain. Blood will therefore be directed away from the outer areas of the body, so the casualty will appear paler than previously and the skin will feel cold and clammy. As blood flow slows, so does the amount of oxygen reaching the brain. The casualty may appear to be confused, weak and dizzy, and may eventually deteriorate into unconsciousness. To try to compensate for this lack of oxygen, the heart and breathing rates both speed up, gradually becoming weaker, and may eventually cease.

Potential causes of shock include: severe internal or external bleeding; burns; severe vomiting and diarrhoea, especially in children and the elderly; problems with the heart.

Signs and symptoms

- *Pale, cold and clammy skin*
- *Fast, weak pulse*
- *Fast, shallow breathing*
- *Dizziness and weakness*
- *Confusion*
- *Unconsciousness*
- *Breathing and heartbeat stopping*

Shock kills, so it is vital that you can recognise these signs and symptoms. With internal bleeding in particular, shock can occur some time after an accident, so if a person with a history of injury starts to display these symptoms coupled with any of the symptoms of internal bleeding (see pages 68-69), advise her to seek urgent medical attention.

Keep the feet supported and higher than the head

Legs in the air for maximum blood flow and hence oxygen to the brain

Lack of oxygen causes weakness and confusion

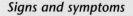

TREATMENT

- *Warmth*
- *Air*
- *Rest*
- *Mental rest*
- *Treatment*
- *Help*

Warmth Keep the casualty warm but do not allow her to get overheated. If you are outside, try to get something underneath the casualty if you can do so easily. Wrap blankets and coats around her, paying particular attention to the head, through which much body heat is lost.

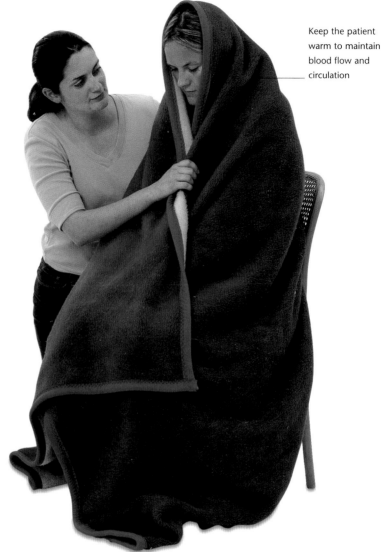

Keep the patient warm to maintain blood flow and circulation

Fainting

A faint is a brief loss of consciousness. Shock is one of the potential causes of fainting but other causes include lack of food, a reaction to emotional news or long periods of inactivity, for example guardsmen standing for a long time in the summer.

To treat someone who has fainted, open the airway and check for breathing (see page 17). If the person is breathing and there are no signs of injury, then the best treatment is to lie her on her back with her legs raised. This puts maximum oxygen back to the brain and speeds up recovery from a faint. If she has not begun to come around after 3 minutes, or if breathing becomes difficult, put her into the recovery position and call for help.

Air Maintain a careful eye on the casualty's airway and be prepared to turn her into the recovery position (see pages 22-25) if necessary, or even to resuscitate if breathing stops (see pages 30-33). Try to clear back bystanders and loosen tight clothing to allow maximum air to the casualty.

Rest Keep the casualty still and preferably sitting or lying down. If the casualty is very giddy, lay her down with her legs raised to ensure that maximum blood and therefore maximum oxygen is sent to the brain.

Mental rest Reassure the casualty but keep your comments realistic. Do not say that everything is going to be fine when it is obvious that there is something seriously wrong. Let the casualty know that everything that can be done is being done and that help has been called for. If she has other worries then try to resolve these.

Treatment Treat the cause of the shock and aim to prevent further fluid loss.

Help Ensure that appropriate medical help is on the way.

ANAPHYLACTIC SHOCK

An allergy is hypersensitivity to a substance (allergen) that is not normally considered to be harmful. Allergies are triggered by the immune system (see pages 210-211), which reacts to the allergen as though it were a harmful substance invading the body. The most extreme response is anaphylaxis, which may result in anaphylactic shock which, if untreated, can kill.

CAUSES OF ANAPHYLAXIS

This extreme allergic reaction has an intense effect on the body, causing a sudden drop in blood pressure and narrowing of the airways that can be fatal. Anaphylactic shock can be caused by anything, but among the most common triggers are: nuts (for those who are particularly sensitive, even touching the trace of a nut can be potentially fatal), seafood, insect stings and bites, and drugs (some people have a very extreme reaction to penicillin, for example).

As with asthma, the number of people suffering allergic reactions appears to be increasing. Whether this is because people are becoming more sensitive to allergens (the substances that cause allergic reactions) or whether we are just becoming better at detecting allergies, nobody is really sure.

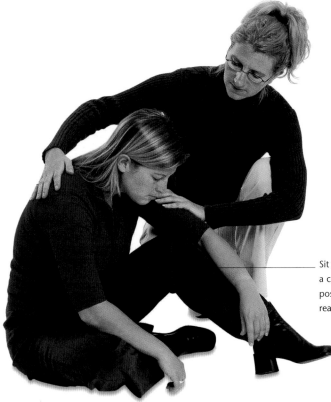

Sit the casualty in a comfortable position and reassure her

Signs and symptoms

One of the main effects of severe anaphylaxis is a constriction of the air passages in a similar way to asthma (see pages 42-43) but generally more severe, preventing the intake of any oxygen at all. There may be a history of contact with a particular allergen, the thing that triggers the attack.

Anaphylaxis can happen very quickly, within seconds. Signs and symptoms include:

- *Difficulty breathing*
- *Pale skin and blue lips*
- *Blotches on the skin*
- *Rapid pulse*
- *Breathing and heartbeat stopping*

TREATMENT

1 *Call an ambulance immediately. The casualty needs adrenaline to counteract the reaction.*

2 *If the casualty is a known sufferer she may have an adrenaline injection. Help her to administer this. If you have been trained and the casualty is unable to do so, you may give the injection.*

3 *Place the casualty in the most comfortable position and reassure her.*

4 *If the casualty becomes unconscious, place in the recovery position (see pages 22-25). Monitor the casualty's breathing and circulation and be prepared to resuscitate if necessary (see pages 30-33).*

Place the casualty in the recovery position

Monitor airway, breathing and circulation

Skin prick test for allergies

Skin prick tests are simple procedures carried out to find out what substances (allergens) cause allergic reactions in an affected person. Extracts of allergens that commonly cause allergic reactions, such as food, pollen and dust are made into didule solutions. A drop of the solution is placed on the skin and the skin is then pricked with a needle. If the person is allergic to the substance a reaction normally takes place within 30 minutes of the test. Several substances can be tested at one time.

Handling an attack

Many anaphylaxis sufferers carry an auto-injector with a measured dose of a known treatment for an attack, most commonly adrenaline. This will often look like a pen. It is easily administered by placing against the skin and clicking the end. Help the person having the attack to find and inject the medication.

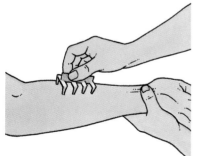

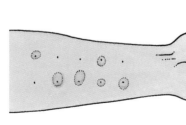

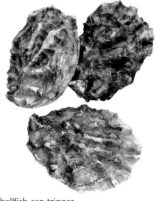

1 *Dilute solutions of substances that a person is thought to be allergic to are placed on the skin, usually the arm, and the skin is then pricked with a needle. Several different allergens can be tested on the skin at the same time.*

2 *An allergic reaction usually takes place within 30 minutes of the test. If the person is allergic to the substance a red weal, indicating a positive reaction, appears at the site where the needle pricked the skin.*

Shellfish can trigger anaphylaxic shock

HEART PROBLEMS

The heart is a muscle that pumps blood around the body, which it does with the help of the thick-walled and muscular arteries and the other vessels of the circulatory system. The heart is controlled by regular electrical impulses that tell it when to contract. Like all other muscles, the heart needs its own blood supply and this is provided by the coronary (heart) arteries. When this blood supply fails to run smoothly, the body starts to experience problems, such as angina pectoris (angina) and heart attack. Either of these may lead to the heart stopping (cardiac arrest).

ANGINA

Throughout life, arteries are clogging up with fatty deposits. As these fatty deposits cause the coronary and other arteries to become narrower, it becomes increasingly difficult for blood to flow around the body. The clogged coronary arteries can just about supply blood to the heart when it is pumping at a normal rate but when the heart rate speeds up, for example because of emotional upset or sudden exercise, the arteries cannot cope with the demand. This leads to an angina attack, a frightening, severe, crushing chest pain that acts as a warning to the casualty to calm down or to rest.

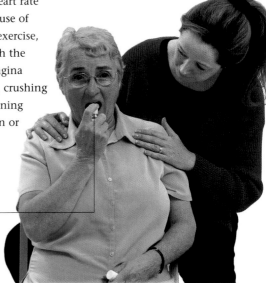

Sit the casualty down and help her to take her medication

Signs and symptoms of angina

- Evidence of recent exertion
- Previous history of angina attacks
- Gripping chest pain, often described by the sufferer as vice-like
- Pain spreading up into the jaw or down into the left arm
- Feeling of pins and needles down the arm
- Shortness of breath
- Dizziness and confusion
- Anxiety
- Pale skin with possible blue tinges
- Rapid, weak pulse

TREATMENT

1 Sit the casualty down and reassure her. This reduces the demands being placed on the heart.

2 Angina sufferers may have medicine that will help relieve an attack. This is often in the form of a puffer or tablet that is placed under the tongue. The drug works by dilating the blood vessels, thereby increasing circulation to the heart. Help the casualty to take this medication.

3 Call an ambulance if the pain does not appear to ease or if the casualty is not a known angina sufferer.

4 If the casualty has regular attacks, listen to what she wants to do next.

RIGHT *If the casualty has suffered a heart attack, move her into a semi-sitting position with her head and shoulders supported and her knees bent to aid breathing. Keep a close watch on her breathing and pulse and be prepared to resuscitate if necessary.*

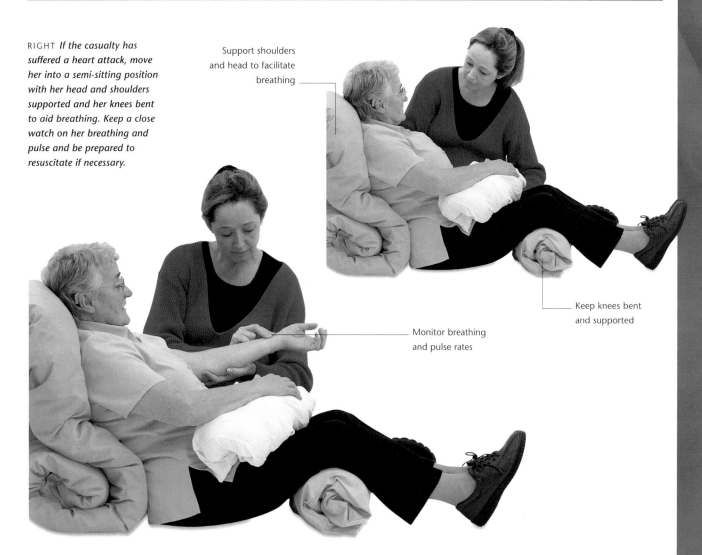

Support shoulders and head to facilitate breathing

Keep knees bent and supported

Monitor breathing and pulse rates

HEART ATTACK

If the coronary artery becomes completely blocked, the area of the heart being supplied by that particular blood vessel will be starved of oxygen and will eventually die. This blockage may be caused by a clot, a condition often referred to as a coronary thrombosis.

The development of advanced cardiac care in hospital and good post-hospital care means that heart attack patients have a good chance of making a full recovery. This is important information to remember when you are reassuring somebody having a heart attack.

TREATMENT

1 *Move the casualty into a semi-sitting position, head and shoulders supported and knees bent, as this is generally the best position to breathe in.*

2 *Reassure the casualty and do not let her move, as this will place an extra strain on the heart.*

3 *Call for an ambulance as soon as possible because the casualty needs hospital care.*

4 *If the casualty has angina medication, let her take this. If you have an ordinary aspirin, give her one to chew (without water).*

5 *Keep a continual check on the breathing and pulse and be prepared to resuscitate if necessary (see pages 30-31).*

Signs and symptoms of a heart attack

These signs and symptoms are generally the same as those of angina – indeed, the patient may initially suffer an angina attack that becomes a heart attack. The key difference is that heart attacks do not always follow physical exertion. While angina sufferers will recover from their attack on resting, heart attack patients do not tend to improve without medical treatment.

STROKE

A stroke occurs when a blood clot or bleeding cuts off the blood supply, and therefore the oxygen, to part of the brain. The affected area of the brain will eventually die. The effect of a stroke depends on how much of the brain is affected and where the clot or bleeding is. Different parts of the brain control different functions, so a clot in the part of the brain that controls speech, for example, will result in slurred or confused speech. Often the signs will be confined to one side of the body.

EFFECTS OF STROKE

If the bleeding or clot is in one of the larger blood vessels supplying a large area of the brain, then the stroke will often be immediately fatal. However, many people do survive such strokes, some making a full recovery, while others may need extensive periods of rehabilitation and support to manage stroke-related problems such as reduced mobility. For more information on strokes, see pages 338-341.

TREATMENT

Monitor airway and breathing and be prepared to resuscitate if necessary (see pages 30-31). Place the person in the recovery position if she becomes unconscious (see pages 22-23). If she is conscious, help her to lie down with the head and shoulders slightly raised. Provide support and reassurance. The person will often be disorientated and may be speaking nonsense if the speech centre is affected. Equally, she may hear what you are saying but not understand it. Speak in a reassuring tone with confidence. Call an ambulance. Wipe any dribbling away from the side of the face and be prepared for the person to be sick.

BELOW *If a person has had a stroke and is still conscious, help her to lie down with her head and shoulders raised. Speak in a reassuring voice and seek medical help.*

Keep the head and
shoulders raised

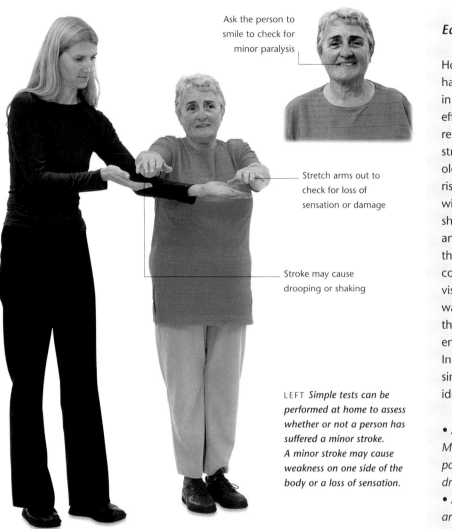

Ask the person to smile to check for minor paralysis

Stretch arms out to check for loss of sensation or damage

Stroke may cause drooping or shaking

LEFT *Simple tests can be performed at home to assess whether or not a person has suffered a minor stroke. A minor stroke may cause weakness on one side of the body or a loss of sensation.*

Signs and symptoms

Any combination of the following may be present. In minor strokes, the signs and symptoms may be very limited.

- *History – the sufferer may have a history of smaller strokes over previous years, or may have been feeling unwell for some days with no known cause*
- *Headache*
- *Blurred vision, partial loss of sight or seeing flashing lights*
- *Confusion and disorientation, often mistaken for drunkenness*

- *Signs of paralysis or weakness, often only down one side of the body*
- *Difficulty speaking; drooping mouth*
- *Dribbling from one side of the mouth*
- *Loss of consciousness (this can be gradual or sudden)*
- *Sometimes the pulse will be full and throbbing, the person's breathing noisy and the skin flushed*

Early recognition of a stroke

Hospital treatments for a stroke have developed tremendously in recent years but their effectiveness relies on early recognition and diagnosis of strokes. Friends and relatives of older people, or those at higher risk of stroke, such as people with high blood pressure, should be aware of the signs and symptoms of stroke listed in the box. Confused behaviour combined with headaches or vision problems are early warning signs, and if noticed the sufferer should be encouraged to visit a doctor. In addition, there is a number of simple home tests that may help identify a minor stroke:

- *Ask the person to smile. Minor strokes often cause minor paralysis. Look for an uneven or drooping smile.*
- *Ask the person to hold both arms out in front of her. Minor strokes often cause minor weakness on one side. There may be damage or loss of sensation on one side. Look for one arm drooping or shaking.*

If you suspect signs of a stroke in a person who otherwise seems well, seek medical advice quickly.

EPILEPSY

Epilepsy is a very common condition, best described as a rogue electrical discharge across the brain. As the body's functions are controlled by electrical impulses this discharge can lead to a number of physical reactions. Many things may start a seizure (fit): tiredness, stress or flashing lights are common triggers. For more information on epilepsy, see pages 336-7.

ABSENCES: MINOR FITS

During a minor fit somebody with epilepsy suffers a brief disturbance in the brain's normal activity, leading to a lack of awareness of his or her surroundings. To the observer it might seem like the person is daydreaming or has suddenly switched off.

There is little for you to do other than to guide the person away from danger and reassure him when he returns to normal. If he is not aware of any similar episodes happening before, advise him to see a doctor.

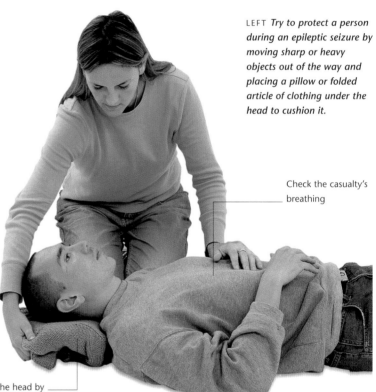

LEFT *Try to protect a person during an epileptic seizure by moving sharp or heavy objects out of the way and placing a pillow or folded article of clothing under the head to cushion it.*

Check the casualty's breathing

Protect the head by placing an article of clothing under it

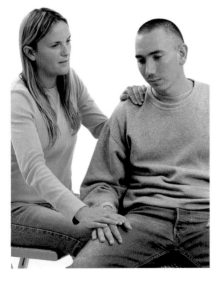

ABOVE *During a minor fit a person may appear to have suddenly switched off. If this happens, stay by the person so that you can reassure him when his behaviour returns to normal. Seek medical advice if this is the first episode.*

MAJOR SEIZURE

This is what most people would recognise as epilepsy, and there are typically four stages:

1 *Many people get a sense that a seizure is likely to occur.*

2 *The electrical impulses lead to a contraction in the muscles that causes the epilepsy sufferer to fall to the ground with a* cry. *This is known as the tonic phase. The casualty's muscles may then go into spasm. This is known as the clonic stage. During this stage the casualty will not be breathing.*

3 *When the convulsion is over, the casualty will be in a state of unconsciousness.*

4 *On recovery from unconsciousness, the casualty will be very sleepy and will want to rest for some time.*

TREATMENT FOR A MAJOR EPILEPTIC SEIZURE

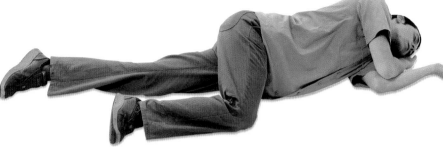

1 During the seizure, do not try to restrain the person. The muscular contractions are so strong during a fit that holding a person down may lead to broken bones – yours and his. Do not attempt to put anything in the mouth. Try to protect the casualty – move sharp objects out of the way, remove constrictions and, if possible, place a soft coat under the head.

2 Once the seizure has finished, check the casualty's airway and breathing and be prepared to resuscitate in the unlikely event that this is necessary (see pages 30-33). Place the person in the recovery position (see pages 22-25).

3 When the casualty comes around, reassure him. He may have lost control of bowel or bladder function so cover him up and, when he is steady on his feet, help him to find somewhere to clean up. He is likely to be very tired so, if possible, find him somewhere to lie down and sleep. Most of all, ask him what he wants to do – most epileptics manage the condition very well and will have their own coping strategies.

INFANTILE CONVULSIONS (CAUSED BY HEAT)

Babies and young children may have seizures induced by a high temperature. This may be the result of an infection or because they are overwrapped and in a warm environment. The signs and symptoms are similar to a major epileptic seizure.

TREATMENT

Make sure that the child is protected from hitting himself on a bed or cot – do not attempt to restrain. Cool down by removing bedclothes and clothing where possible. Sponge the head and under the arms with a tepid flannel or sponge, re-soaking it regularly. When the convulsion is finished, check ABC and take action as appropriate (see pages 20-21). In most cases, the child will want to sleep. Dress him in dry clothes and let him sleep. Call a doctor for advice.

WHEN TO CALL AN AMBULANCE

Generally, neither epilepsy nor infantile convulsion are medical emergencies. However, you should be prepared to call an ambulance if:

- The casualty is injured during the seizure.
- The seizure lasts for longer than 3 minutes.
- There are repeated seizures in a short period of time.
- The casualty does not regain consciousness.

If it is the first seizure, advise the casualty to call his doctor or take him to hospital.

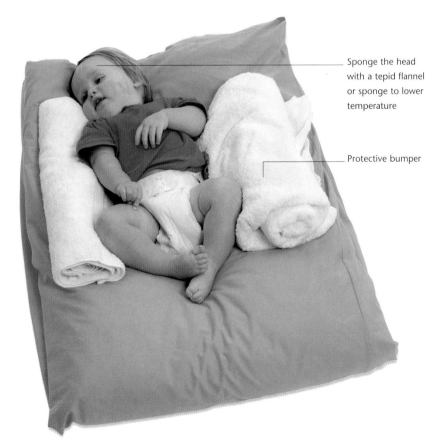

Sponge the head with a tepid flannel or sponge to lower temperature

Protective bumper

UNCONSCIOUSNESS

Unconsciousness is an interruption of normal brain activity. It can happen suddenly or gradually. Unconsciousness can be caused by a range of injuries and medical conditions, as well as by a number of different drugs. An unconscious person may still have some reactions to pain or to commands, for example, or may have no reactions at all.

Whatever the cause or degree of unconsciousness, the immediate emergency treatment remains the same:

● *Assess whether the person is unconscious by gently squeezing the shoulders and asking a question.*
● *Open the airway by lifting the chin, clearing the mouth and tilting the head.*
● *Check the breathing and be prepared to resuscitate if necessary (see pages 30-33).*
● *If breathing, check for life-threatening conditions and then turn into the recovery position (see pages 22-25).*
● *Call for emergency help.*

This may be all that you have time to do before emergency help arrives. However, if you have longer, there are some things that you can do to gather information that may help medical staff with their diagnosis and treatment.

ASSESS THE LEVEL OF RESPONSE

There is an agreed scale for assessing how responsive an injured or ill person is – the Glasgow Coma Scale. A fully alert person will score 15 while somebody who is totally unresponsive will score 3 with several variations in between (see observation chart, pages 182-83). You can help collect information to inform medical staff using some of the checks from this scale.

EYES

Do they:
● *Open without you having to ask the person to open them?*
● *Open on command?*
● *Open if you cause the person pain (this is often done by pinching the earlobe)?*
● *Remain closed?*

MOVEMENTS

Does the person:
● *Understand and follow sensible instructions?*
● *Move only in response to pain?*
● *Not move at all?*

SPEECH

Does the person:
● *Answer questions sensibly?*
● *Answer questions in a confused way?*
● *Make sounds that cannot be understood?*
● *Make no noise?*

Do these checks every 10 minutes and record your answers if you can.

Ask a question loudly and clearly

Gently shake the shoulders

MONITOR AND RECORD BREATHING AND PULSE RATE

Breathing is measured by counting the number of breaths in 1 minute (one breath being one rise and fall of the chest). Pulse rate is measured by counting the number of beats at the pulse at either the neck or the wrist for 1 minute. Take these recordings every 10 minutes and write them down if possible.The easiest place to feel a pulse is the carotid artery in the neck, though you can check the wrist.

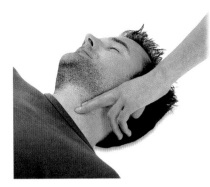

ABOVE *Press the hollow between the windpipe and large neck muscle with two fingers.*

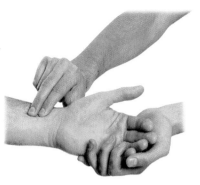

ABOVE *To check circulation, a pulse can be taken at the wrist, though this can be difficult to find.*

EXAMINING THE UNCONSCIOUS PERSON

Your initial check of the injured or ill person will be for life-threatening conditions, particularly serious bleeding (see pages 60-61). If you have more time while waiting for the ambulance, a more thorough check may show up less serious injuries or illness and potential clues to the cause of unconsciousness. This check should never be at the cost of monitoring and maintaining the airway or of keeping the injured person as still as possible. If doing a check of the body, it is sensible to do so in the presence of a third person.

Check the body from head to toe, looking for areas of bleeding, signs of broken bones or burns, or clues as to the cause of unconsciousness.

Potential causes of unconsciousness and some clues to diagnosis

Cause	Clues
Hypoglycaemia *(low blood sugar)*	*Medic alert or card declaring diabetes, diabetic medication.*
Epileptic fit	*Medic alert or card declaring epilepsy. Medication.*
Head injury	*Blood, spinal fluid from ear or nose, dent or bump on the head, uneven pupils.*
Stroke	*Paralysis on one side of the body (may be apparent in somebody with a higher level of consciousness); uneven pupils.*
Heart attack	*Details from bystanders (e.g. collapsed holding his chest), pale skin and blue lips.*
Poisoning or drugs	*Evidence of drugs or poisons, e.g. medicine bottles, syringes, empty canister with poisons label etc. Abnormal heart and/or breathing rate/rhythm.*
Fainting	*Slipped rather than fell, pale before falling. May have epileptic-type movements afterwards.*

DIABETES

Diabetes mellitus is a medical condition where the body is unable to effectively regulate the amount of sugar in the blood. The pancreas (an organ in the body) normally produces a hormone called insulin that regulates blood sugar level. In a person suffering from diabetes this does not happen effectively and as a result blood sugar levels become too high (this is known as hyperglycaemia). Most diabetics control the condition through a combination of diet and injections of insulin. Too much insulin can lead to a condition known as hypoglycaemia (low blood sugar). For more information on diabetes, see pages 408-9.

HYPERGLYCAEMIA

Hyperglycaemia is most likely to occur in an undiagnosed diabetic. Diabetes is generally first noticed in early adolescence or in middle age. If left untreated, a high blood sugar level will lead to unconsciousness and death. Onset may be gradual with deterioration often happening over a number of days.

TREATMENT

During the early stages, encourage immediate contact with the local doctor. If this is difficult, or the condition deteriorates, take or send the person to hospital. Monitor airway and breathing and be prepared to resuscitate (see pages 30-33) if necessary.

Signs and symptoms

Early signs:

- *Wanting to drink a lot (the body is trying to flush sugar from the system)*
- *Passing water regularly (urine may smell sweet)*
- *Lethargy*

As the condition deteriorates:

- *Dry skin and rapid pulse*
- *Deep, laboured breathing*
- *Increasing drowsiness*
- *Breath or skin smells strongly of acetone (like nail-polish remover) as the body tries to get rid of sugar*

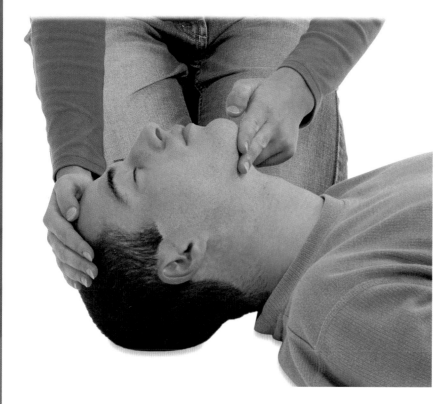

LEFT *A person whose diabetes is not under control may rapidly lose consciousness. Keep the airway open by tilting the head back and lifting the chin and check for breathing.*

HYPOGLYCAEMIA

Low blood sugar level has a quick and serious effect on the brain. Most commonly it is caused by somebody with diabetes either taking too much insulin, or taking the right amount of insulin and then either not eating enough or burning off sugar through vigorous exercise. Less commonly, it can accompany heat exhaustion, alcohol abuse or epileptic fits.

SIGNS AND SYMPTOMS

- *History of diabetes (however, a diabetic suffering a hypoglycaemia attack is often confused or aggressive and may not admit to having diabetes)*
- *Hunger*
- *Feeling faint or dizzy*
- *Strange behaviour: confusion, aggression or even violence*
- *Pale, cold, sweaty skin*
- *Rapid loss of consciousness*
- *Shallow breathing*
- *Evidence of diabetes, e.g. medic alert, sugar solution or syringe in pocket*
- *Evidence of recent heavy exercise or drinking*

TREATMENT

If the person is unconscious, monitor the airway and breathing and be prepared to resuscitate as necessary.

If the person is fully conscious, help him to sit down or to lie down with the shoulders raised. Give something high in sugar and easy to consume, such as chocolate or a sugary drink, to try to restore the body's chemical balance. If this marks an improvement, give more. If the condition does not improve, seek medical advice. Stay with the person until he recovers. Ask his guidance on what he wants to do next. Arrange for some help to take him home or to the doctor. If the condition continues to deteriorate, call an ambulance.

RIGHT *A sugary drink should help to reduce symptoms of low blood sugar but if the condition gets worse seek medical advice.*

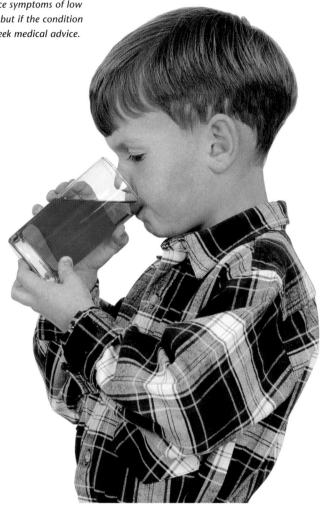

Confusion with other conditions

It is not unusual for diabetes to be mistaken for other common situations such as drunkenness, substance abuse, compression (see *Fractures of the Skull, Face and Jaw*, pages 84-85) or a stroke. The treatment in all these situations is to monitor and maintain the airway, be prepared to resuscitate if necessary, use the recovery position if the person becomes unconscious and seek medical advice or call emergency help.

Do not make assumptions as to the cause of the problem. Instead, look for clues to diagnosis for the medical staff. Somebody who is drunk may also be suffering from head injury; the syringe in a person's coat may be for diabetic medication or for drug abuse. While you do not need to know the cause the medical staff do and any clues that you can hand over could be potentially life saving.

BLEEDING

Blood is carried around the body in a transport system of arteries, capillaries and veins, and any damage to this network results in bleeding. Bleeding can be both external and internal. External bleeding involves a break to the skin surface, known as a wound, which can take many different forms. Internal bleeding is bleeding that occurs inside the body when there is no external injury for the blood to escape from. The most common form of internal bleeding is a small bruise from a minor impact. Heavy impact from car accidents, fights or falls, for example, can lead to serious internal bleeding, which may kill.

How does the body stop bleeding?

When a blood vessel is torn or cut, a series of chemical reactions takes place that causes the formation of a blood clot to seal the injury. Components of the blood known as platelets clump together at the injury site. Damaged tissue and platelets release chemicals that activate proteins called clotting factors. These react with a special protein (fibrinogen) to form a mesh of filaments that traps blood cells. These form the basis of a blood clot that contains white blood cells to help fight infection and specialised blood cells that help promote repair and recovery. Over time, the site will form a scab to protect the wound until repair has taken place. When applying pressure to the site of a wound you are helping the clotting process.

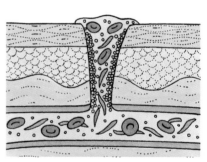

ABOVE *When a blood vessel is damaged it constricts immediately to reduce blood flow and blood loss. Platelets stick to the blood vessel walls near the site of injury.*

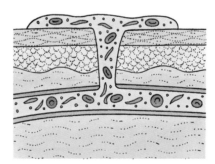

ABOVE *Platelets clump together at the site of injury and along with damaged tissue release chemicals that begin a complex series of reactions involving clotting factors.*

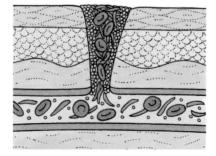

ABOVE *The final part in the chemical process is the conversion of the protein fibrinogen, found in blood plasma, into sticky threads that form a tangled mesh to trap cells.*

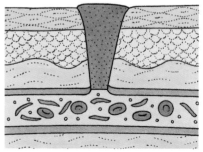

ABOVE *Cells trapped in the mesh form a blood clot at the site of injury. Over time, the clot hardens to form a protective scab over the wound while healing takes place.*

Puncture

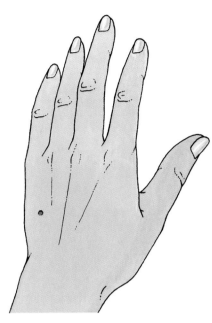

ABOVE *Puncture wounds are holes caused by long objects such as knitting needles. They do not bleed profusely but may carry dirt into body tissues which may cause infection.*

Laceration

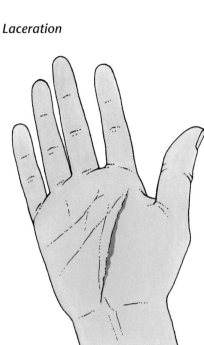

ABOVE *Clean, deep cuts caused by knives or paper are known as incisions. The underlying tissues and tendons may be damaged even though there may be little blood loss.*

Graze

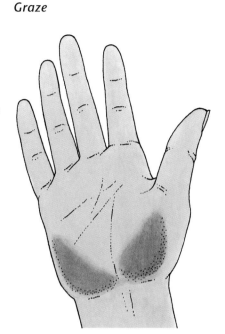

ABOVE *A graze occurs when the top layer of skin is damaged, usually caused by a fall. Grazes rarely bleed much but often have debris embedded within them.*

TRANSPORT OF BLOOD

Arteries have thick muscular walls, which contract. This pushes blood out from the heart under pressure. The blood contained within them is full of oxygen, which has been collected from the lungs, and the main function of the arteries is to take this oxygen-rich blood to the organs and body tissue. Because the blood is under pressure, and is so full of oxygen, arterial bleeding is characterised by bright red blood pumping from an injury. Arterial bleeding is very serious as blood is rapidly lost.

Veins have thin walls and return blood from the organs and tissues to the heart. They do not have muscles of their own and rely on the actions of the muscles around them to squeeze the blood around. To keep the blood moving in one direction around the body, they have a series of one-way valves that ensure a one-way flow. When these valves deteriorate, blood pools up in the veins making them swell up. This weakens the vein wall, resulting in a condition known as varicose veins (see page 395). While the blood loss from a bleeding vein does not tend to be as quick as an arterial bleed, it does nonetheless have the potential to be a very serious and even fatal injury. Bleeding from a vein will seem to flow from an injury and as it has little or no oxygen it will appear to be a dark red.

Capillaries are very thin-walled vessels. Blood is forced through them under pressure, causing the food and oxygen stored in the blood to be pushed out into the body tissues and organs. For more information on blood, see pages 208-209.

TYPES OF INJURY

Small bleeds are very common and rarely need much treatment. Large blood loss may lead, if untreated, to shock and, potentially, death.

Incisions Clean and deep cuts characterised by paper cuts and knives are known as incisions. While these wounds do not tend to bleed a lot, there may be underlying damage to tendons and other tissues.

Lacerations are jagged wounds, which tend to bleed a lot.

Puncture wounds are, as their name suggests, deep injuries caused by a long object such as a knitting needle. They do no tend to bleed a great deal but they carry the risk of infection as dirt can be carried a long way into the tissue. There is also a greater risk of damage to vital organs such as the lungs or liver.

Grazes are a commonplace injury and involve damage to the top layers of the skin. They do not cause major blood loss but are often dirty, as grazes tend to have debris embedded within them.

TREATMENT OF EXTERNAL BLEEDING

Coming across somebody who is bleeding heavily can be very frightening. It may be reassuring to remember that many adults donate up to a pint (570ml) of blood with no ill effects, and yet if this same amount were tipped on to the floor it would look very alarming. Serious shock in an adult tends to develop only after 2 pints (roughly 1 litre) of blood or more is lost from the body, and even this can be effectively treated with good first aid and early hospital care.

TREATMENT

The three main principles of the treatment of external bleeding are:

- *Look*
- *Apply direct pressure*
- *Elevate*

While treating bleeding, it is vital also to treat for shock (see pages 44-45) and to make appropriate arrangements for secondary help.

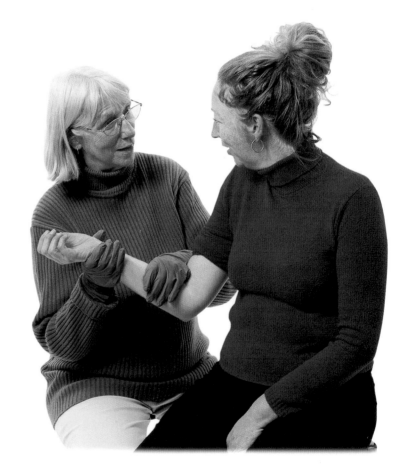

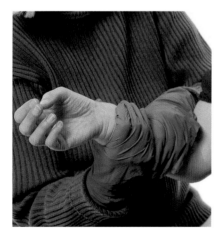

1 *Look at the wound to check how large it is. Check that the wound has nothing in it (known as a foreign body).*

2 *Apply direct pressure to the wound. If the casualty is able to press on the wound, encourage him or her to do so. If not, then apply direct pressure yourself, initially with your fingers and, if you have something to hand, eventually a sterile dressing or a piece of clean cloth.*

Applying direct pressure to the wound enables the blood to clot and therefore stems the blood flow from the cut. Once applied, a sterile dressing (or whatever you have to hand) should ideally be held in place with a firm bandage or improvised bandage such as a scarf or tie.

Protecting yourself

Where possible, you should avoid direct contact with blood or other body fluids such as vomit. This is to protect both you and the person that you are treating. There are several ways of doing this:

• *If available, use gloves. These come in many different sizes and materials (particularly useful if you have an allergy to latex) and should be kept in every first aid kit.*
• *If the person bleeding is able, ask her to apply direct pressure to the injury herself.*
• *Use bandages, dressings or other materials, such as a handkerchief or T-shirt, as a barrier between your hand and the wound.*
• *Keep injuries on your own hands covered with plasters or dressings.*

If you do get blood on your skin, simply wash off well with soap and hot water. Clear up spills of blood or vomit with a bleach and water solution. Clothing that has been stained by blood or vomit should be put through a hot wash in the washing machine.

If you are concerned about the possibility of infection after dealing with body fluids, contact your doctor. It is important to remember that the risk of cross-infection is minimal and that in most instances where you are applying first aid you will be doing so for a member of your own family.

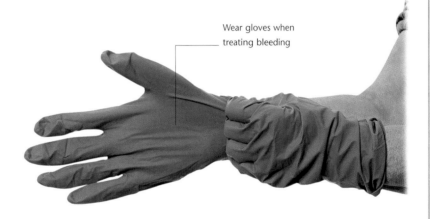

Wear gloves when treating bleeding

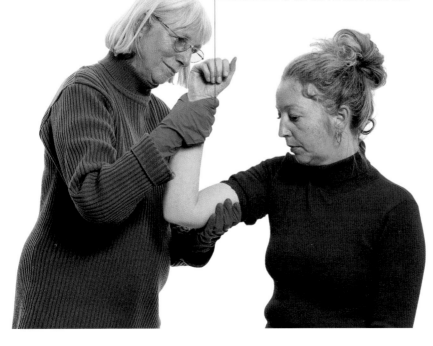

Raise the wound above the level of the heart to stem blood flow

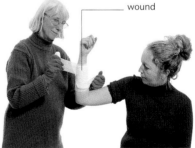

Apply a bandage to the wound

3 *Elevate the wound. If the injury is on an arm or leg, raise the wound above the level of the heart. It is harder for the blood to pump upwards and this therefore reduces the blood flow to the wound and thus the fluid loss from the body.*

4 *Treat for shock (see pages 44-45). Keep the casualty warm and continually at rest. Reassure the casualty.*

BLEEDING FROM THE HEAD OR PALM

Bleeding from the head is usually caused by a blow. The scalp in particular has a rich blood supply and even a small wound can bleed heavily. The palm of the hand is commonly cut while cutting objects or through a fall. Bleeding is often severe as the palm also has a rich blood supply. There are many tendons and nerves in the hand, and wounds to the palm many be accompanied by loss of movement or feeling in the fingers.

HOW TO TREAT HEAD BLEEDS
Treatment should include taking full details of what happened and checking for signs of head injury, such as skull fracture, concussion or compression (see *Fractures of the Skull, Face and Jaw*, pages 84-85).

1 *Help the injured person to sit or lie down.*

2 *Check for any signs of head injury. Treat as appropriate.*

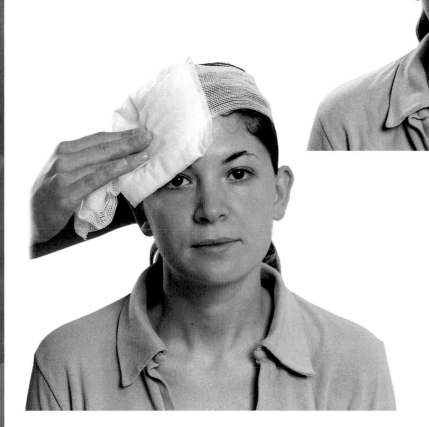

3 *Using a sterile bandage, apply direct pressure to the wound to stop the bleeding.*

4 *Cover the wound with a sterile dressing or a clean pad. Tie this in place with a bandage.*

5 *Take or send the casualty to hospital as soon as possible.*

If the casualty becomes unconscious, monitor and maintain airway and breathing and be prepared to resuscitate as necessary (see pages 30-33).

HOW TO TREAT BLEEDING FROM THE PALM

1 *Help the casualty to sit or lie down. Apply direct pressure to the wound and raise the arm. If the person has had a fall, take care to rule out a broken arm or collar bone before raising the arm.*

2 *Place a sterile dressing or clean pad in the hand and ask the casualty to grip her fingers over it. Bandage the fingers so that they are clenched over the pad. Leave the thumb exposed. If there is an embedded object in the wound, treat the hand flat and bandage around the object. If tendon damage means that the fingers cannot be clenched, bandage the wound with the hand flat.*

3 *Treat for shock (see pages 44-45) if necessary. Keep the casualty warm, at rest and reassure him or her.*

4 *Support the arm in an elevation sling and take or send the casualty to hospital.*

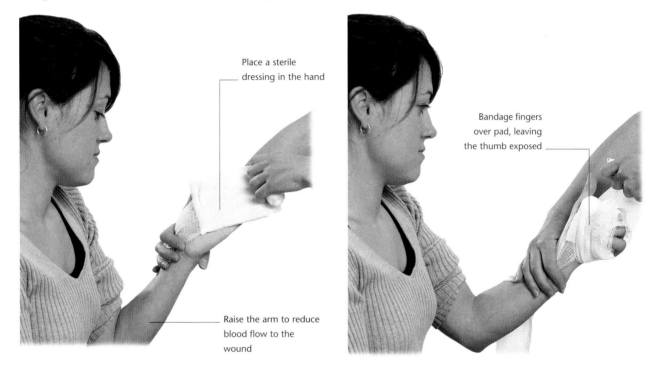

Place a sterile dressing in the hand

Raise the arm to reduce blood flow to the wound

Bandage fingers over pad, leaving the thumb exposed

Signs and symptoms of skull fracture, concussion and compression

Skull fracture
- *Bruising to the eye socket*
- *Pain*
- *A bump or dent in the skull*
- *Straw-coloured fluid coming from one or both ears*
- *Casualty becomes increasingly drowsy and unresponsive over a period of time. Does she respond slowly to questions or commands? Is she having problems focusing?*

Concussion
- *Pale skin*
- *Dizziness, blurred vision or nausea*

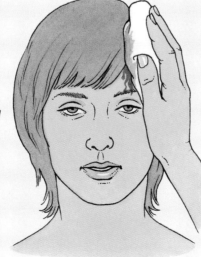

- *Headache*
- *Brief or partial loss of consciousness*

Compression
- *Person becomes increasingly drowsy and unresponsive*
- *Flushed and dry skin*
- *Slurred speech and confusion*
- *Partial or total loss of movement, often down one side of the body*
- *One pupil appears to be larger than the other*
- *Noisy breathing, which becomes slow*
- *Slow, strong pulse*

TREATING CHEST OR ABDOMINAL WOUNDS

The chest wall protects the lungs, heart and other essential organs such as the liver. A puncture wound to the chest can therefore be extremely serious. Wounds to the abdomen (stomach and intestines) are very serious. External bleeding may be severe and internal bleeding is likely, both of which will lead to serious shock. In addition, there may be damage to internal organs and the digestive system.

CHEST WOUNDS

Common complications of penetrating chest wounds include:

• *Collapsed lung (pneumothorax), caused by air entering the space between the chest wall and the lungs. This applies pressure to the lungs, causing them to collapse. The lung can also be damaged directly, causing it to fill with blood.*
• *Tension pneumothorax which occurs when the pressure builds up sufficiently to affect the uninjured lung and possibly even the heart.*
• *Damage to vital organs such as the liver – this will result in severe shock as these organs have a large blood supply.*

1 *Seal the wound using, in the first instance, your hand or the casualty's hand.*

Signs and symptoms of chest wounds

• Difficulty with breathing
• Shock
• Bright red, frothy blood (blood with air in it) being coughed up or escaping from the wound
• Pale skin with blue lips
• Sound of air being sucked into the chest

TREATMENT

2 *Help the casualty into a position that makes it easier for him to breathe. This will usually be sitting up and inclined to the injured side. This allows the uninjured lung maximum room to move and allows blood to pool on the injured side.*

3 *Cover the wound with a dressing and cover the dressing with airtight material,*

such as plastic or foil. Seal this on three sides.

4 *Call an ambulance and treat for shock (see pages 44-45).*

If the casualty is unconscious, monitor and maintain the airway and be prepared to resuscitate (see pages 30-33) if necessary (sealing the wound before resuscitating). Place the casualty injured side down.

TREATING ABDOMINAL WOUNDS

1 *Call an ambulance and help the casualty to lie down in the most comfortable position.*

2 *Consider the position of the wound. If it is vertical – runs down the abdomen – moving the casualty so that he is lying flat on the ground will help bring the edges together, ease discomfort and help reduce bleeding. If the wound is horizontal, gently raising the legs will have the same effect.*

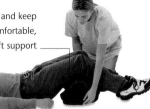

Raise the legs and keep the person comfortable, with a soft support

ABOVE *A horizontal wound can be helped if you raise the casualty's legs and support them with a rolled-up coat or blanket. This action will help close the edges of the wound and slow down the flow of blood.*

Move the person gently into a position where he is comfortable.

Lying flat will bring together the edges of a vertical wound

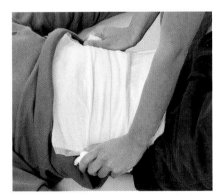

3 *Place a large dressing over the wound and secure in place. Add pads to this dressing as necessary.*

4 *Treat for shock (see pages 44-45).*

Support the wound if the casualty coughs, vomits or needs to be moved into the recovery position (see pages 22-25). Press lightly on the bandage to prevent intestines protruding from the wound. If intestines are protruding, do not attempt to replace them. Cover with a clean piece of plastic film.

Major organs

Damage to any of the body's major organs can be life-threatening and prompt action must therefore be taken to minimise the effects of injuries to the chest or abdomen. Even when external bleeding is slight, the risk of internal bleeding cannot be discounted. Knowing whereabouts in the body the organs are located will help a first aider to assess a situation and decide the most appropriate emergency treatment, as well as give accurate information when the emergency services arrive.

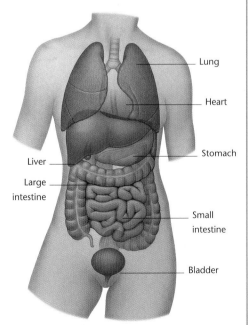

Lung

Heart

Stomach

Liver

Large intestine

Small intestine

Bladder

CRUSH INJURIES, IMPALEMENT AND AMPUTATION

Crush injuries generally result from serious car accidents or explosions. There may be part of the body stuck under heavy debris; several broken bones, multiple external bleeding and much internal bleeding; burns from an explosion; severe shock, and deterioration into unconsciousness. If a person is impaled on an immovable object, treatment is similar to that for a foreign object embedded in a wound (see page 71). An amputation is where a part of the body has been severed. This may occur through a straight and heavy cut or through twisting and pulling under extreme force.

TREATING CRUSH INJURIES

1 *Ensure that it is safe to approach the scene. If in doubt, call the emergency services and wait for help.*

2 *Monitor and maintain airway and breathing and be prepared to resuscitate if necessary (see pages 30-33).*

3 *Treat major bleeding and cover smaller wounds with sterile dressings.*

4 *Keep the injured person still and try to reassure them while waiting for help.*

5 *Treat for shock (see pages 44-45). Keep the person warm and still.*

6 *Make an early call for an ambulance and explain what has happened.*

IF THE INJURED PERSON IS TRAPPED

There are additional risks for the injured person if any part of the body is trapped. Releasing the body may bring on severe shock as fluid leaks to the injured part.

An even greater cause for concern is 'crush syndrome'. Toxins build up around the injury site and are trapped by an object crushing the person. If the object is removed, these are suddenly released into the body, and the kidneys, the organs chiefly responsible for flushing out toxins, cannot cope. This condition can be fatal.

IF THE PERSON HAS BEEN TRAPPED FOR LESS THAN 10 MINUTES

Crush syndrome takes some time to develop. If you can do so, safely remove the object. Treat as for crush injuries above.

IF THE PERSON HAS BEEN TRAPPED FOR LONGER THAN 10 MINUTES

Make an early call for help, explaining the situation. Treat as for crush injuries above and reassure the person.

Monitor and maintain airway and breathing

Remove object if possible

TREATING IMPALEMENT

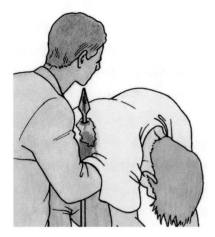

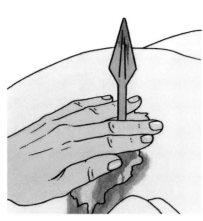

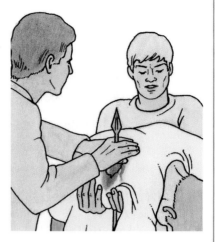

1 Do not attempt to remove the object or to move the injured person.

2 Provide swift assistance for the injured person, supporting his body weight where possible to prevent any further damage.

3 If bleeding is severe, apply pressure around the edges of the wound without pressing on the object.

4 Try to stop the object moving around as much as possible, enlisting bystander support where available.

5 Call an ambulance, making sure that you explain the need for cutting equipment or fire service.

6 Treat for shock (see pages 44-45) as best you can.

TREATING AMPUTATION

1 Your priority is to stop any bleeding at the site of the injury. Apply direct pressure and raise the injured stump. An amputation high on the arm or leg can be accompanied by severe arterial bleeding, particularly if caused by a twisting or tearing movement. Be prepared to apply continuous pressure using several pads as necessary.

2 If the bleeding comes under control, cover the wound with a sterile dressing or clean non-fluffy material tied in place with a bandage.

3 Treat for shock (see pages 44-45) and reassure the person.

4 Call an ambulance, advising that there is an amputation.

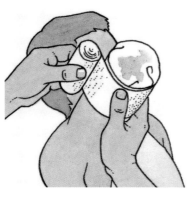

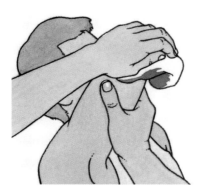

FOR THE AMPUTATED PART

A surgeon may be able to reattach the amputated part.

1 Wrap the part in a plastic bag and wrap the bag in a clean cloth.

2 Place the cloth-wrapped bag in ice and place into a sturdy container. Do not let the ice come into close contact with the amputated part, as this will damage the flesh. Do not wash the amputated part.

3 Label the container with the time of injury and the casualty's name and make sure that you hand it over personally to medical staff.

INTERNAL BLEEDING

Severe internal bleeding is a potentially life-threatening condition. While the blood may not be obvious it is still lost from the circulatory system and the victim is therefore very likely to go into shock (see pages 44-45). Internal bleeding may also cause a build-up of pressure that, in areas such as the skull or around the heart, can cause serious problems, loss of consciousness and, if untreated, lead to death.

STIES OF BLEEDING

Internal bleeding can be very difficult to identify. It is not unusual for internal bleeding to happen slowly, with signs and symptoms showing up days after an accident. It can happen to any part of the body but the richness of the blood supply in the stomach, around the organs such as the liver and the spleen and in the bowel make these sites particularly vulnerable.

Internal bleeding is also likely to accompany some broken bones. The thigh bone protects the femoral artery and if broken may pierce it, causing a large and life-threatening bleed.

TREATMENT

1 *Treat for shock. Keep the casualty warm. Place him in a comfortable position, preferably lying down with the legs slightly raised. Reassure him. Treat any external bleeding or bleeding from orifices.*

2 *Call for an ambulance as soon as possible and explain what has happened.*

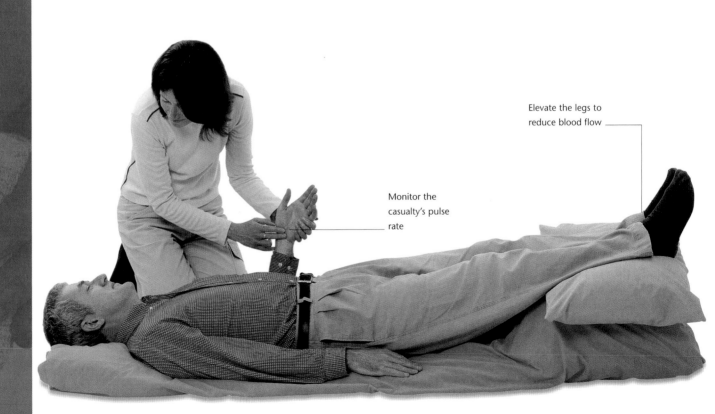

Monitor the casualty's pulse rate

Elevate the legs to reduce blood flow

Monitor and record the person's pulse and breathing rates. This information will be useful for the medical staff in determining the extent of the injury.

If the casualty becomes unconscious, place in the recovery position (see pages 22-25) and monitor airway and breathing. Be prepared to resuscitate if necessary (see pages 30-33).

Bruising

Less serious internal bleeding such as small bruises can be treated with a cold compress to relieve pain and reduce swelling. However, the possibility of further internal bleeding or underlying injury should not be ruled out, particularly if the casualty is known, for example, to have hit his head on a window during a car accident, or has been hit in the stomach by a reversing car. For more information on bruising, see *Minor Wounds*, pages 76-77.

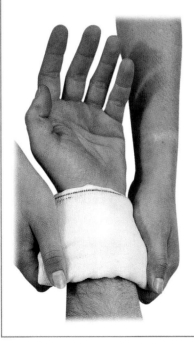

Signs and symptoms

• *The person is known to have had an accident (not necessarily in the immediate past)*

• *Signs and symptoms of shock (see pages 44-45)*

• *Bruising*

• *Boarding – this most commonly occurs where there is bleeding into the stomach area; the quantity of blood combined with the tissues swelling result in a rigidity to the tissues*

• *Swelling*

• *Bleeding from body orifices (see Bleeding from Special Sites, pages 72-73)*

If there is any combination of these signs and symptoms, suspect internal bleeding

Major organs susceptible to internal bleeding

Internal bleeding can happen in any part of the body but the stomach, the liver, spleen and intestines are particularly vulnerable because they have a rich blood supply. Internal bleeding can be very difficult to identify and signs and symptoms may not arise until several days after an accident has occurred.

Liver

Spleen

Stomach

Intestines

EYE WOUNDS AND DIFFICULT PLACES TO BANDAGE

Cuts to the eye can be very frightening and even small, difficult to notice injuries are potentially very serious. However, medical treatments mean that even injuries that appear to be very severe may not necessarily result in the loss of sight in the eye. Do not touch the affected eye.

Signs and symptoms of eye wounds

- *Knowing that something has impacted with the eye – this could be as small as a grain of sand or a splinter*
- *Pain in the eye*
- *Loss or limitation of vision*
- *Bleeding*

TREATMENT

Prevent further injury and get medical help as soon as possible.

1 *Lie the person down, on his back if possible, and hold the head to prevent movement and keep it stable.*

2 *Ask the person to try to keep his eyes still to prevent movement of the injured eye. Ask the person to focus on something to prevent movement.*

3 *Ask the casualty to hold a clean pad over the eye to help prevent movement and infection. If the wait for an ambulance or other further help may take some time, you may wish to hold the pad for the person or to gently bandage it in place. However, as blood loss from the eye area is not likely to be life-threatening, any bandage should be used only to hold the pad in place and not to apply pressure.*

ABOVE *Hold a clean pad over the eye to prevent movement and infection but do not apply pressure by bandaging it tightly.*

Do not attempt to remove any object embedded in the eye. If the object is very long, then gently support it to prevent movement at its base. If small, ensure that the pad you place over the eye does not push it in any further.

Hold the head to prevent movement

TREATING AN OBJECT EMBEDDED IN THE WOUND

The first step in the treatment of any external bleeding is to check the extent of the injury and see if there is anything embedded in the wound.

1 *Apply pressure around the edges of the wound using your hands or the casualty's hands without pressing on the object.*

2 *Replace this pressure with a dressing or clean material and bandage firmly in place, avoiding pressure on the object.*

3 *Raise the injured limb if possible to staunch the flow of blood.*

4 *Prevent longer objects from moving by supporting them with your hands or by packing around the base of the object with blankets, for example.*

5 *Treat for shock (see pages 44-45) and reassure the casualty.*

If the casualty is impaled on something which cannot be moved, support him or her to stop from pulling on the impaled object and causing further damage. Where possible, treat the casualty as described above, and ensure that the emergency services are aware of the need for cutting equipment. For further information on impalement, see pages 66-67.

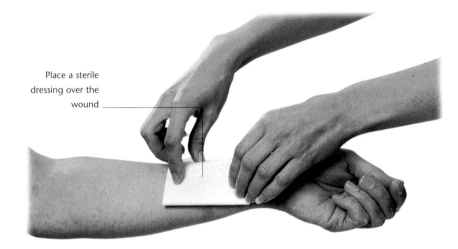

Place a sterile dressing over the wound

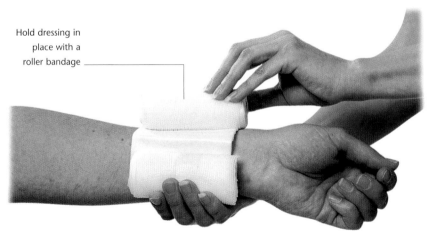

Hold dressing in place with a roller bandage

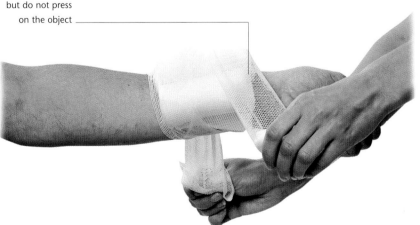

Bandage firmly but do not press on the object

Warning

If there is something stuck into the injury, do not attempt to remove it because:

• *If the object went in at an angle, you may cause more damage pulling it out*
• *You may leave splinters in the wound*
• *The object may be pressing against a vein or an artery, reducing blood loss*
• *You may have mistaken a broken bone for a foreign body*

The principles of applying pressure, elevating and treating for shock (see pages 60-61) still apply.

BLEEDING FROM SPECIAL SITES

Bleeding from bodily orifices includes nosebleeds, bleeding from the ear, mouth, vagina, anus and urethra. It may be an indication of a serious disorder.

NOSEBLEED

Nosebleeds are very common and often the cause is unknown. For general treatment of uncomplicated nosebleed, see *Controlling Bleeding from the Mouth and Nose*, pages 74-75. If the bleed follows a heavy impact to the nose, then assume that there may be a broken nose or cheekbone (see *Fractures of the Skull, Face and Jaw*, pages 84-85).

BLEEDING FROM THE EAR

If the blood from the ear is thin and watery then it is likely that there has been some damage to the skull, and possibly the brain, as the blood is mixing with the fluid that cushions the brain. This is a very serious injury and the emergency services should be called as soon as possible. Keep the casualty as still as you can and gently rest the head, injured ear down, with a clean

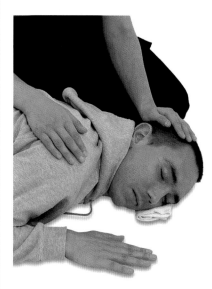

How to treat bleeding from the mouth

1 Lean the person forward and encourage him to spit any blood and/or broken teeth into a receptacle.

2 If the bleed is easy to reach, controlling it may be helped by placing a small dressing over the wound and encouraging the casualty to apply pressure for 10 minutes. If there is a severe bleed from a tooth socket, place a rolled-up dressing, large enough to stop the teeth from meeting, into the mouth and ask the casualty to bite on it. If this does not control the bleeding after 10 minutes, reapply a clean pad.

If the bleeding has not stopped after 30 minutes, or is particularly severe, either take or send the casualty to hospital. There may be damage to the jaw or cheekbone. Cold compresses may relieve this pain and reduce swelling and you may need to support broken bones with pads or your hands (see also *Fractures of the Skull, Face and Jaw*, pages 84-85).

How to treat nosebleeds

1 Lean the person forward and encourage him to spit blood into a handkerchief or some other receptacle.

2 Pinch the nose just below the hard bit at its top and apply firm pressure for 10 minutes (this is the amount of time it takes for a clot to form). If the bleeding has not stopped after 10 minutes, apply pressure for two further periods of 10 minutes. If it is still bleeding then either take or send the casualty to hospital.

Once the bleeding has stopped, advise the casualty not to scratch, pick or blow his nose, not to drink hot liquid and not to exert himself, as all these activities can dislodge the clot and cause the bleeding to start again.

LEFT *If there is blood loss from the ear, keep the casualty as still as possible and rest the head with the injured side down, with a clean pad held over the ear into which the blood can drain.*

RIGHT *A woman with vaginal bleeding needs to be treated sensitively. Provide clean towels or sanitary pads, and keep these for medical staff to check if you suspect a miscarriage.*

pad held over the ear for the blood to drain into. Do not tie this pad in place. Keep a check on the casualty's airway and breathing and be prepared to resuscitate if necessary (see pages 30-33).

If the blood is bright red and is accompanied by earache, deafness, a sudden change in pressure or an explosion then it is likely to be a burst eardrum. Again, keep the injured ear downwards, hold a clean pad in place and seek medical attention.

BLEEDING FROM THE MOUTH

If bleeding from the mouth follows a direct impact to the face it is likely that the bleed has been caused by damage to the teeth, gums or tongue. There may also be damage to the jaw and cheekbones (see *Controlling Bleeding from the Mouth and Nose*, pages 74-75).

Bright red and frothy bleeding from the mouth may be a sign of damage to the lungs (see chest and abdominal wounds, pages 64-65).

Dark red blood being coughed up from the mouth may be a sign of a burst stomach ulcer. Seek urgent medical attention.

BLEEDING FROM THE VAGINA

The most likely reason for vaginal bleeding is menstruation (periods). If this is the case and the bleed is accompanied by cramps then a woman may wish to take her normal painkillers.

A woman complaining of vaginal bleeding not related to her periods should be given privacy and sensitive handling, with gentle questioning to determine the cause. For all vaginal bleeding, provide sanitary pads or a

clean towel where possible. Where the bleeding is potentially pregnancy-related, do not dispose of old pads of any blood loss. Instead, move these discreetly away from the woman to be checked by medical staff.

Bleeding in early pregnancy may be an indication of a miscarriage, but there are a number of other potential causes. Make the woman comfortable and seek advice from her midwife or doctor. If the bleeding is severe and/or she is displaying signs of shock (see pages 44-45), call an ambulance.

In later pregnancy a bright red, painless bleed may indicate a serious problem with the placenta. Make the woman comfortable, call an ambulance and treat for shock.

If the bleeding is as a result of an accident or recent assault, call an ambulance and treat for shock.

BLEEDING FROM THE ANUS

Bleeding from the anus may be bright red and fresh looking. If it follows a recent accident, this may indicate injury to the anus or lower bowel. Treat for shock as appropriate and seek medical help.

Black, tarry blood has been partially digested and indicates a potential injury to the upper bowel. Again, treat for shock as appropriate and seek medical help.

BLEEDING FROM THE URETHRA

Blood in the urine, particularly following an accident, may indicate injury to the bladder or kidneys. It may also accompany a broken pelvis where the bone has damaged the bladder. Treat for shock as appropriate and seek medical help.

CONTROLLING BLEEDING FROM THE MOUTH AND NOSE

There are a number of potential reasons for bleeding from the mouth. If the bleed is a result of direct impact to the face, there are likely to be injuries to the jaw and possibly the cheekbone, as well as to the gums and teeth. It may also be that the bleed follows dental treatment. In the case of nosebleeds, find out what caused the nosebleed so you can establish whether the the nose or cheekbone has been damaged. Many nosebleeds start spontaneously and the cause is never known. The priority with any mouth or nosebleed is to protect the casualty's airway and try to prevent blood being swallowed as this may cause vomiting.

HOW TO TREAT BLEEDING FROM THE MOUTH

1 *Lean the casualty forward and encourage her to spit out any blood and/or broken teeth into a receptacle.*

2 *If the bleed is easy to reach, controlling it may be helped by placing a small dressing over the wound and encouraging the casualty to apply pressure for 10 minutes.*

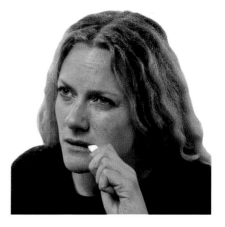

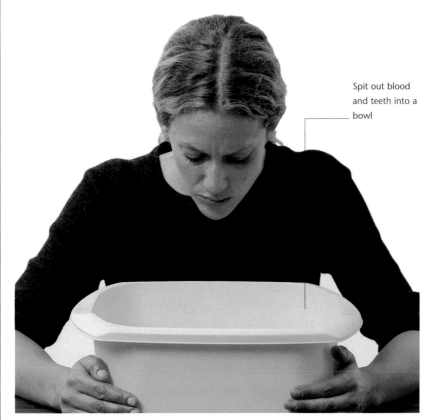

Spit out blood and teeth into a bowl

3 *If there is a severe bleed from a tooth socket, place a rolled-up dressing, large enough to stop the teeth from meeting, into the mouth and ask the casualty to bite on it. If this does not control the bleeding after 10 minutes, reapply a clean pad.*

If the bleeding has not stopped after 30 minutes, or is particularly severe, either take or send the casualty to hospital.

There may be damage to the jaw or cheekbone. Cold compresses may relieve this pain and reduce swelling and you may need to support broken bones with pads or your hands (see also *Fractures of the Skull, Face and Jaw*, pages 84-85).

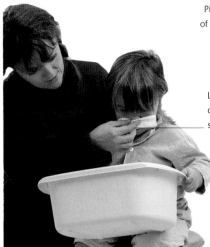

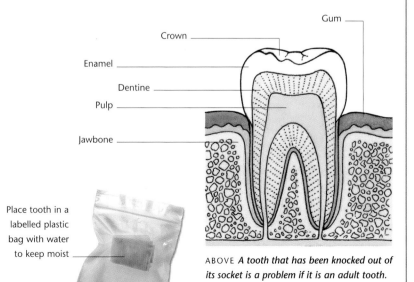

Pinch the bridge
of the nose firmly
for 10 minutes

Lean the casualty
over a bowl to
spit out blood

HOW TO TREAT NOSEBLEEDS

1 *Lean the casualty forward and encourage him to spit blood into a handkerchief or some other receptacle.*

2 *Pinch the nose just below the hard part at its top and apply firm pressure for 10 minutes (this is the amount of time it takes for a clot to form). If the bleeding has not stopped after 10 minutes, apply pressure for two further periods of 10 minutes. If bleeding continues then either take or send the casualty to hospital.*

Once the bleeding has stopped, advise the casualty not to scratch, pick or blow his nose, not to drink hot liquid and not to exert himself, as all these activities can dislodge the clot and cause the bleeding to start again.

If the nose or cheek appears to be broken

Lean the casualty forward and encourage him to spit out blood. Do not pinch the nose. Cold compresses either side of the injury may provide some relief and help to reduce the bleeding.

If a tooth has been knocked out

Adult teeth can sometimes be replanted in the mouth, so it is worth storing the tooth carefully. Do not wash the tooth; instead, place it in a labelled plastic bag with some milk or water to keep it moist, and send with the person to the emergency dentist or hospital. Teeth need to be replanted quickly – go to a dentist or hospital emergency department.

Gum

Crown

Enamel

Dentine

Pulp

Jawbone

Place tooth in a
labelled plastic
bag with water
to keep moist

ABOVE *A tooth that has been knocked out of its socket is a problem if it is an adult tooth. The front teeth are the ones most commonly knocked out, often during contact sports.*

MINOR WOUNDS

Most minor wounds can be treated in the home without the need for further medical attention. First aid treatment can promote recovery and prevent infection. However, further medical advice should be sought if: there is a foreign body embedded in the wound; the wound shows signs of infection; the wound has the potential for tetanus and the injured person's immunisation is not up to date; the wound is from a human or animal bite.

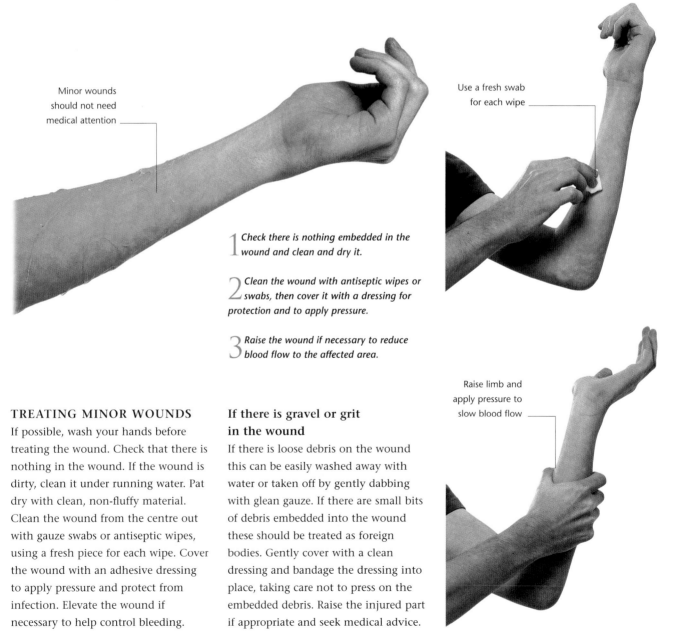

Minor wounds should not need medical attention

Use a fresh swab for each wipe

1 Check there is nothing embedded in the wound and clean and dry it.

2 Clean the wound with antiseptic wipes or swabs, then cover it with a dressing for protection and to apply pressure.

3 Raise the wound if necessary to reduce blood flow to the affected area.

Raise limb and apply pressure to slow blood flow

TREATING MINOR WOUNDS

If possible, wash your hands before treating the wound. Check that there is nothing in the wound. If the wound is dirty, clean it under running water. Pat dry with clean, non-fluffy material. Clean the wound from the centre out with gauze swabs or antiseptic wipes, using a fresh piece for each wipe. Cover the wound with an adhesive dressing to apply pressure and protect from infection. Elevate the wound if necessary to help control bleeding.

If there is gravel or grit in the wound

If there is loose debris on the wound this can be easily washed away with water or taken off by gently dabbing with glean gauze. If there are small bits of debris embedded into the wound these should be treated as foreign bodies. Gently cover with a clean dressing and bandage the dressing into place, taking care not to press on the embedded debris. Raise the injured part if appropriate and seek medical advice.

BRUISING

A bruise is the sign of an internal bleed. Usually caused by direct impact, bruises are sometimes painful but generally heal swiftly with little intervention needed.

A bruise goes through several changes in appearance as it heals and may not appear for some time, even days, after the accident. Initially, the injured part may be red from the impact; over time this may become blue as blood seeps into the injured tissue; as it heals it becomes brown and then fades to yellow.

Severe bruising can also be the sign of serious internal bleeding. If bruising is extensive and is accompanied by any of the following signs and symptoms assume that a serious internal bleed is present. Treat the injured person for shock and seek medical help.

Signs and symptoms of internal bleeding

- *Casualty is known to have had an accident (not necessarily in the immediate past)*
- *Signs and symptoms of shock*
- *Bruising*
- *Boarding – this most commonly occurs where there is bleeding into the stomach area; the quantity of blood combined with the tissues swelling results in a rigidity to the tissues*
- *Swelling*
- *Bleeding from body orifices (see Bleeding from Special Sites, pages 72-73)*

Most bruises, however, are not serious. First aid can reduce pain and promote recovery from an uncomfortable bruise.

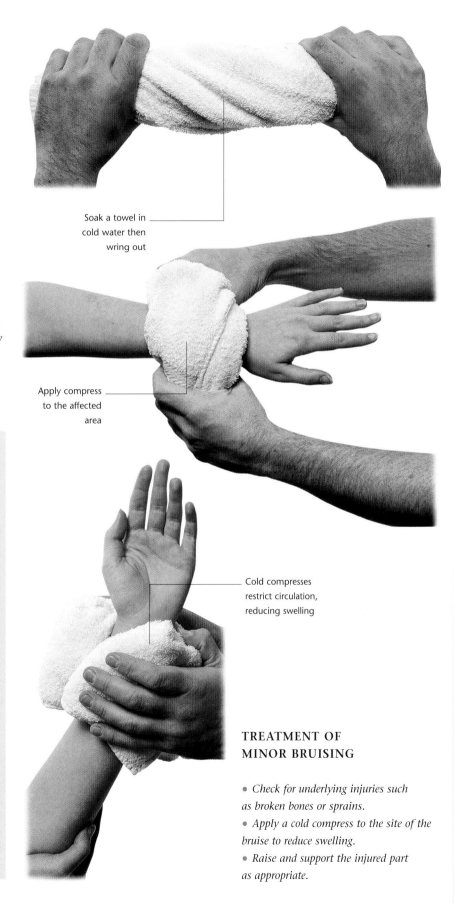

Soak a towel in cold water then wring out

Apply compress to the affected area

Cold compresses restrict circulation, reducing swelling

TREATMENT OF MINOR BRUISING

- *Check for underlying injuries such as broken bones or sprains.*
- *Apply a cold compress to the site of the bruise to reduce swelling.*
- *Raise and support the injured part as appropriate.*

INFECTED WOUNDS

Any injury that pierces the skin can become infected. Infection is caused by germs entering the body, either through the object causing the injury (for example a dirty knife) or from sources after the injury occurred. Cuts, burns, bites, stings and open fractures all carry with them a risk of infection.

PREVENTING INFECTION

There is a number of things that you can do to reduce the risk of infection.

- *When time permits (for example for non life-threatening, less serious injuries), wash your hands thoroughly before treating an open wound.*
- *Wear gloves if available.*
- *Try to reduce direct contact with the open wound – for example, ask the injured person to apply pressure with her own hand if possible.*
- *Cover injuries as soon as practicable.*
- *Do not cough over injuries – turn away and cover your mouth.*
- *Advise the injured person to check that her tetanus immunisation is up to date.*

Signs and symptoms of infection

If the following signs and symptoms develop after an open wound is inflicted, the injured person should seek immediate medical attention:

- *Increased pain*
- *Swelling*
- *Redness around the site of the wound*
- *Discharge from the site*
- *Unpleasant smell from the site of the wound*
- *Red tracks from the site to the heart*
- *Swollen glands*
- *Failure to heal*

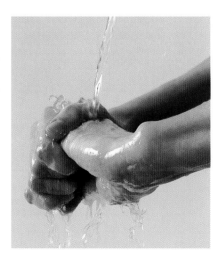

ABOVE *Wash your hands thoroughly under running water before treating an open wound if you have time to do so. This will reduce the risk of transmitting germs into the wound.*

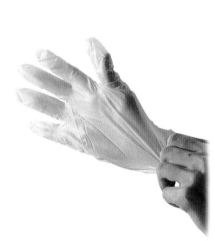

ABOVE *A disposable rubber glove is an ideal barrier method to prevent contamination of a wound. Keep a pair in the top of your first aid box to reduce direct contact with the wound.*

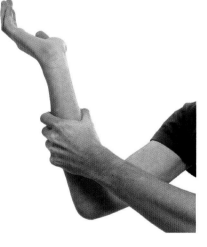

ABOVE *Ask the person who has been injured to apply pressure with her own hand if possible to reduce direct contact with an open wound and lessen the risk of infection.*

TREATING AN INFECTED WOUND

1 *Cover the wound with a sterile dressing and bandage into place.*

2 *Raise the injured part if possible, to reduce swelling and pain.*

3 *Seek early medical advice. Treat for shock if necessary (see pages 44-45).*

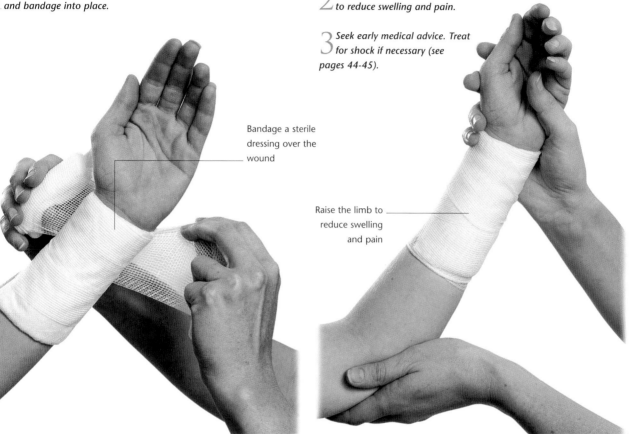

Bandage a sterile dressing over the wound

Raise the limb to reduce swelling and pain

SPECIFIC INJURIES AND THE RISK OF INFECTION

Bleeding wounds

The immediate risk of infection with a serious bleed is minimised as blood leaving the body carries away debris and potential germs. Minor wounds and grazes caused by dirty objects present a greater risk of infection. Puncture wounds are particularly bad as they carry infection deep into the tissue, tend not to bleed a lot and can be difficult to clean. For more information on bleeding, see pages 58-65.

Burns

Infection is one of the biggest concerns with burns. Large areas of skin are often destroyed, leaving the body vulnerable to infection. Unlike cuts, burns are not healed through clotting and can take a long time to heal over. This means that they are open to infection for a long period. After cooling, burns should be covered with a sterile, or very clean, non-fluffy dressing. Alternative dressings include clean sandwich bags or clingfilm. For more information on burns, see pages 104-111.

Open fractures

Infections in the bone take a long time to heal, in some cases requiring extensive surgery and even removal of the infected area. Open fractures, where the broken bone pokes through the skin, carry a particular risk of infection and should be treated with care. Do not touch the ends of the bone. Instead, cover the area as soon as possible with a light, sterile, or very clean, non-fluffy dressing, replacing this with a firmer dressing and bandage as appropriate. For more information on open fractures, see pages 82-83.

Bites and stings

Animal bites and wounds caused by insects may cause infection to the wounded area and certain animals and insects carry specific risks, such as rabies from infected dog bites, for example. Clean and dress the site of the injury and seek medical attention. Check that tetanus immunization is up-to-date. For more information on bites and stings, see pages 130-133.

FRACTURES, DISLOCATIONS AND SOFT TISSUE INJURIES

Fracture is just another word for a broken bone. A dislocation occurs at the site of a joint and is where a bone is fully or partially displaced. Soft tissue injuries include sprains, strains and ruptures. They are often caused in the same way as fractures and generally are hard to distinguish from broken bones.

BROKEN BONES

There are two main types of broken bone. The first is a closed (simple) break or fracture, where the bone has broken but has not pierced the skin. A closed fracture is sometimes difficult to diagnose, even for experienced medical staff, who will usually rely on an X-ray (see pages 454-455) to determine whether or not the bone is definitely broken. The second type is an open (compound) break or fracture, where the bone has either pierced the skin or is associated with an open wound. The greatest risk with open breaks is infection. Both open and closed breaks can result in injury to underlying organs or blood vessels and may also be unstable if the ends of the broken bone are moving around. In young children the bones are not fully formed and may bend rather than break (termed a greenstick fracture).

While it is possible to give some general guidance for the recognition of broken bones, no two people are identical in their response. The first general rule therefore is, if in doubt, assume that a bone is broken and treat as such. Be particularly aware of potential fractures if the accident involved a sharp blow, a fall, a rapid increase or decrease of speed, or a sudden twist.

DISLOCATIONS

The most common sites for dislocations are the shoulders, thumbs and hips. Dislocations are usually characterised by intense pain and an obvious deformity. There may be signs and symptoms similar to a broken bone, including feelings of pins and needles or numbness below the site of the injury, caused by trapped nerves or blood vessels. Do not attempt to replace the bone. Make the casualty comfortable and take or send him to hospital.

SOFT TISSUE INJURIES

Strains are an overstretching of the muscle, leading to a partial tear. Ruptures are complete tears in muscles. Sprains are injuries to a ligament at or near a joint. The signs and symptoms of soft tissue injuries will be similar to the signs and symptoms of a fracture and will generally follow a sharp twisting or stretching movement.

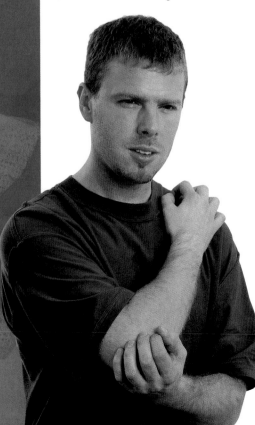

LEFT *If a bone is misshapen, it may be fractured. There is likely to be swelling and bruising. Keep the bone still to reduce pain and swelling and prevent further damage.*

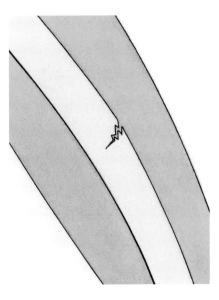

ABOVE *If a long bone in the arm or leg bends it may crack on one side only, known as a greenstick fracture. This type of fracture only occurs in children, whose bones are still flexible.*

Signs and symptoms of broken bones

PAIN This accompanies most, but not all, fractures and is caused by the broken bone ends pushing on to nerve endings

DEFORMITY An injured part may appear deformed, particularly when compared to the uninjured side

SWELLING

TENDERNESS This accompanies most broken bones and can often only be felt when the injured part is gently touched

SHOCK The signs and symptoms of shock (see pages 44-45) will often accompany major fractures in particular. There may be reddening or bruising over the

site of the break, but this often takes some time to appear. You may also hear the ends of broken bone rubbing together, a sound known as crepitus

Another potential sign of a broken bone is a lack of feeling or a 'pins and needles' sensation below the fracture site. This may indicate nerve damage or a reduction in circulation caused by the bone pushing on either the nerves or the blood vessels. The treatment for injuries displaying these symptoms is the same as for any broken bone. However, if you have been trained, applying traction may alleviate the problem

If your casualty is displaying any combination of these signs and symptoms or the nature of the accident suggests that a fracture is likely, assume that a bone is broken

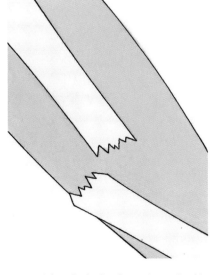

ABOVE *When the broken bone pierces the skin it is known as an open or compound fracture. There is a risk of infection and increased damage to nerves and blood vessels.*

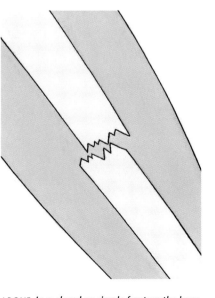

ABOVE *In a closed or simple fracture the bone does not break through the skin. If the break is straight across the bone (usually in the arm or leg) it is known as a transverse fracture.*

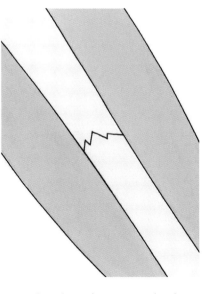

ABOVE *Sometimes a bone may crack rather than break, usually as a result of repeated jarring of a bone such as may occur in the shinbones of long-distance runners.*

HOW TO TREAT FRACTURES

The general rule for treating all broken bones is to keep them still, as this reduces pain and the likelihood of further injury. The risk of infection is also an important consideration in the treatment of open fractures and requires action. Do not give a person who has a broken bone anything to eat or drink in case he needs a general anaesthetic in hospital.

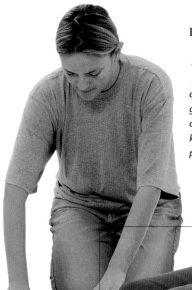

KEEPING A BROKEN BONE STILL

1 *The casualty will often have put the injured part in the position that is most comfortable for him and will generally be guarding the injury and keeping it still. If the casualty has not done this, encourage him to keep still and help him into a comfortable position.*

2 *Once the casualty is still you can help to steady and support the fracture using your hands. By helping the casualty keep the injured part still you enable him to relax. The very act of relaxing the muscles reduces the pull on the broken bones and often alleviates pain.*

Use your hands to
immobilise the
broken bone

3 *If you have to transport the casualty yourself, or if it is going to be a while until help arrives, then you can immobilise the broken bone further with bandages or improvise with coats or blankets, for example.*

The key points to remember with any type of bandaging are:

• *Not to tie the bandage too tightly.*
• *To pad around the site of the break.*

Do not move the injured area unnecessarily.

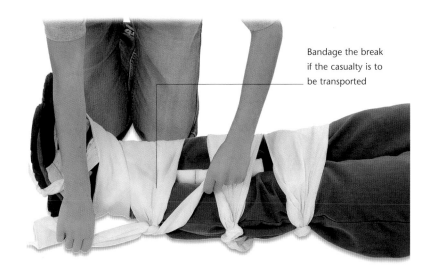

Bandage the break
if the casualty is to
be transported

TREATMENT OF OPEN BREAKS

In the first instance, the wound should be protected using either a sterile dressing or an improvised dressing made from a piece of clean, dry and non-fluffy material. If the bleeding is profuse, or you are going to have to wait some time for further help, this dressing should be held in place using the same principles as you would apply if there were a foreign object in the wound (see page 71).

CHECKING FOR DAMAGE TO CIRCULATION

With any bandaging, you run the risk of cutting off the circulation to the area below the site of the bandage. While this can in part be avoided by not tying bandages too tight and by never using a tourniquet, the nature of wounds means that they swell and this can cause a once satisfactory bandage to become too tight.

There is a number of ways to check whether a bandage is cutting off the circulation:

- *If the skin below the site of the bandage becomes white, grey or blue, or feels cold to the touch.*
- *If the casualty complains of pins and needles or of a lack of circulation.*
- *If the pulse in the limb slows or stops.*
- *If the colour does not quickly return to the skin after the skin is gently pinched or the nail compressed.*

If you notice any of these signs, gently loosen, but do not remove, the bandage until the blood flow returns.

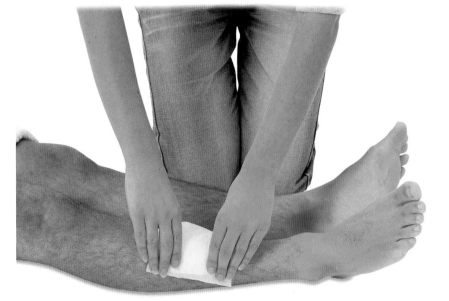

1 *Place the dressing over the wound and build up padding alongside the bone.*

2 *Tie both the padding and the dressing in place, using firm pressure.*

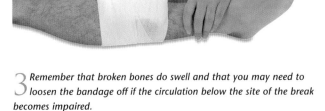

3 *Remember that broken bones do swell and that you may need to loosen the bandage off if the circulation below the site of the break becomes impaired.*

FRACTURES OF THE SKULL, FACE AND JAW

A skull fracture is a very serious injury as it is often associated with some form of damage to the brain. Concussion and compression may both accompany skull fractures. If a casualty has a fracture to the bones of the face or jaw, the airway is your overwhelming priority.

TREATING A FRACTURED SKULL

1 *Keep the casualty still while she is conscious. Encourage her not to move her head.*

2 *Keep a constant check on the airway, breathing and circulation (see pages 18-19).*

3 *Be prepared to resuscitate (see page 18) or turn into the recovery position (see pages 22-23) if necessary.*

4 *Call for emergency help as soon as possible.*

HOW TO TREAT CONCUSSION

1 *Place the casualty in the recovery position if necessary and monitor ABC.*

2 *Call an ambulance if the casualty does not recover after 3 minutes or if there are signs of skull fracture or compression.*

CONCUSSION AND COMPRESSION

Concussion is a shaking of the brain caused by sudden movement of the head. The casualty is likely to be displaying a number of the following signs and symptoms:

- *Pale skin.*
- *Dizziness, blurred vision or nausea.*
- *Headache.*
- *Brief or partial loss of consciousness.*

Concussion in itself is not a serious injury as the casualty will recover when the disturbance caused by the shaking stops. However, because concussion often accompanies violent head movement, there is always the possibility of a skull fracture or more serious, longer-term brain injury, such as compression. It is important therefore that even a seemingly recovered casualty with concussion should seek medical treatment.

3 *Advise the casualty to seek medical advice if recovery appears to be complete.*

4 *Encourage the casualty to keep still while recovering as this reduces dizziness and nausea.*

5 *Be aware of the increased likelihood of neck injuries.*

Compression is a very serious injury that occurs when pressure is exerted on the brain, either by a piece of bone, bleeding or swelling of the injured brain. It may develop immediately after a head injury or stroke, or some hours or even days later.

POTENTIAL SIGNS AND SYMPTOMS OF COMPRESSION

- *Person becomes increasingly drowsy and unresponsive.*
- *Flushed and dry skin.*
- *Slurred speech and confusion.*
- *Partial or total loss of movement, often down one side of the body.*
- *One pupil bigger than the other.*
- *Noisy breathing which becomes slow.*
- *Slow, strong pulse.*

If some or all of these symptoms are present, suspect compression and carry out the following treatment.

1 If the casualty is unconscious, place in the recovery position and monitor airway, breathing and circulation.

2 If conscious, lay the casualty down with the head and shoulders slightly raised, maintaining a close check on the ABC. Call an ambulance, and be prepared to resuscitate.

Warning

Do not give anything to eat or drink – the casualty may need a general anaesthetic in hospital.

HOW TO TREAT FRACTURES OF THE FACE AND JAW

1 *Ensure that any blood in the mouth is allowed to dribble out – encourage the casualty to spit into a bandage or handkerchief.*

2 *Gently remove any teeth or bits of broken bone from the mouth and give the casualty a pad to hold against the injured part for additional support and comfort.*

3 *A cold compress may help to reduce pain.*

4 *Get the casualty to hospital because she will require medical treatment.*

5 *Do not pinch a broken nose to control bleeding – hold a pad under it.*

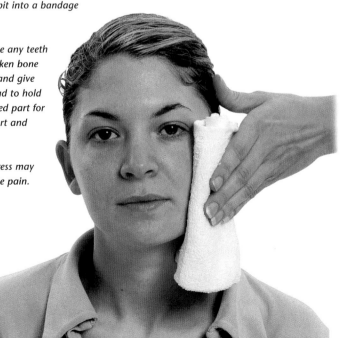

Signs and symptoms of a skull fracture

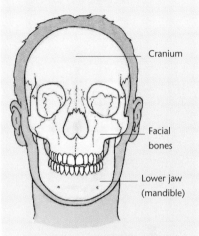

Cranium

Facial bones

Lower jaw (mandible)

Alongside these signs and symptoms consider what happened. Skull fractures may be caused by direct and heavy impact to the head or by indirect impact, for example a fall from a great height on to the feet that may have caused the force to move up the body, stopping when it hit the skull.

- *Bruising to the eye socket*
- *Pain*
- *A bump or a dent*
- *Straw-coloured fluid coming from one or both ears*
- *Deterioration in the level of consciousness of the casualty Does the person respond slowly to questions or commands? Is he having problems focusing?*

If any of these things are present, assume a skull fracture with a potential injury to the brain.

FRACTURES OF THE UPPER BODY

The collarbone can be broken by direct impact. However, it is most commonly fractured by indirect force moving up the arm following a fall on to an outstretched hand, and often happens after a fall from a bicycle or a horse. A broken shoulder often follows a heavy impact to the site of injury. It is therefore important to do a careful examination to rule out back or rib injury.

BROKEN COLLARBONE

Alongside potential swelling, bruising and tenderness above the site of the injury, the casualty is most likely to be supporting the injured arm with the shoulder on the injured side slumped. As the collarbone is close to the skin it is particularly important to look for an open fracture.

TREATMENT

If the bone has pierced the skin, place a light dressing over the wound. Bleeding is likely to be minimal and your main concern is to prevent infection.

Work with the injured person to find the most comfortable position for the arm and for the body as a whole. Generally this will be sitting up with the arm supported at the elbow. The casualty may wish to go to hospital in this position, but she should be offered the option of an elevation sling, which will help alleviate pressure on the collarbone and provide some comfort.

Hold uninjured shoulder

LEFT *A broken collarbone often happens following a fall from a bicycle or a horse rather than direct impact. Use an elevation sling to take the weight of the arm and relieve pressure on the collarbone. It is important to check for an open fracture as the collarbone is close to the skin and may easily puncture it.*

Support elbow to reduce pressure on collarbone

Use a triangular bandage to make an elevation sling

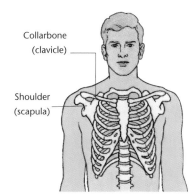

Collarbone (clavicle)

Shoulder (scapula)

Place a bandage around the body for extra support

Keep the arm supported at the elbow

APPLYING AN ELEVATION SLING

The elevation sling has a range of uses. As well as the treatment of a broken collarbone it also provides comfort in the treatment of crushed or broken fingers and hands, relief in the treatment of burns to the arm and is an aid in controlling bleeding through elevation.

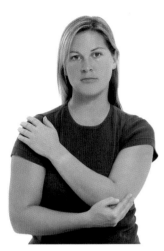

1 *Place the injured arm with the fingers by the collarbone on the uninjured side.*

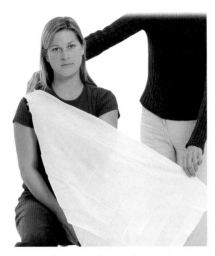

2 *Place the triangular bandage with the point resting at the elbow on the injured side.*

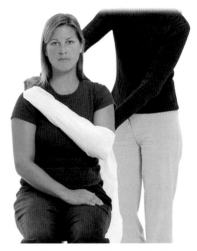

3 *Tuck the bandage underneath the hand and down underneath the injured arm.*

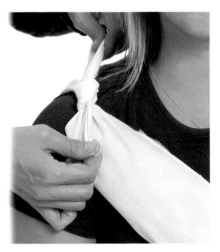

4 *Tie at the collarbone in a reef knot (or a bow).*

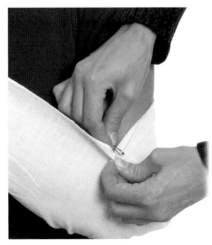

5 *Fasten the spare material at the elbow with a pin or twist it and tuck it away.*

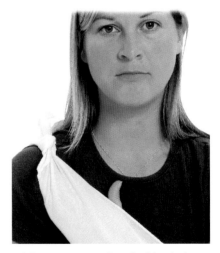

6 *Extra support can be gained by placing a triangular bandage folded into three (a broad fold) around the arm and body.*

BROKEN SHOULDER

If you are confident that the shoulder itself is broken then the treatment is to work with the casualty to find the best position. The application of an arm sling (see *Fractures of the Arm and Hand*, pages 88-89) may provide some support, but more commonly the casualty will want no bandages, settling instead for steady support from another person if available. The pain of the injury may make it necessary to call for an ambulance rather than transporting the casualty to hospital in a car.

Warning

Do not give anything to eat or drink – the casualty may need a general anaesthetic in hospital.

FRACTURES OF THE ARM AND HAND

There are three long bones in each arm – one in the upper arm and two below the elbow. These are among the most commonly broken bones in the body. There is also a number of small bones in the wrist that are vulnerable to breaks. Fractures to the hand or fingers can be extremely painful because of the many nerve endings.

The principles of treatment are, as for all broken bones, to provide support to the injured part and to stop it from moving too much. Most people with a broken arm will be able to make their own way to hospital or health centre, so treatment focuses on providing support that is appropriate when walking and stabilises the injured limb. This can be done with an improvised sling using clothing, or by using a triangular bandage to form an arm sling.

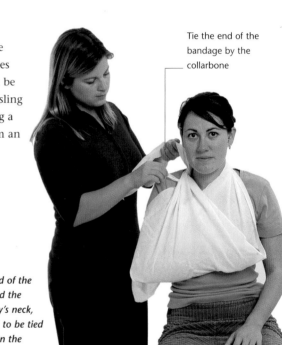

Tie the end of the bandage by the collarbone

HOW TO MAKE AN ARM SLING

1 *Gently place the bandage under the casualty's arm, placing the point underneath the elbow.*

2 *Pass the top end of the bandage around the back of the casualty's neck, leaving a short end to be tied by the collarbone on the injured side.*

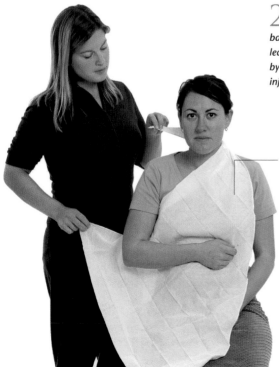

Top end of bandage is put around the neck

3 *Bring the bottom end of the bandage up carefully, ensuring that it fully supports the injured arm. Tie into place with a reef knot or bow.*

4 *For additional support, you can tie another triangular bandage fold into three (a broad fold) around the arm, avoiding the site of the fracture, to stop the arm from moving.*

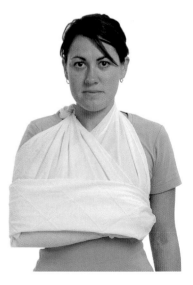

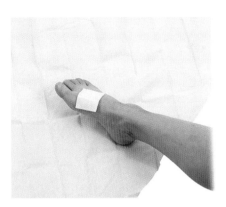

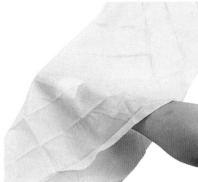

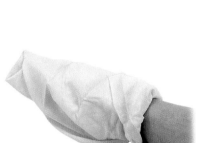

HAND OR FOOT COVER BANDAGE

1 *Fold a hem along the base of the triangular bandage. Place the casualty's hand on the bandage and bring the point down towards the casualty's wrist.*

2 *Cross the two ends of the bandage around the wrist and tie loosely.*

3 *Pull the point of the bandage up over the knot and tuck it away.*

The casualty may then find it comfortable to have the arm in an elevation sling

> ### Warning
>
> Do not give anything to eat or drink – the casualty may need a general anaesthetic in hospital.

TREATMENT

1 *Gently cover any open wounds with a dressing or clean, non-fluffy piece of material. Encourage the casualty to raise her arm. This helps to reduce swelling and bleeding and also provides some pain relief.*

2 *If possible, remove rings and watches before the injury starts to swell. If jewellery has been crushed into the hand or swelling prevents its easy removal, pass this information on as soon as possible to the medical staff as early treatment will be needed to prevent damage to the circulation in the fingers.*

3 *Cover the injured area with a pad of soft fabric or cotton wool (taking particular care if there are open wounds not to get strands of material stuck into the injury). This padding can be held in place with a cover created from a triangular bandage, which can also be adapted for crush injuries to the foot and for burns to the hand or foot.*

BROKEN ELBOW OR AN ARM THAT CANNOT BEND

If the broken bone is on or near the elbow it may not be possible for the casualty to bend the arm, either because of the pain or because the joint is fixed. In this case you need to treat the arm in the position found – do not try to bend the arm.

1 *Help the casualty into the most comfortable position; this will often be lying down on the ground, but it may also be standing up with the arm hanging straight down.*

2 *Place padding around the injured part, both between the arm and the body and on the outside of the arm.*

3 *The casualty will need to be transported by ambulance. Do not attempt to bandage the arm if help is on its way as this will cause further discomfort and may make the injury worse.*

FRACTURED WRIST

In older adults, the wrist may be broken by a fall on to an outstretched hand, causing a break very low down on the radius (one of the long bones in the lower arm) known as a Colles's or dinner fork fracture. Other injuries can break one of the small bones to the wrist or cause a sprain that is particularly difficult to distinguish from a break.

TREATMENT

Provide support and immobilisation in the same way as for a break to the upper or lower arm. Remove watches and bracelets as these may contribute to cutting off circulation to the hand if the injury swells.

HAND FRACTURES

Direct impact may break one or two of the small bones in the palm or fingers. Crushing injuries may break several bones and cause considerable bleeding. In addition the thumb, and even some of the fingers, may become dislocated.

FRACTURES OF THE RIBCAGE

Simple fractures, characterised by bruising and tenderness over the fracture site, are usually confined to one broken rib, with no underlying damage to the lungs or other internal organs. Multiple, or complicated, rib fractures will often result in the casualty having difficulty in breathing, as the chest wall is unable to move effectively. There may also be lung damage. Broken ribs are generally not strapped up because the chest needs to expand normally during breathing to reduce the risk of pneumonia.

TREATING A SIMPLE BROKEN RIB

The best treatment for a simple fractured rib is to put the arm on the injured side into an arm sling and to advise the casualty to seek medical aid.

MULTIPLE BROKEN RIBS

In a case of multiple rib fractures there may also be lung damage, where one or a number of ribs have punctured one or both of the lungs. There may also be an open break on the chest wall where ribs have sprung out. Remember that the ribs extend around the back of the casualty and there may be injuries here as well as on the front. Rib injuries may be accompanied by a sucking wound to the chest, creating a direct passage between the external environment and the lungs.

Warning

Do not give anything to eat or drink – the casualty may need a general anaesthetic in hospital.

TREATING MULTIPLE BROKEN RIBS

1 *Treat any sucking wounds by covering, initially with a hand and then with plastic (see also Treating Chest or Abdominal Wounds, pages 64-65). Treat any open breaks.*

2 *If the casualty is conscious, lay him down. The casualty is most likely to find breathing easier in a half-sitting position.*

3 *Lean the casualty towards the injured side. This allows any blood to drain into the injured lung, leaving the good lung free to breathe.*

Cover wound and help casualty sit comfortably

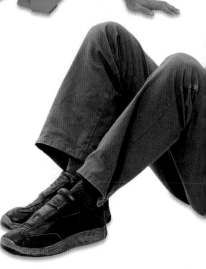

4 *Place the arm on the injured side into an elevation sling.*

5 *Treat for shock (see pages 44-45).*

If the casualty becomes unconscious, monitor the airway and breathing (see pages 18-19) and place the person into the recovery position (see pages 22-25) with the injured side upwards.

Signs and symptoms of multiple broken ribs

- *Chest rises on the injured side as the person breathes out (paradoxical breathing)*
- *Swelling or indentation along the line of the ribs*
- *Open breaks*
- *Difficulty in breathing*
- *Pain on breathing*
- *Shock (as there is likely to be some degree of internal bleeding)*
- *Bright red, frothy blood coming from the mouth and/or nose. (This is an indication of a punctured lung as oxygenated blood is escaping from the respiratory system. There may or may not be an associated sucking wound to the chest)*
- *Sucking wound to the chest*

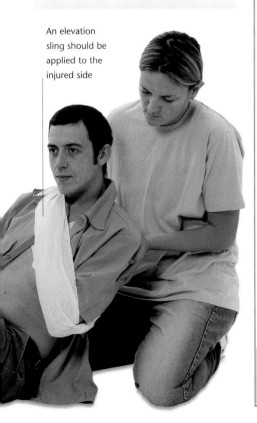

An elevation sling should be applied to the injured side

Back pain

There are many causes of back pain. Among the most serious is damage to the spinal cord (see pages 91-92), which may lead to paralysis or meningitis. More commonly, neck or lower back pain can be caused by muscle sprain or damage to the ligaments or the discs between the vertebrae (the back bones). Broken ribs or damage to the muscles between the ribs at the back may also cause back pain. For more information on back pain, see pages 382-84.

Signs and symptoms
- *Dull or severe pain, usually made worse by movement*

- *Tension in the neck or shoulders*

- *Pain travelling down limbs*

Treatment
- *Check the nature of the incident carefully – if the pain is related to a recent heavy fall or other accident, assume that there may be spinal cord damage and treat as for a broken back (see pages 92-93).*

- *Help the casualty to lie down. Usually the most comfortable position will be flat on the back on a hard surface.*

- *If the symptoms do not ease, advise the casualty to see a doctor.*

If back pain is accompanied by signs of spinal cord damage, such as numbness, pins and needles, or by headaches, nausea, vomiting, fever, or a deterioration in the level of consciousness (e.g. increasing drowsiness), call an ambulance.

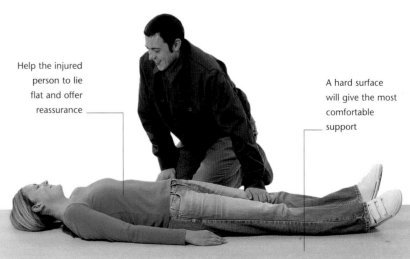

Help the injured person to lie flat and offer reassurance

A hard surface will give the most comfortable support

RECOGNISING BACK AND SPINAL INJURY

The spine is made up of a number of small bones call vertebrae. These form the backbone or spinal column, through which run the spinal cord, the part of the central nervous system connecting all parts of the body with the brain, and major blood vessels. Injuries to the back are caused in a number of ways: through direct impact (such as a heavy blow to the neck or back); indirect impact (landing on the head or feet without bending the legs, thus allowing the force to travel up the body); and when the head is violently thrown forwards and backwards (common in car accidents).

COMPLICATIONS WITH BACK INJURY

The biggest danger with back injuries is the risk of nerve damage. The spinal cord containing the spinal nerves runs down the centre of the vertebrae and fractures can sever or pinch these nerves, leading to partial or full paralysis. If the fracture is high in the neck, breathing may stop. Displaced vertebrae or swelling due to blood loss can also apply pressure to the spinal cord, leading to nerve damage.

Not all broken backs result in immediate damage to the spinal cord. However, the risk of spinal cord injuries is greatly increased if bones are broken, and any suspected fracture of the spine should be treated with extreme care.

Suspect a broken back or potential nerve damage if the accident involved:

- *Rapid slowing down of movement.*
- *A fall from a height.*
- *A sharp blow directly to the back.*
- *Injury to the face or skull (as this often results from the head being thrown backwards and forwards).*

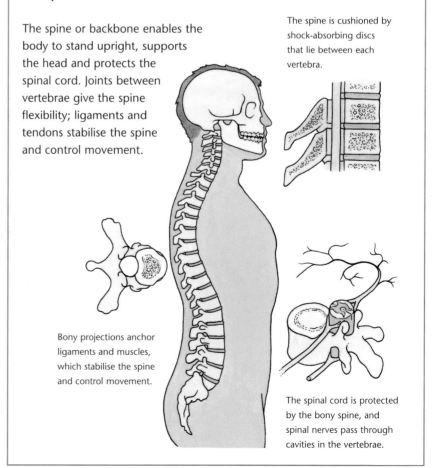

The spine

The spine or backbone enables the body to stand upright, supports the head and protects the spinal cord. Joints between vertebrae give the spine flexibility; ligaments and tendons stabilise the spine and control movement.

The spine is cushioned by shock-absorbing discs that lie between each vertebra.

Bony projections anchor ligaments and muscles, which stabilise the spine and control movement.

The spinal cord is protected by the bony spine, and spinal nerves pass through cavities in the vertebrae.

RIGHT *If spinal injury is suspected, the safest position for a person to be in is with the head, neck and spine aligned. To check alignment, make sure that the casualty's nose is in line with his navel. Keep the head immobilised.*

Casualty's nose should be in line with the navel

Warning

• *Do not give anything to eat or drink – the casualty may need a general anaesthetic in hospital.*
• *Do not move the casualty unless he is in danger or needs resuscitation.*

Signs and symptoms of a broken back

• *Dent or step in the spine, which may indicate a displaced vertebra*
• *Bruising or swelling over the backbone*
• *Complaint of pain in the back*
• *Tenderness over the area of the break*

Signs and symptoms of spinal cord damage

• *Loss of movement below the site of the break*
• *Pins and needles in the fingers or toes or throughout the body*
• *Feeling strange, perhaps 'jelly-like'*
• *Numbness*

If any of these signs and symptoms is present, or if the nature of the accident indicates a potential fracture, assume that a bone is broken and keep the person still until help arrives.

TREATMENT

Any spinal injury is potentially serious and you should seek emergency assistance immediately. The treatment for injuries to the back is to keep the injured person still while monitoring and maintaining airway and breathing. The general rule for dealing with broken bones or spinal cord damage is to keep the casualty in the position that you found him until a doctor arrives, taking particular care to ensure the head is immobilised.

Unless the person is in danger or becomes unconscious and requires resuscitation, do not move him from the position in which he was found. If you have been trained to do so, you can move the head into the neutral position before immobilisation. Remain in this position until emergency help arrives.

1 *If the casualty is conscious and already lying down, leave him where he is. If the casualty is still walking around, support him in lying down on the ground. If you can, put a blanket or coat underneath before you lie the person down.*

2 *Tell the person to keep still until medical help arrives and reassure him.*

3 *Ensure that an ambulance has been called at the earliest opportunity.*

4 *Hold the casualty's head still by placing your hands over the ears and your fingers along the jawline.*

5 *Do not remove your support from the head until help arrives.*

If the casualty is unconscious, maintaining a clear airway is your first priority. See *Unconscious Casualty*, pages 96-97.

IF YOU HAVE TO MOVE THE CASUALTY

The two key reasons for moving somebody with a spinal injury are: to turn the person on to her back in order to resuscitate her; and to turn her into the recovery position if she is unconscious and in a position that does not allow her to maintain a clear airway. For further information, see also spinal injury recovery position, page 93.

Whiplash

This is a common neck injury, particularly after car accidents. It accompanies a sudden impact accident when the person is wearing a seat belt and results from the head being thrown backwards and forwards violently. Whiplash is best described as a neck sprain. It is an injury to the soft tissue in the neck and can result in the need for long-term physiotherapy and the use of a neck collar. Whiplash may not appear until hours or even days after the injury.

It is very difficult to distinguish whiplash from spinal cord damage and a broken neck because the signs, symptoms and potential causes are very similar and the pain of the whiplash injury may be masking other, more serious, problems. For this reason, whiplash should be treated in the same way as other spinal injuries until professional medical staff rule out more serious damage.

LOG ROLL

One of the most effective ways of turning a person over is the log roll technique. Log roll can also be used to turn somebody with a spinal injury on to her side as an alternative to the recovery position. It is also commonly used to move people with other injuries, such as a broken leg or pelvis, on to a stretcher or blanket.

Ideally, six people should be used to carry out this technique, with one person taking the lead and control of the head.

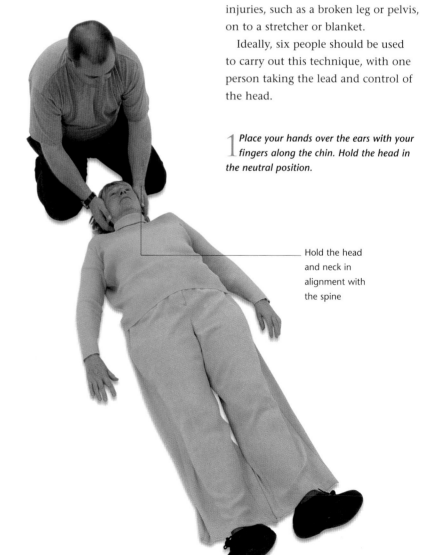

1 *Place your hands over the ears with your fingers along the chin. Hold the head in the neutral position.*

Hold the head and neck in alignment with the spine

Warning

• *Do not give anything to eat or drink – the casualty may need a general anaesthetic in hospital.*
• *Do not move the casualty unless she is in danger or needs resuscitation.*

2 *Ask the supporters to gently move the arms to the side of the body and the legs together.*

3 *Ask the supporters to support the spine and limbs and to follow your commands.*

4 *Roll the casualty like a log, keeping the head and chin in line with the neck and spine.*

Head and neck should be held in alignment

Helpers should be evenly placed around the victim

Move the arms gently to the side and support them

Gently move the legs together and support them

Person at casualty's head instructs other helpers

Helpers slowly roll victim onto her back

If you are by yourself and the injured person is not breathing, do not waste time searching for help. Turn the person as carefully as you can with any help available to you.

NEUTRAL POSITION

The best position for a person with a suspected neck or spinal injury is the neutral position. Here the head is in line with the neck and spine. To move a person into the neutral position, grip the head firmly over the ears and move it slowly into line. Once in this position, do not let go of the support until medical help arrives to take over from you.

Only use this technique if you have been trained to do so.

UNCONSCIOUS CASUALTY

This is a particularly difficult situation to deal with. The casualty's airway is always your first priority. The person may have a broken back that could cause nerve damage and paralysis, but if you do not protect the airway and ensure that the casualty continues breathing, she will die.

TREATMENT

If you come across an unconscious person for whom the nature of the accident or the positioning indicates that she may have broken her back (for example, a bystander tells you the casualty fell, or the person is wearing motorcycle leathers and lying next to a damaged bike), your priority remains to check the airway.

1 *Ask a question to find out if the casualty is conscious. Do not shake the casualty.*

2 *Carry out your ABC checks (see pages 16–20), taking care to tilt the head gently. If the head is already extended a suitable way, do not move it any further. Instead, just use the chin lift and carefully check the mouth.*

3 *If the casualty is not breathing, give rescue breaths (see pages 26–29) and full CPR (see pages 30–33) as needed. Make an early call for an ambulance.*

4 *If you have to roll the casualty on to her back to resuscitate, then you should aim to keep the casualty's head, trunk and toes in a straight line (see log roll, pages 94–95). If possible, get bystanders to help move the casualty over, but do not waste time looking for help because the casualty needs air as soon as possible.*

5 *If the casualty is unconscious and lying in such a way that the head is extended and she is on her side, allowing fluid to drain from the mouth, then leave her alone.*

6 *Hold the casualty's head still by placing your hands over the ears and your fingers along the jawline. Ensure that the airway is monitored.*

If the casualty is unconscious and either the head is not extended or she is not lying on her side, you need to move her into the recovery position. Ideally, with enough bystanders, you should use the log roll (see pages 94–95). If not, be prepared to roll the casualty into the recovery position with all available help.

SPINAL INJURY RECOVERY POSITION

1 *Support the casualty's head as described above. Make yourself comfortable, as you will have to continue to do this until the ambulance arrives.*

Keep the casualty's head supported until help arrives

Bend the furthest
leg upwards and
support the body

Place hands over the ears
and fingers along the jaw

2 *Ask a bystander to put the arm nearest him gently underneath the casualty's body, ensuring that the fingers are flat and the elbow straight. Bring the furthest arm across the body, supporting it at the face.*

3 *The casualty's furthest leg should be bent upwards and the bystander's arm placed on the thigh just above the knee.*

4 *Working under orders from the first aider at the head, the casualty should be gently turned, ensuring that the head, trunk and toes stay in line.*

5 *Once the casualty has been turned over, the neck should continue to be supported while the bystander ensures that the casualty is stable, either by supporting the body himself or by placing coats or rolled-up blankets, for example, around the victim.*

Alternatively, you can use the log roll technique (see pages 94–95).

Warning

Do not move the casualty unless she is in danger or needs resuscitation.

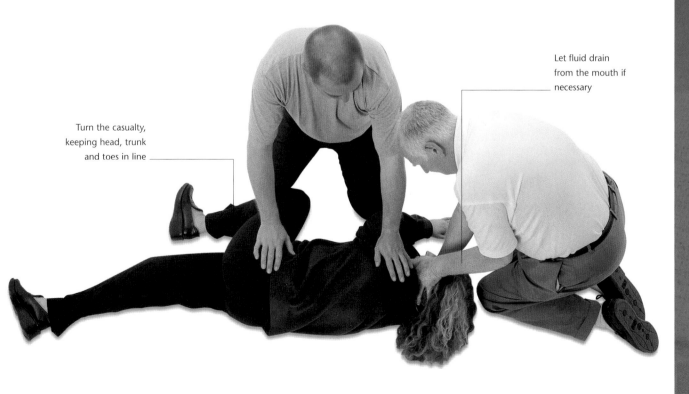

Turn the casualty,
keeping head, trunk
and toes in line

Let fluid drain
from the mouth if
necessary

INJURIES TO THE LOWER BODY

A broken bone in the lower body is a serious injury that requires hospital treatment. The pelvis is a large bone and is generally very difficult to break. Severe impact such as a fall from a height or a car accident are the most common cause in young, fit adults. In the elderly a broken pelvis (or hip) happens more often and can be caused by a relatively minor impact. In healthy adults it takes a major impact to break the thigh bone and there are likely to be other injuries.

Signs and symptoms of a broken pelvis

• *Bruising and swelling over the hip area*
• *Urge to urinate*
• *Blood-stained urine*
• *A sensation of falling apart: the pelvis is like a girdle and a break means that it may not be able to hold itself together*
• *Legs rotate outwards as the support at the pelvis gives*

As the pelvis can also be broken at the back, it is easy to mistake a pelvic fracture for a spinal injury. If in doubt, treat for a broken spine (see pages 92–93).

BROKEN PELVIS

The pelvis protects the urinary system and the biggest danger is that sharp bone ends may burst the bladder, creating the possibility of infection. Internal bleeding is another likelihood with a fractured hip, as the impact required to break the bone is likely to have caused other damage.

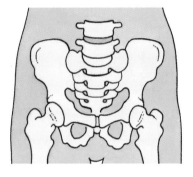

A broken pelvis usually occurs as the result of a fall or a car accident. The main risk is of sharp bone ends puncturing the bladder, creating the risk of infection.

TREATMENT

1 *Call an ambulance immediately and reassure the casualty while you wait.*

2 *This is a very serious condition and it is best to leave the casualty alone because you could easily make things worse.*

3 *If the ambulance will be some time, tie the legs gently together at the ankles and knees using triangular or improvised bandages.*

4 *Treat the casualty for shock (see pages 44–45).*

Gently tie the legs together with a triangular bandage

Place a pillow under the knees for support

FRACTURES OF THE UPPER LEG

The key risk with fractures of the femur (thigh bone) in the upper leg is shock. The thigh bone protects the main artery in the leg, the femoral artery, and if broken may pierce it, causing severe internal bleeding.

A person with a broken thigh bone will require transportation by ambulance. The general treatment is therefore nothing more than to hold the injured part still and treat the casualty for shock. Do not bandage the leg if help is on its way as this is likely to cause more pain and potentially cause further damage.

Support the leg above and below the site of the fracture if possible, placing padding around the broken leg to further help to reduce movement of the injured limb.

If you have been trained in the use of traction then you may apply this gently to the leg to help to reduce pain and circulatory damage.

IF HELP IS DELAYED

If help will be delayed for more than 30 minutes, the injured person may benefit from immobilising the broken leg by using the good leg as a splint.

1 *Apply broadfold triangular bandages under the ankles, knees and above and below the site of the fracture.*

2 *Place padding between the legs to help immobilise them.*

3 *Gently but firmly tie the bandages on the injured side.*

4 *Take care to check the circulation below the bandages to ensure that they do not become too tight as the leg swells.*

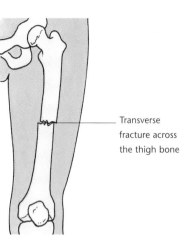

Transverse fracture across the thigh bone

ABOVE *A fractured thigh bone may pierce the main artery in the leg, causing severe internal bleeding. The best treatment is to keep the limb still and treat the casualty for shock.*

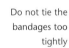

Do not tie the bandages too tightly

Tie a broadfold triangular bandage under the knees

Place a triangular bandage above the site of injury

INJURIES TO THE LOWER LEG

The long bones, the knee and the foot are often injured during sports. There are two long bones in the lower leg. The tibia (shinbone) lies very close to the surface and if broken will often pierce the skin, causing an open fracture. The fibula lies behind the tibia and is more difficult to break and may not obviously affect the ability to walk. The knee is a complex joint vulnerable to fractures of the patella (kneecap), dislocation, strains and cartilage (tissue) injury. It is unusual to break just one bone in the foot – generally, multiple fractures of the small bones in the foot and the toes are caused by crush injuries.

TREATING BROKEN LONG BONES

1 *Help the injured person into the most comfortable position – generally, lying down.*

2 *Examine the injury carefully to see whether there is an open break. If there is a wound, cover gently with a sterile dressing or clean, non-fluffy material, pad around the broken area and tie gently but firmly into place.*

A person with a broken leg is most likely to be transported to hospital by ambulance and the treatment in most settings is therefore limited to steady support and help with immobilisation.

• *Gently support the injury above and below the site of the break. Place padding such as cushions or blankets around the site of the injury.*
• *If you have been trained to do so, applying traction may help alleviate the pain and any potential damage to the circulation.*
• *Treat for shock (see pages 44–45).*

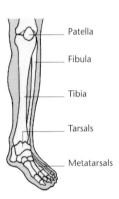

Patella

Fibula

Tibia

Tarsals

Metatarsals

Lower leg bones are often injured during sport. The kneecap is particularly vulnerable to injury.

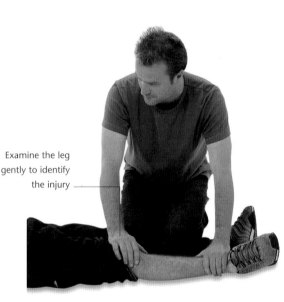

Examine the leg gently to identify the injury

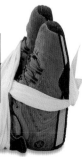

Place padding between the legs to immobilise

Tie the legs together gently at the ankles

Support the leg above the site of the injury

TREATING KNEE INJURIES

In addition to the normal signs and symptoms of bone and soft tissue injuries, there may be an obvious displacement of the kneecap or an inability to bend or straighten the leg.

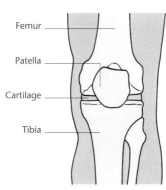

Femur

Patella

Cartilage

Tibia

It may be difficult to identify a knee injury, and treatment for a damaged kneecap, sprains and cartilage injury is broadly the same.

1 *Help the injured person into the most comfortable position. He will generally need to be transported to hospital by ambulance.*

2 *Check the injured area carefully for an open break and treat as appropriate.*

3 *Pad around and under the injured area to provide support, gently tying the padding in place if needed.*

4 *Treat for shock and reassure the casualty until help arrives.*

5 *Do not try to bend the leg because you may cause more damage. Keep it still.*

Tie the padding in place to support the injured knee

Place a pillow under the knee for support

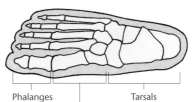

TREATING A BROKEN FOOT

1 *If possible, carefully remove the shoes and socks, tights or stockings as the foot is likely to swell and these items of clothing may damage the circulation.*

2 *Cover any wound with a sterile dressing or clean, non-fluffy material.*

3 *Raise the foot to reduce swelling and pain and support with a large comfortable pad such as a cushion or blanket.*

4 *Wrap the foot in padding. If necessary, this can be held in place with a cover bandage (see fractures of the hand, page 89). A cold compress may further alleviate pain and swelling.*

Take or send the injured person to hospital.

Bones of the foot

Phalanges

Metatarsals

Tarsals

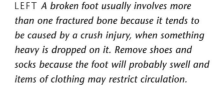

LEFT *A broken foot usually involves more than one fractured bone because it tends to be caused by a crush injury, when something heavy is dropped on it. Remove shoes and socks because the foot will probably swell and items of clothing may restrict circulation.*

Warning

Do not give anything to eat or drink – the casualty may need a general anaesthetic in hospital.

SPRAINS AND STRAINS

Strains occur when the muscle is overstretched, leading to a partial tear. Sprains are injuries to a ligament, a tough band of tissue that links two bones together at or near a joint. Commonly sprained joints include the wrist, knee and ankle.

Signs and symptoms

The signs and symptoms of strains, and more particularly sprains, are very similar to those of a broken bone. There may be pain, particularly on movement, swelling and bruising (usually a little while after the accident). It is often impossible to tell if an injury is a sprain or a fracture without an X-ray (see pages 454–455) and it is not unusual for sprains to take as long a time to heal as a simple break.

If in doubt, treat the injury as a broken bone and seek further medical help.

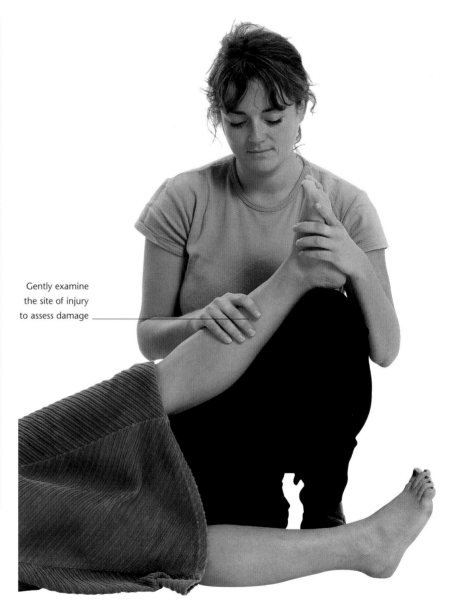

Gently examine the site of injury to assess damage

TREATMENT

The person suffering the injury may often sense that the area is not broken – she may have suffered similar injuries before, particularly if the injury has occurred through sport. If both of you are confident that there is no other injury, then the best treatment is:

- **R**est
- **I**ce
- **C**ompression
- **E**levation

1 *Place the injured part at rest. This prevents any further damage. Help the person into a comfortable position – for a leg injury, this will usually be lying down with head and shoulders supported.*

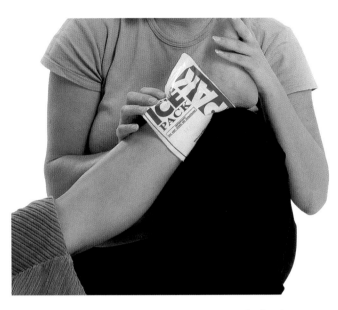

2 *Apply a cold compress. Wrap some ice in a triangular bandage or other clean piece of material and hold gently on the site of the injury. This will help relieve pain and reduce swelling. Do not apply ice directly to the injury as this may damage the skin. Cool the injury for 10–15 minutes, keeping the compress cold with refills as necessary.*

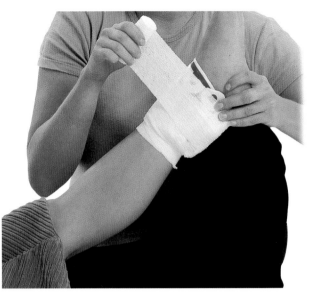

3 *Apply a compressing roller bandage. This will help reduce pain and swelling and will provide support for the injury.*

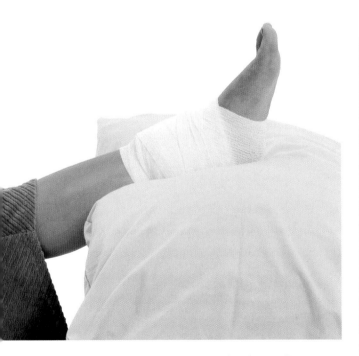

4 *Elevate the injured part. Elevation will help reduce swelling and pain. If the arm is injured, use either the arm or elevation sling as appropriate to provide additional support.*

5 *Seek medical assistance and make sure the casualty keeps the limb raised and supported until help arrives.*

Alternative cold compresses

If ice is not readily available, soak a flannel or other piece of material in very cold water, wring this out and apply to the injury. Replace this every 2–3 minutes as the material warms up. Alternatively, consider the contents of the freezer. Frozen peas, for example, make an excellent cold compress as the bag moulds to the shape of the injury.

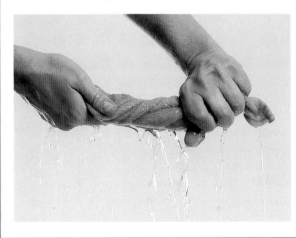

BURNS AND SCALDS

Burns and scalds, a type of burn caused by wet heat, are potentially fatal injuries. They can cause life-threatening shock through serious fluid loss and, if around the face and neck, can restrict breathing.

WHAT ARE THE RISK FROM BURNS?

In burns, fluid is lost in three main ways:

- *Blistering*
- *Swelling around the injury*
- *Directly from the injury*

While the fluid loss may not be visible as liquid lying around the casualty it is nevertheless lost from the blood as a straw-coloured substance known as plasma. Severe burns therefore can and often do prove to be fatal.

The second risk from burns is infection. The damaged tissue provides little or no resistance to infection and serious problems may arise some time after the initial injury. The risk of infection increases with the size and depth of the burn, and the casualty will probably suffer from shock as well.

HOW DO YOU TELL HOW SEVERE A BURN IS?

Many burns are minor and can be safely treated at home or with help from a local doctor or pharmacist.

There are two main things to consider in deciding whether or not a burn needs more urgent treatment:

- *Depth of the burn*
- *Size of the burn*

Depth of the burn

Burns are classified into three types:

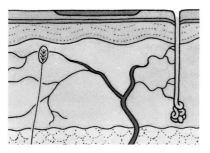 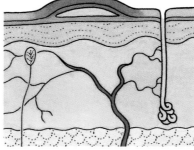 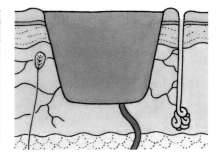

Superficial burns only involve the outer layer of skin and, although often extremely painful, are generally not life-threatening unless a very large surface area of the body is covered. The burnt area is very sore and is usually red and possibly a little swollen. If good first aid treatment is applied and the area burnt is not extensive, then further medical treatment is unlikely to be needed.

Partial thickness burns include the top layers of skin and involve blistering. They are characterised by red, raw-looking skin with blisters that weep clear fluid, and pain. The risk of shock (see pages 44–45) is high with partial thickness burns and any burn of this type needs medical attention. Partial thickness burns covering a substantial percentage of the body can kill.

Full thickness burns involve damage to all the layers of skin, usually including the nerve endings and possibly other underlying tissues and organs. Characterised by charred tissue often surrounded by white waxy areas of dead skin (which may not hurt because of nerve damage), full thickness burns will always need emergency medical attention and in the long term will often require plastic surgery.

Area of the body burnt

Generally, the larger the area of the body covered, the more serious the burn. Any burn to the face or neck needs urgent medical attention. As a general principle, if the casualty has other injuries, appears to be in a great deal of pain, is showing signs and symptoms of shock, is having difficulty breathing, or you have other reasons to suspect that his or her condition is more serious, then call an ambulance whatever the extent or depth of the burn.

BELOW *Prolonged exposure to the sun can cause radiation burn, otherwise known as sunburn. Severe sunburn can result in reddened, painful skin and even blisters.*

Causes of burns

Dry heat	*This is the most common type of burn and includes burns caused by hot objects such as exhausts or by cigarettes or lighters.*
Wet heat	*Also known as a scald, wet heat is generally taken to mean hot water or steam, such as steam from a kettle. However, it can also include other hot liquids such as oil or fat.*
Friction	*When two objects rub together very quickly friction generates heat, causing another kind of dry burn.*
Chemical burns	*Industrial and household chemicals can cause serious burns.*
Electrical burns	*These can be caused by the everyday low-voltage currents found in switches, wires and appliances around the home or from the high-voltage cables scattered around the countryside in the form of power lines, railway tracks and so forth. In rarer cases electrical burns can be caused by lightning strikes.*
Radiation burns	*While this may sound drastic, most of us have suffered some degree of radiation burn at some point in our lives – more commonly known as sunburn.*

HOW TO TREAT BURNS AND SCALDS

The general treatment of all burns is very simple: cool and cover the affected part, and seek appropriate medical help. Before you do anything else, make sure that you protect yourself. This is particularly important at burns incidents. Ensure that the fire is out, that any electrical equipment is safely disconnected or that any chemical spills are not going to affect you.

TREATMENT

1 *Monitor the casualty's airway and breathing (see pages 16–19). This is particularly important if the casualty has burns to the mouth and airway. Be prepared to resuscitate if necessary (see pages 30–33).*

2 *If possible lay the casualty on the ground to help reduce the effects of shock.*

3 *Douse the burnt area with cool liquid. Cooling the burn will reduce the pain, swelling and risk of scarring. Restrict the cool liquid to the injured part where possible because over-cooling could lead to hypothermia, particularly if the surrounding air temperature is low. If applying water from a shower, hose or even a gushing tap, ensure that the pressure is minimal because water hitting burnt skin at speed will add to the pain and the damage.*

4 *Make an assessment about whether or not an ambulance is needed and call for help. If in doubt, call 999.*

5 *Keep cooling the injured part until the pain stops. Often 10 minutes is sufficient but if the casualty still complains of pain after this time then continue with the cooling treatment.*

6 *Remove rings, watches and other potential constricting items as burns swell up. Take care to return these items to the casualty.*

Douse burn with cool liquid for at least 10 minutes

Place a bowl underneath to catch the liquid

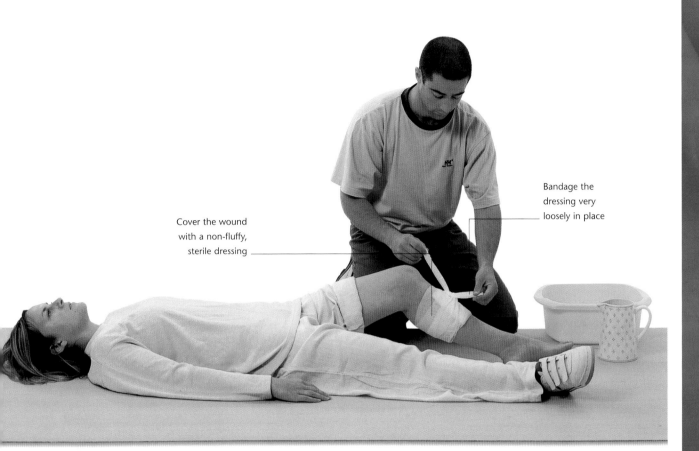

Cover the wound with a non-fluffy, sterile dressing

Bandage the dressing very loosely in place

7 Once the pain has eased, cover the wound to prevent infection. This should be done with a sterile bandage if possible, tied very loosely over the burn. If in any doubt as to whether material may stick to the wound, do not attempt to cover but continue to cool the burns continuously until medical help arrives. If you are having to improvise, any clean, non-fluffy material can be used – ideal examples are clean handkerchiefs, cotton pillowcases or clingfilm.

8 If possible, raise the injured part as this can help to reduce swelling.

Wait with the injured person until help arrives or, if the burn is less serious, accompany her to further medical attention.

• Continue to treat for shock.
• Maintain a check on the casualty's airway, breathing and circulation.
• Keep checking bandages to ensure that they are not too tight.

Warning

• Do not over-cool the casualty.
• Do not apply water under pressure.
• Do not remove burnt clothing if it is sticking to the wound.
• Do not put cotton wool or any other fluffy material on to a burn as it will stick to the injury.
• Do not put any creams or ointments on to a burn as these will need to be removed at the hospital.
• Do not burst blisters as this may increase the risk of infection.

Summary

1 Check for danger

2 Assess ABC (be prepared to resuscitate if necessary)

3 Cool the injured part

4 Make an appropriate decision about what help is required and call for an ambulance if necessary

5 Cover the injured part

6 Treat for shock throughout your treatment of the burn

7 Elevate the injured part if possible

TREATING OTHER TYPES OF BURN

The general principle of treating burns remains to cool and cover the affected area but some types of burn need extra consideration. With burns to the neck and mouth, beyond the risk of shock and infection, the greatest potential problem is the risk of airway obstruction due to swelling. The obvious additional danger with electrical burns is the combination of water as a treatment and electricity as the cause.

TREATING BURNS TO THE NECK AND MOUTH

1 *Check the casualty's airway and breathing and be prepared to resuscitate if necessary (see pages 30–33).*

2 *Call an ambulance and reassure the casualty until help arrives.*

3 *Get the casualty into a position where his breathing is comfortable (this will usually be sitting up).*

4 *Loosen any constriction around the neck to ease breathing. Keep the airway clear.*

5 *Cool any burns continuously – do not attempt to cover.*

6 *Maintain a check on the casualty's airway and breathing.*

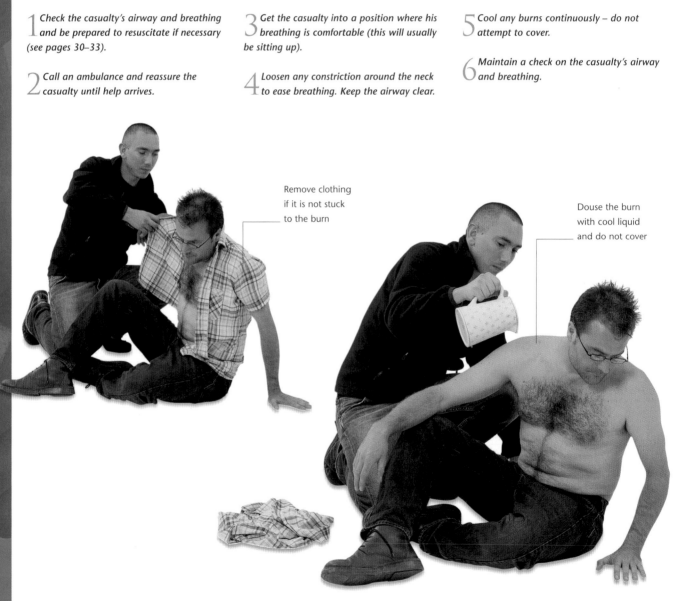

Remove clothing if it is not stuck to the burn

Douse the burn with cool liquid and do not cover

ELECTRICAL BURNS

If a casualty has suffered from an electric shock, do not attempt to touch the person unless you are absolutely certain that he or she is no longer in contact with live equipment. If the person is still attached to an electrical current, your best option is to turn the electricity off at the mains point. If you cannot access the mains, you may be able to turn off electrical equipment at the wall socket but be particularly careful that you do not touch the casualty or any live equipment.

If there is no way to turn the electricity off, you can attempt to move the casualty away from the point of contact using a non-conducting material such as a

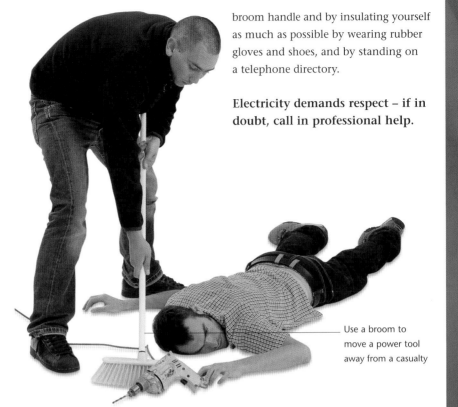

Use a broom to move a power tool away from a casualty

broom handle and by insulating yourself as much as possible by wearing rubber gloves and shoes, and by standing on a telephone directory.

Electricity demands respect – if in doubt, call in professional help.

High-voltage electricity

High-voltage electricity (power lines, railway tracks, overhead power cables etc.) usually kills immediately, causing severe burns, heart problems and potentially even broken bones and internal injuries as the victim is thrown by the shock. If somebody has been hit, your first priority is to keep yourself and other bystanders safe. High-voltage current can jump some distance so keep people back at least 20 metres (66 feet) and call for professional help via the emergency services.

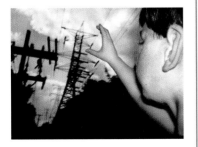

Lightning

Although rare, lightning strikes do happen and can kill. If caught outside in a thunderstorm, seek shelter in a car or building. If there is no shelter, make yourself as low as possible, minimise your contact with the ground by crouching rather than lying and avoid single trees, bodies of water and tall objects.

If a person has been struck by lightning, check their airway and breathing, be prepared to resuscitate if necessary, treat any burns and call for medical help.

TREATING ELECTRICAL BURNS

A casualty suffering from an electrical burn may well have respiratory or circulatory difficulties. An electrical discharge across the heart can make the heart stop beating (see heart attack, pages 392–393) so be prepared to resuscitate over and above the treatment of any burn that may be present.

1 *Make absolutely sure that there is no further risk from the electricity.*

2 *Check to see whether the casualty is conscious. If unconscious, check airway and breathing and take action as appropriate.*

3 *Treat any burns with cold water if safe to do so.*

4 *Cover burns as appropriate with sterile, non-fluffy dressings.*

5 *Seek urgent medical attention. Stay with the casualty and reassure him until medical help arrives.*

CHEMICAL BURNS AND EYE BURNS

While the general rules for the treatment of burns are the same, regardless of the type of burn, there are some additional considerations for chemical burns. The key point when dealing with chemicals is not to contaminate yourself. Chemical spills are not always obvious – some very toxic chemicals look like water – so look for signs such as a HAZCHEM label, empty chemical containers or guidance from bystanders. If in doubt, call the emergency services rather than approach the injured person yourself. Remember that some household substances can cause chemical burns, particularly cleaning materials such as oven cleaner.

TREATING CHEMICAL BURNS

1 If you feel that you can safely approach the casualty, then do so carefully.

2 If necessary, wear protective clothing to protect yourself from contamination.

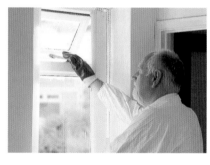

3 Ventilate the room if possible because many chemicals affect breathing.

4 When cooling the burn with water, ensure that the contaminated water runs away from both the casualty and yourself. It may be necessary to flood the injured part for longer to ensure that the chemical is totally washed away. This may take more than 20 minutes.

5 Call an ambulance. Make sure you have mentioned that it is a chemical burn so that additional help can be sent from the fire service if necessary and so that any antidotes can be sent with the ambulance.

6 If possible, remove contaminated clothes from the casualty as these may keep burning, but only do this if you can do it without contaminating yourself or harming the casualty more.

7 Cover the burn with a clean, non-fluffy material as appropriate and tie loosely in place if necessary.

8 Treat for shock (see pages 44–45) and reassure the casualty until emergency help arrives on the scene.

What if the chemical reacts with water?

Some industrial chemicals do react badly with water. Where such chemicals are used, people working with them should have been trained in the use of an antidote. If there is nobody around with this expertise, do not waste time looking for an antidote – apply liberal amounts of water to try to wash the chemical away.

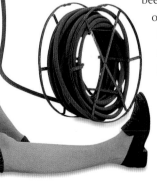

CHEMICAL BURNS TO THE EYE

Chemical burns to the eye can be very serious. Early rinsing of the eye with cold water will help to flush away the chemical and reduce scarring.

TREATMENT

1 Protect yourself, the casualty and bystanders from further contamination.

Signs and symptoms of chemical burns to the eye

• Known exposure to chemical
• Intense pain
• Redness and swelling
• Reluctance or inability to open the eye
• Tears from eye

FLASH BURNS TO THE EYE

Caused by looking into very bright light, flash burns damage the surface of the cornea, the transparent front of the eyeball. Recovery can take some time and in some instances the damage can be permanent (for example, if a person has looked at the sun through a telescope without appropriate protection).

Signs and symptoms of flash burns to the eye

• Known exposure to intense light (which may have happened some time ago)
• Intense pain
• Feeling that there may be something in the eyes
• Redness and watering
• Both eyes affected

TREATMENT

1 Check the history to rule out chemical burns or a foreign body in the eye.

2 Reassure the injured person, and wear gloves to prevent infecting the eye.

3 Place pads over both eyes and bandage in place if it will be some time until medical help arrives. Remember that this will effectively blind the person temporarily so stay with her to reassure and guide.

4 Take or send the person to hospital as she will need medical attention.

2 Hold the affected eye under cold running water for at least 10 minutes to flush out the chemical, allowing the injured person to blink periodically. You may need to hold the eyelid open. Make sure that the water flow is gentle. Do not allow contaminated water to fall across the good eye.

3 Ask the injured person to hold a non-fluffy sterile or clean pad across the eye, tying it in place if hospital treatment may be delayed.

4 Take or send the person to hospital with details of the chemical if possible.

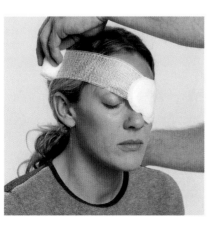

Contact lenses

Where there has been any injury to the eye, encourage the injured person to leave contact lenses in place.

EXTREME COLD

Hypothermia, a condition that occurs when the body temperature falls below the normal range, is caused by a low surrounding temperature and can lead to death. Freezing temperatures cause frostbite, whereby ice forms in the body tissue and destroys it. The risk of frostbite is increased by windy conditions.

CAUSES OF HYPOTHERMIA

Hypothermia (low temperature) occurs when the body temperature falls below the normal range, and can lead to death. The average temperature of a healthy adult is 36–38°C (96.8–100.4°F). Hypothermia occurs when the body's core temperature falls below 35°C (95°F). Survival is unlikely, but not unheard of, below 26°C (79°F).

There are a number of factors that heighten the risk of becoming hypothermic. These include:

- *Age*

The elderly are at greater risk from hypothermia: low mobility combined with poor circulation, a reduced sensitivity to the cold and a greater potential for slips and falls means that an elderly person may develop hypothermia in temperatures that a healthy younger adult could tolerate.

The very young are also at an increased risk as their mechanisms for controlling their own body temperature are poorly developed. They may look healthy but their skin will feel cold and their behaviour may be abnormally quiet or listless.

- *Exposure to wind or rain*
- *Immersion in cold water*
- *Lack of food*
- *Alcohol and drugs*

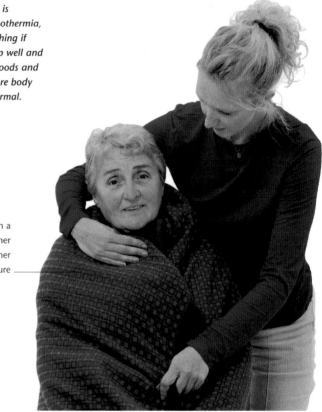

RIGHT *If a person is suffering from hypothermia, replace damp clothing if necessary, wrap up well and give high energy foods and hot drinks to restore body temperature to normal.*

Wrap the person in a blanket to keep her warm and raise her body temperature

Signs and symptoms of hypothermia

Early signs:
- *Shivering*
- *Pale, cold skin*
- *Cold environment*
- *Presence of an increased risk factor as listed left*

As the condition gets worse:
- *No shivering, even though the person is cold*
- *Increasing drowsiness*
- *Irrational behaviour and confusion*
- *Slow, shallow breathing*
- *Slow, weak pulse*

TREATMENT

If the person is unconscious

Open the airway and check for breathing (see pages 16–17). Be prepared to resuscitate if necessary (see pages 30–33). Hypothermia slows the body's functions down before stopping the heart, and it is therefore not uncommon to hear of people with hypothermia being successfully resuscitated some time after the heart has stopped.

If the person is conscious

1 *Improve the surroundings. If the person is outdoors, bring them in or take them to shelter (see Wilderness First Aid, pages 154–155). If the person is indoors, warm the room but do not overheat (25°C/77°F).*

2 *Replace wet clothes with dry warm clothing if possible.*

3 *A healthy adult may be best rewarmed by soaking in a warm bath of 40°F (104°F). Do not use this technique on an elderly person or a child.*

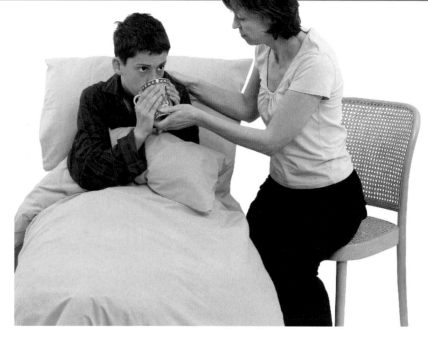

4 *Wrap the person up and give high energy foods and warm drinks. Remember that heat is lost through the extremities so cover the head, hands and feet.*

5 *Check for other conditions or injuries. The confusion caused by hypothermia may mask other signs and symptoms.*

If there is no improvement, or the level of consciousness deteriorates, seek medical advice.

For young children and the elderly, who are particularly vulnerable, always seek medical attention if you suspect hypothermia. Re-warm them slowly.

FROSTBITE

Frostbite occurs in freezing conditions and is the freezing of body tissue at the extremities, most commonly the fingers, toes and earlobes. If it is not treated early enough it can lead to gangrene and to amputation. Frostbitten skin is highly susceptible to infection.

TREATMENT

1 *Remove tight items such as rings and watches that may further damage circulation. Warm the injured part slowly by holding it.*

2 *Get the person to shelter. Do not attempt to thaw the injured part if it is liable to be re-exposed to extremes of cold, as this will do more damage.*

3 *Handle the injured part carefully as the tissue is very fragile and may be easily*

damaged. Do not apply direct heat to the injured part, rub it or allow the injured person to apply pressure to it (for example, do not let the person walk if the toes are affected). Place the injured part in warm water if available. Otherwise continue warming with your hand.

4 *Pat dry and then cover with a light gauze bandage. Remember that the injured part will be exceptionally painful.*

5 *Raise the injured part to help alleviate pain and swelling and allow the injured person to take paracetamol if able to.*

6 *Watch for hypothermia and treat as appropriate.*

7 *Seek medical attention, particularly if the site of the freezing does not regain a healthy colour or is black.*

Signs and symptoms of frostbite

- *Freezing environment*

Early signs
- *Pins and needles*
- *Pale skin*

As the condition gets worse
- *Numbness*
- *Hardening of the skin*
- *Skin colour changes to white, through blue and finally black*

When thawed, the injured part is extremely painful and there may be blistering of the skin.

EXTREME HEAT

Heat exhaustion is a condition resulting from the loss of fluid and salt, usually through excessive sweating. Heatstroke generally occurs rapidly when the brain's temperature regulator fails to work effectively. This tends to occur when the casualty has been in a very hot environment or has a fever caused by a condition such as malaria.

HEAT EXHAUSTION

Heat exhaustion is very similar to shock (see pages 44–45) in that fluid is being lost from the body. It most commonly occurs when a person has been exercising and not replacing fluid content: cyclists and joggers are common sufferers from the condition.

TREATMENT

1 *Lay the casualty down in a cool place and raise her legs.*

2 *If the casualty is conscious give sips of a weak salt solution (one teaspoon to one litre of water).*

3 *Maintain a check on the casualty's consciousness level (see pages 16–17). If it deteriorates, place the casualty in the recovery position (see pages 22–25) and call for emergency help.*

4 *If the casualty's condition improves rapidly, advise her to see a doctor.*

Signs and symptoms of heat exhaustion

- *History of exertion*
- *Pale, cold and clammy skin*
- *Fast, weak pulse*
- *Fast, shallow breathing*
- *Nausea*
- *Dizziness and disorientation*
- *Lapse into unconsciousness*

Give the casualty a cool, salty drink until symptoms have improved

Raise the legs by placing a towel under the feet

HEATSTROKE

In heatstroke, the body becomes very hot very quickly and this condition can be fatal. The signs and symptoms are very similar to those of a stroke (see pages 50–51).

Signs and symptoms

- Hot, flushed and dry skin
- Slow, full and bounding pulse
- Noisy breathing
- High body temperature
- Headache
- Disorientation
- Lapse into unconsciousness

TREATMENT

1 Check airway and breathing (see pages 16–17). If unconscious, turn the casualty into the recovery position. Be prepared to resuscitate if necessary.

2 If the casualty is conscious, move to a cool environment. If this is impossible or the casualty is unconscious, try to cool the environment (use fans, open doors and keep crowds away).

3 Call for emergency help and reassure the casualty if he or she is conscious.

4 Remove outer clothes and wrap the casualty in a cold, wet sheet. Keep it wet. Continue the cooling process. If the body temperature drops, replace the wet sheet with a dry one.

5 Continue to monitor the casualty while you wait for help.

Wrap the casualty in a sheet and keep this wet to reduce heatstroke

Slip slap slop

The treatment for sunburn is detailed under burns (see pages 104–105) but prevention is the best option. Prolonged exposure to the sun's ultraviolet rays can not only cause painful and potentially serious burns (and contribute to heatstroke) but may also in the long term cause skin cancer, particularly if you have fair skin.

The three simple rules for prevention of sun-related problems are:

Slip into a T-shirt — Bare skin burns – keep covered up. This is particularly important for children.

Slap on a hat — The top of the head can burn. Direct sun on the head is also a key factor in heatstroke. Remember that burns can happen even on cloudy days.

Slop on the appropriate sun cream for your skin type — Choose the right cream for your skin and remember to reapply, particularly after swimming. You can still be burnt while wearing sun cream so do not ignore the other precautions.

To help avoid heatstroke, consume liquids regularly in hot weather, avoid alcohol, and ensure that children have regular drinks and trips to a shady area.

DEALING WITH SPLINTERS AND FISH HOOKS

Large objects embedded in a wound, or foreign objects near to a vulnerable site such as the eye, need special care and medical treatment. Smaller debris, such as shards of glass or splinters of wood, stuck into minor wounds can usually be successfully managed at home without further treatment.

REMOVING SPLINTERS

1 If the splinter is fully embedded in the skin clean the wound, cover gently and seek medical attention. If part of the splinter is out of the skin, you may try to remove it with tweezers.

2 Pass the tweezers over a flame to clean them and reduce the risk of infection.

3 Use the tweezers to grasp the end of the object and to gently pull it out at the same angle that it went in. If the splinter breaks off in the wound or is not easy to remove, treat it as you would a larger foreign body (see page 71).

4 Once removed, squeeze the wound to encourage a small bleed, clean the site with soap and water and gently cover with a plaster or dressing as appropriate.

5 Splinters can carry infection into the body so check the site for any signs of infection (see page 78) over the coming days. Tetanus is a particular risk, especially if the splinter was obtained while gardening, so check the date of the person's last tetanus immunisation and seek a booster if necessary.

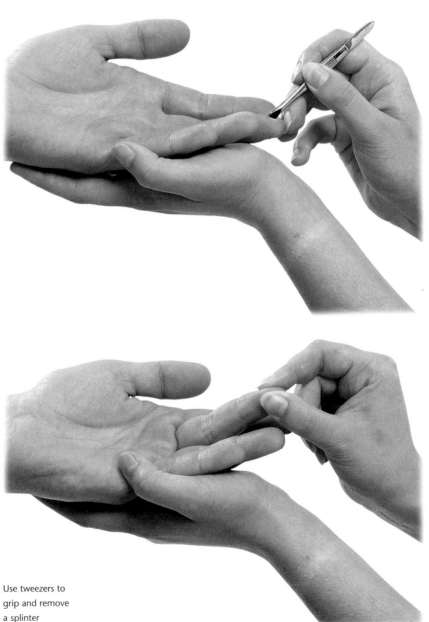

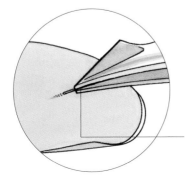

Use tweezers to grip and remove a splinter

FISH HOOKS

While the injuries associated with an embedded fish hook may be relatively minor, they are particularly difficult to remove because of their barbed ends. Only try to remove one if medical help is not readily available, for example if you are on boat.

When medical help is easy to access

1 *Cut the line as close to the hook as possible to prevent it catching on something and causing further damage.*

2 *Pad around the hook until you can bandage over or around it without pushing it further in.*

3 *Seek medical help to ensure there is no underlying damage to the tissues.*

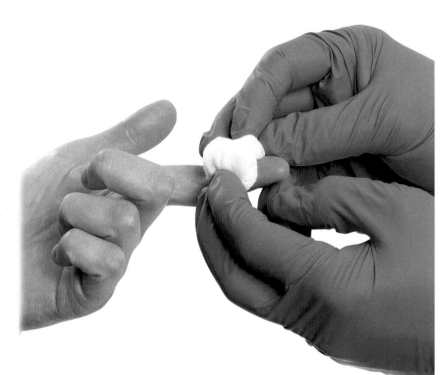

When medical help may take some time to arrive

If you can see the barb

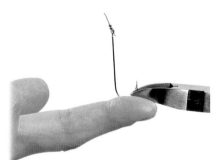

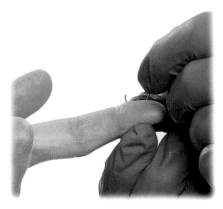

1 *Cut the line as close to the hook as possible.*

2 *Cut the barb away and carefully remove the hook by its eye.*

3 *Clean and cover the wound and elevate if it is on a limb.*

4 *Check the wound for signs of infection over the coming days and check that the tetanus booster is up-to-date.*

If you cannot see the barb

1 *If you are able, push the hook quickly and firmly forward through the skin until the barb can be seen.*

2 *Cut the barb away and then treat as outlined above.*

If the barb cannot be easily removed, do not attempt to remove the hook – instead, treat as for a larger embedded object (see box).

Treating a larger embedded object

• *Do not attempt to remove the object.*
• *Apply pressure to the wound by padding around the base of the object over the top of sterile gauze or a piece of clean material.*
• *Bandage over the padding to apply pressure without moving the object.*
• *If the object is embedded in an arm or leg, elevation may help reduce bleeding and pain.*
• *Seek medical help.*

If the object is very long, provide additional support at its base to prevent it moving.

FOREIGN BODIES

Children are prone to putting objects into their nose, ears and mouth. If left for some time, such objects can cause infection that may result in permanent damage. Young children are also particularly liable to swallow small objects. These usually pass through the system and can be identified in the bowel movement as having safely moved through the body. Larger or sharp objects pose a greater risk of internal injury. If there are signs of difficulty breathing, the object may have gone down the windpipe rather than the tube to the stomach. Call an ambulance and follow the procedures for choking (see pages 34–37).

FOREIGN BODIES IN THE NOSE

The key priority with any object in the nose is the maintenance of a clear airway. If at any time the object appears to be making breathing difficult, follow the procedures for choking (see pages 34–37) and make a call for emergency help.

Signs and symptoms of a foreign body in the nose

- Pain
- Swelling
- Discharge (if the object has been there for some time)
- Breathing difficulties
- A snoring sound on breathing

TREATMENT

1 Sit the child down, and reassure him.

2 Encourage the child to breathe through his mouth rather than his nose.

3 Do not attempt to remove the object as you may push it further in, causing more damage.

4 Take or send the child to hospital so that the object can be removed.

FOREIGN BODIES IN THE EAR

TREATMENT
Do not attempt to remove an object from the ear as you are likely to push it in further, causing more damage, particularly to the ear-drum. Reassure the child and take her to hospital.

Signs and symptoms of a foreign body in the ear

- Pain
- Temporary deafness
- Discharge

INSECT IN THE EAR

Signs and symptoms of an insect in the ear

- Very loud buzzing/ringing noise in the ear
- Pain or discomfort

TREATMENT

1 Sit the person down and reassure him before giving treatment.

2 Lean the person's head towards the unaffected side and pour tepid water into the ear with the aim of floating the insect out.

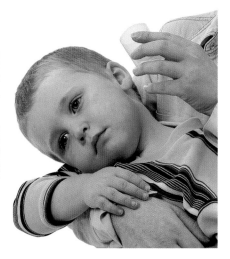

3 If this does not work, take or send the person to hospital as soon as possible.

SWALLOWED OBJECTS

TREATMENT

If the object was very large, sharp or potentially poisonous (for example some kinds of battery), call an ambulance. If the object was small and smooth, take the child to a doctor or hospital as soon as possible.

Signs and symptoms of a swallowed object

- Ask the child or bystanders what happened, and look for other small objects around the child
- Stomach pain

INHALED OBJECTS

It is possible for small and smooth objects to be inhaled into the lungs. This may cause difficulty breathing, particularly if the objects are porous and swell up on contact with body fluids. Small nuts are a particular risk, with the added concern that some people have a severe allergic reaction to them.

Signs and symptoms of an inhaled object

- Choking noises which pass as the object moves into the lung
- Hacking cough
- Difficulty breathing
- Ask bystanders what happened and look around for evidence of bags of nuts, sweets etc

FOREIGN BODIES IN THE EYE

Small items stuck to the white of the eye can be very irritating but are usually easy to remove. If an item is embedded in the eye or is stuck on the coloured part of the eye (the iris), do not attempt to remove it. Cover the eye as appropriate and take or send the person to hospital for treatment.

Signs and symptoms of a foreign body in the eye

- Irritation and/or pain.
- Watering and/or red eye.
- Blurred vision.

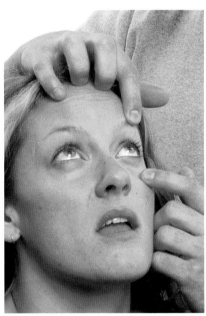

TREATMENT

1 Sit the person down facing the light so that you can clearly see what needs to be removed.

2 Examine the eye by gently separating the eyelids with your finger and thumb. Ask the person to move the eye up and down and from left to right. Allow the person to blink.

3 If you can see the foreign body and it is not embedded or touching the coloured part of the eye, gently wash it out. Tilt the head to one side and run water through the eye, holding the eyelid open. Continue with this treatment for up to 30 minutes, allowing the person to blink regularly.

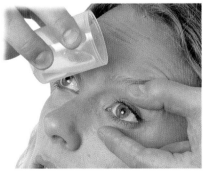

4 If washing does not work and the object is not embedded in the eye, try to remove it with a moist piece of clean material.

5 If you remain unable to remove the object, take or send the person to hospital.

TREATMENT

1 Treat the person for choking if necessary (if the person is unable to take a breath).

2 Call an ambulance as soon as possible and monitor breathing while waiting.

3 Reassure the person and try to find out exactly what was inhaled.

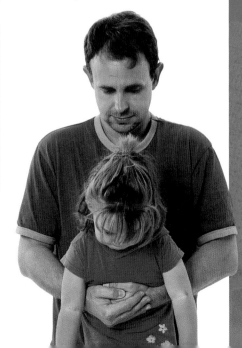

POISONING

A poison is any substance that enters the body and causes temporary or permanent harm. Some substances, such as paracetamol or alcohol, only become harmful to the body when taken in a large quantity. Others, such as some strong weedkillers, need only to be taken in very small amounts to be harmful.

THERE ARE FOUR KEY WAYS IN WHICH POISONS CAN ENTER THE BODY

Method	*Examples*
Eating (ingestion)	*Foods carrying bacteria that cause food poisoning*
	Prescription drugs taken as a deliberate or accidental overdose
	Alcohol in excess
	Household chemicals (children particularly are prone to drinking from chemical containers while playing)
	Plants (these, such as magic mushrooms, may be eaten deliberately when seeking an effect, or by accident)
Breathing in (inhalation)	*Carbon monoxide (in exhaust fumes) Fumes in house fires*
Injection	*Prescription drugs taken as a deliberate or accidental overdose*
	Illegal drugs
	Insect bites and stings
Through the skin (absorption)	*Many industrial chemicals*
	Weedkillers

HOW DO POISONS AFFECT THE BODY?

Different poisons have different effects. The effect is modified by the quantity and the time since exposure.

POTENTIAL EFFECTS OF POISONS

Vomiting This is a key response to many poisons, particularly those that have been eaten, as the body tries to remove the poison from the system.

Impaired consciousness A person may be confused and slowly lapse into full unconsciousness.

Breathing difficulties Poison may eventually cause breathing to stop.

Change in heart rate Some poisons speed up the heart rate; others slow it down. Poisons may eventually cause the heart to stop.

Erratic and confused behaviour

Burns Some poisons burn the skin, some swallowed poisons burn the food canal, bringing the additional risk of swelling around the mouth and throat.

Pain Some poisons will cause pain.

Liver and kidney problems As the liver and kidneys struggle to remove poisons from the body they may become affected themselves.

KEY FIRST AID PRINCIPLES FOR DEALING WITH POISONS

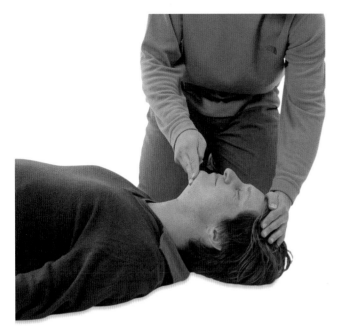

1 Protect yourself and bystanders from the source of the poison by making the scene safe and wearing protective clothing if necessary.

2 Monitor and maintain the casualty's airway and breathing and be prepared to resuscitate if necessary (see pages 30–33).

3 Seek appropriate medical help and help from the emergency services to deal with dangerous substances.

4 Monitor the casualty's level of consciousness and be prepared to turn into the recovery position (see pages 22–23) if necessary.

5 Support the casualty if he vomits and place in the recovery position until medical help arrives.

6 Treat any burns caused by corrosive poisons by flooding the affected area with running water (see chemical burns, pages 110–111).

7 Try to identify the source of the poison because this will help determine appropriate medical treatment.

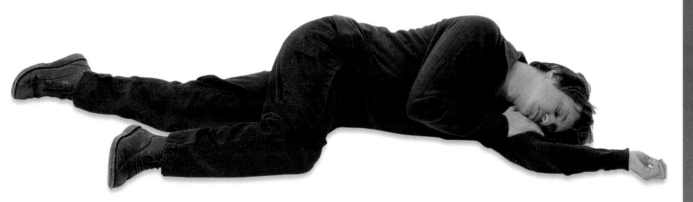

Clues to identifying poisons

The early identification of a poison will help medical staff determine an appropriate course of treatment. Potential clues that you as the first person at the scene of the incident may be able to provide include:

• Medicine bottles/pill containers (do not assume that an empty bottle means that all the pills were taken).

• Samples of vomit: if the victim is sick, try to keep it for inspection.
• Details of what happened from bystanders or from the victim. Useful questions include: What have you eaten over the last 24 hours? Have you taken any medicines or painkillers? Have you been bitten by something?
• Identification of animal or insect: if the poisoning route was a bite, for

example, from a snake or an insect, try to get a description of the creature. If is safe to do so, take the poisonous animal or insect to hospital.
• Chemical containers: be able to describe any HAZCHEM symbol or label if you can get close enough to do so without putting yourself at risk. Do not touch these yourself. Remember that many household substances are toxic.

POISONING FROM HOUSEHOLD CHEMICALS

Many everyday household substances are potentially poisonous if misused. Unfortunately, many admissions to hospital are the result of children drinking household chemicals while playing. Inside the home, cleaning materials are often the biggest risk, while in the garden weedkillers, pesticides and paint stripper are common culprits. Most household chemicals cause problems when they are swallowed. Many are corrosive and together with the effect of the poison also cause burns to the mouth and food canal (digestive tract).

Signs and symptoms

- *Signs of bottles, information from the victim or from bystanders*
- *Burns to the mouth*
- *Vomiting*
- *Pain*
- *Impaired consciousness*
- *Difficulty breathing*

MANAGING SWALLOWED POISONS

TREATMENT
Make sure that it is safe for you to approach. Do not inadvertently kneel in chemicals or otherwise expose yourself to any risk.

1 *Monitor and maintain the airway and breathing (see pages 16–21). Be prepared to resuscitate (see pages 30–33) if necessary.*

2 *Monitor consciousness. If the person becomes unconscious, put into the recovery position (see pages 22–25).*

3 *Call an ambulance and tell the emergency services what has happened.*

4 *Treat any burns (see pages 26–29), wearing protective clothing if necessary.*

5 *Support the person if he is sick and place in the recovery position if necessary.*

6 *Reassure the person while you are waiting for the emergency services to arrive.*

7 *Identify the poison if possible because this will help medical staff determine what treatment is appropriate.*

Do not try to make the person vomit. If a poison burns on the way down to the stomach, it will burn on the way up.

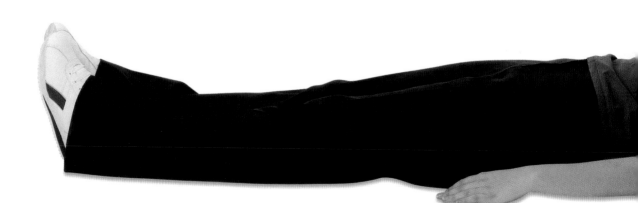

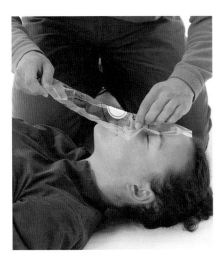

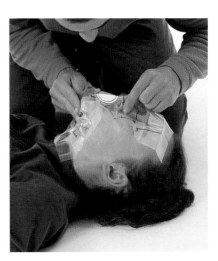

LEFT *You will need to give mouth-to-mouth resuscitation if a person stops breathing but if there are burns to the mouth you must use a face shield or mask to protect yourself.*

RIGHT *Place the plastic face shield or mask over the casualty's face and place the oval tube between the teeth. The shield forms a barrier as you give rescue breaths.*

IF THERE ARE MOUTH BURNS

If the person stops breathing you will need to give rescue breaths (see pages 26–29). However, if there are mouth burns because the poison was corrosive, you must take care not to put yourself at risk. If possible, use a face shield or mask to give the rescue breaths. These should be placed over the casualty's face and the oval tube placed between the teeth. The plastic shield forms a barrier as you give mouth-to-mouth.

If there is no shield available, consider giving rescue breaths mouth-to-nose. Tilt the head and lift the chin as you would normally. Then close the mouth (using a piece of material as a barrier against the poison if appropriate) and seal your mouth around the casualty's nose. Give rescue breaths at the same rate and ratio as you would when giving mouth-to-mouth. Take your mouth away after each breath and open the casualty's mouth between breaths to let the air out.

If the casualty is breathing and conscious, you may provide relief from the burning by giving frequent sips of cold water. This will help relieve pain and reduce swelling.

Prevention of poisoning from household substances

• Put all household cleaning materials and medicines up high out of the reach of children.

• Consider putting any dangerous substances in a locked cupboard.

• Always read instructions for use carefully. Some household chemicals should be used only in a well-ventilated room or with some protective clothing.

• Always store chemicals in the container they came in or a clearly marked alternative. Never store chemicals in drinks containers or unmarked bottles.

• Keep gardening supplies securely in the shed or garage in a locked container.

• Where possible, buy medicines and cleaning materials in childproof containers.

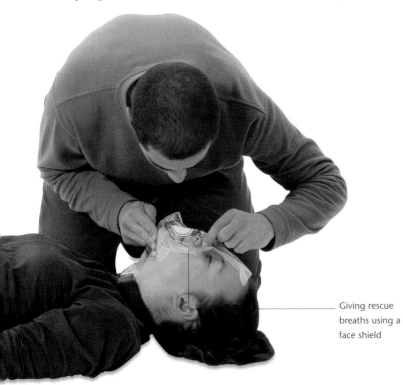

Giving rescue breaths using a face shield

POISONING FROM INDUSTRIAL CHEMICALS

The use of hazardous industrial chemicals is generally strictly controlled and regulated, and staff who work with such substances are aware of the specific first aid and safety requirements. For most people, contact with dangerous industrial chemicals will be through a chemical spill at a road accident or a problem at an engineering plant.

TREATMENT

Many industrial chemicals can be absorbed through the skin or inhaled so it is important not to approach an accident scene unless you are sure you can do so safely. If you are at all unsure of the risk, do not approach the scene. Instead, call the emergency services immediately, giving as much information about the incident as you can. Encourage casualties who can to move away from the source of any danger.

INHALED POISONS

Where possible, remove the casualty from the chemical. If this not possible, then ensure that the area is well-ventilated (open doors and windows).

If in doubt, do not stay in the room yourself. Many chemicals have no odour or obvious effect and you may not be aware that you are being poisoned.

1 *Monitor and maintain the casualty's airway and breathing (see pages 16–21) and be prepared to resuscitate if necessary (see pages 30–33).*

2 *If the casualty becomes unconscious, place him or her into the recovery position (see pages 22–25).*

3 *If the casualty is conscious, help into the most comfortable position. If there are breathing problems this position is most likely to be sitting up.*

4 *Call an ambulance and give as much information as you can.*

POISONS ON THE SKIN

1 *Take every precaution to prevent contaminating yourself. Wear protective clothing if available.*

2 *Wash away the chemical with water, taking care to flush the contaminated water away from both yourself and the casualty.*

3 *Monitor and maintain the casualty's airway and breathing and be prepared to resuscitate if necessary.*

4 *Call an ambulance and reassure the casualty until help arrives.*

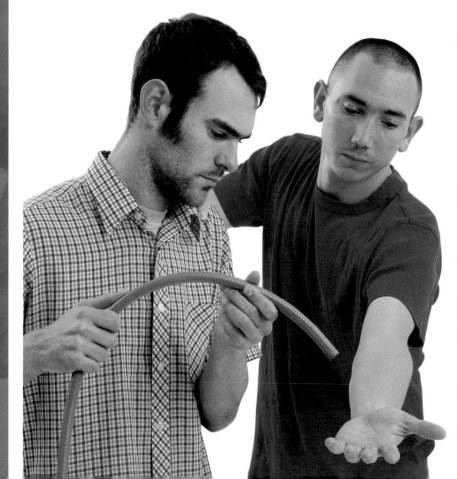

DRUG POISONING

Drug poisoning can be deliberate or accidental. Drugs may be prescription only, illegally supplied, or freely available from a chemist. The signs and symptoms of drug poisoning will vary, depending on the drug that has been taken.

TREATMENT

1 *Keep yourself safe. The effect of some drugs, both legally and illegally supplied, can be to cause aggression or irrational behaviour in the person who has taken them. If this is the case, do not approach the casualty. Call an ambulance instead and explain the situation. They will make a decision about whether the police need to be called.*

2 *Monitor and maintain the airway and breathing (see pages 16–21) and be prepared to resuscitate (see pages 30–33) if necessary, if it is safe for you to do so.*

3 *If the person becomes unconscious, place him or her into the recovery position (see pages 22–25).*

4 *Call for medical help and stay by the casualty until assistance arrives.*

5 *Look for clues as to the cause of the poisoning and inform medical staff.*

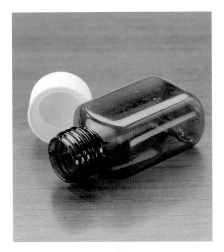

ABOVE *Do not assume that an empty container means all the drugs have been taken, but do pass it on to medical staff.*

Common types of drugs and their effects

Painkillers (analgesics)

Opioids (derived from opium, e.g. morphine, diamorphine (heroin))
Act on the brain and spinal cord to stop the perception of pain. Produce a state of well-being and relaxation. While they have legitimate medical use, they are among the most commonly abused drugs. Side-effects include nausea, vomiting, constricted pupils, constipation and slow and shallow breathing. Overdose may lead to unconsciousness and death.

Non-opioids (e.g. paracetamol)
Act in a similar way to the opioids but with fewer side-effects. Signs of an overdose may not be immediately obvious but if the antidote is not administered swiftly, fatal liver failure can set in, even in an adult who appears to be healthy. Signs include pain, nausea and vomiting.

NSAIDs Non-steroidal anti-inflammatories (e.g. aspirin, Nurofen)
Act at the site of pain to prevent the painful stimulation of nerve endings. While generally safe, they can irritate the stomach lining, causing pain and bleeding, particularly in those susceptible to stomach ulcers.

Sleeping drugs and antidepressants

Benzodiazepines and barbiturates
Act by depressing brain function. Minor side-effects include slow mental activity and drowsiness. Effects of overdose include gradual decline into unconsciousness, shallow breathing and abnormal pulse rate.

Stimulants and hallucinogens

Amphetamines (e.g. ecstasy, cocaine)
Act by stimulating the central nervous system (the brain and spinal cord). Signs include out-of-character behaviour, hallucinations, and energetic sweating, increased heart rate and, particularly with ecstasy in combination with dancing, heatstroke.

ALCOHOL POISONING

Alcohol depresses the central nervous system, which is, the centre of our thoughts, feelings and senses, and responsible for coordinating all movement and body processes. In the early stages of drinking, this creates a relaxed feeling and impression of increased confidence. Continued drinking can affect the ability to make rational decisions and, as consumption increases, slow down breathing and even cause loss of consciousness. The effect of alcohol on the body is affected by factors including weight, body fat and history of alcohol intake. What may be a safe level for one person may have serious effects for another.

EFFECTS OF HIGH INTAKE

There are four key risks following a high alcohol intake:

- *Injury, following poor decision-making and clumsiness.*
- *Vomiting, leading to choking in an unconscious person.*
- *Hypothermia – alcohol dilates the blood vessels, making exposure to the cold a greater risk.*
- *Slower breathing and, ultimately, breathing stopping.*

TREATMENT

1 *Monitor and maintain the person's airway and breathing (see pages 16–21). Be prepared to resuscitate the person (see pages 30–33) if necessary.*

2 *If the person becomes unconscious, place into the recovery position (see pages 22–25). The person is extremely likely to be sick, so watch carefully for signs of vomit and remove from the mouth as needed.*

3 *If the person is conscious, help into a comfortable position and encourage him or her to keep still.*

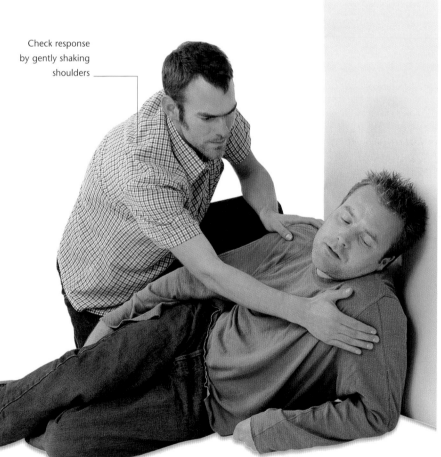

Check response by gently shaking shoulders

4 *Check for additional injury and give treatment as appropriate.*

5 *Protect from extremes of cold to reduce the risk of hypothermia developing.*

If the person is unconscious, you suspect further injury, you are worried that other substances may have been consumed or you have any other doubts as to their condition, call an ambulance. Do not underestimate the risk of alcohol poisoning.

If you do not feel that an ambulance is necessary, ensure that the person is not left alone, that the airway and breathing are regularly checked and that the casualty is in a safe, warm place until he is better.

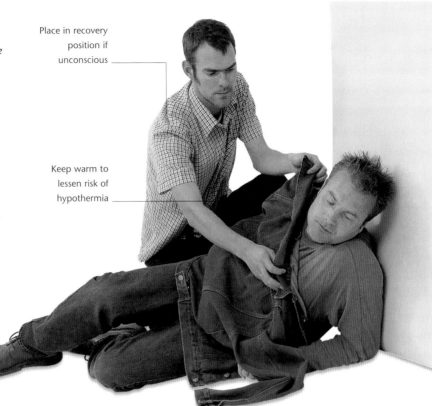

Place in recovery position if unconscious

Keep warm to lessen risk of hypothermia

Long-term effects of alcohol

Drinking alcohol within safe limits may be beneficial for health, helping to protect against stroke and heart disease, but if you have more than a couple of alcoholic drinks a day, there are more risks than benefits.

• *Weight gain: alcohol contains many calories and regular drinkers often put on weight.*

• *Reduced intellectual function: brain cells that control memory and learning are damaged by alcohol. Alcohol is also damaging to mental health causing increased anxiety and depression.*

• *Increased risk of developing many types of cancer (this risk is even higher if you smoke as well).*

• *Increased risk of circulatory disorders such as high blood pressure and stroke.*

• *Reduced fertility in both men and women and damage to the foetus if you drink heavily during pregnancy.*

• *Damage to the liver and other organs; digestive problems such as ulcers.*

Signs and symptoms

• *What has happened. Consider this carefully – a person who has suffered a head injury or stroke may show similar signs and symptoms to somebody who is drunk*
• *Strong smell of alcohol*
• *Lapsing in and out of consciousness. Rousable at first but eventually slipping into full unconsciousness*
• *Red, sweating face*
• *Deep, noisy breathing – sounds of snoring*
• *Strong, fast pulse*

Eventually, breathing may become shallower and the pulse weaker and faster.

FOOD POISONING

There are several forms of food poisoning. Bacterial food poisoning is often caused by bacteria in food that has been poorly prepared. Salmonella is one of the most common culprits and is found in many farm products such as eggs and chickens. Toxic (potentially lethal) food poisoning such as botulism can be due to poisons caused by bacteria in certain types of food, including honey and fish. Some foods are entirely poisonous or have components that are poisonous if not properly prepared (crab and some fish being among the most common culprits).

Signs and symptoms

• *Nausea and vomiting*
• *Stomach cramp*
• *Diarrhoea*
• *Fever*
• *Aches and pains*
• *Signs of shock (see pages 44–45)*

Symptons of toxic poisoning are dizziness, slurred speech and difficulty breathing and swallowing.

When faced with suspected food poisoning, ask what food has been eaten in the last 48 hours. Food poisoning can take some time to show (however, toxic food poisoning tends to act much more quickly). Be alert to the possibility of food poisoning if there is any combination of the following:

• *History of eating food that tasted strange or that was left out in the heat.*
• *Several people who ate together have the same symptoms.*
• *History of eating any one of the common culprits of food poisoning.*
• *History of eating food that was undercooked or reheated.*

TREATMENT

1 *Monitor and maintain the person's airway and breathing (see pages 16–21). If there are any signs of breathing difficulties, call an ambulance.*

2 *Help the person into a comfortable position.*

3 *Call for medical advice on treatment and care.*

4 *Give plenty of fluids to drink, particularly if the person has vomiting and diarrhoea.*

5 *Support the person if he or she vomits, providing a bowl and towel as necessary.*

Do not underestimate food poisoning, particularly in the very young or the elderly. Be prepared to call an ambulance if the condition gets worse.

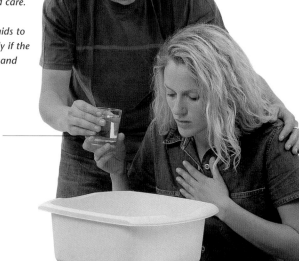

Prevent dehydration by drinking plenty of fluids regularly

Common poisonous plants

Many plants have components that are mildly poisonous if eaten, or that may cause a reaction if they are touched. However, in the UK few are extremely poisonous.

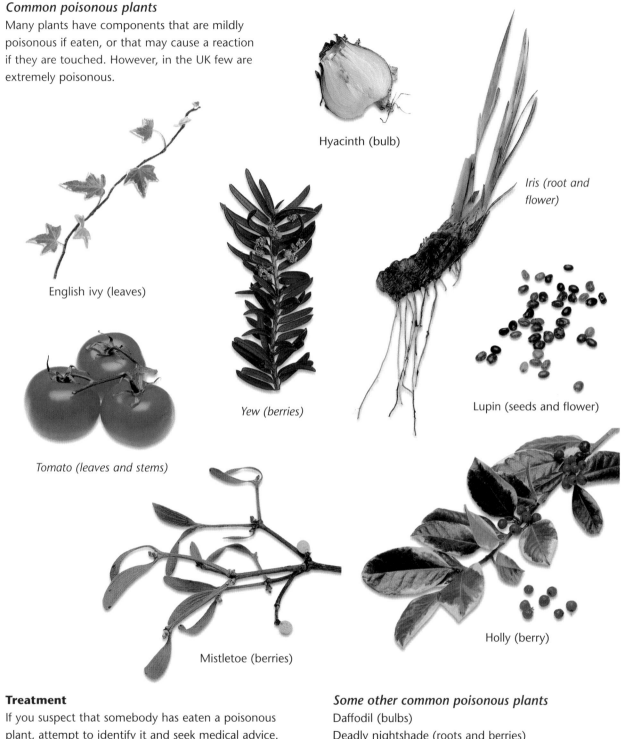
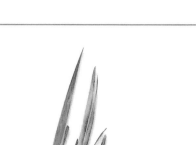

Hyacinth (bulb)

Iris (root and flower)

English ivy (leaves)

Yew (berries)

Lupin (seeds and flower)

Tomato (leaves and stems)

Mistletoe (berries)

Holly (berry)

Treatment

If you suspect that somebody has eaten a poisonous plant, attempt to identify it and seek medical advice. If the person is having breathing difficulties or appears to be lapsing into unconsciousness, call an ambulance. Be prepared to resuscitate (see pages 30–33) if necessary.

Some other common poisonous plants

Daffodil (bulbs)
Deadly nightshade (roots and berries)
English ivy (leaves)
Holly (berry)
Hyacinth (bulb)
Lupin (seeds and flowers)

ANIMAL BITES

There is a risk of infection with a bite and any bite, no matter how small, should be assessed by a doctor as soon as possible to see if a tetanus or rabies injection, or a course of antibiotics, is required. First aid treatment for bites is to keep the wound clean and control any bleeding.

ANIMAL BITES

Any animal bite requires medical attention. Deep bites can cause serious wounds, severe bleeding and tissue damage, while all animal bites can cause infection. Puncture wounds from teeth carry infection deep into the tissue, while scratches are also an infection risk. The human bite is among the most infectious.

TREATMENT

The priority is to ensure the safety of yourself and bystanders. If the animal is still a risk, do not approach it but call the emergency services instead.

For serious wounds

1 *Sit the injured person down to help reduce shock (see pages 44–45).*
2 *Treat any bleeding by:*

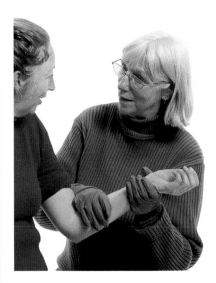

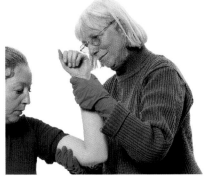

- *Looking in the wound.*
- *Applying direct pressure.*
- *Elevating the site if it is a limb.*

3 *Take or send the person to hospital.*

For smaller wounds and scratches

1 *Wash the wound thoroughly with soap and water.*

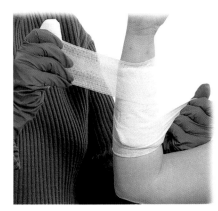

2 *Dry the wound with clean gauze or other non-fluffy material and cover with a dressing.*

3 *Seek medical advice.*

SNAKE BITES

The adder is the only poisonous snake native to the UK. However, some poisonous snakes and lizards are kept as pets and many popular overseas holiday destinations have poisonous wildlife.

TREATMENT

1 *Help the casualty to a position of rest because stress and movement make the effects of the poison worse. If possible, sit them in a position with the heart higher than the site of the bite to discourage blood flow back to the heart.*

Checking for infection

Warn the injured person to watch for signs of an infected wound over the coming days. Seek immediate medical attention if any combination of the following signs and symptoms develops:

- *Increased pain*
- *Swelling*
- *Redness around the site of the wound*
- *Discharge from the site*
- *Unpleasant smell from the site of the wound*
- *Red tracks from the site of the wound to the heart*
- *Swollen glands*

Signs and symptoms of snake bite

The severity of the symptoms will depend both on the species of snake and the time since the bite.

• History of being bitten (may have felt like a scratch)
• Location (warm grassland is the most common site for adders)
• Pain, redness and swelling over the site of the bite
• Puncture wounds or bite marks
• Nausea and vomiting
• Difficulty breathing
• Confusion and eventual loss of consciousness
• Sweating and signs of shock (see pages 44–45)

2 Monitor and maintain the casualty's airway and breathing (see pages 16–19) and be prepared to resuscitate (see pages 30–33) if necessary.

3 Call an ambulance as soon as possible and describe what has happened.

4 Wash the wound and dry it with non-fluffy, clean material.

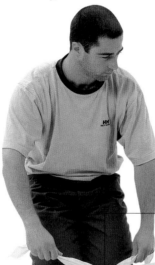

Immobilise the affected area with bandages

5 Lightly compress the wound above the bite with a bandage.

6 If you can do so without putting yourself at risk, identify the markings on the snake.

Tie a compression bandage into place above the wound

Specific infections spread by bites

Rabies
Rabies is an increasingly rare but potentially very serious, even fatal, condition carried by animal bites. Rabies in the UK is particularly rare, but if the bite is from an animal that may have come into the country without going through normal checks, or if you are bitten overseas, then seek immediate medical attention. There is no cure for rabies but early vaccination following a bite can help develop immunity.

Hepatitis B and C
There is a small chance that hepatitis B and C may be transmitted by a human bite. If concerned, seek medical advice. For more information on different types of hepatitis, see pages 406–7.

Tetanus
Tetanus bacteria exist everywhere. However, they carry a particular risk when carried deep into a wound with jagged edges or a puncture wound, as both of these are hard to clean and lead the infection to be buried deeply into the tissue. Animal bites therefore carry a potential risk of tetanus. Tetanus affects the central nervous system (see pages 194–95) and can cause muscle spasms, breathing problems and sometimes death. It is also known as lockjaw because it may tense up the jaw muscles. There is a vaccination for tetanus but immunity is not lifelong and anybody suffering a potentially hazardous injury (e.g. from an animal, while gardening, or any very deep or difficult to clean wound) should seek medical advice on having a booster injection.

INSECT BITES AND STINGS

Insect bites and stings are painful but there are no insects native to the UK that carry potentially fatal venom from a single sting or bite. Biting insects include mosquitoes and fleas; stinging insects include wasps and bees. Stings and insect bites are not usually serious unless there is an allergic reaction. Allergic reactions to stings from insects such as bees appear to be increasingly common and these can be life-threatening. Stings in the mouth or throat are also dangerous as the swelling they cause can block the airway.

STINGS AND BITES

A sting is felt as a sudden sharp pain and appears as a raised white patch on a reddened area of skin. A bite is less painful and usually causes mild discomfort and skin inflammation.

POTENTIALLY LIFE-THREATENING RESPONSES TO STINGS AND BITES

Anaphylaxis

This is an allergic reaction to a substance with which the body is in contact (see pages 46–47). Bee stings are amongst the most common cause. Anaphylaxis can develop within seconds and can be fatal.

Signs and symptoms of a life-threatening reaction

- Difficulty breathing
- Swollen lips, tongue and throat
- Blotchy skin
- Casualty has felt a bite or sting (sometimes this may be described as a scratch)
- Pain, swelling and reddening over the site of the bite or sting

Multiple stings

While one sting is unlikely to cause problems on a major scale for an otherwise healthy adult, several stings may provoke a dangerous response.

Reaction to venom

Insects native to the UK are unlikely to causes problems for an otherwise healthy adult but dangerous insects may be found as pets in the UK or in everyday venues when on holiday overseas.

Stings to mouth and throat

Any sting to the mouth or throat should be treated with care as subsequent swelling may cause difficulty with breathing.

TREATMENT

1 Monitor and maintain airway and breathing (see pages 16–19). Be prepared to resuscitate (see pages 30–33) if necessary.

2 If the casualty is a known sufferer of anaphylaxis, he may have an auto-injector that contains life-saving medicine. Help him to find this as quickly as possible and, if necessary, help to administer it.

3 If the casualty is conscious, help into the most comfortable position (this will usually be sitting up).

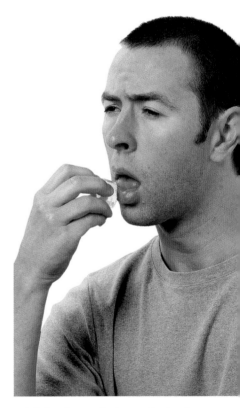

4 If the sting was in the mouth, give the casualty an ice cube to suck or frequent sips of cold water.

5 Call an ambulance and explain what has happened, identifying the insect if possible.

6 Make an attempt to identify what the casualty has been bitten or stung by but do not put yourself at risk.

ORDINARY BITES AND STINGS

Signs and symptoms

• Reddening, pain and swelling over the site of the sting
• Person has felt a bite or sting
• Sting left in the skin (if from a bee)

TREATMENT

1 If you can see the sting, remove it by flicking with the edge of a piece of plastic such as a credit card, or with tweezers. Take care not to squeeze the poison sac at the end of the sting.

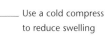

Use a cold compress to reduce swelling

2 Wash the affected area to reduce the risk of infection entering the wound.

3 Apply a cold compress (see page 170) to the site to reduce pain and swelling.

4 Remove rings, watches or anything likely to cause a constriction if the area swells.

5 Advise the casualty to see a doctor if pain persists or there are any signs of infection (see page 130).

Remove the sting by using a piece of plastic to flick it out

FEVER

A person's normal temperature is between 36–38°F (96.8–100.4°F). A fever is said to be when the temperature remains higher than this for some time. Most fevers are caused by infection, either infection associated with diseases such as flu, meningitis or chickenpox or with a local infection, for example following a bite or in an open wound. Most fevers pass with minimal risk but a temperature over 40°C (104°F) can indicate a serious infection and medical advice should be sought. High temperatures, particularly in young children, can cause febrile convulsions (see page 493).

Signs and symptoms of fever

- *Raised temperature*
- *Pale skin (becoming red as the temperature rises)*
- *Feeling shaky and shivery*
- *Increasing aches, pain and headache as the temperature rises*

TREATMENT

1 *Make the person comfortable. Ensure that the surrounding air is cool (open a window or use a fan) and provide the person with cool flannels or sponges. Take care not to overcool.*

2 *Give the person plenty of cool drinks. Encourage the person to sip these slowly to prevent feeling sick.*

3 *Look for any other signs of infection, such as rashes or swollen glands, and seek medical advice if you are unsure of the cause or seriousness of the condition.*

4 *Enable the person to take her usual painkillers. Paracetamol acts as an anti-pyretic, which means that it will help reduce a fever as well as bring pain relief.*

Non-steroidal anti-inflammatories (NSAIDS) such as Nurofen are good for bringing down fever. Children should take medicine appropriate for their age.

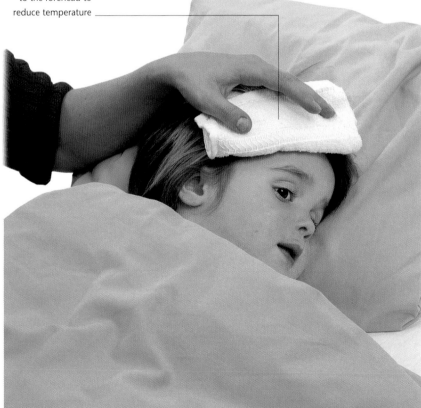

Apply a cold flannel to the forehead to reduce temperature

MENINGITIS

Bacterial meningitis is a potentially life-threatening or disabling condition one of the first signs of which is a fever. It often has a very rapid onset and the sufferer can deteriorate quickly. Signs and symptoms can at first be very similar to conditions such as flu. If in doubt, seek urgent medical attention, if necessary calling an ambulance or going straight to hospital. Early treatment is essential. For more information, see meningitis, page 414–15.

TREATMENT
Seek urgent medical advice.

HEADACHE

Headaches have many causes. Often they can develop for no apparent reason or as a symptom of common illnesses such as flu. Sometimes they are an indicator of a more serious condition such as a head injury, stroke or other serious illness. For more information, see headache, pages 332–33.

TREATMENT

1 *Help the person into a comfortable position in a quiet place. Consider remedies such as dimming the lights, cold compress, fresh air and sips of cold water.*

2 *Check for other signs and symptoms that may indicate a more serious condition and take action as appropriate. Seek urgent medical advice if:*

- *There has been a head injury.*
- *There are signs and symptoms of meningitis.*
- *The person appears confused, drowsy, or there is any fall in the level of consciousness (see pages 54–55).*

3 *Help the person to take her usual painkillers.*

4 *If the pain persists, advise the person to seek medical advice.*

Signs and symptoms of meningitis

Any combination of the following may be present:

- *Fever*
- *Headache*
- *Nausea or vomiting*
- *Stiff neck (pain or difficulty in touching the chest with the chin)*
- *Convulsions*
- *Sensitivity to light*
- *Rash (bleeding under the skin) which does not go away if a glass is pressed against it*

In addition, in babies and young children:
- *The soft spot on the head (the fontanelle) may be stretched tight*
- *There may be floppiness, lack of focus on surroundings*

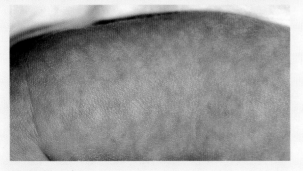

Meningitis rash

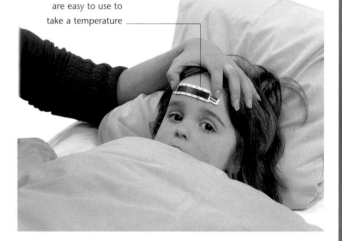

Strip thermometers are easy to use to take a temperature

Taking a temperature

A raised temperature is a sign that the body is fighting off an infection. There are several types of thermometer that can measure the body's temperature, one of the most accurate being a mercury thermometer, in which a narrow column of mercury expands in response to heat and moves up to a point on a clearly marked scale. Take a temperature on the forehead, in the mouth, under the arm or, if you have an appropriate thermometer, in the ear. Do not take a child's mouth temperature if you are using a mercury thermometer – she may bite it and swallow mercury, which is a poison.

EARACHE, TOOTHACHE AND SORE THROAT

Earache can be exceptionally painful. It has a number of common causes, including infection, or as a symptom of other conditions such as flu or tonsillitis. Like earache, toothache can cause agonising pain. Usually caused by a decaying or damaged tooth, it can also arise as a result of problems such as an ear infection or sinusitis, or even from jaw tension. In babies and children, there may be pain and discomfort as their teeth come through. Sore throats can be a sign of infection such as tonsillitis or a symptom of colds and flu. There may be swelling and infection around the throat, or swollen glands visible under the jaw.

TREATING EARACHE

1 *If there is a fever or discharge, seek urgent medical help, as this may be a sign of serious infection or a burst ear-drum. Seek medical advice if there is any loss of hearing. Check the history of the problem to rule out injury to the ear or skull, or the presence of a foreign object.*

2 *Help the person into a comfortable position. A hot-water bottle wrapped in a towel placed on the ear may provide some pain relief.*

3 *Enable the person to take her usual painkillers.*

4 *If the condition persists or gets worse, especially in children, seek medical advice.*

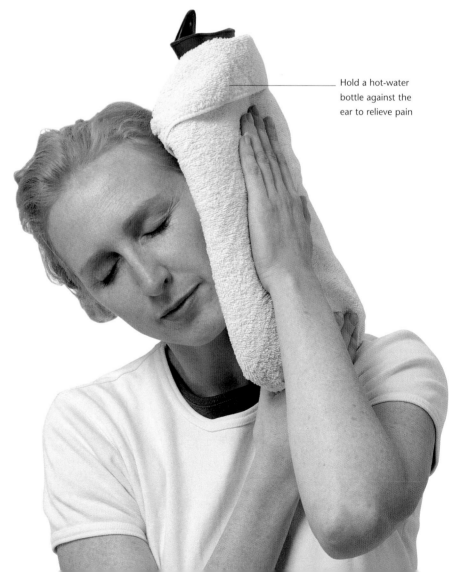

Hold a hot-water bottle against the ear to relieve pain

TREATING TOOTHACHE

1 Check the history of the problem to rule out any injury to the mouth or jaw.

2 Help the person into a comfortable position. The throbbing pain associated with an infected tooth is often eased if the person is sitting up.

3 Enable the person to take her usual painkillers.

4 A hot-water bottle wrapped in a towel or hot compress placed alongside the face may help relieve the pain. Oil of cloves applied to cotton wool and placed on the tooth (not the gums) may also help numb the pain. Children may benefit from teething remedies available from pharmacists.

5 Encourage the person to make an appointment with a dentist.

Dab the tooth with oil of cloves to reduce pain

TREATING A SORE THROAT

1 Check the history of the problem to rule out poisoning or burns.

2 Give the person plenty of cold drinks.

3 Enable the person to to take her usual painkillers.

4 Seek medical advice if the condition persists or if sore throats are recurrent, particularly in children.

Painkillers

When used according to the instructions painkillers such as paracetamol have little risk for a healthy adult. Likewise, medicines such as paracetamol syrup made especially for children can provide safe pain relief.

People in severe pain are at risk from an accidental overdose of painkillers and while paracetamol is generally safe, one of its potential drawbacks is that very few extra tablets are required to risk an overdose.

To reduce the chances of problems with any painkillers:
• Read and follow the instructions carefully.
• Seek advice from your doctor or pharmacist if necessary.
• Do not leave painkillers near the bed while sleeping. It is easy to wake up in pain and forget when the last dose was taken.
• Seek early medical advice if you think that an overdose may have been taken, even if there are no signs and symptoms of a problem. Paracetamol poisoning, for example, does not show up immediately but the antidote needs to be taken as soon as possible.

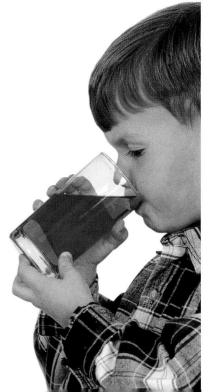

ABDOMINAL PAIN

Pain in the abdomen can range from mild discomfort to agony. There are many causes of abdominal pain. Most are not serious but others may be an indication of serious injury, such as internal bleeding (see pages 68–69), of a potential medical emergency such as appendicitis (see page 406) or a stomach ulcer (see pages 398–99), or of problems with the muscles, for example, a hernia or muscle strain. If stomach pain in an infant is accompanied by fever, diarrhoea or vomiting, seek prompt medical advice. It is important to consult a doctor if there are recurrent bouts of abdominal pain, even if they are short-lived.

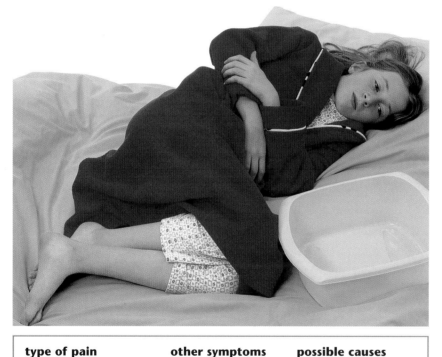

TREATING ABDOMINAL PAIN

1 *Check the history of the pain to rule out recent injury, potential poisoning (see pages 120–129) or an underlying medical condition.*

2 *Help the person into a comfortable position and provide a covered hot water bottle to provide some relief from the pain.*

3 *If the pain is severe or does not ease within half an hour, seek medical advice.*

Seek early medical advice or an ambulance if the pain is accompanied by:

- *Vomiting red blood (a potential burst stomach ulcer).*
- *High temperature (possible infection, such as peritonitis, caused by a burst appendix).*
- *Rigid (inflexible) abdomen (may indicate internal bleeding).*
- *Signs of shock (see pages 44–45).*

type of pain	other symptoms	possible causes
generalised stomach ache	sickness, tearfulness, clinginess	stress
generalised stomach ache	sore throat, fever blocked nose	throat infection, cold
sudden pain causing baby to scream and draw up legs	baby under four months of age	colic
severe pain near navel that moves right	temperature, lack of appetite vomiting	appendicitis

COLIC

Colic is a type of abdominal pain that babies suffer from during the first four months of life, usually in the evening. The baby, who is otherwise well, will suffer bouts of pain during which he screams and draws his legs up towards his stomach. Colic is not an illness and disappears on its own without treatment when a baby is about four months old. The cause of colic is unknown but it is thought to be due to intestinal spasm.

No drugs are needed for colic and the best treatment is to comfort the child. A rhythmic activity such as rocking or taking the child for a drive may pacify him.

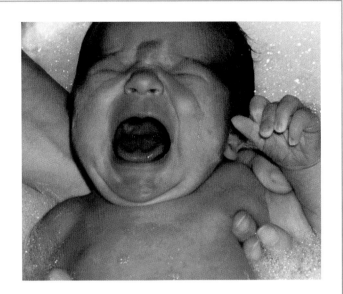

HERNIA

A hernia occurs when part of the abdomen's contents poke through the stomach wall, producing swelling and potentially an obvious lump. Sometimes painful, many hernias will heal by themselves with rest. Others may need to be surgically repaired.

Sometimes the hernia becomes twisted (strangulated), cutting off the blood supply to the protruding part (which is often part of an intestine). This is a potentially serious condition and alongside the swelling the injured person may be vomiting and in extreme pain.

Sites of hernia

Bulging small intestine

hiatus hernia

Inguinal hernia

Femoral hernia

TREATMENT

1 *Get the injured person into a comfortable position. If the hernia is painless, suggest that the victim seeks medical advice as soon as possible. Advise the person not to try to push the hernia back in and do not attempt to do so yourself.*

2 *If the hernia is painful, support the person in the most comfortable position and call a doctor. If the pain is severe or is accompanied by vomiting or signs of shock, call an ambulance.*

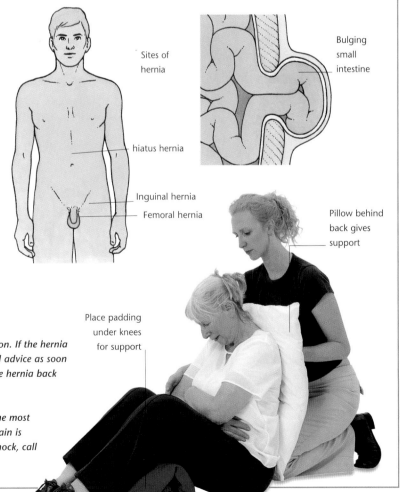

Pillow behind back gives support

Place padding under knees for support

VOMITING AND DIARRHOEA

Severe vomiting and diarrhoea can be very serious, particularly in children and the elderly, who are more vulnerable to the accompanying risk of dehydration. The loss of circulating body fluid can lead to life-threatening shock (see pages 44–45) if it is not replaced.

CAUSES

Likely causes of vomiting and diarrhoea include: food poisoning; viral infections such as gastroenteritis, and sensitivity to a new or unusual food. Vomiting alone can also accompany some medical conditions such as concussion and compression (see skull fractures, page 84) and other injuries.

TREATMENT

1 *Check the person's recent history for clues as to the cause and to rule out underlying injury such as a serious blow to the head.*

2 *Help the person into a comfortable position. If he is vomiting, this will usually be sitting up. Help the person to the bathroom as necessary.*

3 *Help the person to clean himself up and to change clothes as necessary.*

4 *Give bland fluids (except milk) to drink slowly – it is important to keep fluid levels up.*

5 *Seek medical advice if the condition persists. If the person shows signs of shock, seek urgent medical attention.*

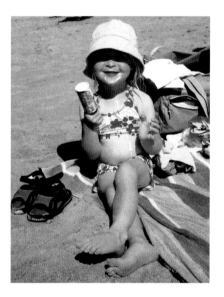

ABOVE *Vomiting and diarrhoea often occur as a result of food poisoning contracted on holiday, particularly if food has been left out in the sun. The complaint is extremely common and the person usually recovers without any treatment other than replacement of vital fluids and minerals. However if the person is a young child or elderly, seek medical advice as soon as possible because these people are at particular risk of dehydration.*

Isotonic drinks

These drinks replace vital fluids and important minerals and sugars in the body. Available to purchase ready made, you can also make your own.

Add
1 tsp salt and
5 tsp sugar
per litre (2 pints) of water or
diluted orange juice

This drink should be taken in short sips as needed.

CRAMP

Cramp is a muscle spasm generally caused by exercising and loss of fluid, for example through heatstroke (see pages 115). However, it can also occur spontaneously, often at night, particularly in older people. Common sites for cramp include the sole of the foot, the calf and the thigh. If the abdominal muscles are affected, the condition is known as a stitch.

TREATING CRAMP
A gentle stretching and massage of the affected area will help to relieve cramp. Give the affected person plenty of fluids and something salty to eat.

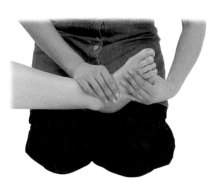

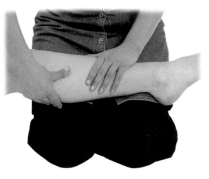

FOR A FOOT
Often if the affected person stands on the foot with the sole flat on the ground this will relieve the pain. If this does not work, accompany this with gentle massage.

FOR THE CALF
Straighten the person's knee and gently push the foot up towards the shin. Massage the affected muscle.

Straighten leg and massage affected muscle firmly

FOR THE THIGH

1 *Straighten the knee and raise the leg if the cramp is in the back of the leg.*

2 *Bend the knee if the cramp is in the front of the thigh.*

3 *Massage the affected muscle firmly.*

HYSTERIA, PANIC ATTACKS AND HICCUPS

The word hysteria has come to mean the extreme behaviour exhibited at time of high emotion. This can be positive emotion, for example delight at a pop concert, or negative emotion, for example the shock of hearing bad news. Hiccups are caused by an involuntary contraction of the diaphragm, the muscle that separates the lung and stomach cavities. They are very common and although not serious can be irritating and tiring if an attack continues.

TREATING HYSTERIA

Although this type of behaviour may appear to be extreme, the affected person's feelings are very real to him or her. Hysteria is often a common, and some would argue, healthy response to situations of high stress.

1 *Speak to the affected person firmly but quietly. Do not shout at her.*

2 *Move the person away from onlookers as subconsciously she may be reacting to the crowd.*

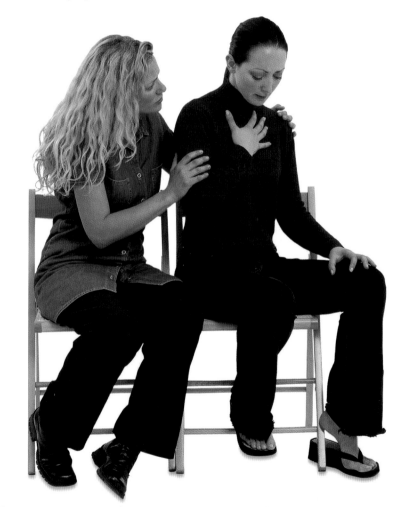

Signs and symptoms of hysteria

• *Screaming, shouting and uncontrollable crying*
• *Hyperventilation (breathing too fast) – this may lead to dizziness and or trembling*
• *An apparent inability to move (the person may appear to be rooted to the spot)*
• *Aggressive behaviour (the person may direct this towards himself)*

3 *Encourage the person to focus on breathing. If she is suffering from the effects of hyperventilation, such as cramps in the hands or dizziness, hand over a paper bag and advise her to re-breathe her own exhaled air.*

4 *Stay with the person until she has recovered.*

5 *Check the person for injury or any underlying medical condition, and treat as appropriate.*

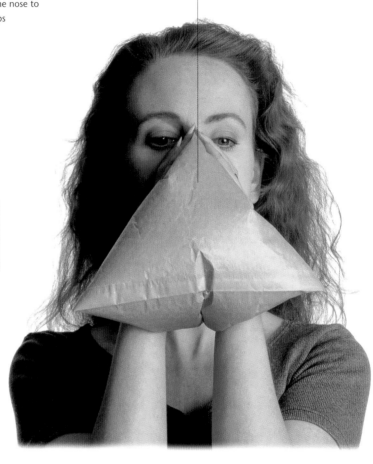

LEFT *Attacks of hiccups usually last for only a few minutes and are not serious. There are many home remedies for treating hiccups, such as holding the breath or drinking a glass of water from the wrong side.*

Hold the breath by pinching the nose to stop hiccups

Hold the paper bag tightly against the mouth

ABOVE *To control hiccups or a panic attack, a person should breathe in and out slowly into a paper bag 10 times then breathe normally for another 10 breaths. This should be continued until breathing is normal.*

Panic attacks

Panic attacks are sudden instances of extreme anxiety accompanied by alarming physical symptoms such as chest pains, breathing problems, sweating, stomach pains, palpitations (awareness of an abnormally fast heartbeat), dizziness and faintness. The best way to treat this is to encourage the sufferer to stay calm and to remember that the attack will soon pass. Rapid, shallow breathing can be helped by breathing into a paper bag. Relaxation exercises can help a person reduce anxiety levels. If a person has frequent panic attacks, she should see a doctor.

TREATING HICCUPS

There are various suggested treatments for hiccups.

• *Give the affected person a paper bag and encourage her to re-breathe her own exhaled air.*

• *Make the person drink from the wrong side of a cup.*

• *Tell the person to hold her breath for as long as possible.*

All these treatments work by increasing the level of carbon dioxide in the blood, which has a positive effect on breathing.

If hiccups persist for more than 30 minutes, or the person is exhausted, seek medical advice.

ALLERGY

An allergy is hypersensitivity to a substance (allergen) that is not normally considered to be harmful. The body's response can be mild but irritating or severe, quick and life-threatening. The most extreme response is anaphylaxis, which can result in anaphylactic shock (see pages 46–47) that, if untreated, can kill. The number of allergy sufferers is increasing in the developed world.

Signs and symptoms

- *Itching skin*
- *Rash*
- *Red, watering eyes*
- *Sneezing*
- *Flushed, warm face*
- *Dizziness*
- *Breathlessness*
- *Swelling, particularly of the eyes, tongue and face*
- *Nausea*
- *Vomiting*
- *Pain and cramps*
- *Increasing difficulty in breathing*
- *The person becomes increasingly light-headed and drowsy*
- *Breathing ceases*

Allergies are often also held responsible for triggering asthma attacks (see pages 42–43) and the skin condition eczema (see pages 372–73).

LEFT *Open the airway by lifting the head and tilting the chin, and monitor breathing.*

BELOW *Help the casualty to take her medication if it is available, and call an ambulance.*

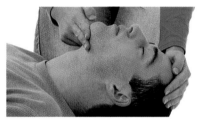

TREATING EXTREME REACTIONS

1 *For extreme reactions affecting breathing, call an ambulance and help the person to take her own medication if it is available.*

2 *Monitor airway and breathing (see pages 16–19) and be prepared to resuscitate (see pages 30–33) if necessary. See also Anaphylactic Shock, pages 46–47.*

CLUES THAT SOMEONE MAY SUFFER FROM ANAPHYLAXIS

- *Carrying auto-injector pen.*
- *Medic alert bracelet or necklace.*
- *Medical card.*
- *Medication such as adrenaline.*

Over-the-counter remedies
Some allergic reactions can be eased with over-the-counter remedies that contain antihistamines, which dilate blood vessels and relax muscles. Seek advice from a pharmacist.

TREATING MILD REACTIONS

Mild reactions usually involve skin irritation, minor swelling and a rash. Some reactions take the form of red irritated eyes and sneezing. If the sufferer shows signs of breathing difficulty or impaired consciousness, assume that the reaction is severe and call for immediate medical help.

Common allergens causing mild reactions include insects bites or stings, long grass, flowers and long-haired animals.

1 *Offer reassurance and find out if the person has a history of allergic reaction.*

2 *Apply a cold compress or calamine lotion to any rash or itchy skin.*

3 *Try to identify the source of the allergy so that it can be avoided. Reactions can become more extreme if the person is exposed to the same allergen in the future.*

4 *Seek medical advice because tests may be needed to identify the allergen.*

Apply a cold compress to relieve itching

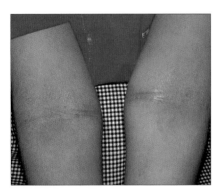

ABOVE *Skin rashes that occur as a result of allergic reaction are often intensely itchy. Calamine lotion and oral antihistamines may help to relieve symptoms.*

Using an auto-injector

If you have been trained to do so, you may help somebody administer her own medicine. Ensure that the medicine belongs to the casualty. Help her to expose an area of skin and to take the lid off the injector. Place the injector on the skin and help the casualty push to administer the medication into the body.

Allergic rhinitis, hay fever and urticaria

If a person experiences an allergic reaction after inhaling a specific airborne substance, the membrane lining the nose, throat and sinuses becomes inflamed, a condition termed allergic rhinitis. This increases mucus production and causes sinus congestion. Symptoms may include blocked or runny nose, itchy, red, watery eyes, sneezing, drowsiness and a sore throat. Depending on the allergen, symptoms may be experienced year-round or seasonally, when the disorder is known as hay fever. Urticaria, also known as nettle rash or hives, is an intensely itchy rash that usually occurs as the result of an allergic reaction. The rash consists of white lumps and red, inflamed areas that may affect the whole body, and usually clears up after a few hours. Treatment for all these conditions depends on the use of antihistamines and avoiding the allergen when possible.

MISCARRIAGE

A miscarriage is the loss of a pregnancy in the first 24 weeks. There are many causes of miscarriage, and for some parents the reason for their loss will never be known. About a fifth of all pregnancies end in miscarriage, most of these before the twelfth week. For further information on miscarriage and emergency problems in pregnancy, see pages 272–273.

Other emergency problems with pregnancy

Ectopic pregnancy

In this circumstance, the fertilised egg has become embedded in the Fallopian tube rather than the womb. As well as ending the pregnancy, this is a potentially life-threatening condition for the mother. The woman will usually have severe pain in the abdominal area, with potential bleeding and signs of shock. Call an ambulance immediately.

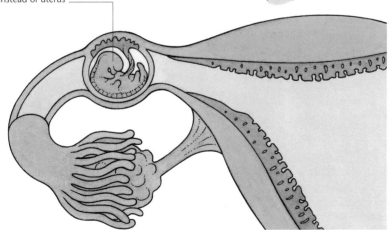

Embryo develops in Fallopian tube instead of uterus

Placenta praevia/placental abruption

A bleed in later pregnancy is more unusual. A painless bright red bleed may be an indicator that something is seriously wrong with the placenta, causing potential life-threatening problems for both the mother and child. Support the mother in a position of rest, call an ambulance and treat for shock (see pages 44–45).

Signs and symptoms

- *Bleeding – this may be light spotting over a number of days and/or a sudden heavy bleed*
- *Period-like pain or pain in the lower back*
- *Potential signs and symptoms of shock, caused by blood loss (see pages 44–45)*
- *Passing the foetus and other products associated with birth (this may just look like a heavy blood clot)*

Many miscarriages can take several days from start to finish and may not start with a heavy bleed or severe pain. Some women who are miscarrying may not have realised that they were pregnant as many miscarriages take place in the first weeks after conception.

Pregnant woman suffering a bleed should always seek early medical advice from their doctor or midwife. An investigation may show that the pregnancy has not ended or that miscarriage is threatened but not inevitable.

TREATMENT

1 Overall, listen to the wants and needs of the woman. She will often be very distressed and scared. Where possible, help her to a position of privacy and if possible, ensure that she is treated by another woman and has support from her partner or friend.

2 If bleeding or pain is severe, or there are signs of shock, call an ambulance.

3 Reassure the woman and offer her a sanitary pad or towel.

4 Keep anything that is passed from the vagina, out of sight of the woman, for medical staff to examine.

Listen to the woman and give reassurance and support

LEFT A woman who has had a miscarriage needs to be treated sensitively. Reassure her and monitor for signs of shock while waiting for an ambulance to arrive.

Support groups

Most women who have a miscarriage do not have problems with subsequent pregnancies but a woman should take time to grieve and talk about her feelings before becoming pregnant again. Group therapy with others who have had the same experience is a good way of helping a woman come to terms with the loss of her baby. The woman's doctor should be able to provide details of appropriate support groups in her area.

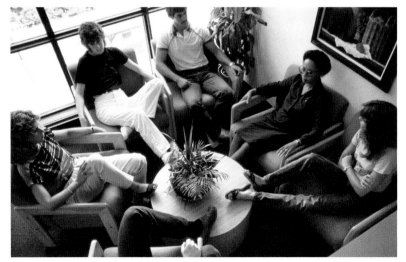

LABOUR

It is important to remember that labour is a natural process and that the emergency first aid role is usually limited to ensuring that the midwife has been called or that the mother is transported safely to the planned place of birth.

Labour is conventionally divided into three separate stages. Although no two labours will be the same, in most cases, labour will progress smoothly. During the first stage, the cervix dilates to allow the baby to pass through. In the second stage, the baby is born. In the third stage, the placenta is delivered.

Labour is generally a long process, with first births particularly taking many hours and even days. However, for some women, particularly those with previous children, labour can be relatively fast. Others may not realise that they are in labour, or even pregnant until the baby is showing (crowning.) In these situations, your role is to seek medical help and to support the natural process until this arrives. For more information on labour and childbirth, see pages 274–275.

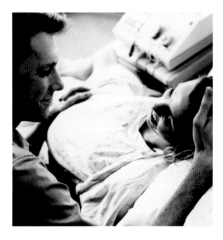

RIGHT *Labour is the culmination of pregnancy, and the help and support of a partner throughout can be invaluable in making it a smoother, more enjoyable experience.*

SIGNS AND SYMPTOMS OF STAGES OF LABOUR

Stage 1

The cervix (entrance to the uterus) gets bigger to allow the baby's head to emerge. This can take many hours or even days. The waters around the baby may break and the plug protecting the uterus from infection may come away. Potential healthy signs and symptoms of the first stage of labour include:

• *Contractions become more painful and more frequent.*
• *Blood-stained discharge (but not bleeding – call an ambulance if there are signs of a heavy bleed).*
• *Waters breaking – this may be a trickle or a rush, or the waters may not break at all. Do not attempt to break them manually.*

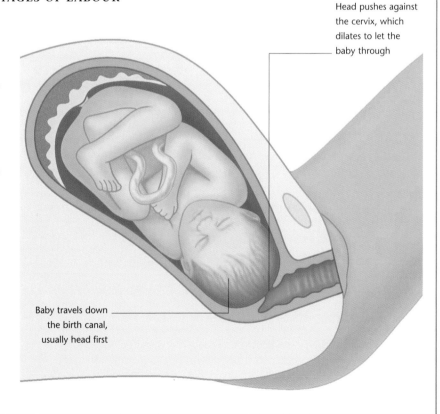

Head pushes against the cervix, which dilates to let the baby through

Baby travels down the birth canal, usually head first

Stage 2

When the neck of the uterus (womb) is as wide as it needs to be, the baby is forced out from the uterus. The vagina stretches to allow the baby to move out from the mother. The mother may feel an urge to push, which may also feel like the need to pass a stool. The vagina may feel painful as it is stretched. The baby's head emerges and is pushed out by ever more frequent and intense contractions.

Make sure the cord is not around the baby's neck. If it is, ask the mother to pant (which will help reduce the urge to push) and try to loosen the cord from around the baby's neck.

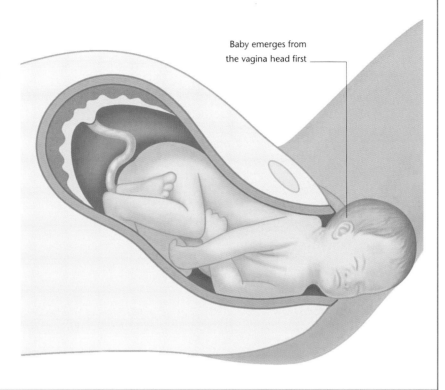

Baby emerges from the vagina head first

Stage 3

During the third stage of labour, the placenta and cord are expelled and the uterus contracts to stop bleeding. There are some mild contractions and bleeding while the placenta and cord are delivered. If there is more severe bleeding, call an ambulance immediately.

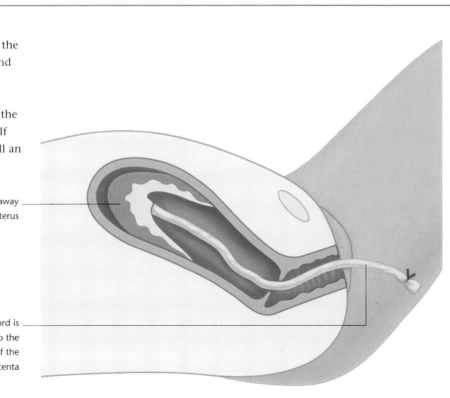

Placenta peels away from wall of uterus

Umbilical cord is attached to the centre of the placenta

EMERGENCY CHILDBIRTH

It is very unlikely that you will have to deliver a child in an unplanned-for situation. Even the second stage of labour can allow enough time for an ambulance or midwife to arrive. However, if you are called upon to help with an emergency birth, take comfort from the fact that there is little that you can do to affect the birth process. Your key role is to support the mother, to ensure that medical help has been called and to care for mother and baby after the birth.

WHAT CAN YOU DO TO HELP?

1 *Ensure that the midwife or doctor has been called. If labour is in the early stages, ask the mother where she wants to be and make arrangements for transport.*

2 *If at any time there is severe bleeding or signs and symptoms of shock (see pages 44–45), call an ambulance.*

3 *Support the mother in her most comfortable position. This will usually be standing or squatting as gravity helps the delivery process. Ask her what she would like you to do to help with the pain. Potential options include a warm bath, rubbing the small of her back and frequent sips of water. Encourage her to breathe out as breath-holding makes pain worse by increasing muscle tension. Most pregnant women will have a pregnancy record. Help her to find this as it contains useful information for both you and the medical staff.*

4 *If labour has progressed to the second stage and birth is imminent, ensure that:*

- *The woman has removed the clothes from her lower body.*
- *The ambulance is on the way – the ambulance control or midwife may give you instructions over the phone.*
- *You and the environment are as clean as they can be.*
- *You have a warm covering for the baby and mother.*

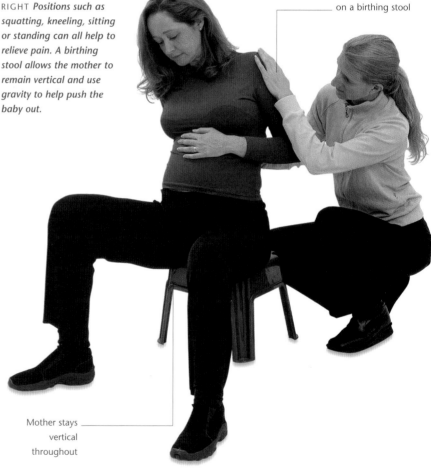

RIGHT *Positions such as squatting, kneeling, sitting or standing can all help to relieve pain. A birthing stool allows the mother to remain vertical and use gravity to help push the baby out.*

Supporting woman on a birthing stool

Mother stays vertical throughout

5 *Help the mother into a position she finds comfortable.*

6 *Support the mother while she pushes out the baby as it descends.*

7 *Support the head and shoulders as the baby appears – this will happen naturally and quickly. Do not pull the baby. If the cord is wrapped around the neck, check that it is loose and gently pull it over the head.*

8 Gently lift the baby and place on the mother's stomach. There is no need to cut the cord. If the baby does not show any signs of movement, check its airway and breathing (see page 17) and be prepared to resuscitate (see pages 32–33) if necessary.

9 Keep mother and baby warm while waiting for the ambulance. The placenta and cord will follow shortly – keep these for the medical staff to check. Gently massaging below the belly button may help stop bleeding.

Wiping the mother's face during labour can be very soothing

Signs that the birth may be imminent

• Contractions less than 2 minutes apart

• Strong urge to push

• Bulging vaginal opening

• Baby's head visible

If the urge to bear down comes on the way to hospital, the mother can try using breathing techniques to avoid pushing.

If the baby is breech (not head first)

The concern with a breech birth is that the largest part of the baby (the head) may not be easily delivered. If the baby is breech a foot, knee or buttock may come out first. If this happens:

1. Ensure that medical help has been called.

2. Allow the birth to continue – do not try to stop the baby coming out.

3. Support the baby's body as it is delivered.

4. If the head is not delivered within 3 minutes of the shoulders, gently raise the baby's legs to the ceiling until you can see the face (do not pull the baby from the mother). Wipe the face clear and encourage the mother to keep pushing until the head is delivered.

WHAT TO DO IF YOU ARE A LONG WAY FROM HELP

Undertaking any journey into wilderness requires careful preparation. When planning a trip you need to take many factors into account, including what you would do in the case of an accident or illness. Most treatments remain exactly the same for wilderness conditions.

PLANNING A JOURNEY

The following are some of the things that you may like to consider when planning your journey as well as some questions that you may like to ask yourself. Take a mobile phone but be aware that network coverage may be poor or non-existent in the area you are visiting.

Location Is the area that you are visiting suitable for all the abilities in your family or group? An area with a reputation for beauty will not necessarily be safe.

Fitness Is everyone in your group fit enough to undertake the trip, or is anyone suffering from any injuries or illnesses? If so, has the person got enough medication?

The right clothes Having the right clothes for the environment that you will be visiting could mean the difference between life and death. Having an outer layer that is windproof, keeps water out, keeps the heat in and allows sweat to evaporate will help the other layers stay dry and function correctly. The next layers should consist of a fleece-type jumper or jacket. A shirt and underwear made of polypropylene will draw moisture away from the skin. Today's modern clothing is designed to be functional even when wet and will dry out surprisingly quickly.

Footwear Choose footwear that supports your ankle, is waterproofed and is comfortable and well worn in. This will help prevent sprains, broken bones and blistering.

Equipment Carry first aid and survival equipment suitable for your route (see *Wilderness First Aid Box*, pages 180–181).

Planning your route Ensure that the route is realistically within the ability of your family or group and achievable in the amount of time available. Always tell someone who is not going with you what your route is, who is going, what time you are starting and what time you will be finishing.

IF FACED WITH A PROBLEM A LONG WAY FROM HELP

If faced with an accident or illness a long way from help, your priorities are:

- *To secure the safety of the whole group.*
- *To treat the injury or illness.*
- *To obtain help.*
- *To seek appropriate shelter.*

Careful preparation is essential.

The biggest decision you will probably have to make relates to obtaining help. If you have not got a mobile phone, or you cannot get a signal, you will have to make alternative arrangements.

If one member of the group is unable to continue, a decision will have to be made to split the group or wait for help as a whole. The decision will depend on a number of factors:

- *Popularity of the route and therefore likelihood of passers-by.*
- *Access to shelter.*
- *Nature of the injury or illness and the speed at which help is required.*
- *Skills of group members in survival and navigation.*
- *Weather conditions.*
- *Time of day.*

If sending people for help, make sure that your equipment is divided appropriately. Ensure that those leaving have good directions and navigation aids and those remaining have sound shelter. If the weather is poor or it is dark, consider waiting until conditions improve. Instead, seek shelter.

Carrying an injured or ill person for help should usually be a last resort as it poses risks to both the person being carried and those lifting and moving him. There is a number of ways in which a stretcher can be improvised.

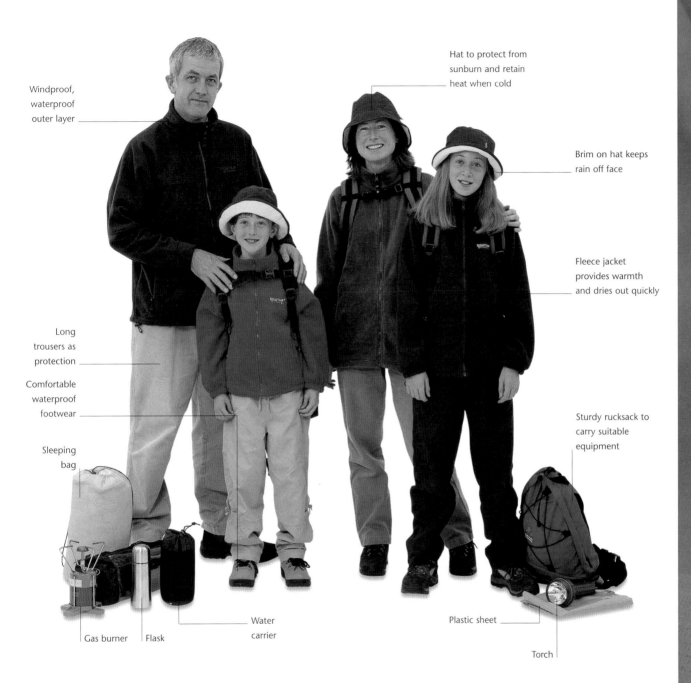

Windproof, waterproof outer layer

Hat to protect from sunburn and retain heat when cold

Brim on hat keeps rain off face

Fleece jacket provides warmth and dries out quickly

Long trousers as protection

Comfortable waterproof footwear

Sturdy rucksack to carry suitable equipment

Sleeping bag

Gas burner   Flask

Water carrier

Plastic sheet

Torch

DIFFERENCES IN TREATMENT

As you are likely to be in wilderness conditions for some time, the following factors should be considered:

● *Maintaining warmth when treating shock (see pages 44–45) or conditions such as hypothermia (see pages 112–113) may require the creation of shelter. Focus on putting blankets or survival bags under the injured person and covering the head, hands and feet as well as putting a blanket over him.*

● *Consider shelter from the sun and the heat and make sure that everyone in the party drinks enough liquid, including the injured person (providing that he is fully conscious).*

● *Be aware that altitude sickness may develop if you are high in the mountains, because of reduced levels of oxygen in the air. Symptoms include tiredness, headache, unsteadiness and nausea.*

● *Broken bones, burns and bleeds swell. Continually recheck bandaging to ensure that it is not cutting off circulation. Loosen and re-tie as necessary.*

● *Consider providing extra bandaging support to broken bones – particularly if the injured person needs to be moved.*

WILDERNESS FIRST AID

Should there be an accident, or a member of your group is taken ill, you have two choices: you either send someone for help or you wait for help to arrive. The decision you make will depend on the weather conditions, the ability to navigate, how far it is to get help and what kind of terrain you will have to cover. Only in the most extreme circumstances should a casualty be left alone, and you should leave the person spare clothing and food. The casualty will also require a whistle and/or torch in order to alert the rescue services. Finally, the person should be told to stay where he is and not move.

GETTING HELP

Whoever goes for help should carry with them enough spare clothing and equipment to deal with any situation that may be faced. The person should also take the following information:

- *The exact location of the injured person or group (this is best done using a six-figure grid reference).*
- *What has happened.*
- *When it occurred.*
- *What injuries or condition they have.*
- *A description of where they are.*
- *Who else is with them.*

Six whistle blasts are a recognised signal for help

Leave a torch with the casualty so he can signal for help

ATTRACTING HELP

There are internationally recognised signals that can be used while out in the wilderness that are easily remembered and require no specialist equipment. Although shouting for help may attract attention, after a while you will become hoarse and tired. Voices do not carry as well as other sounds such as whistle blasts, which can be heard over surprisingly large distances. At night, light can also travel much further than voices and during the day a reflective object such as a mirror can send the rays of the sun a considerable distance.

There are two international signals for help. The first is SOS, which represents the phrase Save Our Souls. Although Morse code is no longer used in everyday life, it is still practiced to summon help in emergency situations. For an audible signal on a whistle, give three short blasts (S) three long blasts (O) and three short blasts (S). With a light signal, give three short flashes (S) three long flashes (O) and three short flashes (S). Alternatively, six blasts of a whistle or six flashes of light in quick succession also mean that help is needed. A red flare also acts as an emergency distress call on water and in the mountains.

RIGHT *You can attract attention by using a torch at night to give three short, three long and three short flashes, an internationally recognised signal for help.*

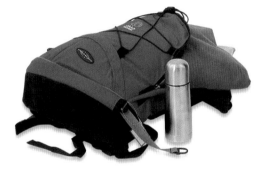

Use a torch to flash an SOS signal to attract help

Communicating with the rescue teams

You may find that you can hear instructions given by a mountain rescue team or similar through a loudhailer from a helicopter but are unable to shout back to them.

There are three ways in which you can communicate that you understood their message:

• *Give three blasts on a whistle in quick succession, repeated after a 1-minute interval.*
• *Give three flashes of the torch in quick succession, repeated after a 1-minute interval*
• *Send up a white flare.*

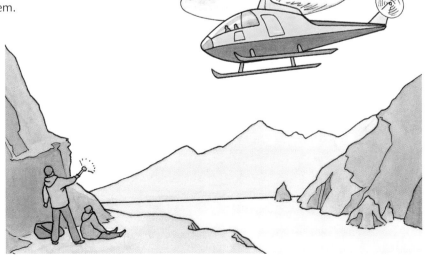

MORE ON BITES AND STINGS

The general guidance for dealing with bites and stings is: to monitor airway and breathing (see pages 16–19); be prepared to resuscitate (see pages 30–33) if necessary; to support and reassure the injured person; to offer relief with a cold compress; and to avoid infection by cleaning and covering the wound. In addition, there are some specific treatments that may be useful for certain types of bites and stings. For more information on bites and stings, see pages 132–33.

Ticks

Ticks are tiny bloodsucking creatures found in long grass that attach themselves to animals and humans firmly by embedding their mouthparts into the skin. Ticks cause discomfort and can transmit disease. Although simple to remove, great care should be taken as the mouthparts could remain in the skin if removed incorrectly. Use a flat-ended pair of tweezers or gloved fingers and grasp the tick at its head end, as close to the skin as possible. Using even pressure, pull the tick straight up, avoiding twisting and squeezing the tick's body. Once it has been removed, clean and cover the bitten area.

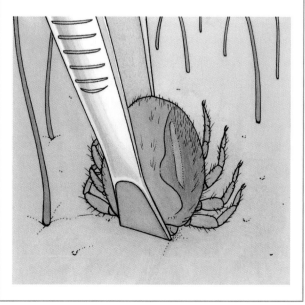

Mosquitoes

Mosquitoes are found all over the UK and are small airborne insects. They feed on animals, including humans, by injecting a minute amount of anaesthetic and a chemical that stops blood from clotting and then sucking blood from their host until they are full. Unfortunately this can leave a small inflamed area that is uncomfortable but not life-threatening. This can be easily treated by a cold compress.

In many countries mosquitoes carry malaria, which can be fatal. Should you visit countries that have malarial areas, you must seek advice from your doctor on how to protect yourself and which antimalarial drugs are best suited to you.

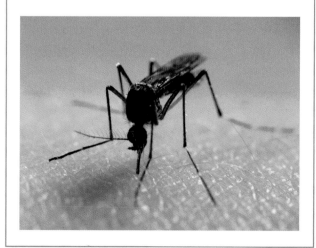

Jellyfish

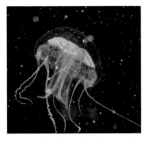

There are very few species of jellyfish that are poisonous in the waters around the UK. However, there are plenty overseas, and some do find their way to our coastal waters. Generally those that are poisonous have long tentacles that sway freely beneath their bodies and contain stingers that inject chemicals into anyone that should come too close. Although not normally fatal, they can cause extreme pain that leads to panic, especially in children,which can lead to further danger in the water.

These stings can be treated by calming the casualty and then applying alcohol or vinegar to the affected area for a minimum of 3 minutes or until the pain subsides.

Should the victim suffer a severe allergic reaction (see pages 144–145), emergency medical aid should be sought.

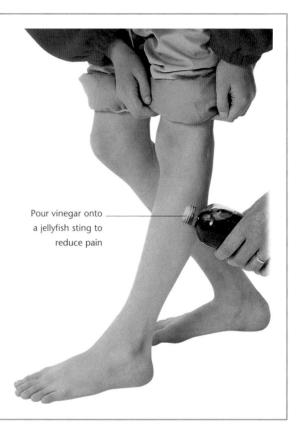

Pour vinegar onto a jellyfish sting to reduce pain

Weaver fish

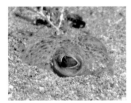

Weaver fish are found all around the UK but are particularly prevalent in some areas of the south coast. They are small fish that bury themselves at the very top of the sand, usually in shallows where they hunt. They have sharp spines on their dorsal fin that can inject poison into anyone who steps on them.

Although the pain is extreme, it can be quickly relieved by placing the affected area in a bowl of water as hot as the sufferer can stand for 20 minutes or until the pain subsides. Make sure you test the hot water with your elbow first because otherwise you may scald the skin.

If the casualty suffers a severe reaction, emergency medical aid should be sought.

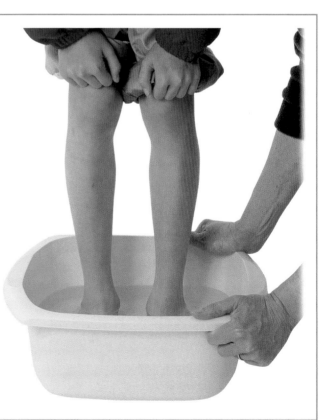

AVALANCHE AND SNOW SURVIVAL TECHNIQUES

Over the years, remote and faraway places have become more accessible and, although as much care as possible is taken whenever there is snow on a mountain or slope, an avalanche is always possible. Find out the local emergency signals for 'avalanche warning' and 'avalanche imminent' and heed them. Many avalanches are caused by a skier going off-piste or ignoring local warnings. Make sure that you are wearing appropriate clothing for the mountain and that you have at least a whistle as a rescue aid. Leave details of your route with a local contact.

SURVIVING AN AVALANCHE
If caught in an avalanche, try to hold on to an immovable object for as long as you can as the more snow that passes you, the less likely you are to be buried when it comes to a halt.

If at all possible, try to work your way to the side of the flow by using a swimming or rolling motion, keep your mouth shut and try to cover your mouth and nose with the top of your jumper, sweater or anorak while continuing the swimming motion.

When you come to a stop, create yourself an air space by folding your arms in front of your face and chest while the snow comes to a halt. Orientate yourself by spitting and feeling which way it falls. Try to move one hand upwards and if you feel air, and you are able to, dig your way out. Otherwise, save both your air and your energy until help arrives.

There are various avalanche beacons. These are small, portable transceivers, which are a worthwhile investment for those regularly in the mountains.

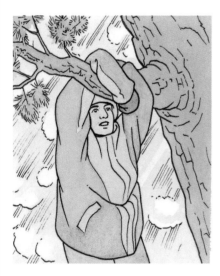

ABOVE *Holding on to an immovable object such as a tree when caught in an avalanche will increase your chances of survival because you are less likely to be buried by snow.*

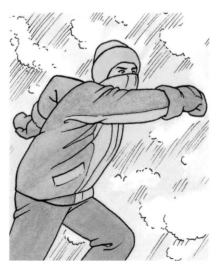

ABOVE *Use a swimming or rolling motion to try to work your way to the side of the snow fall. Try to cover your mouth and nose with your jacket, scarf or jumper.*

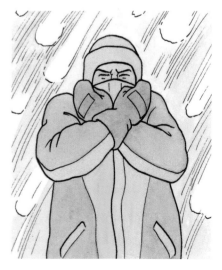

ABOVE *Make an air space for yourself by folding your arms in front of your face and chest. Move one hand upwards and try to dig your way out if you can feel air.*

HYPOTHERMIA

Hypothermia is the lowering of the body's core temperature to 35°C (95°F) or below. The best treatment for hypothermia is prevention. As the body's temperature drops there may be signs and symptoms that, if recognised early enough, can prevent an easily treatable condition becoming fatal. In the outdoors it is important to watch out for these signs in the group that you are with and to take early action to prevent deterioration. For more information on hypothermia, see pages 112–13.

TREATMENT

Once recognised, the treatment for hypothermia is to rewarm the casualty to the body's natural temperature. However, this needs to be done with care as rough handling could lead to a heart attack in some people.

1 *Try to provide a warm, dry environment. Lay the person at risk down, ensuring that he is insulated from the ground, and gently remove any wet items of clothing, replacing them with dry ones as you go. As we lose almost a third of our body heat through our heads, this should be covered as quickly as possible. If the person is able, sips of a warm drink may be taken, although this should not be relied upon and other warming techniques will need to be employed.*

Signs and symptoms of descent into hypothermia

Core body temperature	Sign/symptom
36°C (96.8°F)	*Sensation of cold, stumbling, personality changes, mild confusion*
35°C (95°F)	*Slurred speech, poor coordination, no memory of events (on recovery)*
33°C (91.4°F)	*Shivering disappears and is replaced by stiff muscles*
31°C (87.8°F)	*Pupils become dilated, loss of consciousness*
30°C (86°F)	*Unconsciousness*
29°C (84.2°F)	*Muscle stiffness disappears*
23°C (73.4°F)	*Breathing stops*
18°C (64.4°F)	*Death*

2 *Try to get the casualty into a sleeping or survival bag and cuddle up close, reassuring him all the time. Closely monitor the casualty's progress by continuing to talk to him, noting down any changes in the level of consciousness (see pages 54–55).*

3 *Although space blankets or silver foil blankets are useful when used with other equipment, they work by reflecting the person's own body heat. If the casualty is cold, they will reflect the cold, making the situation worse. They should therefore never be relied upon on their own.*

4 *If you have a tent or survival shelter available, set this up and get inside as soon as possible. Take care to ensure that other members of your group do not succumb to the cold.*

Use your own body to keep the casualty warm

Get the casualty into a survival bag to keep warm

COLD WATER SURVIVAL TECHNIQUES

Today there are many different pursuits that can be undertaken on water, often by people with limited experience. Under appropriate supervision most water sports are perfectly safe, although the combination of weather, unpredictable water and inexperience can lead to difficulties. The biggest danger from the water is drowning. There are simple measures that can help prevent this situation, such as wearing a personal flotation device or having rescue equipment to hand.

PREPARING FOR ACTIVITY WHERE IMMERSION IN COLD WATER IS A POSSIBILITY

On average, the temperature of the sea around the UK is about 15°C (59°F), making it some 22 degrees cooler than our bodies (body temperature is 37°C/98.6°F). Water conducts heat approximately 25 times faster than air, meaning that heat will be lost rapidly from the body. Hypothermia is therefore a big risk following immersion in cold water, particularly if you are not wearing appropriate clothing. If you know that there is a risk that you will be immersed in water for some time, always wear proper protective clothing such as nylon underwear, a thick layer of fleece, a dry suit and a head covering.

Always undertake water sports under appropriate supervision and consider the many sources of information about the conditions of the water that you are visiting, such as the coastguard, beach offices, sailing and diving clubs and local water-sports shops.

In the water alone
Should an accident occur, and you find yourself in a situation where you may be in water for some time, there are some simple but effective ways of staying as warm as possible.

Cover your head with a hat or hood – remember that one-third of your body heat is lost through your head.

Blasts on a whistle, or the release of flares, will alert others to your situation.

Inflate your personal flotation device, if you have one.

Bring your knees up to your chest and wrap your arms around them, making yourself into a ball. This exposes less skin area to the water, which slows down the cooling process and buys you valuable time.

In the water as a group

If there is more than one person in the water then there are additional steps.

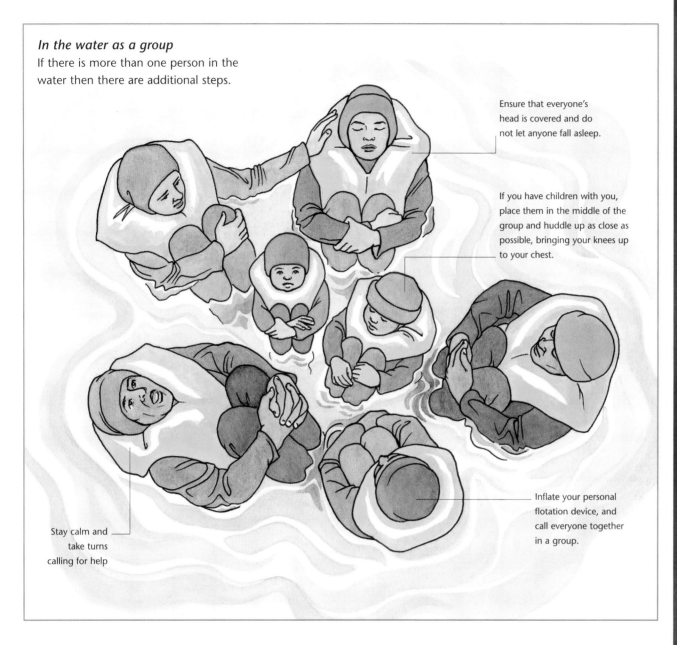

Ensure that everyone's head is covered and do not let anyone fall asleep.

If you have children with you, place them in the middle of the group and huddle up as close as possible, bringing your knees up to your chest.

Inflate your personal flotation device, and call everyone together in a group.

Stay calm and take turns calling for help

Cold shock

Falling into cold water can almost literally take your breath away. This is known as cold shock. The body's response to this sudden immersion in cold water causes the breathing and heart rate to soar. Although this is normally not a problem, when the water is less than 15°C (59°F), sudden immersion can cause the heart to beat at rates of 150–180 beats per minute and the breathing rate to rise to 60–90 breaths per minute.

This may completely incapacitate a young fit person, and in a less fit or older person cause heart attack or stroke.

When safely out of the water, treat the victim for hypothermia (see pages 112–13) and call for emergency help. Monitor and maintain the airway (see pages 16–19) and be prepared to resuscitate (see pages 30–33) if necessary.

STRETCHER IMPROVISATION

In certain extreme circumstances it may be necessary to transport a person who is sick or injured to a place of safety, or to move from somewhere such as a windy river back into shelter when the casualty is only able to offer you limited or no help. This should not be undertaken lightly as there is great risk of injury to both yourself and the person being carried. Should you find yourself in such a situation, there is a number of techniques whereby a stretcher can be quickly improvised.

METHOD 1: BRANCH AND CLOTHING

1 *Select two strong branches that will extend by about 30 cm either end of the person to be carried. Ensure that the branch is tested for rot and that any sharp parts are cut away. It is also worth checking for moss at each end as this will make any grip slippery. Although the branches do not have to be exactly the same size, it will obviously help if they are roughly the same length. It is vital that they are capable of holding the weight of your casualty.*

2 *Now select some clothing that is strong as this will bear the weight of the casualty. Items such as jumpers and good quality cotton T-shirts are ideal. You should not forget yourself – do not give away clothing that may mean you are at risk from the weather.*

3 *Slide the clothing on to the poles with the poles coming through the arms of the garment. Place the next piece of clothing on to the poles in the same way and overlap the first item. Place enough pieces of clothing on to the poles to ensure that the casualty's head and legs will be supported.*

You could also use this kind of system using a large plastic survival bag instead of clothing. These can be bought relatively cheaply from most camping and outdoor shops.

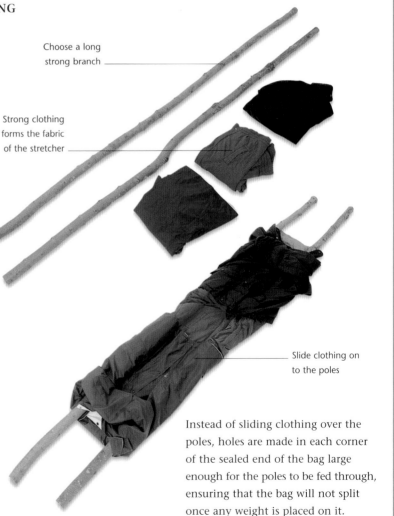

Choose a long strong branch

Strong clothing forms the fabric of the stretcher

Slide clothing on to the poles

Instead of sliding clothing over the poles, holes are made in each corner of the sealed end of the bag large enough for the poles to be fed through, ensuring that the bag will not split once any weight is placed on it.

METHOD 2: CARRYING A SURVIVAL BAG

1 It is possible to use the survival bag as a stretcher without damaging it. Lay the bag out and, depending on how many people you have to help with the carry, collect stones large enough for each person to grip. Next, using string or rope, tie the stones at each corner of the bag and at each side in the middle. If stones are not available, items of clothing such as hats, socks or gloves can be used in their place.

2 There are definite limitations to this kind of stretcher. The polythene is relatively easy to split, especially on rough ground and when wet can be extremely slippery. Therefore care should be taken when picking the stretcher up and you should always take things slowly.

3 If you do not have a survival bag handy, then the flysheet of a tent will do instead. However, bear in mind that rocks and stones may damage the fabric.

Lay the survival bag flat on the ground to use as a stretcher

Find several stones large enough to be gripped

Wrap the ends of the survival bag around the stones to form handholds.

LOADING AND CARRYING A STRETCHER

Consider carefully whether the benefits of moving somebody will outweigh the risks. If you are able to seek appropriate shelter and send or call for help, it is generally considered safer to stay where you are, particularly at night or if the weather is bad. Alongside the danger of getting lost or falling, carrying a stretcher comes with the risk of damaging the backs of those carrying it.

PREPARATION FOR LOADING AND CARRYING

Consider the following:

- *Have you got enough people to lift the casualty safely on to the stretcher?*
- *What are the conditions of the ground underneath your feet? Are you liable to slip or sink or is it on a steep slope? Will the ground move?*
- *Does everyone involved understand what you are doing and how you are planning to do it?*
- *Do you or anyone else in your party have any injuries or conditions that could be greatly worsened by the lift?*
- *Are there any other factors that may hinder or prevent you from safely carrying out the lift?*

Try to eliminate or reduce any of the conditions that the answers to these questions identify as a risk. If in doubt, do not attempt to lift the stretcher and seek shelter while awaiting help.

GETTING A PERSON ON TO THE STRETCHER

It may be possible for you to lift the person directly on to the stretcher. Ideally this should be done with a minimum of two people. Bring the stretcher to the casualty and lay it down as close as you can without it being in your way. Decide who will take the top half and who will take the bottom half of the person to be lifted.

1 *Sit the person up and ask her to cross or fold her arms across her chest.*

2 *Squatting behind the casualty, slide your hands under her arms, taking hold of her wrists or lower arms.*

3 *Ask your partner to squat beside the casualty and pass their arms under her thighs, taking hold of the legs.*

4 *The person at the head end takes control and will determine the timing of the lift. When ready, working together and keeping your backs straight, rise slowly and move the casualty on to the stretcher.*

SURVIVAL BAG/FLYSHEET TECHNIQUE

If you are using the survival
bag/flysheet technique, it will be
easier to put the stretcher underneath
the casualty before you add either the
poles or stones. The easiest way
for this to be done is to use one of
two methods:

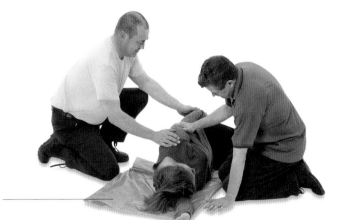

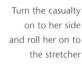
Turn the casualty
on to her side
and roll her on to
the stretcher

Method 1
*Lay the bag/flysheet next to the casualty and
gather up approximately half of the fabric on
the side closest to her placing it as close as
you can to body. Turn the casualty on to her
side and place the bundle as close as you can
to her body and gently roll her back. Now pull
the remainder of the bag/sheet out from the
sides. You are then ready to add the poles or
stones.*

Method 2
*Concertina-fold the top and bottom ends of
the bag towards the centre with one person
on each side of the casualty, placing the
folded bag/sheet under the hollow in the small
of her back (if you need more room you can
gently lift her hips). Together, pull the bottom
part down towards the casualty's feet and
then the other half of the bag/sheet can be
pulled up towards her head. You can then add
the poles or stones.*

Fold both ends of
the bag and unfurl
when the casualty is
placed on top

Keep your back straight
when lifting a stretcher

LIFTING
The following principles will reduce
your risk of injury when performing
any lift or moving and handling.

1 *Stand with your feet shoulder-width apart,
with one foot slightly in front of the other.*

2 *Bend at your hips and your knees,
not at your back. Keep your back
straight but not rigid.*

3 *Get a secure grip of the
casualty. Raise your head.*

4 *Use your strongest muscles
(in your thighs) to lift,
keeping your elbows close
to your body.*

One person should take
the lead at all times –
usually the person guiding
the head. Take regular
breaks as needed and
move slowly and carefully.

ONE- AND TWO- PERSON CARRIES

If moving an injured or ill person is absolutely necessary, encouraging him to move by himself is by far the best approach, minimising risk to both you and him. However this is not always possible. There is a number of dangers inherent in lifting and moving people and it should not be undertaken lightly. The following techniques require no real equipment and in an emergency situation can be very effective.

ONE-PERSON CARRIES

The human crutch

If you find yourself in a situation where the injured person has, for instance, sprained an ankle and is having difficulty in walking, this technique will provide additional support if nothing else, such as a walking stick or crutch, is available.

1 *Stand on the person's injured or affected side, pass her arm around your neck and grasp her hand or wrist.*

2 *Place your other arm around her waist and grasp her clothes, preferably the top of the trousers or a belt.*

3 *Move off with your inside foot first, walking at the casualty's pace.*

The drag

This technique is really for extreme emergencies and will be effective only over short distances as it is very labour-intensive. Its key use is in moving people from very hazardous areas quickly.

1 *Crouch behind the casualty. Carefully pull him towards you. Stop, take a step back and pull the casualty towards you again.*

2 *Repeat this procedure until you have reached your destination.*

Human crutch

Piggy back

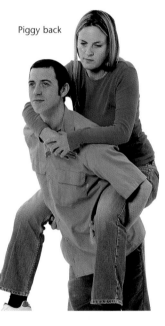

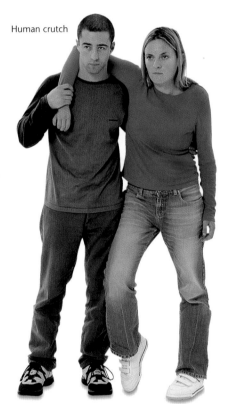

Drag

Piggy back

Although this is an effective carry, how far you will be physically capable of moving the casualty will depend on her size and weight. It also reduces your ability to carry your own equipment, particularly if you are hiking with rucksacks.

1 *Crouch in front of the casualty with your back towards her and ask her to put her arms over your shoulders.*

2 *Grasp the casualty's thighs, pull them in towards you and slowly stand up, remembering to keep your back straight.*

TWO-PERSON CARRIES

It is far easier for two people to control and move someone. However, these techniques do have their limitations, even with two people, and require a little practice.

Two-handed seat carry

1 *Crouch down, facing each other on either side of the injured person.*

2 *Cross over your arms behind the casualty and grab hold of her waistband or belt.*

3 *Pass your other hands under the casualty's knees and grasp each other's wrists.*

4 *Bring your hands towards the middle of the casualty's thighs.*

5 *Get in close to the injured person and stand up slowly; you are now ready to move off.*

Cross arms and grab waistband

Pass other hands under knees and grasp wrists

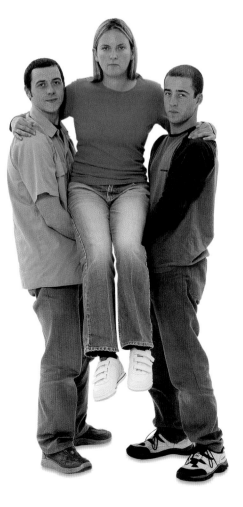

Four-handed seat carry

The two-handed and, in particular, the four-handed seat carries can only be used with conscious people as they require the person being carried to have some control over her body and give some assistance to the rescuers.

1 *With the person to be carried standing close to you, first hold your left wrist with your right hand, and ask your carrying partner to do the same.*

2 *Now link hands, taking hold of your partner's right wrist. This should form a square.*

3 *Allow the casualty to gently sit back on to your hands and get her to place her hands around your shoulders.*

It should be noted that this is extremely strenuous and awkward for the rescuers.

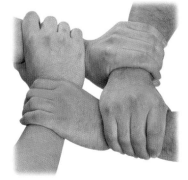

HELICOPTER RESCUE

Helicopters have saved many lives since their introduction as a rescue tool. As well as being used to evacuate people from ships and mountains and rescue people from the sea, they are being utilised by numerous ambulance services all over the UK to transport seriously ill or injured people to hospital. Although they are an effective life-saving tool, they can also be extremely dangerous if safety precautions are not followed. Should you find yourself in a situation where you or a member of your group is to be rescued by helicopter, the following simple precautions should be taken.

1 *The pilot will select the best area for the helicopter to land but if there is an obvious clear area that you believe they may wish to use, try to clear it of any obstructions such as loose debris. Assemble everybody to the windward of the landing site, as the helicopter will approach into the wind. You must be at least 50 metres (165 ft) away from the landing point.*

2 *If it is not obvious where you are, wave some bright clothing or shine a torch so that the pilot and crew can see you. While the helicopter lands, stay still, holding on to any loose items of clothing or baggage. If you are on the beach you may find it more comfortable to cover your face because of the downdraft caused by the aircraft, which will stir up the sand.*

3 *Once the helicopter has landed, under no circumstances approach it until you are signalled to do so by the pilot. When you are told to move towards the aircraft, approach in the direction that is indicated by the pilot. This will normally be from the front and to the pilot's right-hand side. This is so that you remain in the pilot's sight at all times. Follow any instructions you are given by the crew exactly.*

RIGHT *Gather together everyone who is to be rescued and assemble windward of the landing site because the helicopter will approach into the wind.*

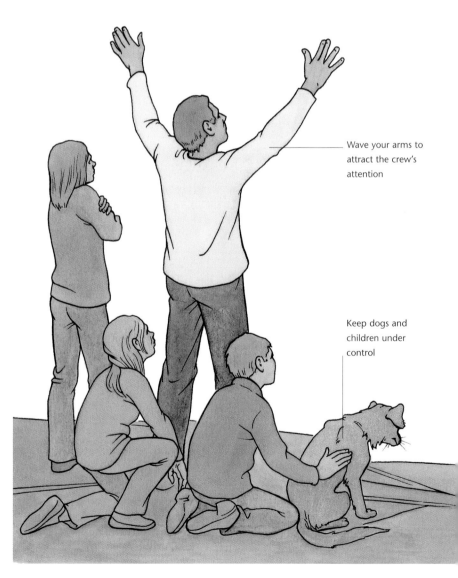

Wave your arms to attract the crew's attention

Keep dogs and children under control

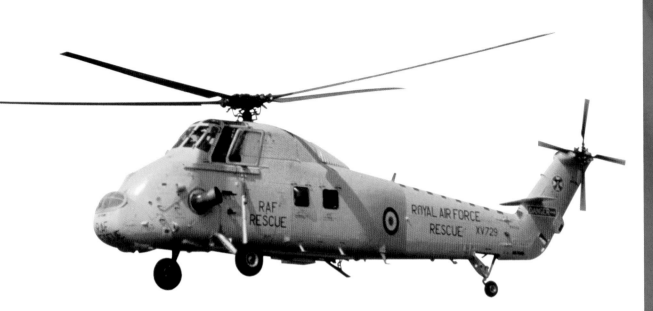

LEFT *Sometimes a person will need to be winched to safety but care must be taken not to touch the winch lines because they carry an electrical charge and could deliver a shock.*

ABOVE *A helicopter will be used in an emergency such as evacuating people from ships and mountains, and to take people in remote areas to hospital.*

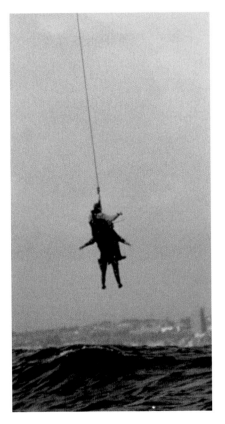

RESCUE BY WINCH

If you are being rescued from a winch, for example you are being taken off a boat, do not touch the winch lines until they have reached the ground as they carry a static electrical charge until they have been earthed.

Search and rescue

In addition to the fire, police and ambulance emergency services, the UK has a number of specialist organisations that operate search and rescue services in more hostile conditions.

Mountain Rescue Teams provide a rescue service to anyone who finds themselves in difficulty in hills and mountainous areas. These highly trained volunteers are well-equipped with specialist vehicles, helicopters and medical resources. They are on duty 24 hours a day and are contacted through the usual emergency agencies.

Emergencies at sea are dealt with by the Coastguard, the Royal National Lifeboat Institution (RNLI) and the Royal Air Force which operates a fleet of Sea King rescue helicopters. As well as participating in search and rescue operations, the RNLI runs a public education programme on water-safety as well as training programmes for beach lifeguards.

The RAF's search and rescue (SAR) service covers the whole country as well as a large area of sea. Working closely with the other emergency services, the SAR rescues approximately 1,500 people a year. The RAF is also active in rescues on land and is responsible for five Mountain Rescue Teams (MRTs) in different parts of the country.

To summon any rescue service you should phone 999 or 112.

USING DRESSINGS AND COLD COMPRESSES

A dressing is a piece of material that covers a wound to protect it from infection or to staunch bleeding. Cold compresses are used to reduce swelling and relieve pain. They are particularly useful for sprains and strains.

COLD COMPRESSES

There are three main types of cold compress:

- *Ice pack*
- *Cold pad*
- *Chemical pack*

APPLYING AN ICE PACK

Do not apply ice directly to the skin.

1 Wrap a bag of crushed ice in a clean piece of material such as a triangular bandage or tea towel.

2 Apply to the injured part for up to 20 minutes, securing in place as necessary.

3 Replace the ice as needed.

Items from the freezer compartment such as frozen peas make a good alternative to crushed ice.

APPLYING A COLD PAD

1 Soak a pad such as a flannel or folded triangular bandage in cold water. Wring it out so that it does not drip.

2 Apply to the injured area for up to 20 minutes, securing as necessary.

3 Wet the pad as needed to keep it cool.

4 If the wound is bleeding, tie the bandage firmly directly over the site of the injury to ensure maximum pressure.

5 Check the circulation below the site of the bandaging (see page 173).

USING CHEMICAL PACKS

Cool packs are available from most chemists or sports shops. They contain chemicals which, when mixed together, usually by twisting or tapping the surrounding plastic bag, become cold. The pad can then be used in the same way as an ice pack.

1 Follow the instructions on the pack.

2 If the pack is damaged, do not use it as the chemicals may leak on to the skin.

Chemical packs are ideal for situations in which you may be some distance from water or ice.

Types of dressing

There are various prepacked varieties of dressing available:

Non-adhesive These usually have one shiny side made of a material that minimises the risk of the dressing sticking to the wound. Generally more expensive than ordinary dressings, they are good for burns and grazes.

Gauze or lint These are backed by a layer of cotton wool padding. They come in various sizes, often with a bandage attached. The larger ones are particularly useful for managing major bleeds.

Adhesive dressings or plasters These are available in a variety of sizes and are used for smaller cuts. There are specially shaped plasters for fingers, heels and elbows, blue plasters for food handlers, fun plasters for children and plasters for a range of skin tones. To ensure maximum cleanliness, use individually wrapped plasters rather than cutting one from a long roll.

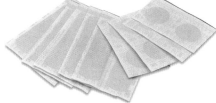

APPLYING A DRESSING

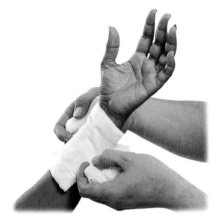

1 *Remove the wrapping, taking care not to touch the dressing. Place the dressing gently over the wound.*

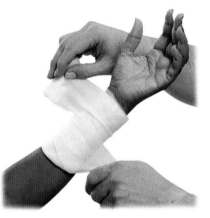

2 *Wind the bandage around the dressing, covering the entire pad.*

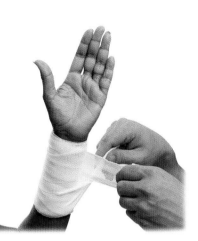

3 *Secure the bandage in place with tape, a bow or a reef knot.*

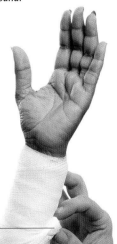

Check that the bandage is secure but not too tight

Improvised dressings

If you do not have a pre-packed dressing available, use a piece of clean, non-fluffy material such as a clean handkerchief, a freshly washed pillow case for burns covering a large surface area, or a clean plastic sandwich bag or piece of clingfilm for smaller burns.

Holding dressings in place

Dressings can be held in place:

• *With a bandage – either one attached to the dressing or a separate one. Triangular, tubular and roller bandages can all be used to hold dressings in place.*
• *With tape. Take care not to stick tape to the wound. Do not tape all the way around a limb as this may damage circulation.*
• *By the injured person. Injuries to the face, for example, are particularly hard to bandage and the dressing may be better held in place by hand.*

If using tape (or an adhesive dressing or plaster) ask the injured person if he or she is aware of any allergy to plaster. If there is a history of allergy, use an alternative method of securing the dressing.

WHEN USING DRESSINGS

• *The dressing should be larger than the area that is being treated.*
• *Place non-adhesive dressings shiny side down.*
• *If bleeding comes through the dressing, do not remove it. Place another dressing on top of it.*
• *For larger bleeds or for large burns, use additional layers of padding on top of the dressing.*
• *Check that the seal on a pre-packed dressing is not broken as this will mean that the dressing is no longer sterile.*

To reduce the risk of infection

• *Wear gloves if possible.*
• *Open the dressing as close to the wound as possible.*
• *Do not touch the wound or the dressing.*
• *For smaller wounds, wash your hands if possible before dressing the wound.*

BANDAGING

Bandages have three key uses: applying pressure to bleeding wounds; covering burns and providing support and immobilisation for broken burns, sprains and strains. The three main types are triangular, roller and tubular.

TYPES OF BANDAGE

Triangular bandages Made from cloth or from paper, these are exceptionally versatile. When they are made into a pad they can be used as a cold compress or for padding. When folded up they can be used to provide support or pressure; when unfolded they can be used as a support sling or cover bandage.

Roller bandages Used to provide support or secure dressings in place.

Tubular bandages Larger ones are used to support joints or hold dressings in place, smaller tubular bandages are ideal for finger injuries.

GENERAL PRINCIPLES OF BANDAGING

1 *Work with the injured person, explaining what you are doing.*

2 *Work in front of the injured person where possible and from the injured side if you can.*

3 *Bandage firmly over bleeding and securely over broken bones, but not so tight as to damage circulation below the site of the injury.*

4 *When passing bandages around an injured person, use the body's natural hollows such as the knees, ankles, neck and small of the back to slide the bandages gently into place.*

TYING A REEF KNOT

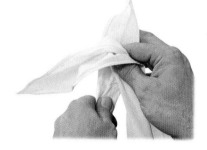

1 *Pass the right end of the bandage over the left and tuck it under.*

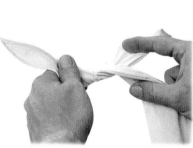

2 *Bring both ends alongside each other.*

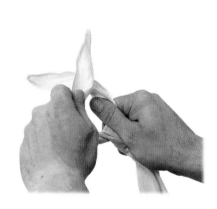

3 *Pass the left end over the right and tuck it under.*

When you tie a bandage, it is best to do so with a reef knot. Reef knots lie flat, so they do not press into the injured person, and are easy to untie. Alternative fastenings include tying a bow, using a safety pin, securing with tape or using a clip.

4 *Pull both ends firmly to complete the knot.*

5 Be aware that most injuries swell – check regularly to ensure that the bandage is still comfortable. Also, check that the bandage remains firmly secured, particularly if the injured person has to move, as this can loosen the bandage.

6 Secure bandages with tape, clips, a bow or a reef knot.

7 Make sure that bandages, especially knots, do not press into the skin, by placing padding between the bandaging and the skin as necessary.

Checking circulation

Bandages can cut off circulation, particularly as the injury swells. Check circulation below the site of the bandaging immediately after treatment and every 10 minutes thereafter.

Signs and symptoms of reduced circulation

- Pale skin, becoming blue
- Skin feeling cold to the touch
- Injured person complains of pins and needles or loss of feeling
- Weak or slow pulse in an injured limb
- Slow capillary refill below the site of the bandage (see below)

1 Look and feel for the signs and symptoms of reduced circulation. When bandaging, leave an area of skin exposed below the site of the injury to enable regular checks of circulation.

2 Ask the injured person to report any tingling or loss of feeling.

3 Gently squeeze the skin or the nail bed below the site of the injury and bandaging until the colour goes from the skin. When pressure is released, the colour should return swiftly (colour returns as the small blood vessels, the capillaries, refill with blood). If colour does not return quickly, circulation may be restricted.

If there are signs that circulation is restricted, gently loosen the bandage(s). If the bandage is covering a wound or burn, do not remove dressings. If it is supporting a broken bone, take care to support the injury as you loosen and re-tie the bandage.

APPLYING TUBULAR GAUZE

These bandages come in several sizes. The smallest size is used to hold dressings on to fingers and toes. It comes with its own applicator and is best secured with tape.

1 Cut two and half times the length of the finger or toe to be bandaged and push all of this on to the applicator.

2 Place the dressing over the wound. Slide the applicator over the finger or toe.

3 Hold the gauze at the base of the finger or toe and pull the applicator upwards, covering the finger or toe with one layer of gauze.

4 Above the finger or toe, twist the applicator twice and then push it back down, covering the finger or toe with another layer of gauze.

5 Tape the gauze in place.

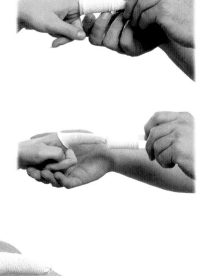

ROLLER BANDAGES

Roller bandages are used to secure dressings or to provide support, particularly to sprains and strains. They are usually made of cotton, gauze or linen and are secured in place with pins or tape.

TYPES OF ROLLER BANDAGE

There are three key types of roller bandage:

Open-weave best used for applying light dressings

Conforming used for securing dressings and providing support

crepe used for support, particularly for joint sprains

Roller bandages come in a variety of sizes. For an adult, the following are the recommended sizes:
Finger: 2.5 cm (1 in); **Hand:** 5 cm (2 in); **Arm:** 7.5–10 cm (3-4 in); **Leg:** 10–15 cm (4-6 in)

HOW TO APPLY A ROLLER BANDAGE

1 *Partly unroll the bandage.*

2 *Place the unrolled end below the injury and do two complete turns around the limb to secure the bandage in place.*

3 *Bandage up the limb, using spiral turns. Be aware that conforming and crepe bandages mould to the shape of the body and while they should be applied firmly, take care not to over-stretch the bandage as this may impair circulation.*

4 *Finish off with a single turn and secure in place. Secure with tape, clip or by tying off.*

5 *To tie off a roller bandage, leave enough bandage to do two complete turns of the limb. Cut down the middle of the bandage. Tie a knot at the bottom of the split and place both ends around the limb, one in each direction. Tie them in a bow or a reef knot.*

TRIANGULAR BANDAGES

These are amongst the most versatile of all items of first aid equipment. Usually made of washable calico, they are also available in a disposable paper form. In its open form, a triangular bandage can be used as a sling or as a cover bandage.

USING A TRIANGULAR BANDAGE

Making a broad fold to support broken bones or hold dressings loosely in place

1 *To make a broad fold, fold the point to the base of the bandage.*

2 *Fold the bandage in half again. This is a broad fold.*

Making a narrow fold to control bleeding

1 *To make a narrow fold, fold a broad fold in half again. This is a narrow fold.*

TO USE AS A COLD COMPRESS OR PADDING OR TO APPLY PRESSURE WITH A DRESSING

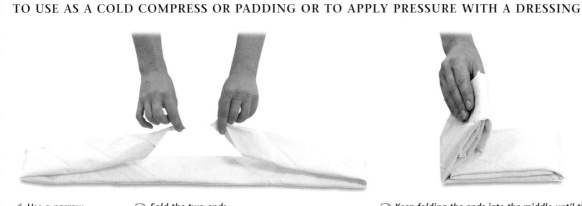

1 *Use a narrow fold bandage.*

2 *Fold the two ends into the middle.*

3 *Keep folding the ends into the middle until the size is appropriate for use. Bandages are best stored in this way in a plastic bag in a dry place.*

FIRST AID BOX FOR THE HOME

Most pharmacies and major supermarkets supply ready-made first aid boxes for the home. Alternatively, you may wish to put together your own first aid kit to best meet the needs of your family.

STORING FIRST AID EQUIPMENT

The equipment should be stored in a waterproof box clearly labelled in an easy to access position. The European symbol for first aid is a white cross on a green background.

WHAT SHOULD BE IN THE KIT?

Consider carefully the needs that you might have in the home for first aid equipment. Your kit should be able to provide you with equipment to do the following tasks:

- *Manage major bleeding*
- *Cover minor wounds and burns*
- *Clean small cuts and grazes*
- *Provide support for strains, sprains and broken bones*
- *Provide cover for large burns*
- *Apply a cold compress*

In addition, you may want to store over-the-counter remedies with your kit, such as painkillers and spares of family medications.

Numbers of each item will be influenced by the number, age and activities of people in the home. Very young children, for example, will have lots of small knocks and scrapes to their bodies and would therefore benefit from a copious supply of brightly coloured plasters. Sports-mad teenagers may be more at risk of sprains and strains.

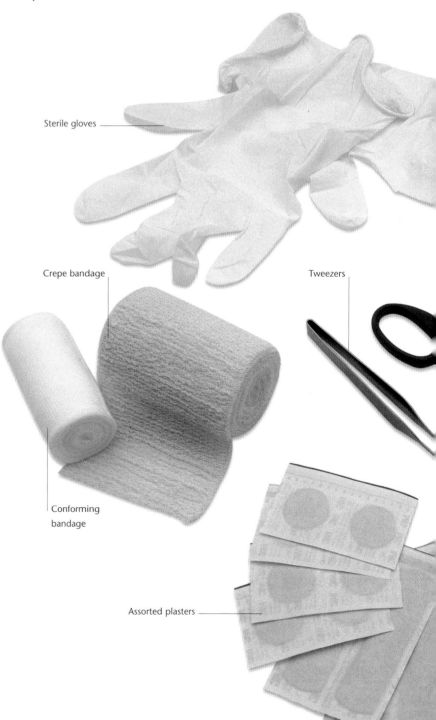

Sterile gloves

Crepe bandage

Tweezers

Conforming bandage

Assorted plasters

POTENTIAL EQUIPMENT

Small, medium and large dressings
These are sterile pads with bandages attached that can be used to control major bleeding and cover minor wounds.

Triangular bandages
These are an extremely versatile piece of equipment. Folded into a pad, they can be used as a cold compress or as padding around a painful area. They can provide cover to burns or large grazes and support broken bones. See also *Triangular Bandages*, page175.

Plasters
For small wounds.

Non-adhesive sterile dressings (various sizes), safety tape, adhesive tape and hypo-allergenic tape
Dressings can be cut to size and used to covers grazes, burns and small wounds.

Gauze swabs
For use with water to clean wounds.

Roller bandages, compression bandages, tubular bandages
For use in providing support to sprains and strains.

Disposable gloves
For use in managing body fluids.

Blunt-ended scissors

Tweezers

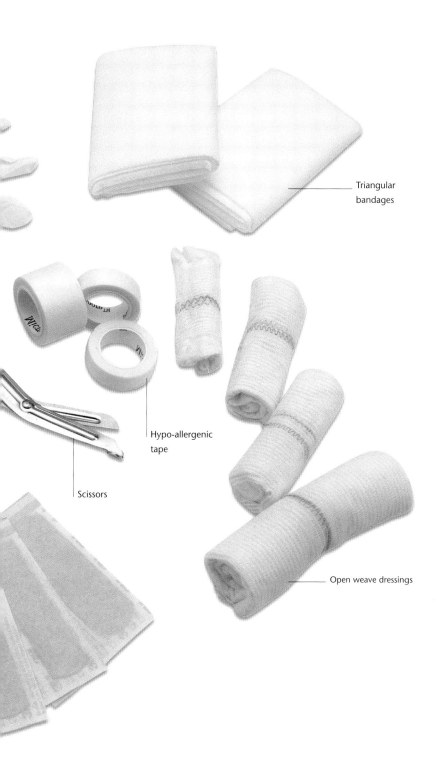

Triangular bandages

Hypo-allergenic tape

Scissors

Open weave dressings

Maintaining your kit

Make sure that you have a system for replacing equipment when it has been used and check dressings and medicines regularly to ensure that they are in date and undamaged.

FIRST AID BOX FOR THE CAR

More than 3,000 people are killed on the roads in the UK each year, with thousands of accidents every day. Carrying simple first aid equipment in your car can help to protect you at the scene of an accident and provide you with the tools to carry out necessary first aid procedures. In addition, a well-stocked first aid box can provide many items needed to ensure comfort on long journeys.

PROTECTING YOURSELF

Many people are injured while helping at the scene of a road accident. If you stop to help, make sure that you are clearly visible to oncoming traffic. Use your car as a warning signal and consider carrying a combination of the following equipment:

- *Hazard warning triangle*
- *High visibility jacket or strap*
- *Torch*

Keeping the injured person warm

- *Blanket(s)*

There may be little that you can do for many seriously injured victims other than treat for shock (see pages 44–45). Keeping the person warm is an important part of this treatment and can be potentially life-saving. Carry at least one blanket in your car. In addition to its value in treating shock, it can also be used as padding for broken bones or to keep family members warm if your car breaks down in freezing conditions.

TREATING INJURIES

Space is often in short supply in the boot of a car so a first aid kit should be kept to the minimum. The following provides a basic guide for a car first aid kit:

- *4 assorted sterile dressings, small, medium and large*
- *2 triangular bandages*
- *Plasters or non adhesive dressings and hypo-allergenic tape*
- *Gloves and face shield*
- *Note pad and pen*

FAMILY JOURNEYS

In addition to carrying equipment for major emergencies, you may wish to include useful items for family travels.

These include:

- *Sick bags*
- *Face wipes*
- *Wound cleaning wipes (when water is not available)*
- *Cold pads (these are cold compress ice packs made from chemicals that get cold when you break the seal; see also page 170)*
- *Over-the-counter remedies such as paracetamol for common ailments*

STORING YOUR FIRST AID BOX

If storing your first aid box in the main part of the car, ensure that it is either made of a soft material or that it is firmly bolted down to prevent it becoming a dangerous missile if the car stops suddenly. The container should be waterproof and clearly labelled.

Open weave dressings

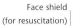

Face shield (for resuscitation)

On a boat

The guidance for cars applies equally well to boats. In addition, the boat first aid boxes may include:

• *Strong pliers for cutting away fish hooks*
• *Treatments for common marine creature bites and stings*
• *Sun cream and relief for sunburn*
• *Spares of medications for crew members*

Boats should always carry appropriate communication devices and rescue flares as well as standard rescue and survival equipment such as life jackets and life ring.

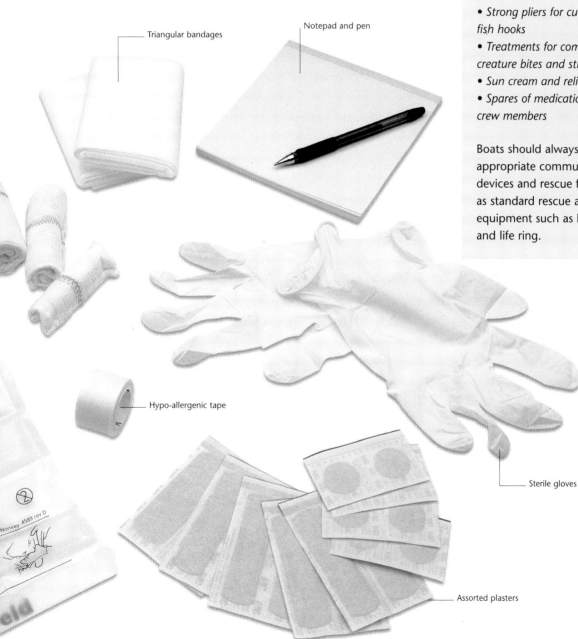

Triangular bandages

Notepad and pen

Hypo-allergenic tape

Norway 4589 rev D

Sterile gloves

Assorted plasters

WILDERNESS FIRST AID BOX

If planning a journey away from towns and easy access to medical treatment, consider carefully what equipment to take with you. As you will be carrying the first aid box yourself it should contain lightweight essential supplies. If you are out in wild country with a guide, check what equipment will be brought for the group (guides often have extended training in emergency skills) and what items you should bring personally.

KEEPING WARM AND PROVIDING SHELTER

This is often the first priority for an injured person in a wilderness situation. Useful equipment includes:

- *Survival bags: tough polythene body-size bags that can be used as protection from the elements. Often brightly coloured, they are also a useful signalling tool*
- *Sleeping bag/tent/floor mat*
- *Complete spare set of clothes*
- *Method of warming up hot drinks or food*

SIGNALLING FOR HELP

If an accident happens, the best advice is usually to stay put and call for help. Consider taking a combination of the following:

- *Mobile phone (but check network coverage in the area that you are going to be in)*
- *Whistle*
- *Mirror*
- *Torch*
- *Rescue flare*

PROTECTION FROM THE ELEMENTS AND WILDLIFE

When shelter is limited and you are exerting yourself walking, both heatstroke and heat exhaustion are real risks (see pages 114–15). Keep your head covered and wear cool clothes that allow sweat to evaporate from the body. Drink regularly and try and keep out of the sun during its hottest time (around midday). Remember too that insect and animal bites are common.

The following may be useful additions to your kit:

- *Insect repellent creams*
- *Over-the-counter remedy for insect stings*
- *Sun cream and sunburn remedy*
- *Sunglasses*

TREATING INJURIES

Restrict first aid equipment to a minimum to keep weight down. The following should cover most key emergency situations:

- *4 assorted sterile dressings: small, medium and large*
- *2 triangular bandages*
- *Plasters or non-adhesive dressings and hypo-allergenic tape*
- *Conforming bandages to fit ankles and knees (this bandage may enable a person with a sprained ankle to carry on walking to safety)*
- *Gloves and face shield*

OWN MEDICATION

It is important to know the medical requirements of all group members and to ensure that sufficient supplies of medications are carried for the trip (including extra in case conditions delay return times).

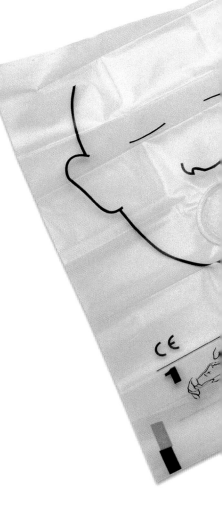

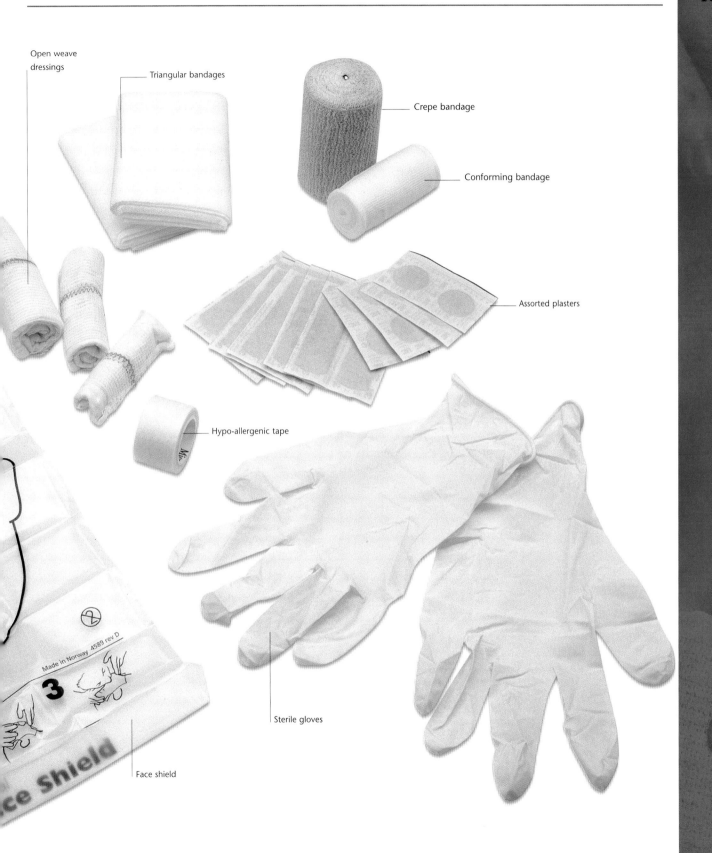

Open weave dressings

Triangular bandages

Crepe bandage

Conforming bandage

Assorted plasters

Hypo-allergenic tape

Sterile gloves

Face shield

Made in Norway 4589 rev D

3

ce Shield

OBSERVATION CHART/ CASUALTY RECORD

Administering first aid treatment to a casualty is an enormous responsibility. When help arrives it is important to pass on as much accurate information as possible. This will enable the professionals to make a swift assessment of the casualty's condition and to decide on the next most appropriate course of action. While waiting for help to arrive, aim to make regular checks on the patient and, if the circumstances allow, record your findings.

An observation chart/casualty record has two main purposes:

● *To provide information to the health professionals to help them to make an accurate diagnosis of the casualty's condition. The Glasgow Coma Scale is a widely used score that helps to provide information on whether a casualty's condition is improving or deteriorating over time.*

● *To meet legal requirements. If you are acting as a first aider in the workplace or in any other formal setting check the recording requirements of your role.*

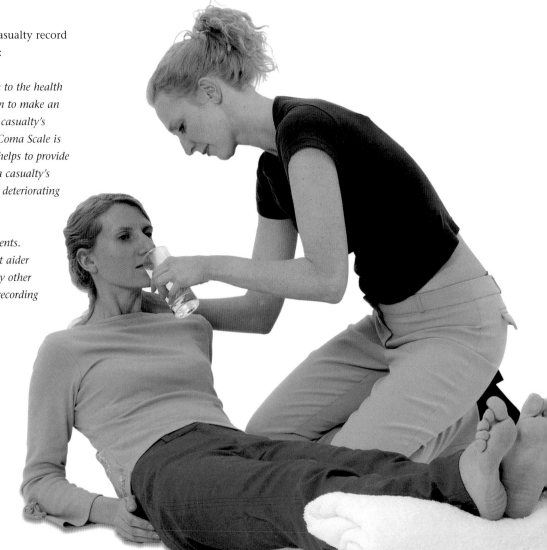

RIGHT *Check on progress at regular intervals, keep the casualty comfortable and offer reassurance*

Date . . . .

Brief history of incident . . . .
. . . .

Brief details of the casualty's signs, symptoms and medical history . . . .
. . . .

Name of casualty . . . .

Brief details of treatment given . . . .
. . . .

GLASGOW COMA SCALE (Measuring the level of response)

Put the appropriate score in the column after each check

		Record at 10 minute intervals	10	20	30	40
Eyes	Open spontaneously 4					
	Open to speech 3					
	Open to pain 2					
	No response 1					
Speech	Responds clearly to questions 5					
	Seems confused 4					
	Responds inappropriately 3					
	Incomprehensible sounds 2					
	No response 1					
Movement	Obeys commands 6					
	Points to pain 5					
	Moves from pain 4					
	Bends in response to pain 3					
	Stretches in response to pain 2					
	No response 1					
	Total (out of 15)					

RECORDING PULSE AND BREATHING RATES (Where possible record pulse and breathing rates every 10 minutes.)

Record at 10 minute intervals	10	20	30	40
Pulse rate – beats per minute				
Description (weak, strong, regular, irregular)				
Breathing – breaths per minute				
Description (noisy, quiet)				

CONTACT DETAILS OF FIRST AIDER

You may wish to include your contact details in case medical staff have questions on the scene, care of the casualty or the casualty's condition that
may help with the diagnosis and treatment of the casualty.. . . . .
. . . .

PART TWO

THE WELL BODY

CONTENTS

INTRODUCTION

Human beings are designed to be capable of withstanding physical and psychological stress. We can adapt to survive in a wide range of environments, and may live our lives at altitude or in cold or hot climates and still continue to function. The body consists of various systems that interact with each other and renew and repair themselves, and has its own built-in defence system to protect us from harm. Many minor illnesses or injuries are automatically dealt with by the body without us even being aware of feeling ill in the first place. But when something more serious upsets the normal workings of your body, you become ill.

The first part of this section describes the major body systems that the body can be divided into and their basic functions. If you have a fundamental knowledge of the structure and function of the various parts of your body it will help you to have a greater understanding of why illnesses happen.

Each major body system has a particular part to play in the way your body works and they are controlled by the body's control centre, the nervous system. When you are healthy all these systems work in harmony to enable you to go about your daily life without a hitch. Why something goes wrong depends on many factors. In the past, the majority of deaths were caused by infectious disease. Improvements in medical care, public health measures and the introduction of vaccination has meant that infectious diseases pose a far less serious threat to health in the West today. But disease has not been eliminated: infections have instead been replaced by a number of illnesses that are often preventable and that are mostly associated with lifestyle.

The second part of this section shows how your lifestyle affects your present and future health. All aspects of life, including where you live, what you do for a living, your method of transport and what you do in your spare time have implications for health. The main ones discussed in this section are diet, exercise, stress, relaxation and sleeping, aspects of your lifestyle over which you can exert some control. Smoking has an article to itself, because it is the single most damaging lifestyle choice affecting health.

Diet is the most important factor in living a long and healthy life, and many unpleasant and serious illnesses are linked to what you eat and drink. Advice is given on what you should be eating to ensure a healthy, low-fat, high-fibre diet and what should be avoided or consumed in moderation. Closely linked to diet is weight. Obesity levels are escalating, and this section will show you how to maintain a healthy weight.

Exercise is the second most important factor for good health. Regular exercise benefits physical and mental health, keeps you flexible and mobile into old age and promotes a feeling of well-being by increasing the body's level of feel-good hormones.

Learning how to relax and deal with stress will help you stay mentally and emotionally well. Finally, a good night's sleep is essential for your health.

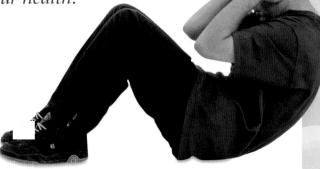

HOW THE HEALTHY BODY FUNCTIONS

The functioning of the human body has been compared to all manner of machines, but the reality is that no machine ever invented or designed comes close to the huge complexity that is man or woman. Every second of the day, in billions of individual cells in the body, a vast array of chemical, electrical and mechanical reactions are taking place without a hitch, allowing us to go about our daily lives.

POWER SUPPLY

Probably the most important feature that distinguishes the body from mere machines is its ability, through the reproductive organs, to produce children. However, in some respects, the way the body works has some passing similarities to machines, in that certain functions are common to both.

Without power, most machines would cease to function, and there is no doubt that this is the case for the human body.

BASIC REQUIREMENTS

Two essential elements are required for life – nutrients and oxygen – and if either were in limited supply for any length of time, the body would die.

The body requires nourishment to fuel the many chemical reactions taking place within the body, and to maintain and build new cells, replacing those that die off each day. Food and drink are processed by the digestive system and absorbed into the body, providing the nutrients and water that must be present for life to continue.

Equally essential for life, oxygen from air is breathed in via the respiratory system and transported to the lungs, where it is absorbed into the surrounding blood vessels.

CIRCULATORY TRANSPORT

The presence of food in the stomach and air in the lungs would be of no consequence without a means of conveying them to the parts of the body where they are needed. The heart and blood vessels form a transport network that supplies oxygen and nutrients to the tissues, collections of specialised cells that perform certain functions in the body. Blood rich in

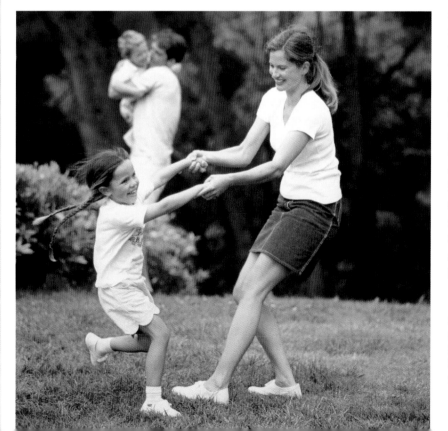

LEFT *Every second of the day, countless unseen chemical, electrical and mechanical processes take place to enable the various interactive systems of your body to renew and repair themselves, and sustain life.*

oxygen from the lungs reaches the heart, which pumps it around the body, picking up nutrients absorbed from the digestive system on the way. Blood then returns to the heart and is transported to the lungs to have its oxygen levels topped up.

Like all machines, there are waste products and poisons produced as fuel and oxygen are consumed. Unused food products leave the digestive system in the form of faeces. By-products of chemical processes in the cells, such as carbon dioxide, are removed via the bloodstream and breathed out though the lungs. Other chemicals in the blood are filtered out by the kidneys, and removed from the body as urine.

COMPLEX ACTIVITIES

The human body gathers information about its environment through the sense organs – the eyes, ears, nose, taste receptors on the tongue and touch sensors in the skin. This information is conveyed through a hugely complex system of nerves to the body's control centre, the brain. The brain is the seat of conscious thought, emotion, memory and countless other functions, such as coordinating movement through the bones, muscles and joints. The brain is also responsible for many bodily functions that are automatic and beyond conscious control, such as sweating. This is often in association with the endocrine system, a series of glands that communicate through chemical messengers called hormones.

The human body also has a built-in security system, designed to repel germ and chemical warfare. It has physical and chemical barriers at the entrance to the digestive and respiratory systems, in addition to the protective skin. There is also the internal immune system, a highly efficient destroyer of all manner of bacteria and viruses.

Major body systems

The body consists of various systems that interact with each other to sustain life and enable chemical, mechanical and electrical reactions to take place. Each body system has a particular function, such as respiration, and comprises highly specialised organs and tissues.

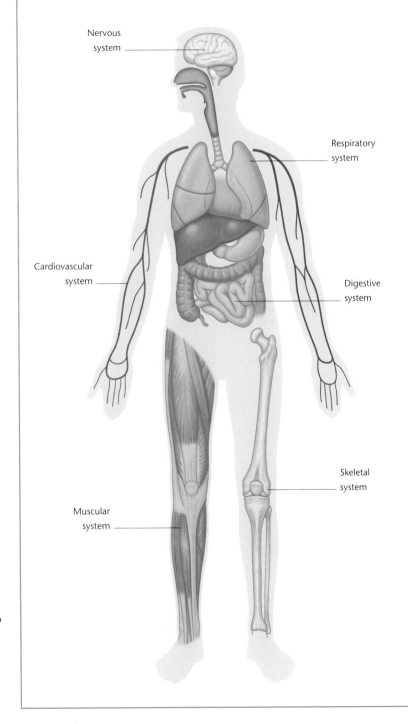

Nervous system

Respiratory system

Cardiovascular system

Digestive system

Skeletal system

Muscular system

HEART AND CIRCULATION

The circulatory or cardiovascular system consists of the heart and blood vessels, and is responsible for supplying all of the body's tissues and organs with blood. The circulatory system also carries various waste products to the liver and kidneys for processing and elimination from the body. At the centre of the system, almost literally, is the heart, a powerful muscular pump that beats more than 100,000 times per day to send oxygen and nutrients around the body.

HEART

The heart has distinct halves, each with an upper chamber (atrium) and lower chamber (ventricle). Each of these four chambers is connected to one or more blood vessels. The two upper chambers, or atria, receive blood returning under low pressure from the veins. The two lower chambers, the ventricles, pump blood from the atria out through the arteries, under high pressure, around the body. Compared to the ventricles, the atria are less muscular and have thinner walls.

In a typical beat of the heart, blood passes from the two atria through one-way valves into the corresponding ventricle. The ventricles then contract powerfully, forcing blood out through narrow openings, guarded by more valves, into the arteries.

The left ventricle empties into the aorta, the body's main artery, about the diameter of a garden hose, transporting blood rich in oxygen to organs and tissues. The right ventricle pumps blood low in oxygen through the pulmonary arteries back to the lungs, where oxygen levels are renewed.

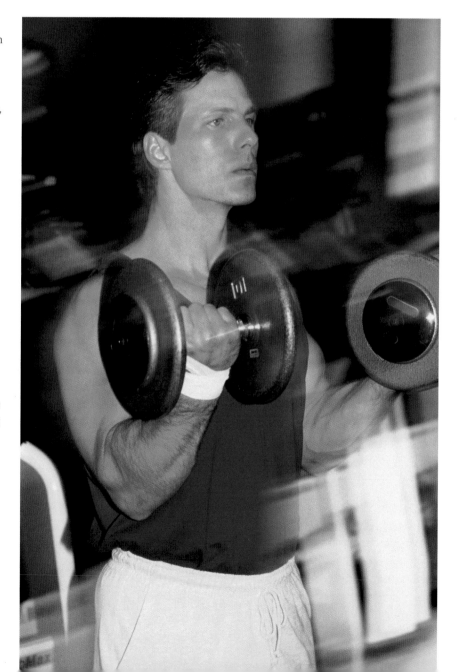

RIGHT *Both heart and lungs benefit from regular exercise, which strengthens the heart and helps reduce blood pressure.*

The heart and circulatory system

The heart pumps blood around the body in a network of arteries (red) and veins (blue).

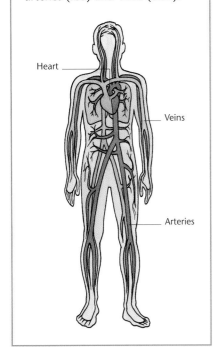

Heart

Veins

Arteries

How the heart functions

Blood flows through veins into the heart's upper chambers (atria) and is pumped into the arteries by the lower chambers (ventricles). The right side pumps deoxygenated blood from the body to the lungs; the left side pumps oxygenated blood to the body.

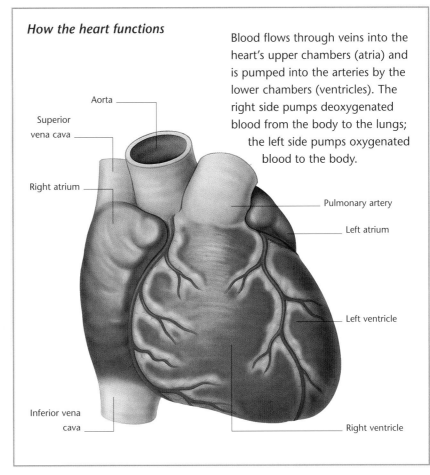

Aorta

Superior vena cava

Right atrium

Inferior vena cava

Pulmonary artery

Left atrium

Left ventricle

Right ventricle

In a lifetime, it is estimated that the average heart beats more than 2.5 billion times, and each of these beats sends a pressure wave through the arteries, causing their walls to expand. Each beat involves a sequence of contractions of the four chambers of the heart, controlled by electrical impulses that spread throughout the heart muscle. The heart rate and the volume of blood pumped with each heartbeat are not under conscious control, but function automatically.

BLOOD VESSELS

The ventricles of the heart pump blood into thick-walled blood vessels known as arteries. Arteries are strong, elastic vessels that are able to withstand the high pressures generated within them by the forceful action of the heart, the elasticity allowing the artery to expand as a pressure wave of blood passes through its interior.

Blood destined for the lungs leaves the right ventricle through the pulmonary artery. Blood that supplies the rest of the body leaves the left ventricle via the body's largest blood vessel, the aorta. All arteries divide into progressively smaller vessels, eventually becoming very fine branches known as arterioles. As the arteries divide, the pressure within gradually diminishes.

The very finest arterioles become capillaries, the smallest blood vessels in the body, having walls that are a single cell in thickness. The exchange of oxygen, nutrients and waste products, such as carbon dioxide, takes place between blood and tissues through the walls of these microscopic capillaries.

There are around one billion capillaries in the human body and, if these were laid end-to-end, they would cover a distance of approximately 100,000 km (62,000 miles).

Blood passes through the capillaries and drains into small veins, known as venules. These merge to form veins, which return blood to the heart through two large vessels called the superior and inferior vena cava, which drain into the right atrium. Blood pressure in the veins is significantly lower than in arteries, and veins have thin walls to let them expand and hold large volumes of blood. Many veins run through muscles, and when the muscles contract this encourages blood flow through the veins back to the heart. Veins contain one-way valves to stop blood flowing in the wrong direction.

RESPIRATORY SYSTEM

The respiratory system includes the nose, mouth, throat, windpipe, branching airways and lungs. Its main function is to deliver oxygen from the air to the bloodstream and to remove carbon dioxide from the blood and return it to the lungs to be breathed out. It also warms and filters the air we breathe, and assists in speech production by providing air for the voice box and the vocal cords. The average adult breathes in and out between 18 and 20 times per minute, and every day about 150 cubic metres (490 cubic feet) of air, the equivalent of a balloon about 7 metres (23 feet) in diameter, passes through the respiratory tract.

BREATHING PROCESSES

Breathing, or respiration, has two phases: inhalation, or inspiration, in which air is sucked into the lungs, and exhalation, or expiration, where the air is forced back out of the lungs. The main muscle for breathing is the diaphragm, a large dome-shaped muscle separating the chest and abdominal cavities. When the diaphragm contracts, it flattens, enlarging the chest cavity, causing air to rush into the lungs. Relaxation of the diaphragm allows the chest cavity to return to its normal size, forcing air out of the lungs.

Breathing is an automatic process, controlled by a part of the nervous system called the brainstem. This control is so strong that it is impossible to stop breathing for any significant length of time.

MOUTH AND NASAL PASSAGES

During respiration, air enters the body through the mouth and the nasal passages. The nose filters the air that we breathe: its lining – the mucous membrane – has thousands of tiny hairs that move waves of mucus back towards the throat. Dust, chemical

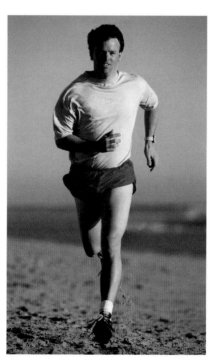

ABOVE *Aerobic exercise increases the efficiency of gas exchange in the lungs and improves the working of the respiratory muscles.*

particles and bacteria are trapped in the mucus, carried back towards the throat and swallowed out of harm's way. The mucous membrane warms and moisturises the air breathed in. The nose is also the site of organs of the sense of smell.

THROAT

Once air has entered the body through the nose and mouth, it passes through the throat or pharynx, a muscular tube connecting the back of the nose and the mouth with the voice box. The throat also forms part of the digestive system. Within the walls of the throat are the tonsils and adenoids, collections of tissue that help to trap and destroy many infectious organisms that enter the airways.

VOICE BOX

The voice box or larynx consists of rings of dense tissue called cartilage, some of which can be seen in a structure known as the Adam's apple, which in men sticks out at the front of the neck just below the chin. Within the voice box are two sheets of fibrous material that stretch across the rings of cartilage. These are the vocal cords, and their main function is voice production. Air from the lungs passes across the vocal cords, causing them to vibrate, and these vibrations are modified by the tongue, palate and lips to produce speech. Sounds vary according to the position of the cords. The vocal cords also prevent food entering the lungs.

Respiratory system

Every body cell requires a constant supply of oxygen in order to survive. Air is breathed in and out via the respiratory system. This enables oxygen to be taken into the body, and carbon dioxide, the cells' waste product, to be released. The respiratory system includes the nose, mouth, throat, windpipe, branching airways and lungs, and the diaphragm and various muscles. Breathing is controlled by the respiratory centre in the brain.

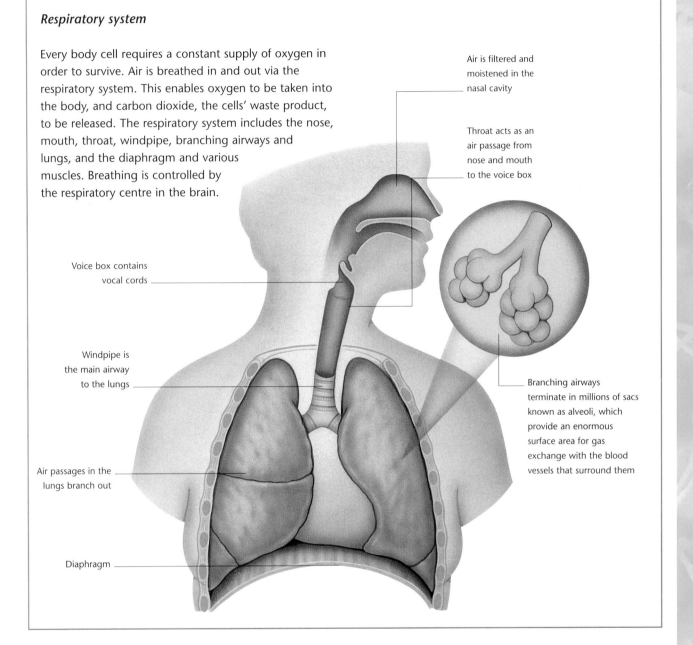

Air is filtered and moistened in the nasal cavity

Throat acts as an air passage from nose and mouth to the voice box

Voice box contains vocal cords

Windpipe is the main airway to the lungs

Air passages in the lungs branch out

Diaphragm

Branching airways terminate in millions of sacs known as alveoli, which provide an enormous surface area for gas exchange with the blood vessels that surround them

WINDPIPE AND BRANCHING AIRWAYS

Once air has passed through the voicebox, it enters the windpipe, or trachea, which branches into two main air passages, each leading to a lung. Within each lung, these air passages divide, branch and subdivide into thousands of tiny air passages. At the end of the tiniest air passages are balloon-like sacs called alveoli.

ALVEOLI AND GAS EXCHANGE

Rather like the capillaries (tiny blood vessels) that surround them, alveoli have walls only one cell thick, allowing the rapid transmission of oxygen from air to the bloodstream and equally rapid diffusion of carbon dioxide from blood into the lungs to be breathed out. Efficient gas exchange is enhanced by the huge surface area of the alveoli, and the fact that at the site of gas exchange, the distance between air and blood is only one-thousandth of a millimetre. There are more than 700 million alveoli in the lungs, and their internal surface area is about the size of a tennis court. After crossing the walls of the alveoli into surrounding tiny blood vessels, oxygen binds with haemoglobin in red blood cells. Carbon dioxide is released from blood plasma into the alveoli and breathed out.

BRAIN AND NERVOUS SYSTEM

The nervous system is the most complicated system in the body, an extensive, intricate network of structures that activates, coordinates and controls all the functions of the body. It is divided into the central nervous system, comprising the brain and the spinal cord, and the peripheral nervous system, which branches to every part of the body and includes the cranial nerves (twelve pairs of nerves that arise within the skull) and the spinal nerves.

AUTONOMIC NERVOUS SYSTEM

Many of the body's activities, such as the beating of the heart, or the flow of digestive juices, are automatic and not under conscious control. Part of the peripheral nervous system, known as the autonomic nervous system, is responsible for these functions. The autonomic nervous system consists of a series of cranial and spinal nerves that supply the internal organs. It is further subdivided into the sympathetic and the parasympathetic nervous systems, which balance each other. Generally, the sympathetic system stimulates, for example speeding up the pulse rate, while the parasympathetic system has a calming action, for example slowing the pulse rate.

Electrical messengers

A minute gap, the synapse, separates each nerve cell, or neurone, from the next. Messages carried as electrical impulses 'jump' the gap between neurones when a chemical called a neurotransmitter is released from the end of the axon.

The nervous system

The nervous system is divided into two parts. The central nervous system (CNS) comprises the brain and spinal cord. The peripheral nervous system (PNS) comprises various nerves that transmit signals between the CNS and the rest of the body.

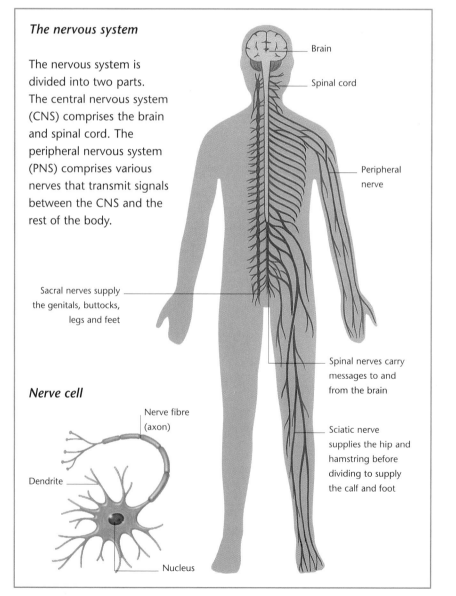

Brain

Spinal cord

Peripheral nerve

Sacral nerves supply the genitals, buttocks, legs and feet

Spinal nerves carry messages to and from the brain

Sciatic nerve supplies the hip and hamstring before dividing to supply the calf and foot

Nerve cell

Nerve fibre (axon)

Dendrite

Nucleus

BRAIN

This is the portion of the central nervous system contained within the skull, and weighs about 1400 g (3 lb) in adults. It is divided into three main parts: the cerebrum, the cerebellum and the brainstem.

The cerebrum is the largest part of the brain, and is a mass of convoluted grey and white matter divided by a deep fissure into two halves or hemispheres, which are linked by a thick band of nerve fibres. The cerebrum is responsible for most of the 'higher' functions of the brain, such as understanding the messages that the senses are sending to the brain (sensory interpretation) and initiating movement (motor actions). It is also the seat of many mental activities such as logical thought and emotions.

The cerebellum is situated towards the back of the skull, and again is divided into two hemispheres. It is mostly responsible for coordinating movement. The brainstem connects the rest of the brain with the upper part of the spinal cord, and performs motor, sensory and reflex functions, automatic responses to certain stimuli, such as withdrawing your hand from a hot surface before you become aware of the heat.

The left side of the brain controls the right side of the body, and in 90 per cent of the population is the dominant hemisphere for speech and writing. The left hemisphere is also thought to be more analytical. The right side of the brain interprets visual stimuli and sounds other than speech, such as music. Here lies our ability to think visually and to use our imagination.

SPINAL CORD

The spinal cord lies inside a canal within the backbone, and extends to the small of the back. This is about 1 cm (½ in) thick, and approximately 45 cm (18 in) long. Arising from the

Brain areas – map of cerebral cortex

The intricately folded outer layer of the cerebrum is the cortex, the part of the brain that processes complex information. Areas each have specific functions and have been mapped.

- Premotor cortex
- Broca's area (speech)
- Motor cortex
- Sensory cortex
- Auditory cortex
- Visual cortex
- Cerebellum

RIGHT *When playing a computer game, the nervous system is under conscious control and the brain responds to thoughts and visual stimuli to trigger appropriate hand movements.*

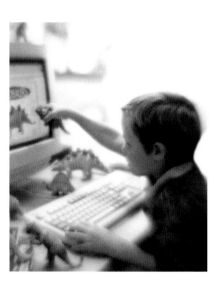

spinal cord are 31 pairs of spinal nerves, which, along with the 12 pairs of cranial nerves, form the peripheral nervous system.

HOW NERVE CELLS COMMUNICATE

Nerve cells communicate with each other by way of electrical signals or impulses, travelling at up to 400km (250 miles) per hour, allowing information to be processed, assessed and acted upon within milliseconds. A single nerve cell may connect with hundreds of others, and the junction between these cells is known as a synapse. The synapse is, in reality, a gap between the nerve cells, and the electrical impulse travels across the gap by way of specific chemical messengers known as neurotransmitters.

The nerve cells of the body branch out to supply every muscle and particle of skin, as well as all of the internal organs such as the heart, intestines and lungs. Many of these nerves are bundled together like rope, carrying messages from the periphery, through the spinal cord to the brain. Similar messages travel back from the brain to the nerve fibres in the muscles to initiate movement, for example.

BONES, MUSCLES AND JOINTS

The human adult skeleton is made up of 206 bones, connected by ligaments, muscles and tendons to provide a framework to support the body and give mobility. Although the bones themselves are tough, hard, rigid structures, the various types of joint between the bones allow for an enormous range of movement. The skeleton also provides a protective cage to help shield some of the body's vital organs from injury.

BONES

Bone is a living tissue, constantly being renewed throughout life. Babies are born with 270 soft bones, but many, for example, those of the skull, will have fused together by the age of twenty. There are a few differences between male and female skeletons: male bones are generally larger and heavier, and the female pelvis is wider to allow for childbirth.

All bones have a hard, solid outer layer, but many of the larger bones have a spongy interior to reduce their density. Some of the long bones, the breastbone (sternum) and the pelvis, also have cavities within them which

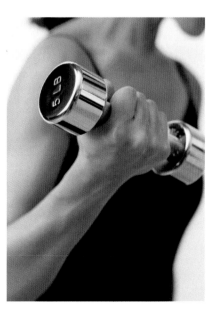

contain marrow. Bone marrow manufactures red and white blood cells (see pages 208–9), which pass into the bloodstream.

MUSCLES

Muscles are composed of millions of tiny protein filaments capable of contraction and relaxation to produce movement. There are three types of muscle within the body: skeletal, smooth and cardiac.

Skeletal muscle is the most abundant tissue in the body, comprising up to 40 per cent of a man's weight. It is attached to bone by tendons, flexible cords of fibrous tissue, and is under the conscious control of the brain. The muscle is supplied by a nerve that conveys electrical signals from the brain, causing the cells within the muscle to contract, producing movement.

The largest skeletal muscle is the latissimus dorsi, a flat muscle in the back; the smallest, at just 1.2 mm (1/20 in), is the stapedius in the middle ear, which activates one of the three small bones that transmit vibrations from the eardrum to the inner ear.

LEFT *Both muscle size and strength can be significantly increased by carrying out regular exercise that involves pushing against resistance or lifting weights.*

Smooth muscle is found in many of the internal organs of the body such as the intestines, the bladder and the walls of arteries. Cardiac muscle is found in the heart, powering the action of the circulatory pump. Both smooth and cardiac muscles are known as involuntary muscles because their actions cannot be consciously controlled.

JOINTS

A joint is a junction between two or more bones. Joints have a variety of forms and functions: some have little or no movement, for example those between the bones of the skull. Others, such as the shoulder joint, are freely moveable in a range of directions.

The vast majority of the body's joints are known as synovial joints, because they contain synovial fluid within a capsule around the joint, which lubricates the internal surfaces of the joint. The ends of the bones that meet in a synovial joint are covered in cartilage, a smooth, tough, slippery material that allows the bones to glide across each other in a frictionless manner, reducing wear and tear on the bones. The joint capsule binds the bones of the joint together.

Joints are classified according to where the bones meet and the range of movement permitted. Plane joints are

RIGHT The human skeleton is a rigid framework that supports and protects the body. The different joints allow the bones to bend and swivel and the muscles fixed to the bones allow movement.

The skeleton

Skull (cranium)

Carpal

Clavicle

Scapula

Radius

Ulna

Rib

Vertebral column

Sternum

Pelvis

Pubis

Thigh bone (femur)

Kneecap

Fibula

Tibia

Tarsal

almost always small and permit a sliding or gliding movement, such as the joint between the clavicle and the shoulder blade (the acromioclavicular joint). Hinge joints, such as the elbows, move in one direction, allowing only bending or straightening. Ball-and-socket joints, such as shoulders and hips, are where a rounded head fits into a cup-shaped socket, allowing movement in a number of directions. Saddle joints, such as the joint at the base of the thumb, permits movement in two different directions. Condyloid joints, such as the knuckles, also allow movement in two directions, but one direction is much freer than the other. Finally, pivotal joints allow rotation. The most important of these is at the top of the neck, where the first vertebra of the spine pivots on the second, allowing the head to turn to either side.

Synovial joint

In a synovial joint, the ends of the adjoining bones are covered with cartilage to enable easy movement and the bones are linked by a fluid-filled capsule that lubricates the joint.

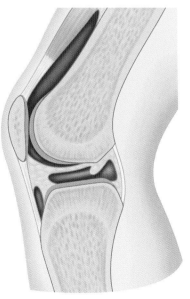

DIGESTIVE SYSTEM

The digestive system is the collective name given to a group of organs that work together to break down the food we eat into simple components that the body's cells can absorb, and then to eliminate the waste products of digestion from the body. Digestion includes mechanical and chemical processes.

FOOD BREAKDOWN

Food consists mainly of water and nutrients that the body needs in order to sustain life. Food has to be broken down in a process known as digestion into molecules small enough for the body to absorb. Digestion begins in the mouth, where food is physically broken down by the grinding action of the teeth (mastication). Lubrication for chewing is provided by saliva, discharged into the mouth from three pairs of glands. These glands also produce enzymes, chemicals that help to digest the starchy elements of food. Once the food has been chewed and pulped into a ball of food (bolus), it is propelled to the back of the throat by

Peristalsis

Contracted muscle

Relaxed muscle

Ball of food

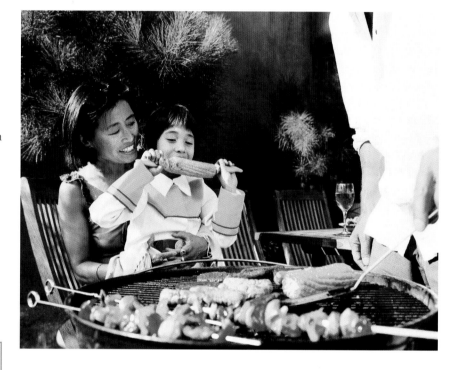

ABOVE *The anticipation of food stimulates the production of digestive juices in the mouth, which is an important precursor to the process of breaking down food.*

the tongue and swallowed, entering the oesophagus (gullet).

OESOPHAGUS AND STOMACH

The oesophagus is a muscular tube that carries food from the throat to the stomach. A bolus is propelled downwards by a powerful, rhythmic contraction of the smooth muscle in the wall of the oesophagus known as peristalsis, which is so forceful in the oesophagus that it is possible to swallow upside down. Muscular contractions continue to move food throughout the length of the digestive tract.

The stomach is a muscular sac-like structure with a number of functions.

Firstly, it continues the process of breaking down food into absorbable nutrients by producing digestive juices. Secondly, it produces a powerful acid to sterilise the contents of the stomach, along with a layer of mucus to prevent the acid damaging the stomach lining. Finally, it acts as a storage area to allow our standard three meals a day to be utilised gradually. Food spends up to five hours in the stomach before being squirted into the small intestine.

SMALL INTESTINE

The small intestine is a muscular tube more than 6 m (20 ft) long, which loops back and forth across the abdomen. The first part of the small intestine is the duodenum, which receives partly digested food from the stomach along with digestive juices from the pancreas and bile from the gallbladder (produced by the liver but stored in the gallbladder) to break down food even further. Pancreatic juices contain bicarbonate to neutralise the acid produced by the stomach, and the pancreas also produces insulin, which regulates the level of sugar in the blood.

The second part of the small intestine is the jejunum, where the majority of nutrients are absorbed into the bloodstream, and the final part is the ileum, where the rest of the nutrients are absorbed. To aid absorption, the inner layer of the small intestine is covered in millions of finger-like projections called villi, which increase its surface area to about twice the size of a tennis court.

LARGE INTESTINE

Food then enters the first part of the large intestine, the caecum. Attached to this is a small pouch that has no function, but can cause lots of problems: the appendix (see appendicitis, page 406). The large intestine, or colon, is divided into the ascending, transverse, descending and sigmoid colons. By the time food reaches the ascending colon, it consists of a watery slurry with little or no nutrients left in it. The large intestine reabsorbs water, then compacts and compresses the residual waste into faeces to be eliminated from the body. Faeces are stored in the lowest part of the digestive system, known as the rectum. From the rectum, the faeces (stools, or motions) are expelled through the anus.

Digestive system

The digestive system is a series of hollow organs that connect to form a long tube from the mouth to the anus. This tube has muscular walls that propel food along it and break it down. Digestion is complete when nutrients have been absorbed into the bloodstream and waste products eliminated through the anus.

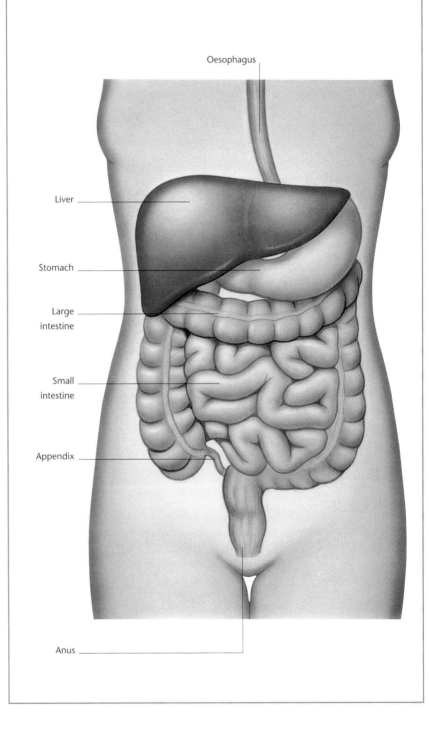

Oesophagus

Liver

Stomach

Large intestine

Small intestine

Appendix

Anus

KIDNEYS AND URINARY SYSTEM

The urinary tract consists of the kidneys, two ureters (narrow tubes connecting the kidneys to the bladder), the bladder and the urethra (a tube that drains the bladder). The basic function of the urinary system is to act as a filtration plant for the body, allowing waste and poisonous chemicals to be extracted from the bloodstream and eliminated from the body as urine.

KIDNEYS

The kidneys are a pair of organs located on either side of the abdomen at about the level of the small of the back. Every hour of every day, they receive more than 57 litres (100 pints) of blood through the renal arteries, representing about a quarter of the total output of the heart. This level of blood supply is maintained all the time because the purifying action of the kidneys is absolutely essential for the continuation of life. Although we have two kidneys, it is possible to survive with only one functioning kidney.

In addition to their filtering action, removing dangerous waste chemicals from the blood, the kidneys are also responsible for maintaining fluid balance within the body. By monitoring fluctuations in levels of salts and sugar in the blood, the kidneys are able to alter the amount of fluid lost as urine, thus preventing dehydration. They can compensate for excess fluid intake by increasing urine output. The kidneys also produce hormones, one of which helps to control blood pressure.

More than 99 per cent of the fluid that passes through the kidneys is returned to the blood, along with glucose (sugar), salts and minerals. The urine that is produced in the kidneys dribbles slowly down to the bladder, 24 hours a day, through the ureters. The ureters are very narrow muscular tubes, which connect the kidneys to the bladder, and are about 30 cm (12 in) long, but less than 6 mm (¼ in) in diameter.

BLADDER

The bladder is a muscular sac that stores urine, and receives between 1–2 litres (2–4 pints) per day, depending on

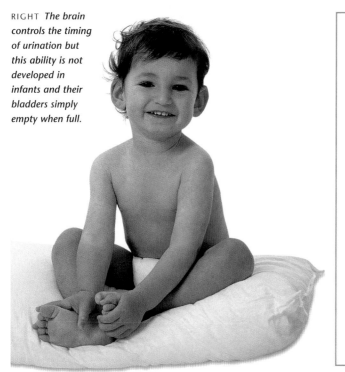

RIGHT *The brain controls the timing of urination but this ability is not developed in infants and their bladders simply empty when full.*

How the kidney works

The cortex contains filtering units called nephrons.
The medulla contains groups of urine-collecting ducts.
The pelvis collects urine and funnels it into the ureter.

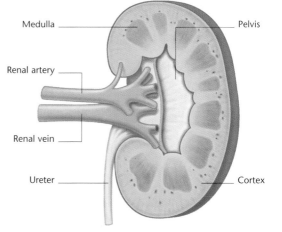

Medulla

Renal artery

Renal vein

Ureter

Pelvis

Cortex

the body's state of hydration. The bladder stretches, and stores urine until it is convenient to dispose of it. The average human bladder is able to comfortably accommodate 0.5 litre (1 pint) of urine before it is emptied.

When the wall of the bladder is stretched past a certain limit, nerves send signals to the brain and the desire to urinate is felt. Older children and adults can control the timing of urination; infants cannot and their bladders simply empty when full. Contraction of the muscular bladder wall forcibly expels urine through the urethra into the outside world. During this contraction, the openings of the ureters, high on the bladder wall, are closed, ensuring that there is no flow of urine back up the ureters towards the kidneys. Urine is sterile – free from infective particles – until it leaves the body.

URETHRA

The urethra is the lowest portion of the urinary tract, and transports urine from the bladder to the outside of the body. It has a comparatively thick layer of smooth muscle in its wall. There is a number of mucus-secreting urethral glands, which discharge secretions into the urethra, keeping it moist and preventing it from drying out.

In women, the bladder is located in front of the uterus and vagina, and for this reason, the urethra is only about 4 cm (1½ in) long. Its only role is to drain the bladder. In men, however, the bladder is positioned just in front of the rectum. The urethra, which is about 20 cm (8 in) long in the male, has an additional function, providing the route for the ejaculation of semen during orgasm. The urethra passes through the prostate gland, receives fluid from glands called the seminal vesicles, and then empties through the penis.

Differences between male and female urinary tracts

The urinary tract is different in men and women. In men, the urethra passes through the prostate gland, transporting urine or semen to the penis. In women, the bladder sits under the uterus. A short urethra (which is more prone to infection than the longer male urethra) carries urine to the entrance at the front of the vagina so it can be released from the body.

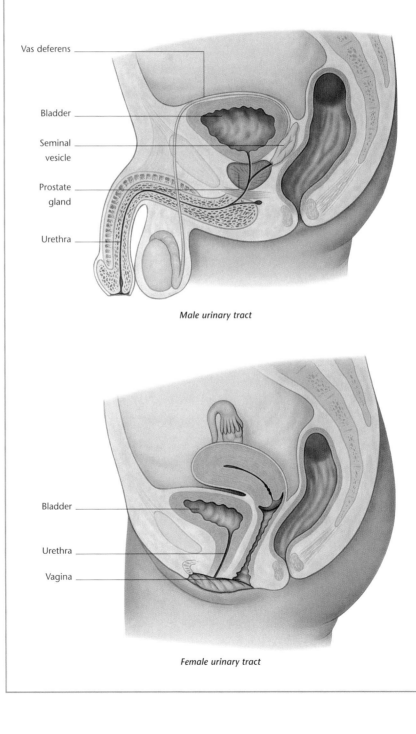

Vas deferens

Bladder

Seminal vesicle

Prostate gland

Urethra

Male urinary tract

Bladder

Urethra

Vagina

Female urinary tract

ENDOCRINE SYSTEM

The endocrine system is responsible for the implementation of a wide variety of processes within the body. It consists of a collection of glands that produce hormones (chemical messengers), which are involved in the regulation of normal bodily functions such as metabolism, growth, sexual development and reproduction. The hormones manufactured by the endocrine glands travel in the bloodstream to target organs and tissues.

PITUITARY GLAND AND HYPOTHALAMUS

The centre of the endocrine system is the pituitary gland, which is located in the skull just behind the bridge of the nose, and is about the size of a pea. The pituitary gland produces a wide range of hormones that have an effect on the other glands within the endocrine system. It is regarded as a vital link between the nervous system and the endocrine system, and is under the

BELOW *The pituitary gland manufactures growth hormones, which stimulate the growth of bones and muscles, particularly in childhood. Hormone levels fluctuate throughout life.*

control of the hypothalamus, a collection of nerve cells located in the area of the brain just above the pituitary gland.

The hypothalamus receives information from the body via the nervous system, and can reply to this in two ways. It can release hormones of its own, which then act on the front (anterior) lobe of the pituitary gland, or it can stimulate the rear (posterior) lobe of the pituitary gland by nerve impulses.

In response to stimulation by the hypothalamus, both lobes of the pituitary gland release hormones of their own into the bloodstream, and these travel to the other glands making

up the endocrine system. These include the thyroid gland, the adrenal glands, the pancreas, the ovaries and the testes. Some of the hormones from the pituitary gland also have effects on organs in the body such as the kidneys.

THYROID AND PARATHYROID GLANDS

The thyroid gland sits in the neck just below the Adam's apple. It produces the hormone thyroxine, which regulates the body's metabolic rate (the speed at which it uses energy). If the thyroid gland is overactive (see *Hyperthyroidism*, pages 410–11), the heart rate speeds up; calories are burnt

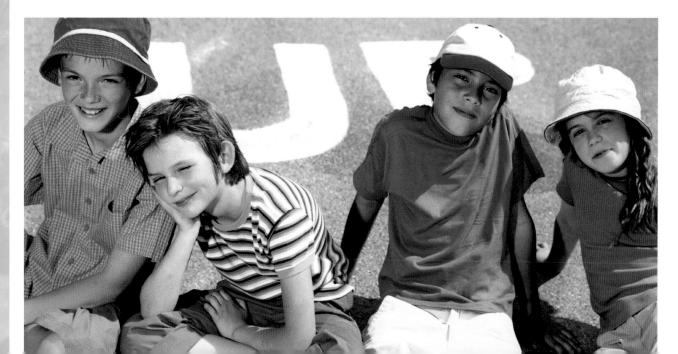

more quickly, leading to weight loss, and the person feels anxious. Under-activity results in a slowing down of physical and mental functions (see *Hypothyroidism*, page 411).

The parathyroids are two pairs of oval glands located just behind the thyroid that maintain the level of calcium in the blood. Calcium is essential for correct functioning of nerve and muscle cells, and is involved in blood clotting.

ADRENAL GLANDS

The adrenal glands rest on pads of fat above each kidney, and are about 5 cm (2 in) long. Each gland consists of an outer area called the cortex, and an inner area known as the medulla. The cortex produces the body's own natural steroids, important in the control of salt and sugar levels in the blood. The medulla is part of the sympathetic nervous system (see page 194) and produces adrenalin, a hormone that raises the pulse rate, blood pressure and blood sugar in response to stress.

PANCREAS

The endocrine portion of the pancreas is responsible for producing hormones that have an effect on the level of sugar in the blood. Insulin lowers levels by promoting the uptake of sugar into the tissues. Glucagon increases levels by stimulating sugar production in the liver. The hormones are manufactured in an area of the pancreas called the islets of Langerhans.

Other glands affected by pituitary gland hormones include the thymus, which is involved in the development of the immune system, the sex glands, and the pineal gland. The exact function of the pineal gland, which is located in the brain, is not fully understood, but it is thought to play a role in the regulation of natural body rhythms and sleep patterns via a chemical called melatonin.

How the endocrine system works

Hormones are produced by a number of glands, collectively called the endocrine system. The hypothalmus conveys information from the nervous system to the pituitary gland. Hormones are released from the pituitary gland into the bloodstream, and act on other hormone-producing glands around the body.

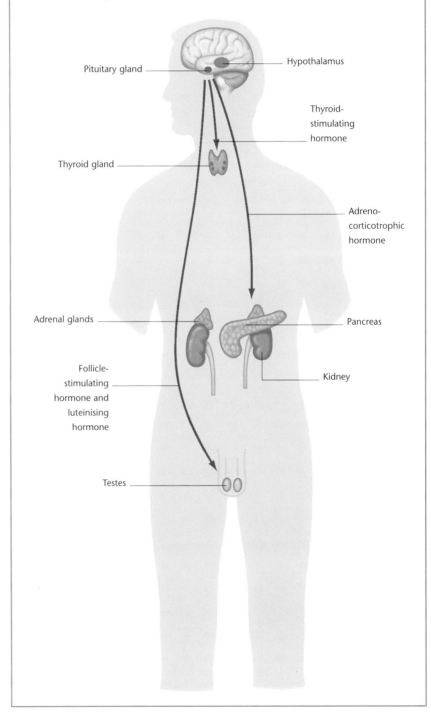

Pituitary gland

Hypothalamus

Thyroid-stimulating hormone

Thyroid gland

Adreno-corticotrophic hormone

Adrenal glands

Pancreas

Follicle-stimulating hormone and luteinising hormone

Kidney

Testes

FEMALE REPRODUCTIVE SYSTEM

The female reproductive system is a collection of structures that allows the production of eggs (ova) for fertilisation by the male, and provides a safe environment in which a fertilised egg can develop and mature. Conception occurs when the egg fuses with a male sex cell (sperm). When the foetus is fully developed, birth takes place, after a pregnancy of around nine months' duration.

AN INTERNAL SYSTEM

In contrast to the male reproductive system, the female system is mainly internal. It consists of the ovaries, uterus or womb, the Fallopian tubes, the vagina and the vulva. The breasts are also generally regarded as belonging to the reproductive system because of the role they play in breastfeeding the newborn baby.

OVARIES

The ovaries are two glands lying within the pelvic cavity next to the Fallopian tubes. Essentially, the ovaries have two roles. The first is to act as a storage centre for the female sex cells or eggs. A newborn baby girl has about 60,000 eggs present in her ovaries at birth.

Every one of these eggs has the potential to develop for fertilisation, but it is likely that during a woman's reproductive life only about 500 will ever mature. Usually, the reproductive system allows a single egg to develop for fertilisation each menstrual cycle.

The second function of the ovaries is to produce the two female hormones, oestrogen and progesterone. These hormones are essential for the development of visible sexual characteristics such as breasts and pubic hair, and they are also involved in the menstrual cycle.

UTERUS

The uterus is a muscular, hollow organ lying within the pelvis, between the bladder and the lower end of the colon. When an egg is released from an ovary, midway through a menstrual cycle, it is collected in one of the Fallopian tubes. These tubes have a funnel-like end with

numerous finger-like projections that catch the egg. The egg moves through the Fallopian tube into the upper part of the uterus.

If the egg is fertilised, it becomes embedded in the wall of the uterus, where, over the next nine months, it receives nutrients and oxygen through the placenta. During pregnancy, the uterus expands from its usual 7.5–10 cm (3–4 in) to accommodate a baby weighing around 3.2 kg (7 lb). The muscular wall thickens considerably, and during labour, the forcible

---

Structure of the breast

Breast milk is produced in glands called lobules which increase during pregnancy. Ducts collect and transport milk to the nipple.

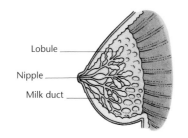

Lobule

Nipple

Milk duct

RIGHT *The main function of breasts is to provide milk for a baby. The number of milk-producing glands increases during pregnancy and after the baby is born they can produce about a litre (2 pints) of milk a day.*

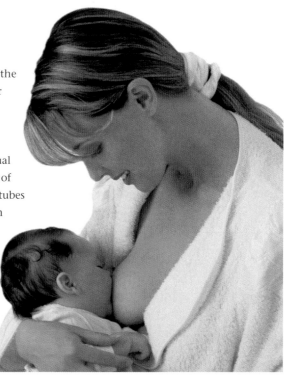

Female reproductive system

The central role of the female reproductive system is to produce eggs for fertilisation and provide a safe environment in which a baby can mature. Female sex cells (eggs or ova) are stored in the ovaries. Once a month, an egg matures and is released into the Fallopian tube in a process known as ovulation. It takes five or six days for an egg to travel along the Fallopian tube to the uterus. If the egg has been fertilised it will attach itself to the wall of the uterus and develop into a baby. If the egg has not been fertilised it will disintegrate and be expelled from the woman's body along with the lining of the uterus during menstruation.

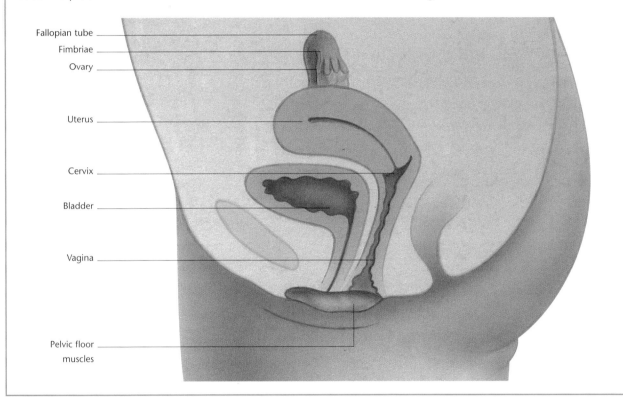

Fallopian tube
Fimbriae
Ovary
Uterus
Cervix
Bladder
Vagina
Pelvic floor muscles

contractions of these muscles lead to the birth of the baby.

The lining inside the uterus is influenced by the hormones produced by the ovaries. If the egg is not fertilised by a sperm, the lining of the uterus, along with the unfertilised egg, passes out of the woman's body during menstruation (a period).

VAGINA

The vagina is a muscular tube that extends from the neck of the uterus (the cervix) to the external genitalia or vulva. The vaginal walls have the potential to stiffen during sexual arousal as the blood supply is increased. The vagina acts as a receptacle for the penis during intercourse. Its other roles are as a canal though which the baby moves during birth, as well as a channel for the products of menstruation.

VULVA

The vulva is the collective name for a number of structures that make up the external genitalia. It comprises the major and minor labia, or lips, which enclose the vagina and the urethra. At the upper end of the vulva is the clitoris, a small, sensitive organ that corresponds to the penis in the male, and becomes engorged and swollen during sexual arousal.

BREASTS

The breasts are two milk-producing glands that protrude from the chest wall. They are present in both sexes, but are poorly developed in the male. Each breast is composed of about twenty lobes that radiate out from the nipple. These lobes contain milk-producing glands that empty through small ducts into the nipple. The main function of the breasts is to provide nourishment for newborn babies.

MALE REPRODUCTIVE SYSTEM

The male reproductive system is a collection of organs that are designed to manufacture, store and then transfer the male sex cells (sperm) to the female to fertilise her sex cells (ova). The male reproductive system is mostly external and consists of the penis and scrotum, testes, prostate gland and various tubes that connect the system. Fertilisation may occur during intercourse, when sperm are ejected from an erect penis into the female vagina.

TESTES AND SCROTUM

The testes are the male sex glands, responsible for the production of sperm and the male hormone, testosterone. They are kept cool by being suspended outside the body in the scrotum, a sac divided into two lying just below the penis. The scrotum is covered by a layer of wrinkled skin, overlying a layer of smooth muscle. The testes are located in this rather vulnerable spot because the temperature required for optimum sperm production is a few degrees lower than body temperature.

The testes produce several million sperm a day, which equates to about 12 trillion during an average lifetime. Each sperm takes around ten weeks to mature, and as many as 400 million are released during every ejaculation of semen.

EPIDIDYMIS AND VAS DEFERENS

When sperm are transported away from the testis, they enter the epididymis, a tightly coiled thin tube, approximately 6 m (20 ft) long, connected to smaller tubes within the testis. The whole structure lies on top of the testis and sperm remain here for several days.

BELOW *Puberty is the time when sexual maturity develops, caused by an increase in sex hormone activity. In boys, rapid growth takes place, the voice deepens, muscles develop, genitals grow and body hair develops.*

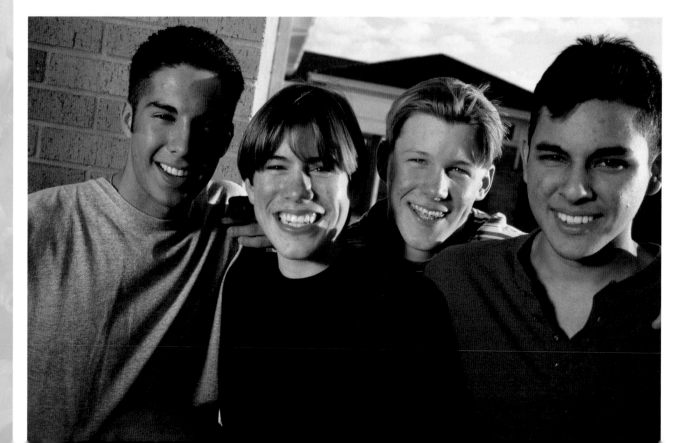

When sperm arrive in the epididymis, they are not yet fully mature, are unable to swim, and are incapable of fertilisation. While the sperm are stored in the epididymis, they receive nourishment, and by the time they leave they are fully mobile.

From the epididymis, sperm pass into a muscular tube known as the vas deferens, which follows an intricate course passing alongside the testis, then entering the abdominal cavity, before joining with small tubes from a pair of glands called the seminal vesicles. The vas deferens and the tubes from the seminal vesicles form an ejaculatory duct, which passes through the prostate gland before emptying into the urethra (see page 201).

PROSTATE GLAND

The prostate gland is just over 2.5 cm (1 in) round and lies under the bladder in front of the rectum. It surrounds the first part of the urethra, the tube leading from the bladder through which urine and semen are transported. The gland has an outer portion, which produces secretions that form part of the semen, and an inner area, which manufactures fluid that helps to keep the interior of the urethra moist.

PENIS

The penis is the main external organ of the male reproductive system, and contains three columns of spongy tissue and many blood vessels. The urethra extends through one column of spongy tissue, enlarged at the end to form a bulbous tip called the glans penis. This is extremely sensitive, and is usually covered by the foreskin until the penis becomes erect.

RIGHT *Each sperm has a long tail that enables it to swim inside the female reproductive tract so that it can reach and fertilise an egg. Sperm is produced continually from puberty onwards.*

The rest of the shaft of the penis is composed of two more columns of spongy tissue, which in turn are surrounded by tough, fibrous material, and the whole shaft is covered with skin. During sexual arousal, the spongy columns of the penis become engorged with blood, leading to an erection, whereby the penis becomes enlarged and firm. The erect penis is inserted into the female vagina, and at the moment of orgasm, semen is ejaculated from the urethra, allowing the chance of fertilisation.

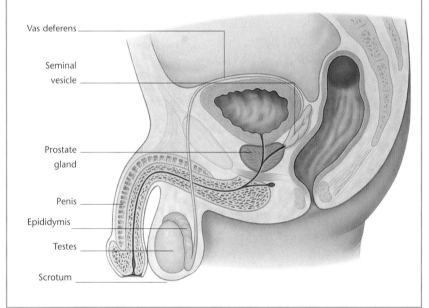

Male reproductive system

The male genitals – the penis, scrotum and testes – are externally visible but inside the body there is also an extensive network of tubes, ducts and glands that manufacture and transport sperm.

Vas deferens

Seminal vesicle

Prostate gland

Penis

Epididymis

Testes

Scrotum

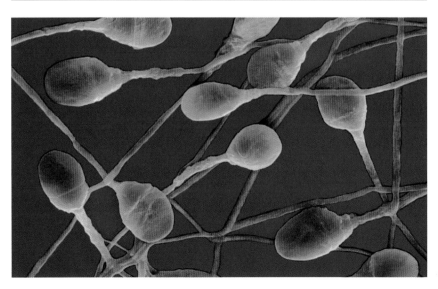

BLOOD AND THE LYMPHATIC SYSTEM

Blood flows through the arteries and veins and is the body's main means of transport. It carries oxygen from the lungs to the tissues, and transports carbon dioxide from the tissues to the lungs. Blood transfers nutrients, salts and hormones to organs, and takes waste products to the organs of excretion. The lymphatic system runs almost parallel to the circulatory system. It collects excess fluid from the tissues and returns it to the blood, and filters out foreign bodies.

BLOOD

Blood varies in colour, from bright red in the arteries to a duller red in the veins. The average adult has around 5 litres (roughly 8–9 pints) of blood. The body can replace blood volume rapidly, taking only a couple of days to make up 0.5 litre (1 pint), for example after blood donation.

COMPONENTS OF BLOOD

Blood consists of two parts: fluid and cells. Plasma is the straw-coloured fluid part and makes up about 55 per cent of the total volume of blood. The other 45 per cent consists of red and white blood cells and platelets. Plasma is mostly water but it also contains other important substances. Red blood cells, the most numerous blood cells, give blood its colour because they contain a red pigment known as haemoglobin. The main function of red blood cells is to transport oxygen around the body. White blood cells are mainly concerned with the body's defence systems, fighting off infection. There are six different types of white blood cell, each having a specific role. Platelets are about a third of the size of red blood cells and are involved in blood clotting; after an injury, they clump together to stop bleeding.

BLOOD GROUPS

Depending upon chemicals called antigens present on the surface of red blood cells, every person's blood can be grouped as either A, B, AB or O. Other chemicals in the blood, such as the Rhesus factor, further differentiate blood groups. The most common blood group is O-positive, which occurs in 38 per cent of the UK population, and the rarest is AB-negative, which occurs in 1 per cent of the population.

FORMATION OF BLOOD CELLS

Bone marrow is a soft, jelly-like substance found in the cavities of certain bones in the body, including

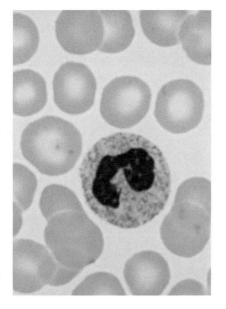

ABOVE *White blood cells are the main components of the body's immune system and there are several different types. This picture shows an eosinophil, which can ingest foreign bodies.*

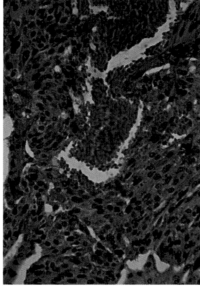

ABOVE *When a blood vessel is damaged, chemical reactions lead to the formation of a blood clot, consisting of clumped-together platelets, at the site of the wound to seal the injury.*

Composition of blood

Blood is the vehicle by which an immense variety of substances is transported around the body. It consists of red blood cells, white blood cells and platelets suspended in a liquid medium, plasma. Red blood cells transport oxygen around the body and pigments within them give blood its colour. White blood cells form part of the body's immune system and fight infection. Platelets form blood clots by clumping together and releasing chemicals that promote clotting to stop bleeding in the case of injury. Plasma consists of water, nutrients, hormones, salts and proteins.

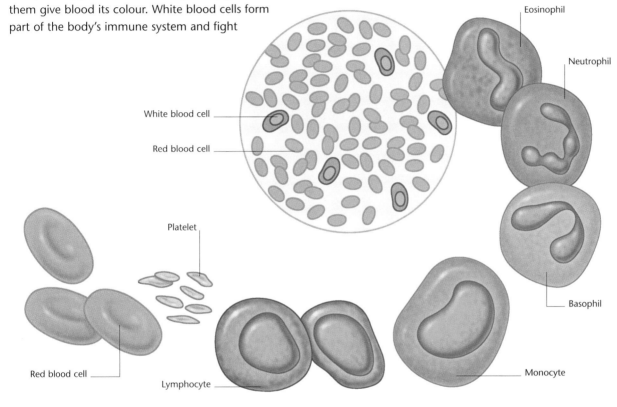

Eosinophil

Neutrophil

White blood cell

Red blood cell

Basophil

Platelet

Red blood cell

Lymphocyte

Monocyte

the pelvis, skull, breastbone, long bones of the arms and legs, ribs and back bones (vertebrae). Red and white blood cells and platelets are all manufactured in the bone marrow from a single type of cell known as a stem cell.

Whereas red blood cells have a life span of about four months, bone marrow replaces all the platelets in the blood every ten days. Red blood cells are destroyed by special white cells called macrophages, and about 180 million are broken down every minute. The iron from the destroyed cells is transported to the spleen to be recycled.

THE LYMPHATIC SYSTEM

Lymph is a milky body fluid that contains lymphocytes (white blood cells involved in fighting off infection), proteins and fats. Excess fluid that leaks out of the bloodstream is mopped up by the lymphatic system and returned to the blood via two large vessels, the right lymphatic duct and the thoracic duct, maintaining the body's fluid balance.

The lymphatic system comprises a network of lymph vessels, lymphatic tissue and lymph nodes. Its main functions are to filter out organisms

that may be causing infection, to manufacture lymphocytes, and to drain fluid and protein from the tissues to prevent them swelling. Lymph vessels have small oval structures called lymph nodes scattered along their length. Most of these are located in the neck, armpit, groin and abdomen.

The spleen, found in the upper part of the left side of the belly (abdomen), is the largest organ in the lymphatic system. It produces some white blood cells, stores blood, breaks down old red blood cells and also returns iron to the bloodstream.

IMMUNE SYSTEM

The immune system is a collection of organs, blood cells and proteins called antibodies that work together to ensure that the human body is in a position to defend itself against attack by micro-organisms such as viruses and bacteria. It comprises the thymus gland, the spleen, the bone marrow and the lymphatic system, including the lymph nodes. Without it we would not survive even the most minor infection.

PHYSICAL AND CHEMICAL PROTECTION

Although not strictly part of the immune system, the skin and the linings of the digestive and respiratory tracts provide physical and chemical protection against invading organisms. Secretions such as oil (sebum) from the skin, saliva and mucus all have an antibacterial function. In addition, the digestive system has its own colony of micro-organisms, known as intestinal flora, which helps prevent more dangerous germs from flourishing.

WHITE BLOOD CELLS

How the immune system works is an extremely complicated process, involving specialised white blood cells that can eat foreign particles, or destroy

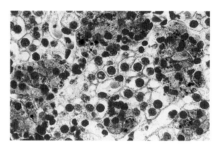

LEFT *A phagocyte is a type of white blood cell that engulfs a foreign body and destroys it.*

them with chemicals. Other white cells recognise foreign protein fingerprints on the surface of bacteria or viruses, and stimulate the production of antibodies, which stick to the surface of the invading cells, making them easier targets for destruction. Associated with this process is a number of specialised chemicals produced by the body, and which are present within the blood and tissue fluids.

The white cells involved in the immune system are manufactured in the bone marrow (see pages 208–9). Unlike red blood cells, which are carried along in the bloodstream, white blood cells are free to roam to all regions of the body to perform their function.

There are a number of different types of white blood cell within the blood, of which the most important are the lymphocytes. Around half of the lymphocytes migrate through the bloodstream to an organ called the thymus gland, situated in the neck, where they develop into T-lymphocytes, or T-cells. The remaining lymphocytes are known as B-cells. Both cell types

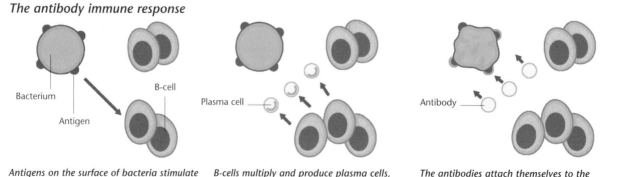

The antibody immune response

Bacterium

B-cell

Antigen

Plasma cell

Antibody

Antigens on the surface of bacteria stimulate the surface of white blood cells called B-cells.

B-cells multiply and produce plasma cells, which produce antibodies.

The antibodies attach themselves to the antigens in the bacteria, and destroy them.

travel to areas of the lymphatic system, particularly the lymph nodes and spleen, where they remain until required to spring into action.

INFLAMMATORY RESPONSE

If foreign organisms breach the body's physical and chemical barriers, the first line of defence is the inflammatory response. White blood cells known as neutrophils, or phagocytes, are often the first on the scene of an area of inflammation (characterised by redness, swelling and pain), and they literally eat invading bacteria by a process known as phagocytosis. Alternatively, some of these cells release chemicals that poison the invading germs.

ANTIBODY IMMUNE RESPONSE

B-cells can recognise proteins on the surface of foreign cells and can target invaders. These proteins are known as antigens, and the B-cells manufacture their own proteins, called antibodies, which either attach to the invader and destroy it, or act as chemical messengers to other white blood cells and chemicals in the bloodstream, leading to destruction. Some B-cells memorise the invading germ, allowing rapid reactivation of the body's defences if the infection turns up again.

T-CELLS

T-cells are not involved in direct contact with invading cells, but are still very much a part of the first-line defences. They come in three different types: killer T-cells that produce chemicals to destroy cells, helper T-cells that prod the B-cells into action, and memory T-cells, which retain a profile of the invaders to protect the body against the germ in the future. Besides their action against invading viruses, T-cells are also involved in preventing the growth of the body's own abnormal cells such as cancer cells.

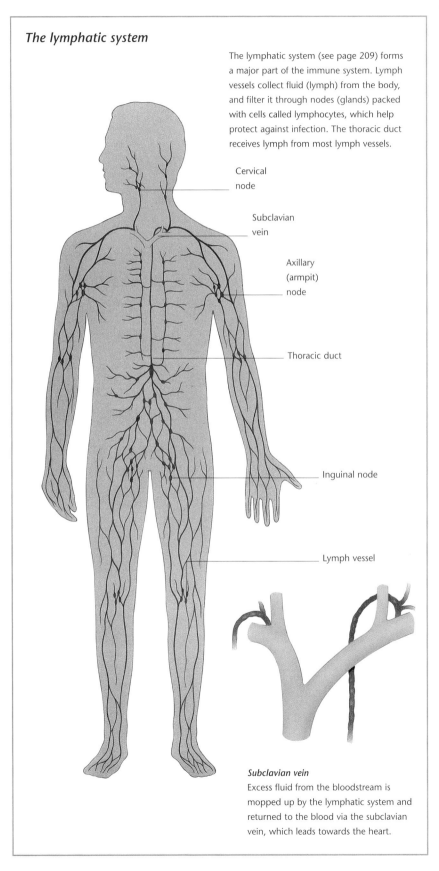

The lymphatic system

The lymphatic system (see page 209) forms a major part of the immune system. Lymph vessels collect fluid (lymph) from the body, and filter it through nodes (glands) packed with cells called lymphocytes, which help protect against infection. The thoracic duct receives lymph from most lymph vessels.

Cervical node

Subclavian vein

Axillary (armpit) node

Thoracic duct

Inguinal node

Lymph vessel

Subclavian vein
Excess fluid from the bloodstream is mopped up by the lymphatic system and returned to the blood via the subclavian vein, which leads towards the heart.

EYES AND VISION

The eyes are located in two sockets either side of the nose, and are responsible for our ability to see the outside world. Each eyeball is a roughly spherical structure with a tough outer coat known as the sclera, or white of the eye, enclosing a number of components that receive light rays, which are focused on to a light-sensitive layer. The image formed is converted into electrical signals that travel along the optic nerves to the part of the brain responsible for sight.

EYEBALL AND EYELIDS

The eye is filled with a combination of watery and jelly-like fluids to prevent it collapsing in on itself. Eyes are protected by eyelids, which can close together to prevent harmful objects entering the eye, and by tears, produced in tear glands located above each eyeball. Tears wash away dust and dirt, and contain an antibacterial ingredient that helps to prevent infection. Eye movement is controlled by three pairs of muscles attached to the white of the eye, which allow it to rotate.

CORNEA

The cornea is a transparent window joined to the edges of the white of the eye. It bulges forward slightly and lets light enter the front of the eye. The cornea is transparent because it contains virtually no cells or blood vessels; it begins the process of focusing light rays.

IRIS

The coloured part of the eye is the iris, which has a black opening in its centre known as the pupil. The iris contains muscles that enable it to control the amount of light entering the eye by contracting or relaxing, thereby altering the size of the pupil. This is a very important role, as the light-sensitive part of the eye is susceptible to damage by bright light.

LENS

Lying immediately behind the iris is the main focusing apparatus of the eye, the lens. The lens has an outer, elastic capsule that is held in place by a number of slender fibres known as suspensory ligaments. These are connected to the ciliary body, which forms an internal ring around the front chamber of the eye. The actions of muscles within the ciliary body alter the shape of the lens, allowing focusing on distant and near objects in rapid succession.

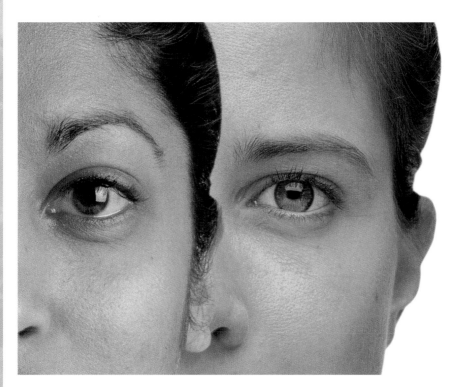

LEFT *The coloured part of the eye, the iris, gets its appearance from the number of pigments it contains – brown eyes have significantly more pigments than blue eyes.*

RETINA

Behind the lens is a gel-filled cavity that comprises most of the eye. Lining the inside of the back of the eye is the retina, where the light rays focused by the cornea and lens are received. Here, light-sensitive cells, called rods and cones because of their shape, convert light into electrical signals in a pattern corresponding to the visual matter.

Rods are sensitive to low levels of light but produce an image in grey only, whereas cones perceive colours and fine detail. The most sensitive area on the retina is the macula, where the central part of the image forms.

OPTIC NERVE AND VISUAL CORTEX

Nerve fibres leave the retina in a huge bundle at the optic disc, where they enter the optic nerve. This transmits a slightly different image from each eye to the part of the brain responsible for sight (the visual cortex at the back of the brain), where the images are combined and interpreted to provide a three-dimensional picture. The brain is able to process this highly complex information without conscious thought.

Visual pathways

Electrical signals from the retina travel along the optic nerves to the brain. Each eye sees an object from a slightly different angle and the brain receives two views, which it integrates into a complete picture.

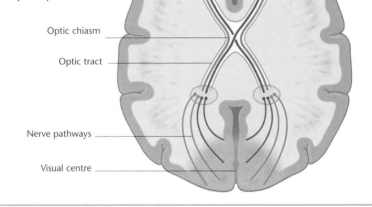

Optic nerve

Optic chiasm

Optic tract

Nerve pathways

Visual centre

Action of the pupil in daylight and darkness

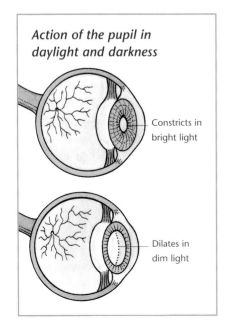

Constricts in bright light

Dilates in dim light

Structure of the eye

Each eyeball has a tough outer coat (sclera). The cornea lets light enter the eye, the amount controlled by the pupil, and the lens focuses rays. The retina converts light into electrical signals and transmits these to the brain.

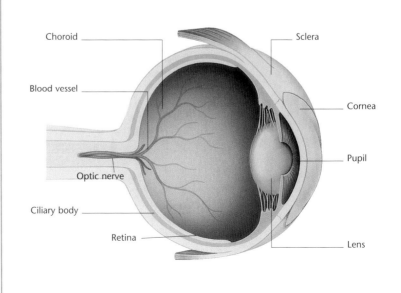

Choroid

Blood vessel

Optic nerve

Ciliary body

Retina

Sclera

Cornea

Pupil

Lens

EARS, HEARING AND BALANCE

The ears are incredibly versatile organs that have a dual function, providing our sense of hearing, as well as allowing us to maintain our balance. The ear is divided into three areas: the outer, middle and inner ear. The outer and middle ears are responsible for collecting and transmitting sound waves to the inner ear, where the sounds are analysed and interpreted. The inner ear also contains the structures concerned with balance.

OUTER EAR

The outer ear gathers and channels sound to the interior part of the ear. It consists of the pinna or auricle, a funnel-like structure that is the only visible part of the ear, and the ear canal. The auricle is composed of cartilage and folds of skin, and funnels sound waves into the entrance of the ear canal.

The ear canal is about 2.5 cm (1 in) long, and its entrance is guarded by a number of stiff hairs that help prevent larger objects entering the canal. The skin inside the canal produces wax from specialised sweat glands, which gives further protection against foreign bodies. Stretched across the inner end of the ear canal is a circular, taut piece of fibrous tissue covered in a thin layer of skin, called the eardrum or tympanic membrane. Sound waves travel down the ear canal to the eardrum. Changes in air pressure triggered by sound waves cause the eardrum to vibrate, transmitting sounds to the middle ear.

MIDDLE EAR

Separated from the outer ear by the eardrum, the middle ear is a tiny cavity that contains the three smallest bones in the human body. This chain of bones is linked to form the ossicles, each bone named according to its shape. Lying against the inner surface of the eardrum is the hammer (malleus), which transmits vibrations to the anvil (incus), and finally to the third in the chain, the stirrup (stapes). These bones amplify the sound so that the last bone, the stapes, pushes against a tiny membrane, called the oval window, which lies in the wall dividing the middle and inner ear.

Leading from the middle ear to the throat is a passageway called the Eustachian tube, which allows air pressure on either side of the eardrum to be equalised by swallowing. This is essential for normal hearing.

INNER EAR

The inner ear is a complex system of linked structures buried deep within the bones of the skull. It consists of a network of tubes and chambers called the labyrinth. The first part of the

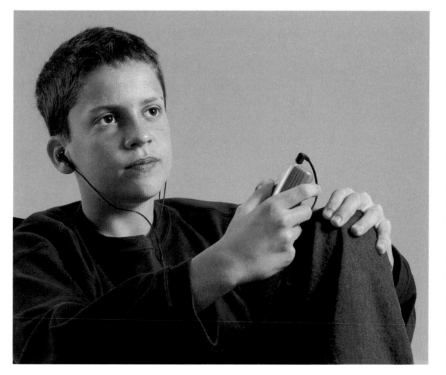

LEFT *The loudness of the sounds we hear depends upon the power of the sound waves, which is measured in decibels (dB). Even brief exposure to noises over 120 dB can damage hearing.*

Structure of the ear

The ear contains separate organs of hearing and balance. Sound waves travel from the outer ear along the ear canal to the eardrum. In the middle ear, vibrations from the eardrum are transmitted by three tiny bones – the malleus, incus and stapes – called the ossicles. In the inner ear, the cochlea contains the receptor for hearing. Balance is also controlled by the inner ear, where three semi-circular canals monitor the smallest changes in movement.

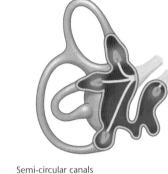

Semi-circular canals

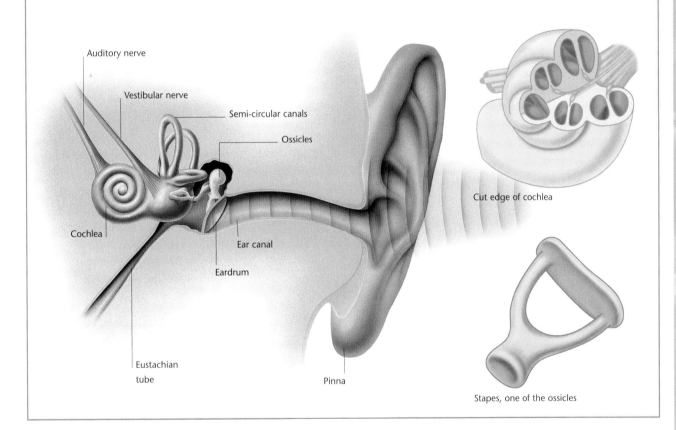

Auditory nerve

Vestibular nerve

Semi-circular canals

Ossicles

Cochlea

Ear canal

Eardrum

Eustachian tube

Pinna

Cut edge of cochlea

Stapes, one of the ossicles

labyrinth, the cochlea, is concerned with hearing; the second part, the vestibular apparatus, is responsible for maintaining balance.

Once the stirrup pushes against the oval window, pressure waves are transmitted to the cochlea, a fluid-filled tube that is coiled around so that it resembles a snail's shell. Inside the cochlea are thousands of sound-sensing hair cells projecting from a membrane.

Sound waves moving through the thick fluid within the cochlea cause specific parts of the membrane to vibrate, depending on the number of vibrations per second (the sound frequency). The hair cells are linked to nerve fibres that transmit electrical signals along the auditory nerve to the part of the brain responsible for interpreting sound.

The second, larger part of the inner ear is the vestibular apparatus, made

up of three semi-circular canals, and the vestibule, comprising two fluid-filled sacs. Their main function is to maintain balance, as well as coordinating eye and head movement. Once again, the structures are filled with sensitive hairs that can detect movement and determine the head's orientation – where it is in space. The vestibular structures are linked to the brain by the eighth cranial nerve.

FIVE SENSES

The human body is capable of experiencing many thousands of different sensations through the five major senses of sight, smell, taste, hearing and touch. Many of our most pleasurable moments, along with some of our worst experiences, are due to our perception of our surroundings through the nervous system's interactions with the environment.

SMELL

Smell is one of the chemical senses, the other being taste. Smells are detected in the nose, as air is drawn in through the nostrils during the action of inhalation. The roof of each nostril is lined with mucous membrane containing about five million olfactory or smell receptor cells, capable of distinguishing more than 10,000 different odours. Nerve fibres from these receptors pass through minute holes in the skull to the olfactory bulb, the end of the olfactory nerve. From here, olfactory nerves transmit electrical signals carrying information gathered by the nose to the brain.

The sense of smell has a number of functions. It allows for continuous sampling of the air breathed in to determine immediate danger, for example, detecting smoke. Smell can also detect danger over long distances, acting as an early warning system. Smell is intimately involved in our appreciation of food and our interaction with each other (everyone has an individual odour). Emotions such as fear, excitement, sexual arousal and our memories of events can all be communicated by smell.

TASTE

Taste is the other chemical sense, detected by special structures known as taste-buds. The majority of these are located on the tongue, lying in recessed pits, with a few on the back of the throat and the roof of the mouth. Each bud contains sensory receptor cells, on which tiny hairs generate nerve impulses that travel to the part of the brain concerned with interpreting taste. There are approximately 10,000 taste-buds, capable of detecting four basic tastes: bitter, sweet, sour and salt. Each of these types of receptor is located on a particular part of the tongue. Sweet and salt receptors are mainly on the tip of the tongue, sour tastes are mostly picked up on the sides and bitter is towards the

The olfactory system

When scent molecules are inhaled and enter the nose they are absorbed by tiny filaments called olfactory receptors. Nerve fibres from these filaments stimulate the olfactory bulb, which then transmits electrical signals along the olfactory nerve to the centres of smell in the brain.

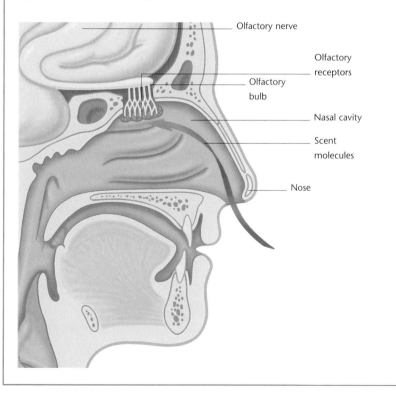

Olfactory nerve

Olfactory receptors

Olfactory bulb

Nasal cavity

Scent molecules

Nose

Sensory receptors in the skin

Sensory nerve receptors are found all over the body but most are in the skin. They detect touch, pain, pressure, vibration and temperature, sending messages about them to the brain.

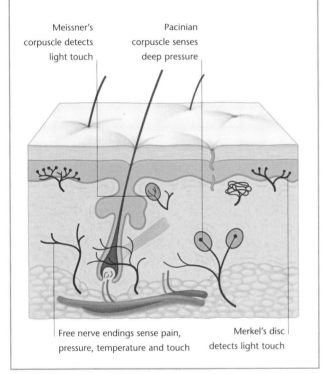

Meissner's corpuscle detects light touch

Pacinian corpuscle senses deep pressure

Free nerve endings sense pain, pressure, temperature and touch

Merkel's disc detects light touch

Taste-buds

Food and drink dissolved in saliva comes into contact with taste-buds on the tongue. Each bud contains tiny hairs that generate electrical signals which travel to the part of the brain that interprets taste.

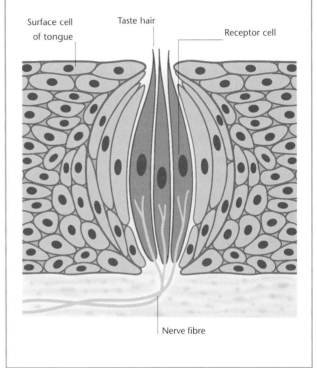

Surface cell of tongue

Taste hair

Receptor cell

Nerve fibre

back. All tastes are a combination of the four basic tastes. Much of our perception of taste depends on our sense of smell, which is thousands of times more sensitive than taste.

HEARING

The ears are the organs responsible for conveying sounds from the outside world to the area of the brain responsible for their interpretation. The outer ear gathers sound waves and funnels them to the eardrum, which vibrates to transmit information through the three small bones of the middle ear to the cochlea in the inner ear. The cochlea is the organ where sounds are heard. Information from the cochlea is converted into electrical signals and passed on to the brain, where sound appreciation takes place. Rather like smell, hearing can act as a warning system, as well as allowing us to recall pleasurable memories and emotions. See also *Ears, Hearing and Balance*, pages 214–15.

SIGHT

Sight depends upon the reception of light rays from objects by receptor cells on the retina of the eye. The two types of receptor cells are rods and cones. Rods are responsible mainly for night vision. Cones detect one of the three basic colours – red, blue or green – and provide detailed and colour vision. A slightly different image is received from each eye, allowing the brain to give a three-dimensional image with depth of field and contrast. For more information on sight, see *Eyes and Vision*, pages 212–13.

TOUCH

The whole surface of the skin is covered by millions of nerve endings, the most sensitive areas being the fingertips, the areas around the lips and eyes, and the nipples. In humans, touch sensitivity is particularly high on hairy parts of the body, such as the face and genitals.

Different types of nerves pick up heat, cold, pain, light and heavy pressure (or touch), and convey the sensations via electrical signals that travel through the spinal nerves to the brain and spinal cord.

SKIN, HAIR AND NAILS

The skin is the largest organ in the human body, and covers the whole of the body, protecting its inner organs and tissues from the outside environment and helping to regulate body temperature. Hair and nails, protective plates that cover the ends of the fingers and toes, grow from the skin and provide extra protection from the outside world.

SKIN

Making up about 12 per cent of the body's weight, the skin is a waterproof barrier and has an average surface area of about 2 m² (11 ft²). It consists of two connected layers, the inner one being the dermis and the outer one the epidermis. The skin is a living organ and its cells are replaced continually, moving up to the surface as the outermost cells are lost through normal wear and tear.

The epidermis is made up of dead skin cells that are packed with a tough protective protein called keratin. It also contains the skin pigment melanin, which protects us from the harmful effect of ultraviolet light. The dead cells that are lost from the epidermis are the main component of house dust.

The dermis is a thick, durable tissue that is rich in blood vessels and nerves, and also contains sweat glands and hair follicles. The skin's nerves can sense a multitude of stimuli and provide us with our sense of touch. Sweat glands help to keep the body cool and produce a slightly salty secretion (sweat) that helps to reduce the number of bacteria on the skin. The skin also contains sebaceous glands that produce oils to maintain the suppleness of the skin.

The depth of the dermis and epidermis varies in different parts of the body, being thickest on the soles of

How hair grows

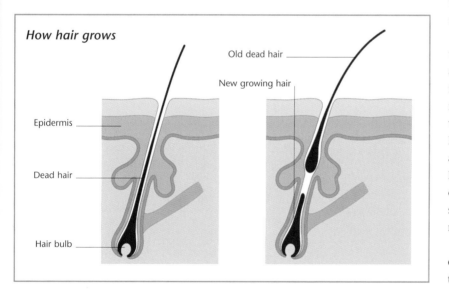

Old dead hair

New growing hair

Epidermis

Dead hair

Hair bulb

Nail structure and growth

Nails are formed from keratin, the tough protein that also makes up hair and skin. They grow from the matrix, which lies beneath a fold of skin (the cuticle). The growing nail slides forward over the nail-bed, an area rich in blood vessels.

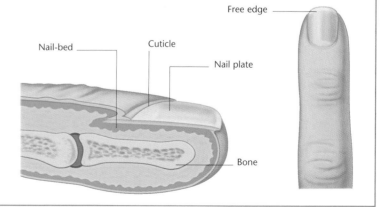

Free edge

Nail-bed

Cuticle

Nail plate

Bone

the feet and the palms of the hands. It is thinnest on the eyelids, where flexibility and lightness are necessary. The surface of the dermis is uneven, pushing up into the epidermis to create ridges in the skin. These are most pronounced on the fingertips where they are arranged in a swirling pattern, creating fingerprints that are unique to a particular individual.

Underneath the dermis, and not strictly part of the skin, is a layer of fatty tissue that provides insulation, acts as a source of energy in times when food is not available and cushions the body's organs against the shocks of everyday movement.

HAIR

All hairs develop from a group of cells at the bottom of a tube-like depression in the skin called a hair follicle. As these cells grow, they move away from the base of the follicle, and as they lose contact with the blood vessels that supply the follicle, they die. The remains of these epidermal cells constitute the shaft of a hair.

Each hair follicle has a sebaceous gland that produces oils to help keep the skin supple. In addition, all hair follicles have a tiny bundle of smooth muscle fibres attached, known as the arrector pili muscle, which contracts to cause the hair to stand upright in the follicle under certain conditions. This gives rise to goose bumps.

Only a few areas of the body's surface are completely hairless – the palms of the hands, the soles of the feet, the lips, nipples and some parts of the external genitalia. Thousands of years ago humans needed thick body hair to keep warm, but this has been lost over time.

NAILS

In a similar fashion to hair, nails are formed from dead epidermal cells and consist of the tough protein keratin. They cover the end of each digit to prevent injury. Nails develop from an active growth layer known as the nail-bed and are pushed out from under a fold of skin known as the cuticle. Fingernails take about six months to grow, whereas toe-nails take twice as long. Medical, nutritional and physical problems can cause changes to the colour, thickness or shape of the nails.

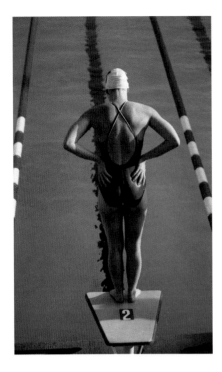

RIGHT *Special blood vessels in the skin help to regulate body temperature. If the body is too cold, the blood vessels narrow and the arrector pili muscles contract, pulling on the skin to to form goose bumps. The erect hairs trap an insulating layer of air next to the skin. Skin itself is waterproof and a layer of fat underneath it provides extra insulation.*

Structure of the skin

The skin consists of an outer layer of dead cells that is constantly shed, called the epidermis; and a strong, elastic tissue containing blood vessels and nerve endings, called the dermis. The skin is cooled by sweat released from sweat glands in the dermis.

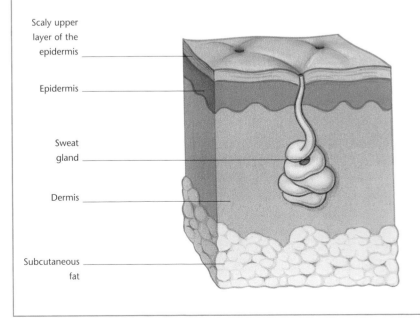

Scaly upper layer of the epidermis

Epidermis

Sweat gland

Dermis

Subcutaneous fat

LOOK AFTER YOURSELF

Your health is greatly influenced by your lifestyle. The Ancient Greeks recognised that how people lived was connected to how they felt and the illnesses they developed, and today this link is even clearer. Most people understand that to enjoy a healthy lifestyle they must not smoke; should drink alcohol only in moderation; should exercise regularly; and must eat a balanced diet that is low in fat, high in fibre and includes plenty of fresh fruit and vegetables. Putting this advice into practice can be difficult. Furthermore, the stresses and strains of modern living can seriously affect physical and mental well-being.

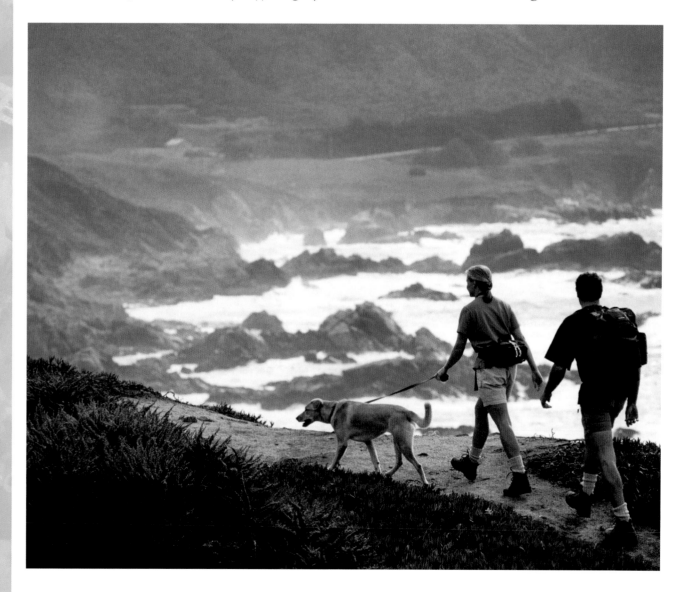

DIET

Study after study has shown that many different diseases are linked to what you eat and drink. The basic advice on diet has remained unchanged for many years: fresh fruit and vegetables and carbohydrate-rich foods should form the bulk of the diet, with moderate amounts of protein and fats. You should also include plenty of water in your diet. Most people in the UK eat too much food, especially too much fat, sugar and salt.

FITNESS

Next to diet, exercise is the most important factor in leading a long and healthy life. Research has shown that people who exercise regularly live longer and are less at risk of developing long-term disease than those who do not. Regular exercise is beneficial for physical and mental health; it improves the efficiency of your breathing, helps to keep you flexible and mobile and promotes feelings of well-being by increasing the production of chemical compounds known as endorphins that act as natural antidepressants. You do not need to exercise for hours every week to get these health benefits. Being moderately active for half an hour a day, or for an hour every other day, is enough. Exercise by playing a sport, going to the gym or taking a brisk walk, or through vigorous activity such as energetic housework, which burns up as many calories as water aerobics.

RIGHT *Meditation is one form of stress-beating relaxation. Focusing your mind brings calm, enabling your muscles to become less tense and your blood pressure to drop.*

LEFT *Walking is a form of exercise that benefits both the body and mind. It can be enjoyed by people of all ages and can range from a gentle stroll to an invigorating hike.*

ABOVE *Food is essential for good health and you need to choose fresh, nutritious food to obtain the maximum number of nutrients. Choose lean types of protein such as fish and bulk out meals with plenty of vegetables.*

STRESS

Stress is a physical or mental demand that causes the body to become flooded with stress hormones that produce physical changes in the body, such as a pounding heart, sweating and tense muscles. A certain degree of stress is not necessarily a bad thing: it provides the spur to achieve, for example. But when stress is long-term, it can cause you to experience symptoms such as headaches and feelings of anxiety, even when the source of stress is not there. The best way to get the better of stress is either to change your circumstances or the way you feel about them. If what is making you stressed cannot be changed, you will find it easier to deal with if you develop new interests in other parts of your life.

RELAXATION

Relaxation is a set of easily learned skills that enable you to reduce the physical and mental effects of stress and enhance your well-being. Everyone can benefit from learning how to relax. When you are relaxed, your mind becomes calm, your blood pressure goes down, and all your muscles become less tense. There are many different relaxation techniques, including controlled breathing, yoga and meditation. Just lying down in a quiet, darkened room and tensing and relaxing all your muscles from your head to your toes is one of the best and simplest methods. Another technique is to spend a few minutes imagining yourself in a beautiful, peaceful place.

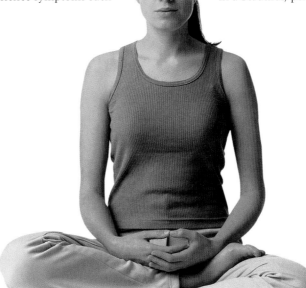

FOODS FOR FITNESS

Healthy eating should not just be a New Year's resolution but something you enjoy doing every day. In our society, many people are eating their way to serious illnesses such as diabetes, many cancers, digestive system disorders, and heart and circulatory diseases. Obesity can also cause mental distress. Eating the right foods will make you look better, feel healthier, avoid many illnesses and probably even live longer – recent government statistics indicate that obesity, on average, shortens life by nine years.

SENSIBLE EATING

A balanced diet that is low in fat, high in fibre and contains plenty of whole grains and fruit and vegetables will give you all the energy and nutrients you need. Cutting down on foods that are high in fat, such as meat and dairy products, and sugars, while boosting your intake of rice, pasta, bread, pulses and fresh fruit and vegetables will help you avoid a number of different diseases.

PLAN FOR HEALTH

When you switch to a healthier diet, it will take time to get used to a new way of eating. Your aim is to replace a high-calorie, high-fat diet with new, healthy habits. Start by keeping a record of what you eat, counting the portions of fruit and vegetables you have every day. You will also need to get to know what nutritionists mean by a portion: it is probably smaller than you are used to. Try new foods, particularly fruits, vegetables, grains and pulses, and change the way you cook, steaming or grilling food rather than frying. For a while, you will have to make a conscious effort to change, but soon you will have the healthy eating habit.

VITAMINS COUNT

Many people worry that they are not getting enough vitamins and minerals. If you do not eat at least five servings of fruit and vegetables every day, or if you always eat the same ones, you may not be. Choose green, orange and yellow fruit and vegetables (broccoli, carrots, sweet potatoes, melons and oranges, for example) because they contain antioxidants and other nutrients that seem to help fight cancer and illness. Women need a lot of iron and calcium and if they cannot obtain these from the foods they eat, they may need to take supplements.

LEFT *As well as being sweet and delicious, fruit is full of fibre, vitamins, minerals and carbohydrates. Nutritionists recommend that you eat two to four servings of fruit a day.*

WATER

If you are what you eat, then make sure you drink lots of water because it comprises 70 per cent of your body. Water takes nutrients to the cells and removes waste products. You need to drink at least 2 litres (3½ pints) of water a day just to replace what is lost in urine, bowel movements, exhaled breath and sweat. Drinks such as coffee and tea, although they contain water, are not as good as drinking plain water because they contain diuretics which make you excrete water. It is almost impossible to drink too much water.

Eat smart

• Eat a low-fat, high-fibre cereal with skimmed milk and fruit instead of a cooked breakfast.
• Eat a variety of fruit and vegetables every day.
• Use meat in small quantities as a topping, rather than making it the main dish at mealtimes.
• Stock up on healthy snacks: snacking is not bad for you, as long as the snacks are nutritious and low in fat.
• Make two or three healthy changes to your diet, such as using semi-skimmed instead of full-fat milk or switching from butter to low-fat margarine.
• Increase the amount of fibre in your diet by choosing whole grains and eating fruit and vegetable peel where possible.
• Eat smaller portions and do not have seconds: if you wait ten minutes you will probably find that you are full.
• Eat regular meals. People tend to overeat if they go for long periods without food.

Healthy eating

The amount of food you need to eat each day depends on your age, sex and activity levels. Carbohydrates should form the bulk of the diet.

CARBOHYDRATES About 60 per cent of the diet should be made up of carbohydrates, such as bread, cereal, rice and pasta, for example. Carbohydrates make you feel full and provide energy. Adults need between 6–11 servings of these foods each day. One serving equates to 1 slice of bread, 28 g (1 oz) dry cereal or 100 g (3½ oz) cooked rice, pasta or pulses.

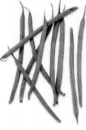

VITAMINS AND MINERALS Fruit and vegetables contain vitamins and minerals that are essential for good health. They are also a good source of carbohydrates. Eating a wide variety of fruit and vegetables ensures that you get all the nutrients you need. You should aim for two to four servings of fruit and three to five servings of vegetables a day. One serving equates to 1 medium apple, 175 ml (6 fl oz) of fruit or vegetable juice, 15 grapes, 1 medium baked potato or 140 g (5 oz) of raw vegetables.

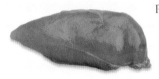

PROTEINS Protein is essential for building and repairing cells in the body and needs to be eaten daily. Excess protein is converted into fat. Everyone needs about two or three servings a day of protein, which is found in meat, poultry, fish, eggs, nuts and pulses, but most of us eat more than that. A serving equals 60–90 g (2–3 oz) of cooked lean meat or fish, 100g (3½ oz) cooked pulses or 1 egg.

FATS Although fats are essential, no more than 30 per cent of your daily calorie intake should come from fats. At 9 calories per gram, fat has more than double the calories of carbohydrates or protein. Switch to low-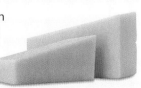fat dairy products and healthier fats, such as sunflower or olive oil. Avoid animal fats, which contain saturated fat and are bad for your heart. Try to limit your intake of foods that are high in cholesterol (see page 230), such as shellfish and eggs.

CARBOHYDRATES

Most of the foods you eat should be carbohydrates, also called starches and sugars. These foods give you long-lasting energy, as well as fibre, vitamins, minerals and sometimes protein. Carbohydrates are found in starchy foods such as rice, bread, pasta, potatoes, pulses, cereals, flour and sugars. They are divided into two groups: simple carbohydrates or sugars, and complex carbohydrates, made up of starches and dietary fibre.

SOURCES OF CARBOHYDRATES

Carbohydrates include most of the food you eat every day, from orange juice, breakfast cereal and toast in the morning, to the bread in your sandwich at lunch, to the vegetables that accompany your meat at dinner, to the biscuit you have with a cup of tea before bed. Almost all foods contain some carbohydrates, but plant foods have the highest amounts. Dairy products are also rich in carbohydrates.

WHAT CARBOHYDRATES DO

Carbohydrates provide energy. Inside the body, carbohydrates are broken down into blood sugar (glucose). This sugar is carried throughout the body in the bloodstream to all body cells, where it provides energy for cell growth and repair. What cannot be used by the body immediately is stored in the liver and muscles as glycogen. When more energy is required, the body can quickly convert glycogen to glucose. However, the muscles and liver can store very little glycogen, so any excess sugar is converted and stored as fat. This can be broken down later to give energy, but if it is not needed it remains in the body as excess weight.

Complex carbohydrates also contain vitamins, minerals and fibre. Vitamins and minerals are absorbed into the bloodstream and ensure continuing good health, while fibre, which has no calories because it cannot be absorbed by the body, keeps the digestive system healthy and is passed out as waste.

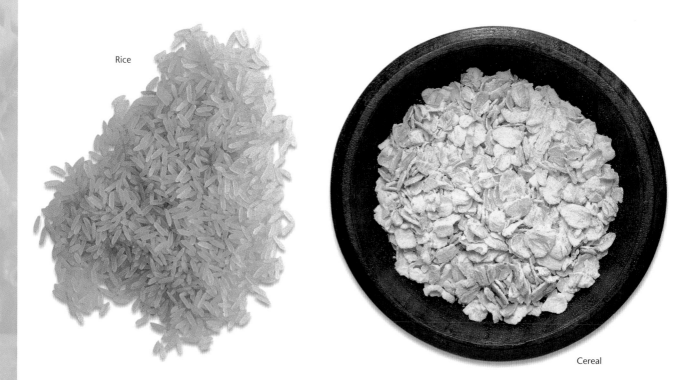

Rice

Cereal

CARBOHYDRATES AND WEIGHT CONTROL

Perhaps because carbohydrates can be turned into fat, many people believe that carbohydrates will make you fat, and that to lose weight, you should cut out bread and potatoes and eat high-protein foods like meat instead. In fact, carbohydrates can help you lose weight, so long as you do not add extra fat to them. A 140 g (5 oz) baked potato has fewer calories than an 85 g (3 oz) lean steak: the potato has no fat but even lean meat contains some fat.

ALL CARBOHYDRATES ARE NOT THE SAME

As well as being generally more nutritious than simple carbohydrates, some complex carbohydrates are better for you than others. The difference lies in the amount of vitamins and minerals as well as fibre that is in the carbohydrate. Wholegrain products are more nutritious than refined products because they contain the bran and the germ. Refined foods are quick to digest, leaving you feeling hungry sooner, while unrefined grains are digested slowly and provide sustained energy. If you drink water with your meals, the fibre will swell in your stomach, making you feel even fuller.

Daily carbohydrate intake

Nutritionists recommend obtaining 60 per cent of your daily calorific intake from carbohydrates, but most people in the UK get only 40 per cent, of which too high a proportion comes from sugary foods. Eating more complex carbohydrates will give you more vitamins, nutrients and fibre while making you too full for fatty, sugary snacks.

6–11 servings of grains (of which at least 3 should be whole grains)
2–4 servings of fruit
3–5 servings of vegetables
2–3 servings of dairy products

SEE BOX ON HEALTHY EATING, PAGE 223, FOR INFORMATION ABOUT SERVINGS.

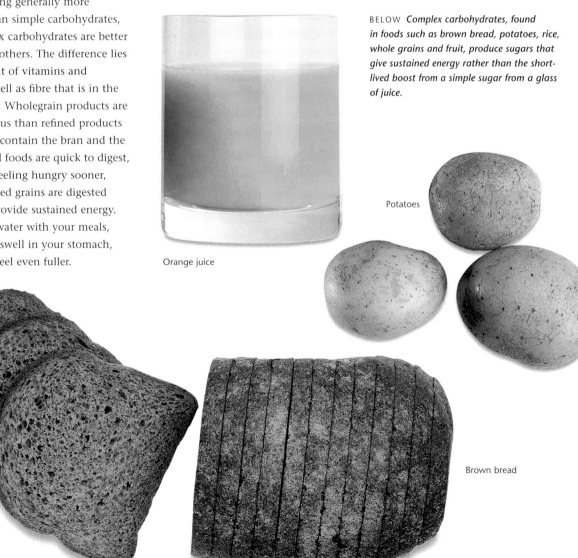

BELOW *Complex carbohydrates, found in foods such as brown bread, potatoes, rice, whole grains and fruit, produce sugars that give sustained energy rather than the short-lived boost from a simple sugar from a glass of juice.*

Orange juice

Potatoes

Brown bread

SUGAR

Sugar is a carbohydrate found in foods such as milk, fruit and honey, as well as in sweets and desserts. Sugar has a bad reputation, and can cause tooth decay and weight gain, but some foods that are high in sugar, such as milk and fruit, are very good for you because they contain vitamins and minerals as well as sugar. Where sugar deserves its bad reputation is in the so-called empty calories it contains – those that come without beneficial nutrients. A piece of fruit might have the equivalent of a teaspoon of sugar, but since it also contains vitamins, minerals and fibre, the calories it contains are far from empty.

SUGAR CONSUMPTION

People in the developed world are eating more sugar than they did in the past. For example, people in the UK now get 17 per cent of their calories from sugar, as opposed to about 10 per cent only 20 years ago. Carbonated (fizzy) soft drinks such as cola account for one-third of the added sugar in some people's diets.

SUGAR AND TOOTH DECAY

Refined sugar is the major, but not the only, cause of tooth decay. Other sugars, such as those from fruit or milk, also play a role. The enzymes in your saliva turn starch to sugar, so even bread becomes sweet as you chew it. The longer sweet foods stay in your mouth and the more they stick to your teeth, the worse they are for the teeth. Foods such as raisins are just as bad for dental health as sweets like caramels. If you consume sweet, sticky foods, rinse your mouth with water or brush your teeth afterwards.

READ THE LABEL

Sugar comes in many different forms, both naturally and as refined products. All sugar is the same: brown sugar is no

Getting the best from sugar

Sugar is an excellent source of energy, but be sure that you are eating your sugar in a nutritious package such as fruit, not as empty calories like a soft drink.

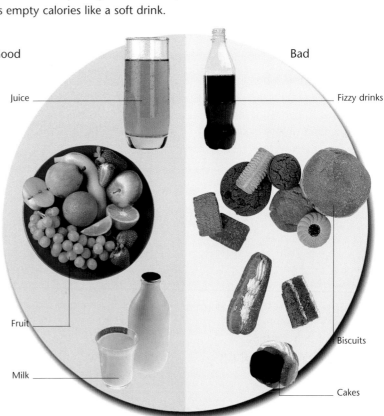

Good

Bad

Juice

Fizzy drinks

Fruit

Biscuits

Milk

Cakes

RIGHT *A sweet tooth is usually acquired in childhood, and although a link between hyperactivity and sugar has not been proven, sugar is bad for dental health.*

better for you than white sugar, nor is honey any better than table sugar. Processed foods often contain sugar, even if you cannot see it listed in the ingredients. It might be hidden under a different name: barley malt, brown sugar, cane sugar, corn sweetener, corn syrup, dextrose, fructose, glucose, honey, invert sugar, lactose, maltose, maple syrup, sorbitol or sucrose.

Artificial sweeteners

Over the years there have been many cancer scares involving artificial sweeteners. In tests on laboratory animals some artificial sweeteners caused cancers, leading to a ban on cyclamates and to health warnings about saccharine. But later studies showed that people who used these products did not have any more cancers than the general population. Pregnant women, however, should not use saccharine. Aspartame is another sweetener and, although there have been health scares, it is generally considered to be safe. You should take artificial sweeteners in moderation: if there are any health risks they are most likely to apply to heavy users, such as people who drink lots of diet drinks. Bear in mind that artificial sweeteners perpetuate a sweet tooth.

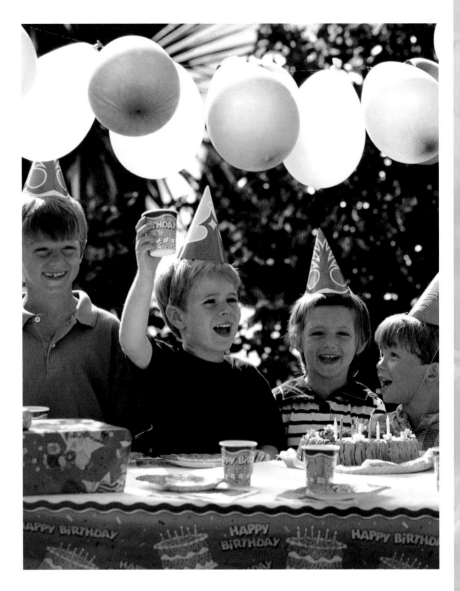

Does sugar make children hyperactive?

Anyone who has ever seen children running around at a birthday party might think they were high on sugar, but research has not shown any link between eating sugar and hyperactivity. It is the excitement of the party, not the sugar rush, that gets children going. Only about 1 child in 100 is affected by sugar. If you think that your child is affected, ban all sugar for three days, then give your child a sweet snack and watch what happens over the next 2–3 hours. If there is no really dramatic change in your child's behaviour, sugar is not a problem. Most studies show that, far from making children hyperactive, eating lots of sugar makes them sleepy.

PROTEIN

Protein is one of the body's essential building blocks and must be obtained daily from food as it is not stored in the body. The amino acids found in protein build, repair and maintain body tissue. But although protein is essential, you only need a relatively small amount to stay healthy. A small chicken breast about the size of a deck of cards contains all the protein you require. Most of us eat much more protein than this, which does no harm and is simply excreted from the body in urine. However, what is harmful are the saturated fats that often come with protein-rich foods. Even lean minced beef contains some saturated fat.

SOURCES OF PROTEIN

A wide variety of foods contain protein. Protein-rich foods include meat, poultry, fish, eggs, dairy products such as milk, cheese and yogurt, pulses and soya products, seeds (such as sunflower, pumpkin and sesame) and nuts (including peanuts, almonds and cashews). Some vegetables and all grains also contain protein. With so many sources to choose from, protein deficiency in people who eat a varied diet is highly unusual.

MAKING LOW-FAT PROTEIN CHOICES

The problem with protein is that protein from animal sources also contains fat, particularly saturated fat. To eat healthily, the protein-packed foods you eat should be low in fat.

When shopping for meat, choose low-fat cuts and trim off all visible fat. Take the skin off poultry – most fat is under the skin. White meat is lower in fat than red meat. When choosing mince, read the label and buy the leanest variety. To help cut down on fat why not try using recipes that normally call for beef or lamb, but substitute turkey, which is much lower in fat. Because turkey is less fatty, it is also drier, so you will need to add more of a low-fat tomato sauce or gravy to your recipe or finished dish.

By choosing low-fat dairy products, you can enjoy the benefits of dairy products (in addition to protein, they contain calcium and vitamin D) without the disadvantages of the large amounts of saturated fat they often contain. If you use full-fat cheese in cooking, buy mature rather than mild cheese since a smaller amount will give you the same flavour.

VEGETARIAN AND VEGAN DIETS

Both vegetarian and vegan diets can provide adequate amounts of protein so long as they are varied and include a mixture of protein-rich foods. Vegetarians, more precisely called

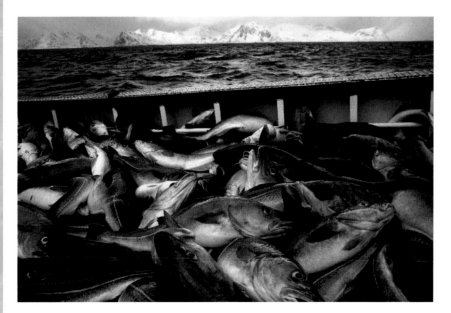

LEFT *Fresh fish is an excellent source of complete protein, containing the eight essential amino acids which combine to make different kinds of protein to form material for body cells.*

Sources of protein

Our bodies break down protein, and so need constant new supplies of protein to replace it. Luckily, protein is found in many different foods, so there is no need to worry that you are not getting enough protein or getting the right protein. All foods from animals contain protein, including fish, meat, eggs, milk and dairy products. These foods are high in protein (about 15–40 per cent protein by weight). Many plant foods also contain protein. Cereals, beans, lentils and peas are made up of about 3–10 per cent protein. Even vegetables contain some protein but it makes up less than 3 per cent by weight. Pregnant women and children up to the age of 18 need to eat slightly more protein.

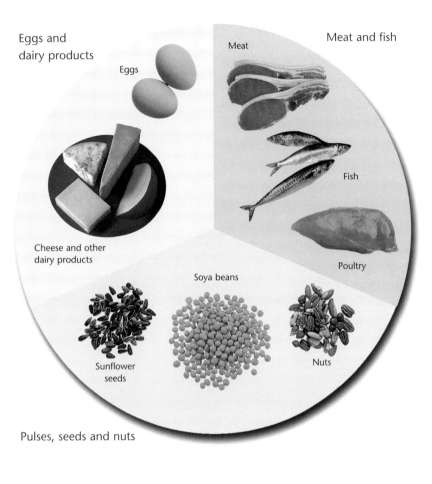

Eggs and dairy products

Eggs

Meat

Meat and fish

Fish

Cheese and other dairy products

Poultry

Soya beans

Sunflower seeds

Nuts

Pulses, seeds and nuts

ovo-lacto vegetarians, eat eggs and dairy products as well as fruit, vegetables, beans and grains. They can easily get enough protein. Vegans do not eat any animal products and therefore need to make sure that they get adequate amounts of protein.

The problem for both vegans and vegetarians is not that they are not eating protein, but rather that they are not eating complete proteins. Proteins are made up of chains of amino acids. The proteins in fish and meat contain complete chains. The proteins in other foods, except soya beans, contain incomplete chains of amino acids, so you need to eat a variety of them to form complete chains in the body. Combining proteins from dairy products or starchy foods with beans or nuts produces a complete protein. For example, beans on toast, walnuts and yogurt, and vegetarian chilli and rice all make up complete proteins. It is not, however, necessary to eat these foods at the same time, or even in the same meal. By eating a variety of protein-rich foods, vegetarians and vegans will get all the protein their bodies need for healthy cell growth and tissue repair.

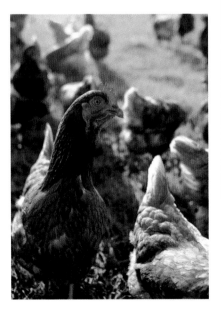

RIGHT *Choose organic meat to avoid possible contamination with hormones and antibiotics, routinely given to intensively reared livestock.*

FATS

Fat is an essential part of the diet and the most concentrated source of energy. Without fat, the body would not be able to absorb vitamins A, D, K and E, which are fat-soluble, and the cells would not be able to form membranes, the protective coats that control the passage of substances in and out of the cells. Fat is only harmful when you eat too much of it. It has twice as many calories as protein or carbohydrates, and eating lots of saturated fats will raise blood cholesterol levels. Some fats are easy to spot, but there are many other fats hidden in foods such as biscuits and cakes, sauces and dressings.

TYPES OF FAT

There are three different types of fats: saturated, unsaturated and trans or hydrogenated fats. Saturated fats are solid at room temperature and are found in meat and dairy products, as well as coconut oil. Unsaturated fats are liquid at room temperature and are either polyunsaturated (such as sunflower oil, corn oil and safflower oil) or mono-unsaturated (such as olive oil). Trans fats are artificially produced and often found in butter substitutes, and shop-bought biscuits and cakes. Most nutritionists recommend that you eat very little fat but most people consume far more than they need.

CHOLESTEROL

Cholesterol is a waxy, fat-like substance that is found in all body cells. The body manufactures it in the liver from saturated fats, so you would have plenty of cholesterol even if you never ate any foods that contained it. Cholesterol is present in foods such as egg yolks, shellfish, meat and dairy products. A high cholesterol level puts you at higher risk of a heart attack. But to make matters more confusing, there are two types of cholesterol in the body: one is good (HDL, or high-density lipoprotein) because it takes cholesterol out of the body by picking up molecules of cholesterol and taking them to the liver where they are broken down, while the other is bad (LDL, or low-density lipoprotein) because it deposits cholesterol in the arteries where it builds up, narrowing them, and causing heart and circulatory problems. Diet is the main influence of cholesterol's production and by eating less of the foods high in cholesterol and, more importantly, by eating fewer saturated fats, you should be able to keep your cholesterol level down and so reduce your risk of heart disease.

THE GOOD FATS

Omega-3 oils and mono-unsaturated fats are good for you. Omega-3 oils are found in fatty fish, such as mackerel, salmon and herring; these oils reduce the risk of blood clots by thinning the blood slightly. Omega-3 oils are also thought to protect against arthritis, and some studies suggest that they may prevent depression and improve mental function in older people.

Mono-unsaturated fats are found in high concentrations in olive oil and canola oil. Eating fatty fish once or twice a week, and switching from butter to olive oil, while cutting down on meat and saturated fats could help protect you from heart disease.

Can certain foods lower your cholesterol level?

Many people claim that garlic can lower your cholesterol level, but recent studies have not shown a clear link between a high intake of garlic and a low cholesterol level. Soya products, however, have been proven to lower cholesterol levels. Because they are potent antioxidants, soya helps fight heart disease, as does garlic, which thins the blood slightly. Despite the inconclusive evidence, eating more garlic and more soya products (such as tofu and soya beans) will not hurt you and may even help.

Balancing the fat equation

Fats are absolutely vital for health in small amounts and are the most concentrated source of food energy, containing twice the amount of calories as proteins or carbohydrates. Overall, not more than 30 per cent of the calories you eat should come from fat. However, most of us eat diets that are much higher in fat than this. As well as eating fewer fatty foods, changing the balance of fats in your diet can help you stay healthy. Only about one-third of your fat calories should come from saturated fats which are found in coconut oil, butter, cheese and meat. Another third should come from mono-unsaturated fats which are found in the following oils: canola, olive, peanut, walnut and almond. The remainder should come from polyunsaturated fats which are found in fatty fish and canola, walnut, flaxseed and soybean oils. These polyunsaturated oils are rich in Omega-3 fatty acids which may help protect you from heart disease. Eating fatty fish once or twice a week is also beneficial.

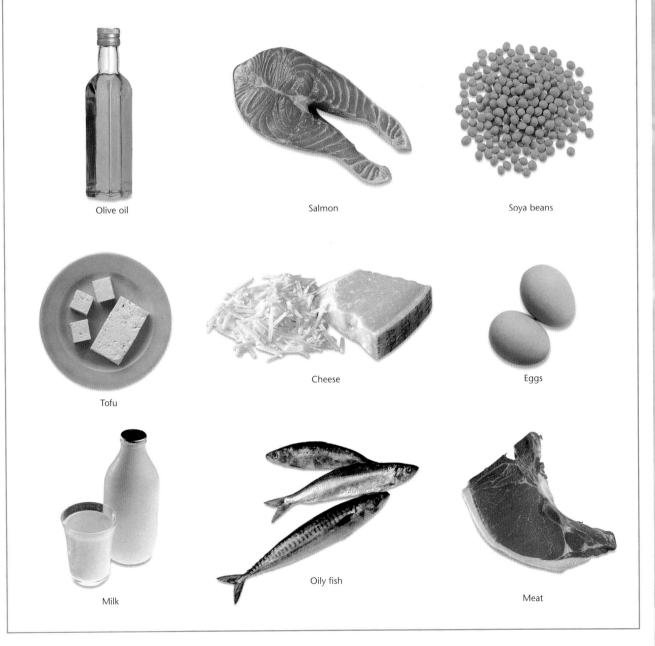

Olive oil

Salmon

Soya beans

Tofu

Cheese

Eggs

Milk

Oily fish

Meat

VITAMINS

The body needs vitamins to stay healthy, and a varied diet usually gives you all the vitamins you need. Vitamins have to come from food since they are not manufactured in the body. There are 13 essential vitamins and each one has a special role to play within the body, helping to regulate processes such as cell growth and repair, reproduction and digestion.

ESSENTIAL VITAMINS

The 13 essential vitamins are divided into two groups: fat-soluble and water-soluble vitamins. Vitamins A, D, E and K are fat-soluble and can be stored by the body. The B vitamins and vitamin C are water-soluble; except for vitamin B_{12} they cannot be stored in the body.

Vegetables that fight cancer

One group of vegetables has been singled out as a cancer-beater. It contains the members of the cabbage family (the cruciferous vegetables) and include bok choy, broccoli, brussels sprouts, cabbage, cauliflower, collards, kale, kohlrabi, mustard greens, radishes, rocket, rutabaga, turnip, turnip greens and watercress. Researchers think that they fight off cancer (particularly that of the colon and rectum) because they contain beta-carotene, fibre and vitamin C. Some people dislike eating these vegetables because they can smell strongly when cooked. To reduce the odour, eat them soon after you buy them, do not overcook and do not store leftovers for more than a day.

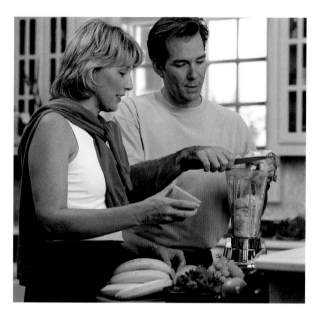

LEFT *Juicing fresh fruits and vegetables just before you consume them is an excellent way of getting the most vitamins from your food, as vitamins are destroyed by heating, water and exposure to air.*

If you have too much of these vitamins, they are excreted in urine; if you have too little, there are no stored supplies to fall back on.

SUPPLEMENTS

Most people can get enough vitamins by eating a varied diet and do not need to take a vitamin supplement. Others, however, do not eat a varied diet and may become deficient in some vitamins. Elderly people in particular may not eat enough different kinds of food and may benefit from a vitamin supplement. Women of child-bearing age who are considering having children, or who are pregnant, should be sure to take folic acid supplements in order to prevent certain birth defects, and may also require iron supplements. A vegan diet lacks vitamin B_{12}, which is present only in animal products or in synthetic form. Yeast extracts fortified with vitamin B_{12} should be consumed to make up for this.

Some research suggests that the body uses up more vitamins when it is under stress, either from illness or daily life. Many people therefore take vitamins when they are busy, feeling run down or have a cold coming on. Smoking and drinking alcohol make it harder for the body to absorb vitamins, so if you smoke or drink heavily you should either pay special attention to your diet or take a vitamin supplement.

Vitamins

Vitamin	Source	What it does for you
Fat-soluble vitamins		
Vitamin A	Fortified milk, eggs, cheese, liver, fish oil, carrots, margarine	Growth; night vision; protects the linings of the digestive, urinary and respiratory tracts; antioxidant
Vitamin D	Fortified milk, oily fish, egg yolks	Helps absorb calcium and phosphorus for healthy bones and teeth
Vitamin E	Vegetable oils, nuts, seeds, wheat germ, green leafy vegetables	Helps form blood cells; antioxidant
Vitamin K	Spinach, broccoli, milk, eggs, cereals	Helps blood to clot
Water-soluble vitamins		
Vitamin B_1 (thiamin)	Pork, pulses, seeds, nuts, fortified bread, cereals, yeast extract	Needed for muscles and nervous system to function; aids digestion
Vitamin B_2 (riboflavin)	Milk, yogurt, meat, nuts, leafy green vegetables, whole grains, lentils	Aids hormone production; keeps eyes, skin and nerves healthy
Vitamin B_3 (niacin)	Meats, fish, pulses, whole grains, nuts	Needed for production of some hormones; forming red blood cells; converting food to energy
Vitamin B_5 (pantothenic acid)	Nuts, yeast extract, organ meats, wheat germ	Helps release energy from food, helps form antibodies
Vitamin B_6 (pyridoxine)	Chicken, fish, eggs, brown rice, bananas, whole grains	Helps formation of red blood cells and making of proteins; fights infection
Vitamin B_{12}	Meat, fish, cheese, eggs, milk	Helps formation of red blood cells; maintenance of nervous system
Biotin	Wholegrain bread, yeast extract, brown rice, dairy products	Promotes healthy hair, skin and nerves; helps produce energy
Folic Acid	Fortified cereals, dark green leafy vegetables, fruits, pulses, yeast extract, fortified bread	Helps form new cells; helps prevent birth defects in foetus and may reduce risk of miscarriage
Vitamin C	Citrus fruits, green vegetables, fortified cereals, potatoes	Needed for healthy skin; fights cell damage, particularly during stress and illness; antioxidant

MINERALS

Minerals play vital roles in growth and metabolism, and enter the body through the foods we eat. Broccoli, grown in calcium-rich soil, is full of calcium, and shellfish are good sources of copper and magnesium. Most people get sufficient minerals by eating a varied diet, with plenty of fresh fruit and vegetables and dairy products, and some meat, fish and shellfish. Women may need extra calcium and iron, while almost everyone would benefit from eating less salt.

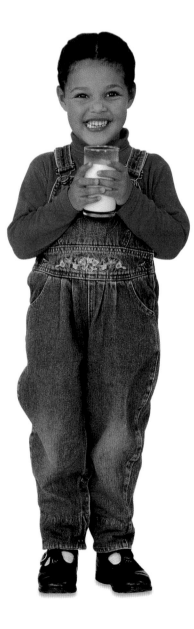

LEFT *A glass of milk is a good source of calcium, a mineral that is essential for the development of strong, healthy bones and teeth in children.*

FUNCTION OF MINERALS

The body cannot function without minerals, even though some of these are only needed in minute amounts. Minerals regulate many processes in the body, balancing fluid, helping muscles contract and aiding the nervous system. They make bones and teeth strong and help metabolise vitamins. The body needs about 20 different minerals, and the chart (right) gives information on what they do for the body and in which foods they are present. If you are eating a balanced diet, you probably do not need a mineral supplement. If you eat lots of fast foods or a very restricted range of fresh foods, a vitamin and mineral supplement might be a good idea.

SALT

For many years, doctors have warned against eating too much salt (also called sodium). Salt raises blood pressure in some people, and in older people and those with heart disease a low-salt diet is recommended. Because there is so much salt in packaged and convenience foods, making up 75 per cent of the salt in the diet, most people consume more salt than necessary. Some manufacturers are now adding less salt to foods: commercial bakeries have reduced the amount of salt in bread, for example. Cut down on salt by reading labels carefully and choosing products with less salt and by adding less salt in cooking.

CALCIUM AND IRON

The body needs lots of calcium and iron. Most men probably get sufficient amounts but most women do not. Women lose iron when they menstruate and need plenty of calcium (1000–1500 mg per day) to keep their bones strong and prevent the development of osteoporosis (see page 389) after the menopause. Pregnant women require extra calcium and iron to nourish their developing babies. Children need calcium to build strong bones and teeth. Dairy products, greens, dried beans and sardines with bones are all good sources of calcium. If you are not getting enough calcium in your diet, take a calcium supplement. Iron can be difficult for the body to digest but vitamin C can help – try drinking a glass of orange juice along with your breakfast cereal.

Minerals

Mineral	Source	What it does
Calcium	Milk, dairy products, green leafy vegetables, tofu, sardines and salmon with bones	Forms and maintains bones and teeth; needed to help muscles contract and nerves to function; aids blood clotting
Chromium	Wholegrain cereals and bran, brewer's yeast, calf's liver	Along with insulin helps the body metabolise sugar
Copper	Shellfish, nuts, seeds, pulses, liver, whole grains	Helps form skin and tissues; essential for heart function; used in production of energy and formation of red blood cells
Iodine	Salt, fish, seaweed	Aids function of thyroid gland
Iron	Meat, poultry, fish, cereals, fruit, green leafy vegetables, whole grains	Helps to take oxygen around the bloodstream and to form red blood cells; helps to resist stress and disease
Magnesium	Nuts, pulses, whole grains, green vegetables, bananas	Aids metabolism of food and communication between cells; helps maintain heart rhythm
Phosphorus	Milk, meats, poultry, fish, cereals, pulses, fruit	Helps keep bones and teeth strong; helps body release energy; aids kidney function
Potassium	Dried fruit, vegetables, pulses, red meat	Needed by nervous system and for muscles to contract; helps regulate blood pressure and keeps skin healthy
Selenium	Seafood, kidneys, liver, cereals, grains	Helps stop cells from being damaged; keeps heart muscle healthy
Sodium (salt)	Table salt, vegetables, many prepared foods	Maintains body's fluid balance; helps control heart rhythm; some bottled water helps nerves transmit messages and muscles contract
Zinc	Red meat, poultry, oysters, eggs, pulses, nuts, milk, yogurt, wholegrain cereals	Needed for sperm production; growth and production of energy; aids immune system, healing and blood clotting

FIBRE

Calorie-free and capable of lowering your risk of disease, fibre is good for you, but in the West we still only eat about half as much fibre as we should. All fibre comes from plants. It is the part of the plant that cannot be digested and so it passes out of the body in the faeces (stools). There are two types of fibre: soluble, which combines with water to form a kind of gel in the intestines, and insoluble, which does not bind with water. Insoluble fibre consists of the tough parts of vegetables, such as potato skins, celery strings, the pips in strawberries and other fruits, and wheat bran and whole grains, while soluble fibre is found in oats, barley, pulses, fruit and vegetables.

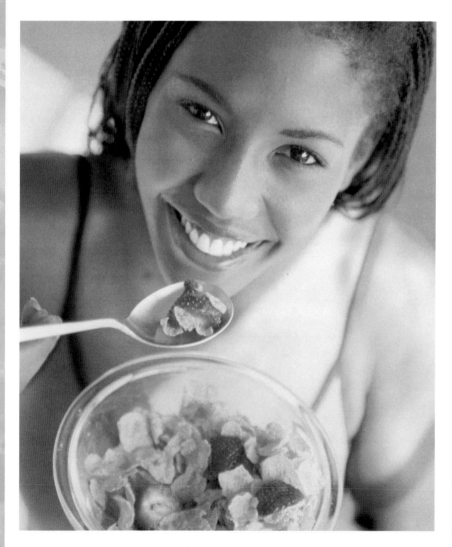

HEALTH BENEFITS OF FIBRE

Fibre helps your body to remove waste more quickly and efficiently by adding bulk to the faeces, decreasing the amount of time potentially harmful substances are in contact with the walls of the intestine. Fibre benefits the digestion and can prevent many diseases and disorders of the digestive tract. A diet high in fibre, assuming that you also drink enough water so that the fibre is soft enough to excrete, will prevent constipation. In countries where people eat a high-fibre diet, cancer of the colon is rare. High-fibre diets can protect against diverticular disease (see pages 400–1), which currently affects about half of those over 60. In this condition, small pockets are formed along the wall of the colon; eating more fibre seems to prevent the formation of these pockets.

Fibre helps fight heart disease because soluble fibre binds with the bad type of cholesterol (LDL, see page

LEFT *High-fibre breakfast cereal and strawberries are good sources of insoluble fibre, which helps material to pass through the digestive system by adding bulk to waste matter.*

Reaching the fibre target

If you eat a bowl of oatmeal and a banana for breakfast, an apple for your morning snack, brown bread with hummus followed by an orange for lunch, and pasta primavera with broccoli and peas for dinner, you will easily reach the target of 25 g (just under 1 oz) of fibre a day, and improve the health of your digestive system.

Food	Amount	total fibre (g)
Oatmeal	small bowl, cooked	3
Banana	1 small	2.2
Apple with skin	1 small	2.8
Wholewheat bread	2 slices	2.8
Chickpeas (hummus)	small serving	5
Orange	1 medium	2
Pasta	large serving, cooked	1.6
Broccoli	1 stalk	2.7
Peas	100 g (3½ oz), cooked	2.9

total: 25 grams of fibre

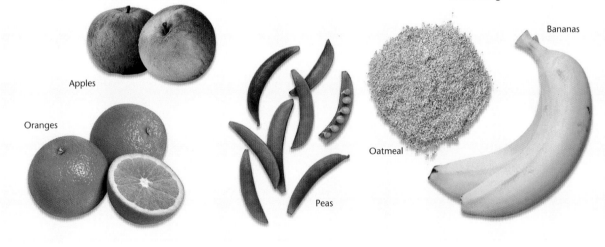

Apples

Oranges

Peas

Oatmeal

Bananas

230), which furs up the arteries around the heart, and this is removed from the body in the faeces. Soluble fibre is so helpful in lowering cholesterol that in the US oatmeal carries a government-approved label, indicating that it can reduce the risk of heart disease. In one recent study, it was found that the more fibre people ate, the lower their risk of having a heart attack. Those who ate the least amount of fibre were 30 per cent more likely to have a heart attack than those who consumed the most fibre.

AMOUNT OF FIBRE

Nutritionists recommend that you eat 25 g (just under 1 oz) of fibre each day, but most people eat only about half of this. Since lots of foods are high in fibre, it is relatively easy to consume the recommended target. Choose wholegrain breads, rice and pasta, and eat fruits and vegetables with their skins on. Also remember that although fruit juices may have the same vitamins and minerals as whole fruit, they do not contain fibre, so eating the whole fruit is better than drinking its juice.

Do not add lots of fibre to your diet suddenly or you might suffer from wind or diarrhoea. Your digestive system needs time to get used to additional fibre in the diet, so increase it gradually over a few weeks, at the same time increasing the amount of water you drink. Your body needs lots of water, about 2 litres (3½ pints or 8 glasses) a day, to help the fibre pass through the digestive system. If you do not drink enough water, the additional fibre in the faeces will make them too dry and you will become constipated.

GOOD ENOUGH TO EAT

With food scares about everything from eggs and salmonella to artificial sweeteners and cancer, many people have become worried about the safety of the food they eat. In many ways, food is safer now than ever before. The ingredients in food are rigorously tested, and refrigeration and freezing make food transport and storage much safer. But despite this, consumers fear that additives and pesticide residues in the food they eat are damaging their health.

COOK WITH CARE

The main cause of food-related illness, food poisoning, is usually due to poor handling in the kitchen. Food poisoning is caused by bacteria present in food, and most cases could have been prevented if the food had been handled properly. The basic rules are to keep cold food cold, to maintain high standards of hygiene and to cook food thoroughly to kill off bacteria.

When shopping, read the labels and make sure the food you buy is not past or near its sell-by dates. At home, store perishable food in the refrigerator. Raw meat and fish and their juices should be kept away from other food; wash chopping boards and counters with hot, soapy water after preparing fish and meat, and be sure to store them at the bottom of the fridge so they cannot drip on other food. Always wash your

hands thoroughly before eating or preparing food. Cook food thoroughly, particularly when you are reheating it in the microwave. Make sure that the centre is really hot, and that the dish is not just bubbling at the edges.

READ THE LABEL

All packaged food carries a list of ingredients, starting with the ingredient of which there is most (by

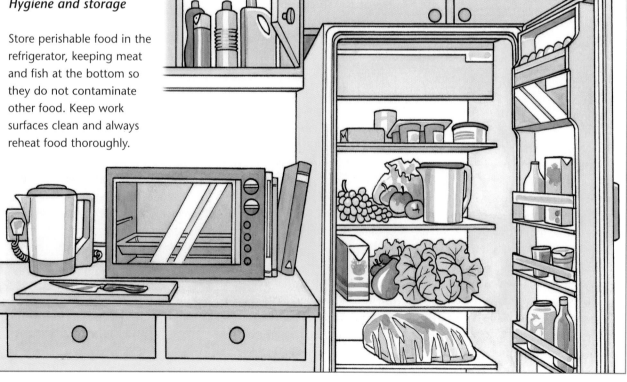

Hygiene and storage

Store perishable food in the refrigerator, keeping meat and fish at the bottom so they do not contaminate other food. Keep work surfaces clean and always reheat food thoroughly.

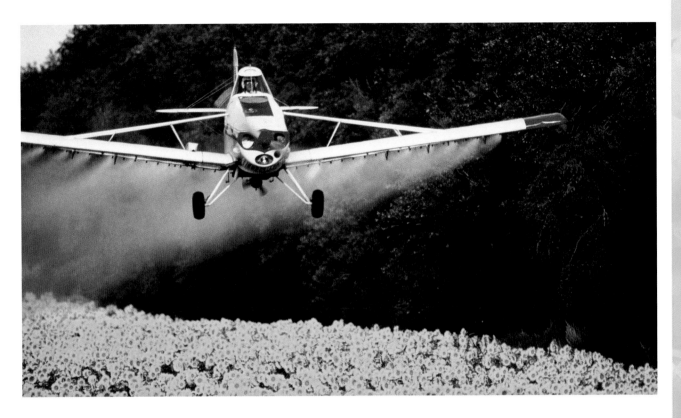

weight) down to the one of which there is least. When comparing foods, choose those where salt, sugar and fat are low down the list. Nutritional information on packaging indicates how many calories there are in 100 g (3½ oz) of the food, as well as telling you the amount of protein, carbohydrates, fat, fibre and sodium. The labels often make surprising reading. For example, you might think that noodles are a low-fat snack compared with chocolate-covered snack bars, but some packaged oriental noodles are made with palm oil, giving them 13 g (½ oz) of fat per bowl, as much as in two small chocolate-covered snack bars.

FOOD ADDITIVES

Any substance that is added to food is a food additive, including natural substances such as salt and yeast as well as artificial substances like synthetic colourings and flavourings. The purpose of additives is to make food

look and taste better and to preserve it so that it keeps for longer. To do this, manufacturers add emulsifiers, stabilisers and thickeners to improve texture, anti-caking agents to keep dry foods from clumping, preservatives to stop food from spoiling, antioxidants to stop food from discolouring or tasting rancid, as well as vitamins and minerals to improve nutritional value, and colourings and flavourings to make food look and taste better. Some of these substances are natural, while others are synthetic. Ascorbic acid (used as a preservative) is a synthetic version of vitamin C, but is chemically no different to the naturally-occurring vitamin C in an orange.

Additives are rigorously tested by the government and should not be harmful. There is no proof that they cause hyperactivity in children or allergic reactions in most adults. Many people feel, however, that they would prefer to avoid additives. To do this, cook food from scratch with fresh

ABOVE *Farmers spray their crops with pesticides to prevent damage but man-made chemicals are harmful to the environment and may cause toxins to accumulate in body tissue.*

ingredients rather than using prepared convenience foods. You will then know what goes into the meals you eat.

ORGANIC FOOD

As fears about food have intensified, the market for organic food has grown. Organic food is grown without pesticides and many people feel that it tastes nicer and is better for you and for the environment. Although the government sets limits on the acceptable amount of pesticide residue in food, there is a growing fear that these limits are too high, and that the cumulative effect of these residues on our bodies may be damaging. In Britain, organic food carries the Soil Association stamp and is widely available in supermarkets, although at present it is more expensive.

FINDING THE RIGHT WEIGHT

More than half of the UK adult population is overweight, and the number of people who are seriously overweight (obese) has doubled in the last ten years to 1 in 5 women and 1 in 6 men. In the UK, this has been mainly caused by a lack of exercise combined with overeating, in particular, eating convenience foods, which are high in saturated fat and carbohydrates. Being the right weight keeps you healthy. For every person, there is an optimal weight that is linked to height, bone structure and amount of muscle. Weight charts are a convenient way to check if your current weight is right for you.

THE DANGERS OF WEIGHING TOO MUCH

Some diseases are caused or made worse by being overweight, including Type II diabetes, heart disease, high blood pressure, stroke, gout, osteoarthritis and gall bladder disease, as well as certain types of cancer, particularly cancer of the colon, rectum and prostate in men and breast, cervical and uterine cancer in women. Carrying a lot of excess weight can also cause back pain and puts extra strain on the joints. For further information on these disorders, see *Section Four: Illnesses*, pages 328–431.

THE DANGERS OF WEIGHING TOO LITTLE

Being significantly underweight can also be a problem. In women, it may cause periods to cease and can contribute to the development of osteoporosis (see page 389) after the menopause. Some people, mainly young women, keep their weight low in order to be fashionable; a few become obsessed with being thin and develop a condition called anorexia nervosa (see pages 352–53), which can be fatal.

BELOW *Waist measurement indicates if you are carrying excess abdominal fat, and if a woman measures more than 89 cm (35 in) or a man 102 cm (40 in) she or he is at increased risk of heart disease.*

How to check if you are a healthy weight

Use your height (in metres) and your weight (in kilograms) measurements to work out your body mass index (BMI), which shows how much body fat you have. Using the graph, draw a line from your height and a line from your weight. The point at which the lines intersect gives your BMI and falls within a range that indicates whether or not the amount of fat you are carrying is bad for your health.

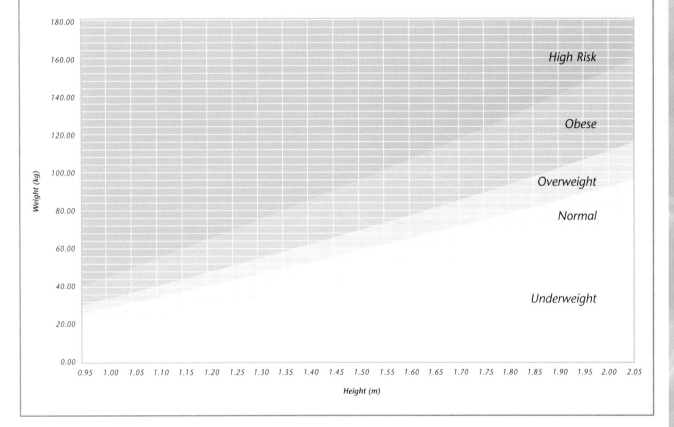

No matter how thin they become, anorexics perceive themselves to be fat. Since they refuse to recognise that they have an illness, treatment is difficult. Sudden unexplained weight loss should always be discussed with your doctor as it may be a sign of serious illness.

APPLES AND PEARS
Although being overweight is bad for anyone's health, it is even worse for those who collect the weight around the stomach and abdomen (apple-shaped) than those who carry the weight on the hips, buttocks and thighs (pear-shaped). Apple-shaped people

are more likely to develop heart disease, high blood pressure or Type II diabetes. You can see whether you are an apple or a pear by working out your waist-to-hip ratio. Measure the hips at their widest point and the waist at its narrowest point. Divide the waist measurement by the hip measurement. Women who have a ratio of more than 0.8 and men with a ratio of more than 1.0 are apple-shaped.

BODY MASS INDEX
Doctors categorise what people weigh as underweight, normal, overweight and obese (more than 20 per cent

overweight). One way to find out where your weight falls on this scale is to calculate your body mass index (BMI), an indicator of body fat. This is reached by dividing your weight in kilograms by your height in metres squared, but you can easily check your height and weight on the axes of the graph above. Draw a vertical line from your weight and a horizontal line from your height. The point at which the lines cross on the graph indicates the range you are in. For example, if you are 1.7 m (5 ft 7 in) tall and weigh 68 kg (150 lb), your BMI is 23.5, within the normal range for your height.

LOSING WEIGHT

Dieting is extremely popular, even though it is rarely effective in the long term. Ninety-five per cent of dieters put the weight back on and gain more. Diets are often dull and hard to stick to, and they do not work quickly enough for most people. The majority of people who are overweight have consumed more calories than the body needs. Small changes in the diet, over a long period of time, can have big results. For example, just eating one additional jam doughnut (290 calories) a day for a year, assuming you did not eat less at some other time or exercise more, will cause you to gain about 4.5 kg (10 lb).

WEIGHT AND GENETICS

A complicating factor in weight gain is that individuals metabolise food at different rates, and as you become older your metabolism slows down and the body uses fewer calories. It is thought there may be a gene that predisposes a person to obesity, which interferes with the body's ability to recognise when it is full, so the brain tells the body to conserve energy rather than use it up.

What is more likely is that eating and exercise habits are passed down through families. In addition, many people eat to satisfy emotional needs rather than hunger, eating when bored, unhappy or under stress, because it makes them feel nurtured. Before attempting to lose weight you should try to identify the reasons why you overeat, perhaps by keeping a food diary, and also realise that losing weight will not solve all the problems you may have.

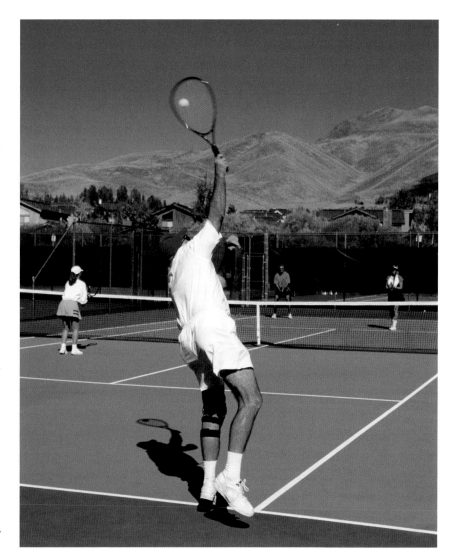

RIGHT *For successful long-term weight loss, you need to incorporate aerobic exercise into your routine so that you burn up more calories, as well as improve your body shape.*

RIGHT *Eating low-calorie foods such as salads can help you cut back on calories – make them more interesting by trying different food combinations and methods of preparation.*

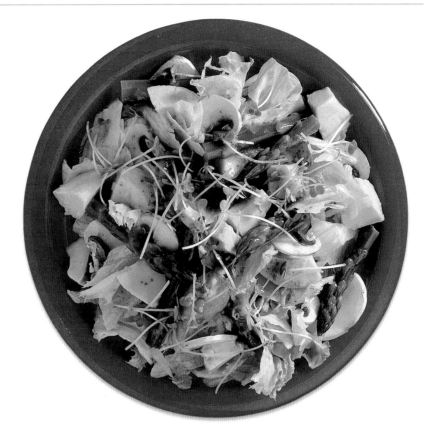

HOW TO LOSE WEIGHT

For long-term weight loss you need to burn more calories than you consume. This means eating at least 500 fewer calories a day while doing some form of aerobic exercise such as brisk walking, jogging or tennis. A sensible target is 2–4 kg (4½–9 lb) a month.

HOW NOT TO LOSE WEIGHT

Fad diets promise quick and easy weight loss, and in the short term they often achieve results. However, these diets are not good for the body – eating only protein-rich foods, cabbage soup, grapefruit and green beans may make you thin but it will not give you the balance of nutrients your body needs to stay healthy. Much of the weight lost in the early stages of these diets is water. Many are so low in calories that they cause the body to go into starvation mode, conserving rather than burning energy, so that the less you eat, the less your body needs and the less weight you lose. These diets fail in the long term because they do not change a person's underlying attitudes and habits about food. Slow, sensible diets may be less glamorous but they

are healthier and the weight you lose is more likely to stay off.

YO-YO DIETING

Losing weight rapidly, then regaining it, then losing it again can become a way of life. This behaviour is termed weight cycling or yo-yo dieting, as you swing between fat and thin. Dieters, particularly those who follow fad diets, often regain the pounds lost and more as well, making another diet inevitable.

This cycle is bad for your self-esteem and some studies have shown that it is bad for your health, too. To lose weight and keep it off you need to make lasting changes to your lifestyle, including following a low-fat, high-fibre diet and exercising more.

BELOW *Rapid weight-loss diets should be avoided because they do not change your underlying eating habits and may deprive your body of essential nutrients, damaging your health.*

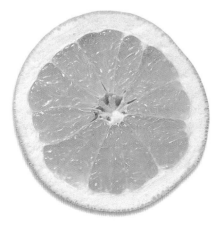

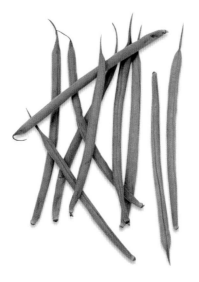

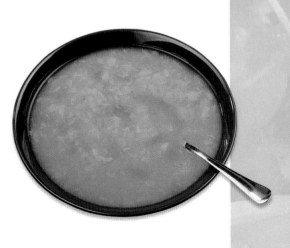

LASTING WEIGHT LOSS

A good weight-loss diet will make you lose weight slowly and steadily, at the rate of 0.5–1 kg (1–2 lb) a week, while eating a diet that is nutritionally balanced. To maintain a certain weight you need to balance the amount of food you eat with the number of calories you burn off.

STEADY WEIGHT LOSS

To lose half a kilogram a week, you will need either to consume 500 calories a day fewer or burn off an extra 500 calories a day. When you have reached your desired weight, you will need to switch from a weight-loss diet to a maintenance diet. Many people find that a specific weight-loss programme helps them to make lasting changes to their eating habits. Good diet programmes also take into account the psychological side of weight gain, helping you examine why you overeat and enabling you to change your behaviour so that you no longer reach for food in times of stress. A good diet programme will not make impossible promises, and you should also check that there are no hidden costs for special foods or literature.

A diet that is low in fat but high in fibre will help you lose weight slowly and safely. It will probably not leave you feeling hungry and it should certainly satisfy all your nutritional needs. In general, you should eat according to the guidelines on pages 242–43, but also cut down on sugars and fats, and eat only lean meats and low-fat dairy products. You will need to exercise more control over portion size, eating less than you may be used to. A diet will be even more effective if eating less is combined with exercising more.

LEFT **Drink plenty of fluid – water contains no calories and will make your stomach feel full, as well as improving the appearance of your skin and increasing your vitality so that you have more energy.**

Tips for low-fat eating

• *Switch to skimmed milk and low-fat dairy products.*
• *Trim all visible fat and skin from meat.*
• *Eat fish or chicken instead of red meat.*
• *Eat smaller portions and think before you have seconds.*
• *Chew slowly.*
• *Eat whole grains such as brown rice and wholewheat bread.*
• *Drink more water.*
• *Keep low-fat snacks handy.*
• *Change your cooking methods: steam, grill or bake food rather than frying it.*
• *Eat 5–9 portions of vegetables and fruit a day but do not add butter or sugar.*
• *Replace sweet snacks and fatty deserts with low-fat, low-sugar options such as yogurt or fruit.*
• *If you drink, cut down on alcohol: not only does it contain calories but it reduces your inhibitions, making you less likely to stick to your diet.*
• *Eat more meals at home – it is very hard to stick to a diet when you are eating restaurant-prepared meals, whether they are take-aways, fast foods or gourmet dinners, and they are more likely to be high in fat.*

Sample daily eating plan

1500 calories a day

Breakfast
125 g (4 oz) strawberries
Large bowl of unsweetened cereal
with ½ sliced banana, if liked
225 ml (8 fl oz) skimmed milk
Coffee or tea

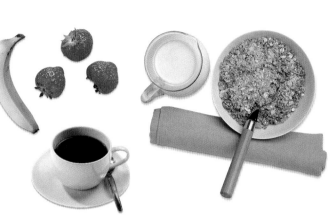

Lunch
Chicken sandwich: 2 slices
wholewheat bread, 55 g (2 oz)
lean chicken breast, with lettuce
and sliced tomato, ½ tsp low-fat
spread or dressing
1 small pot low-fat yogurt
1 apple

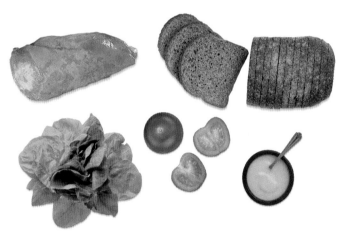

Dinner
85 g (3 oz) grilled fish with
lemon juice
1 medium baked potato
Broccoli
Green salad with low-fat dressing
or lemon juice
Fruit salad (no added sugar)

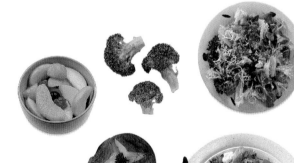

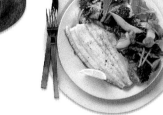

WARNING **See your doctor before starting a diet if
you want to lose more than 10 kg (22 lb), if you have
other health problems or if you are taking medicines.**

WHAT IS FITNESS?

Fitness is the ability to carry out your daily tasks with energy and without getting tired or out of breath. To be fit, you do not have to train like an Olympic athlete but you do have to be active. For optimum fitness, you should work out or exercise at least three times a week.

HOW TO GET FIT

There are literally hundreds of ways to get fit. Different forms of activity benefit the different aspects of fitness – stamina, strength and flexibility – to a greater or lesser extent. Some, such as dancing, swimming or jogging, improve the health of your heart and lungs by making you breathe harder and your heart beat faster. Others, like weight-lifting or doing push-ups, increase muscle strength. Another group, flexibility exercises, include stretching and yoga, and make you more supple and flexible. Daily activities also increase your fitness. For example, walking to the bus briskly is aerobic exercise (builds stamina), carrying groceries is a strength exercise and stretching to reach items on high shelves is a flexibility exercise.

RECOMMENDED LEVEL OF EXERCISE

Health professionals recommend that you exercise vigorously three or four times a week for about 30 minutes each

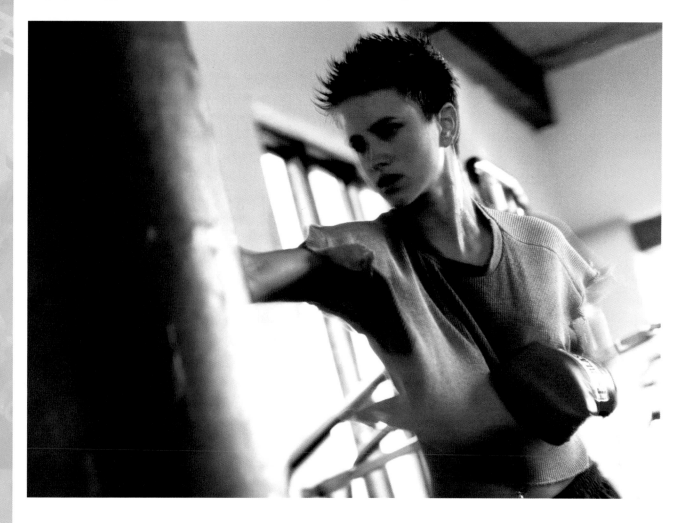

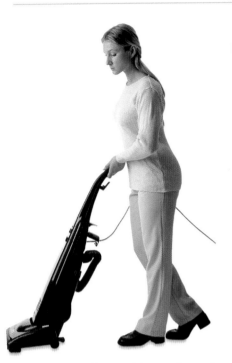

ABOVE *Vigorous housework is a good way of keeping fit and is easily incorporated into your daily routine, helping to keep you active and independent in later life.*

time. The aim of this type of exercise is to make your heart work harder. Ideally you should achieve and maintain your target heart rate (see page 249) for most of this period. However, many studies have shown that even moderate activity is beneficial for health if performed regularly. In one study, sedentary people who did about 30 minutes of moderate physical activity per day, such as vigorous housework or climbing stairs, reaped the same health benefits as others who worked out by swimming, riding a bicycle or running five times a week. The message here is that getting moving now, rather than waiting until you have joined a gym or purchased the right equipment, is the best medicine of all. The best form of exercise is one that you can fit into your daily routine and that you also enjoy doing.

LEFT *Muscle strength, endurance and flexibility all increase when you work out. Bone strength and density also improve, making bones less liable to fracture when you become older.*

How the body benefits from exercise

The benefits of fitness
Both body and mind benefit from fitness. Regular exercise makes you feel and look better. You may even live longer – people in their late thirties who start exercising regularly can add 2½ years to their life expectancy, while even those over 70 who start exercising can add a year to their lives.

Psychological benefits
When you exercise, your brain produces chemicals called endorphins that make you feel better and happier. Exercise can therefore help reduce depression. This feeling of well-being that follows exercise also reduces stress and tension. In addition, exercise increases mental alertness. Some of the symptoms of premenstrual tension can also be relieved by exercising.

Physical benefits
The physical benefits of exercise are great. The more you exercise, the stronger your muscles become. The muscle that benefits most from exercise is the heart. Vigorous exercise increases the heart rate, making the heart pump blood around the body faster, and thereby making the heart stronger and able to pump blood more efficiently. It also lowers blood pressure and reduces cholesterol levels. As the blood flows more quickly around the body, waste is removed from the cells and fatty deposits from the arteries, reducing your risk of developing heart disease and stroke. Other parts of the body become stronger too, including the lungs, which become more efficient.

Exercise makes joints more flexible and bones and muscles stronger. This is particularly important as you age, and for older women exercise is essential. After the menopause, women lose the bone-protecting powers of oestrogen and start to lose bone mass; exercise helps keep this bone loss at bay.

Regular exercise also reduces the risk of developing Type II diabetes, not only by helping to keep your weight down, but more directly by helping the body use sugar more efficiently. Furthermore, some studies have also shown that exercise helps protect against certain types of cancer, particularly of the colon, breast and endometrium (the mucus membrane that lines the womb).

Exercise also helps weight loss because it burns up calories. As an added bonus, as you gain muscle you will burn more calories even when you are resting. This is because muscle burns more calories than fat.

AEROBIC ACTIVITIES

As you exercise, your heart and lungs get a good workout. The health benefits of this are enormous. You will feel more energetic, you may sleep better, and the effect of the endorphins produced by exercise will make you feel better, too. If you have been tense, stressed or depressed, you should notice an improvement in your mood. But many of the most important benefits are unseen: as you exercise you are decreasing your risk of heart disease and stroke. To gain these benefits, you will need to exert yourself for at least 15 minutes at a time without stopping, at least three and preferably five times a week.

TYPES OF AEROBIC ACTIVITY

Any form of exercise that makes the heart and lungs work harder is an aerobic activity. The range of aerobic activities is enormous and includes brisk walking, skating, swimming, cycling, rowing and dancing. Many racquet sports are aerobic; singles tennis provides a particularly good workout. Team sports such as hockey, lacrosse, football or basketball are also good aerobic exercises, so long as you keep moving, as are step and low-impact aerobics classes. When you are walking, you should aim for a quick pace rather than a gentle stroll. A person walking quickly can cover about 5.5–6.5 km (3½–4 miles) in an hour, while someone walking slowly will cover only 3.2 km (2 miles) per hour. Running, jogging and speed walking are all forms of aerobic exercise. Aerobic exercise makes your body more efficient at using oxygen, strengthens the heart and lowers blood pressure.

GETTING STARTED

When you begin exercising, do not push yourself to the limit. As you exercise, you should not be so breathless that you cannot speak.

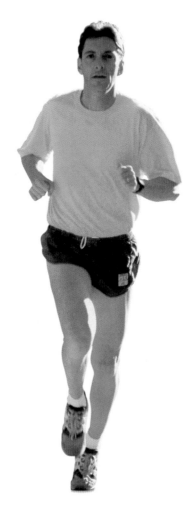

ABOVE *Running and jogging are excellent aerobic activities but it is essential to wear proper footwear to prevent heel damage and avoid making hip and back problems worse.*

Aim for a pace that makes you breathe harder and your heart beat faster, but that still feels comfortable. Start slowly: as you get fitter, you will be able to work harder. If you have not exercised for many years, or if you have any health problems, you should see your doctor for a check-up, particularly if you are over fifty. Should you feel pain at any time when exercising, stop what you are doing. If you do not feel better or if the pain is in your arms or chest, call a doctor immediately. Some muscle soreness and stiffness after exercise, however, is normal and can often be relieved by a hot bath. Do not exercise if you have a cold, flu or fever. Take a couple of days off and begin again when you feel better.

WARMING UP AND COOLING DOWN

Always follow a routine to stretch your muscles before and after exercise. Muscles need time to warm up at the beginning of an exercise session, and to cool down at the end. Instead of starting and stopping abruptly, begin gradually, moving from a gentle walk to a brisker pace or from a slow jog to a more vigorous form of running or

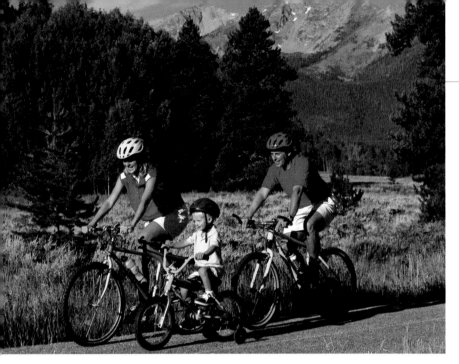

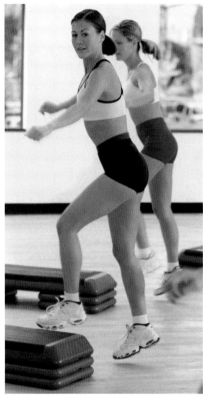

other exercise. Gently stretching your arms, legs, chest and shoulders should also be a part of your warm-up. When you have finished exercising, slow down in the same way until your breathing is nearly back to normal. By warming up and cooling down, you will be less likely to injure yourself and will be able to avoid muscle strain and minimise soreness. Resting between sessions is essential to give your muscles time to recover.

ABOVE AND RIGHT *Aerobic exercise comes in many forms, from step classes to cycling with your family. If you choose an activity you enjoy you are more likely to continue doing it.*

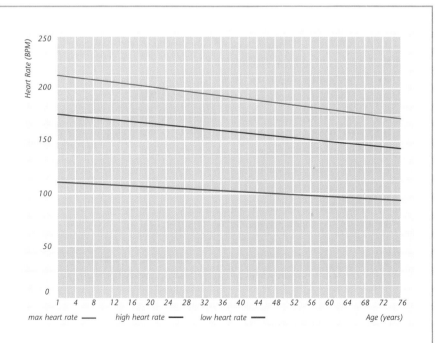

Finding your target heart rate

Your target heart rate is the rate at which your heart should be beating if you are to get the most out of exercise. To find your target heart rate, calculate your maximum heart rate by subtracting your age from the number 220. To calculate the high end of your target heart rate, multiply your maximum heart rate by 0.85. To find the low end of your target heart rate, multiply it by 0.55. As you exercise, you should be working hard enough so that your pulse stays within your target heart rate. There are instruments that attach to a finger and measure your heart rate while you are exercising so that you can tell how you are doing. More simply, however, you can take your pulse at the wrist with your index finger. Count the beats for 10 seconds and then multiply by 6 to find your heart rate per minute. Once you are used to working at your target heart rate, you will know how that should feel and will not need to check your pulse very often.

BUILDING STRENGTH AND FLEXIBILITY

Although aerobic fitness is important, you also need to be strong and flexible for total fitness. Strength exercises (such as weight-lifting) make your muscles stronger, while flexibility exercises (stretching) make your joints and muscles more supple. Being both strong and flexible means that you are less likely to hurt yourself by pulling a muscle or putting out your back when exercising or simply going about your daily activities. Before beginning either strength or flexibility exercises, warm up by jogging on the spot for five or ten minutes. You are less likely to pull or tear a warm muscle, and you will find that it is easier to stretch once your muscles are warm.

THE PERFECT PUSH-UP

Push-ups build strength in your shoulders (deltoids), the backs of your upper arms (triceps) and in your chest (pectorals). Because you need to tense your muscles to keep your body in a straight line as you do a push-up, you are also exercising muscles in the abdomen, hips and back.

1 *Lie on your front with your hands flat on the floor and slightly wider than your shoulders, your arms pressing down, your feet together and your knees locked.*

2 *Breathe in and push yourself up, keeping your body in a straight line from your ankles to your shoulders.*

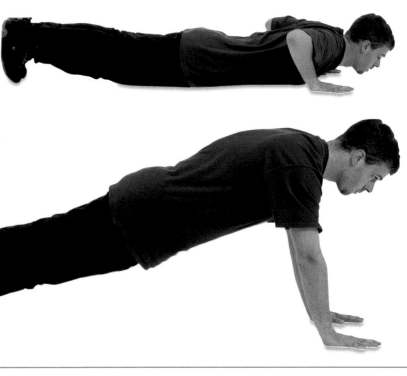

3 *Breathe out and lower yourself down so that your chest almost touches the floor.*

4 *Repeat as many times as you can to make up a set. Rest and do another two or three sets.*

Variations

If you cannot do even one push-up, start with the half push-up – with your knees rather than your toes on the floor.

STRONGER IS HEALTHIER

Exercises that make your muscles stronger are not just for body-builders. They are essential for women because they prevent bone loss and therefore osteoporosis, for older people whose muscles can waste due to inactivity, and for anyone who wants a lower cholesterol level or increased protection from diabetes. Strength exercises also make you look better – they help reduce body fat and make you look trimmer. Stronger muscles may also alleviate low back pain, particularly if you exercise your stomach muscles since they can then take some of the strain off your aching back.

HOW TO BUILD MUSCLE

To build muscle, the muscles need to be worked at their maximum capacity.

One way to do this is by lifting weights. To find out what weight will make your muscles work to their maximum capacity, find a weight that you can lift eight times in a row – if it feels easy, the weight is too light; if you cannot lift it eight times, the weight is too heavy. To give your muscles a workout, you will need to lift the weight eight times, called a set, rest, then repeat twice more. You can either buy equipment (dumb-bells, ankle weights), or you can improvise with heavy tins of soup. Two of the best strength exercises, push-ups and sit-ups, do not require any equipment at all, just your own body weight.

Joining a gym gives you access to machines that help you build up all the different muscle groups. You will be shown how to use the machines and what weights and exercises are best for you. If you are over 40, see your doctor before you start.

REACH FOR FITNESS

Stretching is a great way to reduce stress, feel better and possibly even avoid injury as you exercise. The key to safe stretching is to reach until you have gone as far as you comfortably can, then hold that position for a count of 10 or 20. This is much better for you than ballistic stretching, where you bounce to force the muscle to stretch, increasing the chances of a muscle strain or tear. Stretching should feel good – there is no need to go for the burn – and knowing when to stop is essential for exercising safely. Stop at once if you think you have overdone it.

SUPER SIT-UPS

Sit-ups tighten the stomach muscles and trim the waist, working the rectus abdominus (a long muscle running down the stomach) and the external and internal obliques (muscles that run diagonally in a v-shape across the bottom of your abdomen).

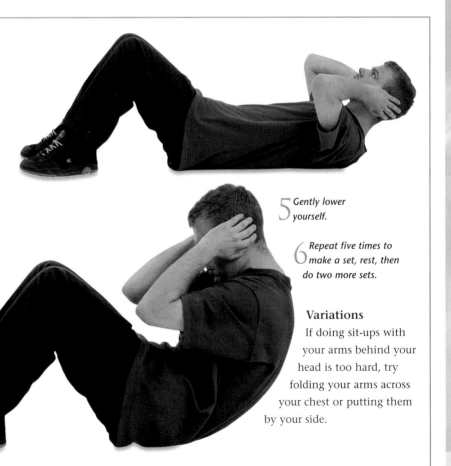

1 Lie on your back with knees bent and feet on the floor.

2 Place your hands on either side of, or behind, your head.

3 Tighten your stomach muscles so that your lower back presses on the floor and your upper body lifts up.

4 Use your stomach muscles to bring your head and torso up towards your knees. You do not need to go all the way to the knees; instead stop at a 45-degree angle.

5 Gently lower yourself.

6 Repeat five times to make a set, rest, then do two more sets.

Variations

If doing sit-ups with your arms behind your head is too hard, try folding your arms across your chest or putting them by your side.

EXERCISE FINDER

The best form of exercise is one that you enjoy and will therefore do regularly. Rowing might burn a lot of calories and use the greatest number of muscle groups, thereby making you fitter faster, but if you do not like it or if you find going to the gym to use the rowing machine too much trouble, you will not do it often enough to reap the benefits. Dancing to Top of the Pops might not fit most people's idea of exercise, but it is a good form of aerobic exercise that burns almost as many calories as cycling.

Brisk walking

Rate: about 6.5 km/4 miles per hour
Calories burned per hour: 300 per hour on level ground
Good for: aerobic fitness, weight bearing, legs
Advantages: can be done anywhere, any time, no equipment needed
Disadvantages: does not work the upper body

Appropriate clothing and footwear

Whatever form of exercise you choose, you need the right clothing. If you are exercising outside, dress in layers so that as you warm up, you can stay cool by removing a layer. There are many new fibres that take moisture away from your body, making you less sweaty and less likely to become chilled on a cold day or overheated on a hot day. The right shoes are the key to preventing strains and sprains. Specialist sporting goods stores can advise you on the right kind of shoes for your sport.

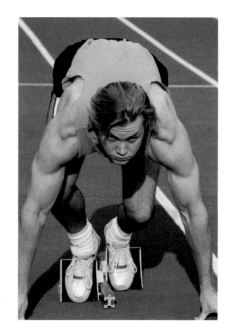

Running is good for cardiovascular fitness.

Additional information: up to 50 per cent more calories burned if you walk uphill or on sand at the same pace, and about 10 per cent more if you swing your arms like a race walker or carry hand weights

Running

Rate: moderate
Calories burned per hour: 800
Good for: cardiovascular fitness, weight loss

Advantages: easy, inexpensive
Disadvantages: does not work the upper body; can injure muscles and joints if you do not warm up properly
Additional information: in cold or rainy weather, you can run on a treadmill. Wherever you run, be sure to warm up before beginning

Cycling

Rate: moderately fast
Calories burned per hour: 400–700
Good for: heart and circulation, legs and upper back and shoulders
Advantages: fun, no lessons needed; a good way to get around
Disadvantages: not much fun in bad weather; stop and start city riding will not give you a sustained level of aerobic workout
Additional information: wear a helmet

Ballroom dancing

Rate: fast (polka or jitterbug)
Calories burned per hour: more than 400 calories
Good for: aerobic fitness
Advantages: fun, sociable
Disadvantages: you need a partner and lessons
Additional information: even moderately fast dancing burns 250–300 calories an hour

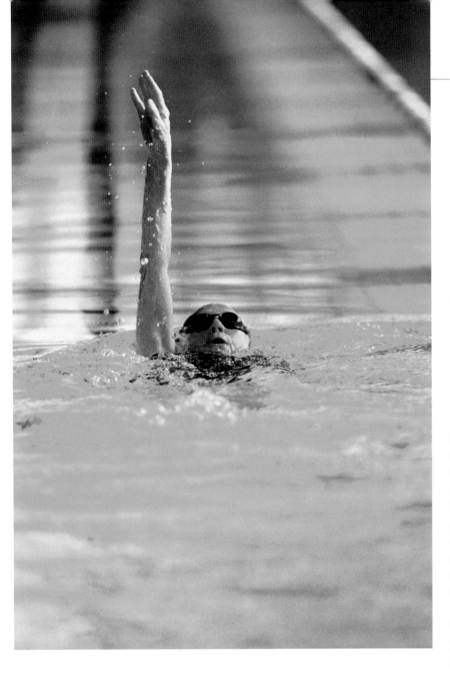

Swimming works all major muscle groups.

Maintain fluid intake

When you are exercising you need to make sure that you do not become dehydrated. As you exercise, you lose fluids both as you sweat and as you breathe out. Drink a glass of water before exercise, and one afterwards even if you do not feel thirsty. Sports drinks are no better for you than water unless you regularly work out for very long periods of time.

Calories burned per hour: 450
Good for: heart and lungs, flexibility, legs, back, shoulders and neck
Advantages: fun, sociable
Disadvantages: need a skating rink
Additional information: although there are few injuries, falling down is common, so older people who are new to the sport should wear padding and take lessons

Tennis (singles)

Rate: fast and vigorous
Calories burned per hour: 450
Good for: cardiovascular system, arms and legs
Advantages: fun, sociable, minimal equipment needed
Disadvantages: can cause tennis elbow
Additional information: Doubles tennis does not make you run hard enough to improve cardiovascular fitness

Skipping rope

Rate: moderate
Calories burned per hour: 650
Good for: cardiovascular and muscular endurance, agility, co-ordination and strength
Advantages: simple equipment; can be done anywhere; easy to learn

Swimming

Rate: vigorous front crawl
Calories burned per hour: 600
Good for: all the major muscle groups, cardiovascular fitness, flexibility
Advantages: minimal equipment, easy
Disadvantages: you need to go to a swimming pool
Additional information: does not put stress on the back; the best stroke for losing weight and increasing cardiovascular fitness is the front crawl

Exercise bike

Rate: moderately fast (24–32 kph/ 15–20 mph)
Calories burned per hour: 400–700

Good for: heart and circulation, legs
Advantages: year-round, no instruction is required
Disadvantages: you need to own an exercise bike or go to a gym; does not tone the upper body
Additional information: a good way to start if you are out of shape, because you can set the pedalling resistance to a level that suits you and then increase it as you get fitter

Ice skating

Rate: moderate

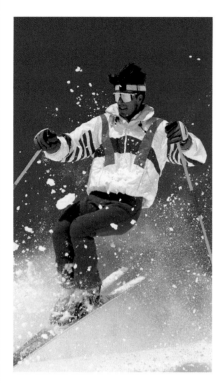

Downhill skiing is great exercise for the legs.

Disadvantages: raises your heart rate too fast and too high, unless you are already very fit
Additional information: wear shock-absorbent trainers with heel support

Table tennis
Rate: quick
Calories burned per hour: 450
Good for: cardiovascular system, agility and coordination
Advantages: fun, sociable
Disadvantages: need special equipment
Additional information: to get more out of the game, work hard, reaching and stretching for the ball. Keep moving and do not stop between points

Cross-country skiing
Rate: vigorous
Calories burned per hour: 600–900
Good for: both upper and lower body, making the workout better than running or cycling

Advantages: fun, not hard to learn
Disadvantages: winter only, in snow-bound areas
Additional information: has a lower risk of injury than downhill skiing

Downhill skiing
Rate: moderate
Calories burned per hour: 420
Good for: legs, thighs, stomach muscles, balance
Advantages: fun, exhilarating
Disadvantages: seasonal, expensive, risky, needs specialist equipment and tuition
Additional information: skiing is safer today than ever before because of improvements in the equipment

Squash
Rate: fast and vigorous
Calories burned per hour: 600–850
Good for: cardiovascular fitness
Advantages: easy to learn, fun, sociable
Disadvantages: you need to be fairly fit before you start
Additional information: you must wear eye protectors because the ball travels at up to 225 kph (140 mph); the court

is small so it is easy for your opponent's racket to hit you by mistake

Water aerobics
Rate: intermediate
Calories burned per hour: 250
Good for: various muscles, depending on exercise routine
Advantages: buoyancy means there is little stress on joints and muscles
Disadvantages: you need to visit a swimming pool
Additional information: helpful for those recovering from hip or back injuries as well as being suitable for pregnant women

Rowing
Rate: moderate
Calories burned per hour: 450
Good for: cardiovascular fitness, muscles in legs, abdomen and torso
Advantages: provides a complete workout and uses lots of calories
Disadvantages: you need to own a rowing machine, visit a gym, or join a boat club
Additional information: rowing may make a bad back worse

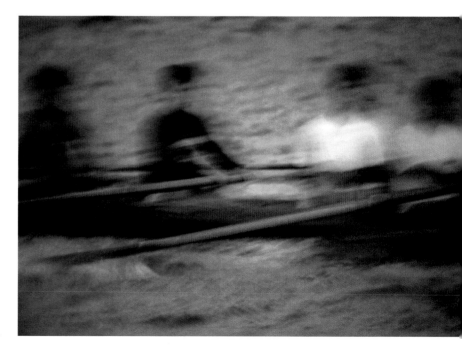

Rowing provides a complete workout.

EXERCISE EVERY DAY

Exercise is not just something you do in a leotard at an exercise class or in a jogging outfit on a track, it is already part of your everyday life. You can get even more out of this if you look for ways to spend rather than save energy as you go about your day. For example, instead of taking the lift, climb the stairs; walk the children to school instead of driving. By making a number of small changes such as these to your habits, you can greatly increase the amount of exercise that you take.

USE YOUR MUSCLE POWER

The modern world is full of labour-saving devices. While washing machines, electric lawn mowers and food processors mean we have more time to spend enjoying ourselves, they also mean that we are using up less energy and therefore getting fatter. One way to burn up calories is to turn back the clock by shutting off some of these electric helpers from time to time and use your own muscle power instead.

HOUSEWORK

Around the house, try making bread by hand rather than in a bread machine or food processor. Sweeping, washing floors and windows, vacuuming and shampooing carpets all use lots of

Calories used up in various household tasks (per hour)

Ironing	145
Cleaning	250
Sweeping	160
Brisk walking	300
Climbing stairs	380
Raking leaves	300
Heavy digging	380
Mowing the lawn with a manual mower	420

energy and will give you a good workout. Instead of going to the car wash, wash your car by hand. Use a push lawnmower rather than an electric or petrol-powered mower: an hour of this uses up the same number of calories as a game of tennis. Other garden work, such as weeding, digging and raking, is also good for you, but do not try to do it all at once. To get fitter, you need to do an hour or so a day rather than several hours on a Saturday, which will only make you feel exhausted and sore.

LEISURE

Spend some of your leisure time being active. You could go bowling or take a walk instead of going to the cinema. When you send the children out to play, go with them and kick around a football, or play tag or frisbee – if you play hard, you will burn off 320 calories in an hour. If you have a dog, make it happy with longer walks and more playtime with a ball or frisbee. It will be good for both of you.

Many different studies have shown that people who include some form of activity in their daily life, even if it is only gardening, housework or gentle strolling, have much healthier hearts and are therefore at much lower risk of heart disease than people who are inactive. In one large study of 40,000

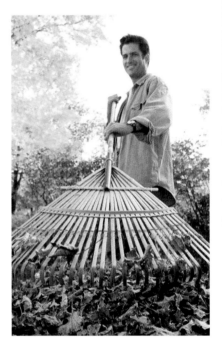

ABOVE *People who exercise regularly live longer than those who do not. Gardening is considered to be a good form of aerobic activity when you put some effort into tasks like raking leaves, digging over the soil or mowing the lawn.*

nurses and other female health professionals, women who walked even at a gentle pace for as little as an hour a week were less at risk of developing heart disease. Even if you feel exercise is not for you, or that you are too busy to go to the gym, you can still enjoy many of the health benefits of exercise simply by becoming more active.

STAYING MENTALLY AND EMOTIONALLY WELL

Being healthy includes mental and emotional well-being, as well as physical health. Stress, emotional pain, anxiety, fear, unhappiness and sorrow come into everyone's life at some point. Each person deals with these difficult emotions in different ways, depending upon individual personality and circumstances. Understanding yourself and your reactions can help you deal with difficult situations by knowing when you need support, be it from family and friends, a minister of religion or a counsellor, and learning when you need to take time out, whether it is in the form of a deep breath or a long walk, massage or meditation.

FEELING GOOD ABOUT YOURSELF

Self-esteem is the feeling that you are worth loving and taking care of. You can foster your sense of self-esteem with affirmations – positive phrases about yourself that you repeat either silently or aloud – and by seeking the company of loving and supportive people. Positive thinking can also help you enjoy life more. There is a number of books on the subject that can help you learn to see difficulties as challenges or opportunities. Research has proven that those who have an optimistic outlook do not get ill as often as pessimists.

STRESS AND YOU

For better or worse, stress is part of life. It can be good, as in the busy but exciting build-up to Christmas, or bad, as in being bullied at work. When you are under stress, your body undergoes a specific series of reactions called the fight-or-flight response, in which the muscles tense, heart rate and blood pressure increase and you breathe faster. At the same time, you perspire more and your digestion slows down. Our ancestors needed this response so that they could put all their energy into running away from physical danger. We still respond in this way to any situations that alarm us, but today most of these concern things like traffic jams or too many bills coming at once from which we cannot physically run.

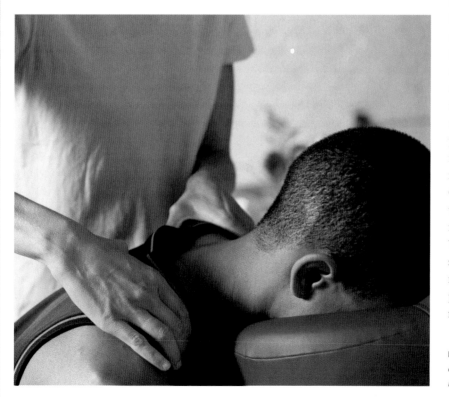

LEFT *Therapeutic massage is a simple and effective way to promote general well-being, release tension and reduce anxiety.*

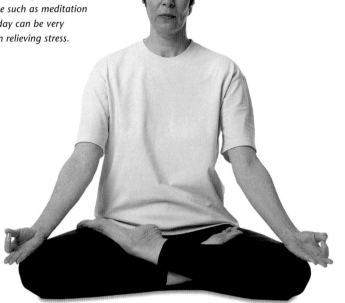

RIGHT *Practising a relaxation technique such as meditation twice a day can be very helpful in relieving stress.*

Stress-busting tips

• *Take regular exercise. This releases adrenalin, which builds up in the body when you are stressed, and produces endorphins, natural painkillers that reduce anxiety.*

• *Learn a relaxation technique. Meditation, breathing exercises or yoga will help you relax and unwind.*

• *Take control of your life. Being out of control is stressful. Try either to change your circumstances or to cultivate outside interests.*

• *Recognise stress. Talk to a friend or just acknowledge how you feel to yourself.*

• *Avoid sugary snacks, alcohol or cigarettes when you become stressed. These contain harmful chemicals that will make you feel worse in the long run.*

If the fight-or-flight response is activated again and again without the physical release of flight, stress-related medical problems, such as stomach pain or anxiety, can result.

There is a number of techniques for relieving stress. Many are based on relaxation. You can teach yourself to relax by learning to meditate or by progressively tensing and relaxing your muscles as you lie quietly. The old stand-bys of taking a deep breath or counting to ten when you feel your blood pressure rise can also help. Getting more exercise is another proven way to relieve stress.

All of these techniques, however, only relieve the symptoms of stress. Researchers have found that the most common cause of stress is feeling out of control. For this reason, it is not managers in high pressure jobs who are under most stress, but the people who work for them, particularly those who are under a lot of pressure to perform but have little control over decisions.

There are two ways to take back control. One is to change your situation, perhaps by getting a different job.

Another is to change the way you act in your situation or the way you feel about it. If one part of your life is making you stressed, you could try getting more out of another part of your life. So if you have a dull job that you cannot change, take up a hobby or get involved in a community project.

WHEN TO GET HELP

There are times when self-help is not enough and you need professional help. See your doctor if you notice physical symptoms such as headaches, back pain, stomach pain, insomnia, exhaustion or sexual problems; behavioural symptoms such as smoking and drinking more, grinding your teeth, becoming bossy and hypercritical; emotional symptoms like crying, anger, depression or feeling on the edge; or mental symptoms such as forgetfulness, constant worry, losing your sense of humour or your ability to concentrate or make decisions.

RIGHT *Having a network of people you are close to, such as friends or family, is important for your emotional well-being and sense of self-esteem.*

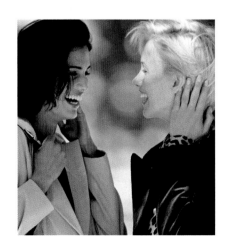

GIVING UP SMOKING

Stopping smoking may be difficult, but it is the best thing you can do to improve your health: as soon as you stop your body starts to heal itself, no matter how long or how much you have smoked. The health risks of smoking are well known, yet millions of people keep puffing away; 29 per cent of men and 27 per cent of women in the UK smoke. When you are trying to quit smoking, remind yourself of how bad smoking is for you in order to motivate yourself to quit.

THE DANGERS OF SMOKING

With each cigarette you smoke, you are reducing your life expectancy by 5½ minutes. Smoking increases risk of heart disease, respiratory problems such as emphysema, and cancer. Lung cancer now kills more men and women than any other form of cancer. The babies of women who smoke are more likely to have a low birth weight and are 40 times more likely to die in the first month of life. They are also more likely to die of Sudden Infant Death Syndrome. Children of smokers have more respiratory problems, including bronchitis and asthma.

AN ADDICTIVE HABIT

Although smokers know that their habit is killing them, they find it hard to give up. The nicotine in cigarettes is physically addictive, producing a high, particularly with the first cigarette of the day. Smokers develop a need for a particular nicotine level and smoke to maintain that level. For this reason, light cigarettes are not better for you; you simply smoke more of them or inhale more deeply to keep nicotine levels up. Cigarettes also provide emotional relief, with many smokers using them to relieve stress, manage anger or fight feelings of boredom or frustration. Some people also smoke because it suppresses the appetite.

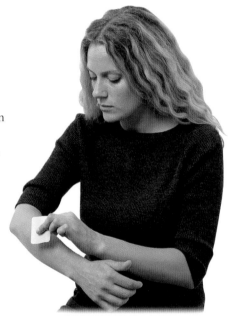

ABOVE *Nicotine patches reduce nicotine cravings and may be recommended by your doctor to help you through the early weeks of withdrawal.*

HOW TO QUIT

There are many ways to quit smoking, from complementary therapies to nicotine patches, tablets and gums, to self-help groups, hypnotism and how-to books. The main thing is to decide to stop and then to set a quit date. You should also choose a time when you will not be stressed. Most people find that setting a date and then stopping completely rather than cutting down gradually works best.

When you quit, be prepared to feel symptoms of nicotine withdrawal, such as irritability, sleeplessness, tiredness, hunger, coughing, and inability to concentrate, as well as cravings for cigarettes. Most of these symptoms will soon disappear. You can fight them by getting more sleep, avoiding stress, and also simply by pampering yourself.

Smoking is a habit, so changing your daily routine for a while will help you break for the habit. For example, if you are used to having your first cigarette with your coffee in the kitchen, switch to tea and have it in the living room. In your first weeks as a non-smoker, avoid situations where you would normally smoke, such as pubs, and instead go to places where smoking is not allowed, such as the cinema or shops.

Most cravings for cigarettes pass in about three minutes, so while you wait for a craving to pass, do something else such as making a cup of tea or polishing your shoes. Many people reward themselves by adding up all the money they are saving by not buying cigarettes and use it to buy themselves treats. And if you slip up and have a cigarette do not get angry with yourself, just resolve to quit again. It takes most people three or four tries before they can finally quit.

Acupuncture

An acupuncturist uses points in the ears to help you overcome your cravings for a cigarette. He or she may leave a stud in your ear, which you can press when you feel that you need a cigarette. Although conventional medicine does not understand how this works, some people have found that it has helped them stop smoking.

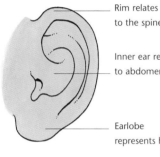

Rim relates
to the spine

Inner ear relates
to abdomen

Earlobe
represents head

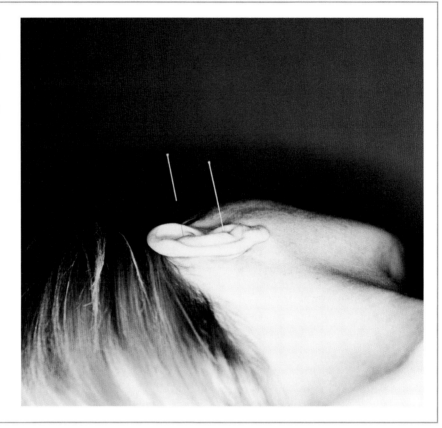

How to quit smoking

• *Set a quit date.*
• *Ask your friends and family for their support and help.*
• *Remind yourself of why you are quitting.*
• *Choose a nicotine medication and find out how to use it.*
• *Find and use strategies to deal with cravings for cigarettes.*
• *Change your habits so that you are not tempted to smoke.*
• *Keep low-fat snacks handy.*
• *Invent rewards for not smoking.*

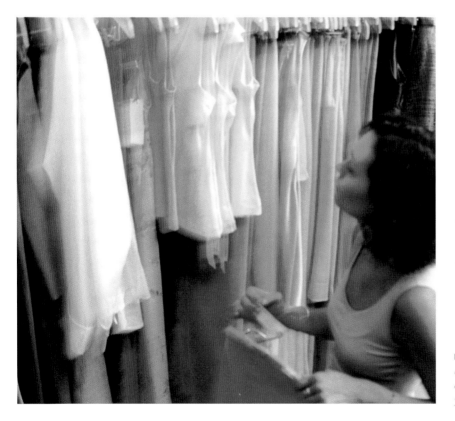

LEFT *Using reward systems – such as saving up the money you would have spent on cigarettes to buy yourself a treat – can help you stay off cigarettes in the early weeks.*

SLEEP

Sleep is a great healer of both mental and physical ills, but there are times when it can be hard to fall or stay asleep. It is possible to have a sleep disorder that causes you to fall asleep without wanting to (narcolepsy), but the most common sleep problem is not being able to fall asleep or to sleep without waking. Feeling exhausted and as though you have not had enough sleep can be a sign of illness or depression. If you are constantly tired, without any obvious reason such as shift work or broken nights with a new baby, consult your doctor.

INSOMNIA

More than 40 per cent of adults experience insomnia at some point during the course of a year. For most of these people, insomnia is caused by events in daily life such as jet-lag, anxiety, stress, such as being too busy at work, or by emotional trauma, such as a death in the family. With time, falling asleep usually becomes easier.

For other people, however, insomnia becomes a way of life, persisting for months or years. Chronic insomnia is a learned behaviour. Lack of sleep makes the person tired during the day, so he or she drinks coffee to stay away or takes naps, both of which make sleep at night more difficult. Anxiety about being able to sleep makes it hard to relax and fall asleep.

There is a number of techniques for solving the problem. All of them rely not on sleeping pills, which are ineffective, habit-forming and even dangerous in the long term, but on improving sleep habits and making lifestyle changes.

OTHER SLEEP PROBLEMS

Sleep apnoea occurs when breathing suddenly stops, often hundreds of times a night. The sleeper is not aware of this, although he or she wakes up to start breathing, then falls asleep over and over again all night long. In addition to making you feel tired, sleep apnoea forces your heart to work overtime, possibly leading to heart disease. The condition is more common in overweight men: half of those with collar sizes over 17½ have sleep apnoea. If you suspect you have

Melatonin

Each night, the body produces the hormone melatonin, which regulates the sleep/wake cycle. When you are jet-lagged your sleep/wake cycle is disturbed. Some people find that taking melatonin before bed helps them sleep better when they have crossed a number of time zones, and therefore adjust to the new hours of sleeping and waking more quickly. It is not recommended for insomnia.

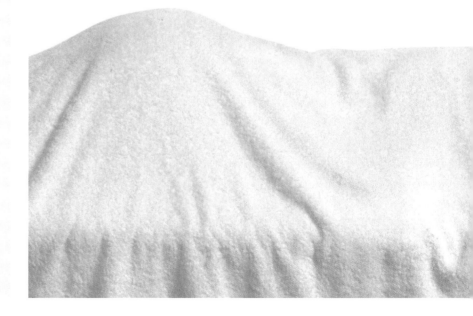

Complementary remedies for a good night's sleep

A number of herbal remedies have been used for centuries to help people sleep. Drinking a cup of herbal tea made with any of the following herbs might make you sleep better: lemon balm, chamomile, hops, passion flower or valerian. Pregnant women should not use any herbal remedies without their doctor's approval. The scent of lavender is also sleep-inducing: try adding lavender oil to bathwater.

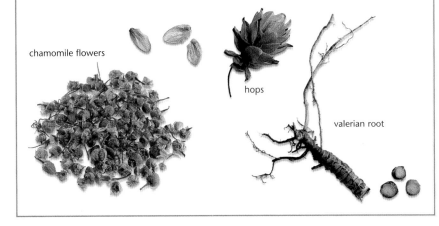

chamomile flowers

hops

valerian root

Learning to get a good night's sleep

If you are having trouble sleeping, whether temporarily or for a longer period, put these rules into practice and you should find yourself sleeping better.

- *Go to bed and get up at the same time every day, even at weekends.*
- *Do not drink coffee, tea or cola after 10 am: the caffeine stays in your body for 16 hours.*
- *Do not go to bed unless you are tired.*
- *Avoid drinking alcohol late at night: it might make you sleepy to begin with, but it will wake you up later.*
- *Exercise during the day.*
- *Do not use your bedroom for anything other than sleep or sex*
- *Avoid napping.*
- *If you really cannot sleep, get up and do something, then go back to bed when you are sleepy.*
- *Do deep-breathing and relaxation exercises in bed to help you fall asleep.*

this condition, possibly because you feel tired all the time, see your doctor.

One in four adults snore often and almost half of all adults snore some of the time. You are more likely to snore if you are overweight. Women snore more in late pregnancy and after the menopause. Snoring disturbs your own sleep and it certainly disturbs your partner's. Since you are most likely to snore when sleeping on your back, sew a tennis ball or rolled-up sock to the back of your pyjama top. This will force you to sleep on your side.

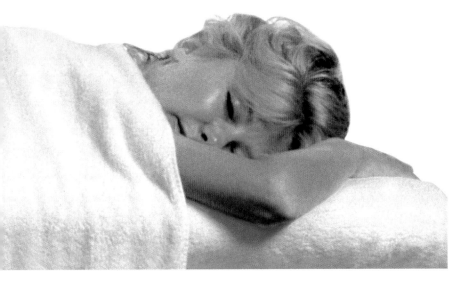

LEFT *A good night's sleep is often the best way to recover from illness or deal with stress, and regular sleep is essential for your physical and emotional health.*

PART THREE

FAMILY
HEALTH

CONTENTS

INTRODUCTION

This part of Family Health describes all major aspects of health throughout the various stages of life, from conception to old age. Your susceptibility to particular illnesses changes as you age and your health needs will alter accordingly. By the age of fifty, cancer and heart and lung diseases rather than accidents or infections are the major threat to life. However, throughout your life you can help to reduce the risk of illness and premature death by following a healthy lifestyle, by having appropriate immunisation and by having relevant screening for diseases. As an adult you have responsibility for your own health but the habits of healthy living are learned in childhood. Ultimately, good health is in your own hands.

Throughout this part of the book, in-depth articles discuss normal growth and development in your body, from the time an egg is fertilised by a sperm through the various stages of infancy, childhood, adolescence, adulthood and old age. Your health is also affected by your sex, and separate sections describe the different concerns for male and female health.

In the section on pregnancy, birth and child development, you will gain an understanding of how conception occurs, why infertility arises, and possible solutions, and how the foetus develops. Staying healthy in pregnancy, pregnancy-related illnesses and the process of giving birth are also discussed.

Having a new baby to look after can seem an overwhelming task, but articles will guide you through the various stages of infancy, giving you detailed information on breastfeeding and baby care, what developmental check-ups your baby will have and the immunisation programme you should follow. Articles on child development cover all aspects of the growing child, its physical and emotional development, from teething to tantrums, and common illnesses the child is vulnerable to at different ages. Articles on adolescence describe what puberty entails, the emotional problems your child may encounter, such as eating disorders, and how you can help.

Women and men have profound physical differences and are prone to particular illnesses because of their sex. The section on the well woman discusses all aspects of female health, from menstruation to menopause. Female health problems are highlighted, and there is specific information on how women can safeguard their health. Menopause is a time of life that has a profound effect on women, and ushers in a whole new set of health considerations. Hormone replacement therapy helps many women through this time of life. Men have their own section which covers the lifestyle factors they are likely to be affected by, the male-specific illnesses they may encounter, and how to self-examine for testicular health.

Sexual health articles discuss the advantages of long-standing, loving relationships for mental and physical well-being. They also cover sexually transmitted diseases, with a chart of main illnesses, symptoms and cures. Finally, there is a section on what happens to your body in old age, how to look after yourself, and common illnesses.

THE BEGINNING OF LIFE

Conception occurs if an egg (or ovum) produced by the ovary is fertilised by a sperm, and is then successfully implanted in the lining of the uterus (womb). Every woman is born with all the eggs she will need for a lifetime. Although, from early in life, eggs are lost through monthly ovulation, or natural wastage, by the time a woman reaches the menopause she will generally have more than a thousand eggs still present in the ovaries.

FERTILITY

Each month, a complicated sequence of hormonal changes and physical events in a woman's body leads to the release of an egg from the ovaries, known as ovulation. The egg is released from a swelling, or follicle, on the surface of the ovary, and after ovulation, the empty follicle forms a structure called the corpus luteum. The corpus luteum releases a hormone, progesterone, which helps to prepare the uterus for an implanted egg if fertilisation is successful. If conception does not take place, then the level of progesterone falls, leading to menstruation.

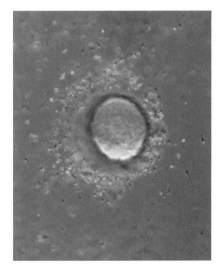

ABOVE *Of the small number of sperm that finally arrive at the egg, only a single cell will penetrate the egg and fertilise it.*

Getting ready for pregnancy

There is a number of simple lifestyle, dietary and general health measures that can help improve readiness for pregnancy and may increase fertility.

DIET Eat a healthy, well-balanced diet to meet all vitamin and mineral requirements (see Foods for Fitness, pages 222–23). Avoid foods made from unpasteurised milk, such as soft cheeses, because of the risk of listeria, an infection that can damage the foetus. Liver products, such as pâté, which are high in vitamin A, can also cause foetal abnormalities.

FOLIC ACID SUPPLEMENTS Take 0.4 mg daily, starting 4 weeks before conception and continuing for the first 12 weeks of pregnancy, to reduce the risk of spina bifida.

WEIGHT Lose excess pounds if overweight.

ALCOHOL AND TOBACCO Reduce consumption or abstain from drinking. Stop smoking: this improves general health, improves fertility and reduces the risk of having a small baby.

IMPROVE FITNESS LEVELS Thirty minutes of brisk exercise three times a week will significantly improve stamina and reduce blood pressure.

RUBELLA Make sure you are immune to rubella (German measles; see page 291). This can be confirmed by a blood test. Vaccination can be arranged, but pregnancy must be avoided for three months afterwards.

REST Get as much rest and sleep as possible.

STRESS Try to reduce stress levels, and in particular try not to put yourselves under pressure in a race to conceive.

Female reproductive organs

Most of the female reproductive system is internal, lying within the lower part of the abdomen. The ovaries, which store and release eggs, are situated either side of the uterus. An egg released from an ovary is guided by the fimbriae into a Fallopian tube, where it is slowly propelled towards the uterus by gentle contractions and the rhythmic waving of tiny hairs in the tube's lining.

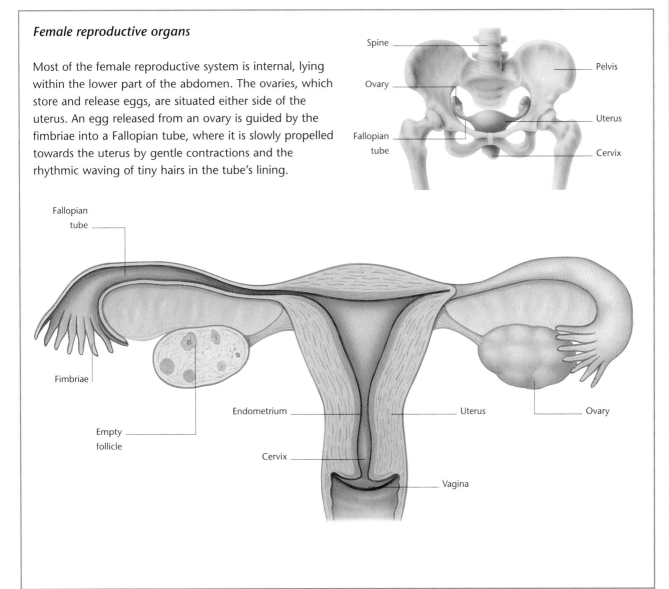

Spine

Pelvis

Ovary

Fallopian tube

Uterus

Cervix

Fallopian tube

Fimbriae

Empty follicle

Endometrium

Cervix

Vagina

Uterus

Ovary

MEN AND CONCEPTION

The male role in conception is to produce an adequate number of healthy, mobile sperm, and to introduce the sperm into the woman's vagina during sexual intercourse. A man does not start to produce sperm until puberty, but thereafter, until around the age of seventy, the average male produces about 5,000 sperm every minute.

Sperm are mixed with other fluids and chemicals produced by the prostate gland and the seminal vesicles to form semen, which is discharged from the penis during ejaculation (see Male Reproductive System, pages 206–7). Each ejaculate contains up to 200 million sperm cells, all with varying degrees of mobility. Only the most active will penetrate the neck of the womb (the cervix), swim through the womb and reach the egg.

CONCEPTION

Fertilisation takes place in one of the paired Fallopian tubes, the structures that transport the egg from the ovaries to the uterus (see Female Reproductive System, pages 204–5). For conception to occur, sexual intercourse has to take place almost immediately after ovulation, which occurs once every menstrual cycle. Although sperm can survive for up to 72 hours inside the female body, eggs have a shorter life span of no more than 24 hours. Ovulation takes place 14 days before the onset of the next period, which means it is easy to predict if the menstrual cycle is regular, but difficult if periods are irregular.

INFERTILITY

Infertility is a common problem, and it is estimated that one in ten couples will experience some difficulty during attempts to conceive. Infertility may be primary, where conception has never occurred, or secondary, when one partner has been involved in producing a successful pregnancy previously. The problem is exclusively female in around 30–40 per cent of cases, wholly male in 10–30 per cent, and 15–30 per cent is due to problems in both partners. Only in around 5–10 per cent of couples, with the high level of investigations available, is infertility truly unexplained.

MALE INFERTILITY

It is rare for sperm to be completely absent, and most cases of male infertility are due to poorly performing sperm (sperm dysfunction). This can occur in reduced or normal sperm counts, and often the cause of the dysfunction cannot be determined.

Sometimes it can be caused by previous viral infections, such as mumps, or previously undescended, or damaged testicles. Occasionally, sperm dysfunction can be caused by the presence of sperm antibodies, which attack the sperm. There are virtually no effective treatments for sperm dysfunction.

FEMALE INFERTILITY

Failure to ovulate is often associated with absent or infrequent periods. With the exception of early menopause (see page 312), nearly all causes of ovulation failure can be treated. Damage to the tubes, or pelvic adhesions (bands of scar tissue binding pelvic organs together) usually happen as a result of pelvic infection, often sexually transmitted, or previous surgery, such as removal of the appendix. Infection often damages the lining of the Fallopian tubes, making success rates for achieving pregnancy after surgery for tubal blockage less than 50 per cent.

Endometriosis, a condition where tissue resembling the lining of the womb is found at other sites in the body, particularly the pelvis, is a common cause of infertility. When present to any extent within the pelvis, the ovaries and Fallopian tubes can become densely bound in adhesions (see Endometriosis, page 423). Unexplained infertility, where all investigations are normal, usually means that the couple have simply been unlucky so far, and the majority will conceive naturally within two to three years.

Sperm count

When seen under a microscope, each millilitre of semen in a normal sperm count contains at least 50 million sperm. There are fewer than 20 million in a low sperm count, reducing the chances of fertility.

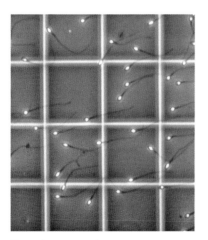

Normal sperm count

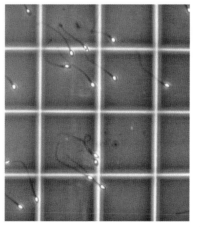

Low sperm count

RIGHT *In-vitro fertilisation involves collecting eggs from the ovary and injecting them with sperm in the laboratory. The eggs are returned to the uterus when they have been fertilised.*

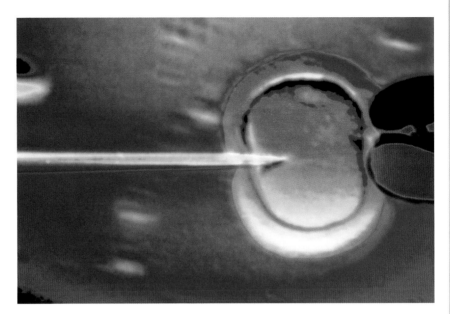

INFERTILITY TREATMENTS

Before tests and treatments are carried out, your doctor will ask you about your state of health, your lifestyle, your medical history and menstrual cycle. If the woman is not ovulating, blood tests to check the levels of certain hormones may be carried out and drugs may be prescribed to stimulate ovulation.

Ovulation failure is initially treated using a drug called clomiphene, taken at the beginning of the menstrual cycle. There is a slight increase in the rate of twin pregnancies using clomiphene. If clomiphene fails, or in some cases of unexplained infertility, drugs that mimic the body's own hormones, called gonadotrophins, are given by injection. Complications include over-stimulation of the ovaries, and multiple pregnancies.

In-vitro fertilisation (IVF) involves stimulating the ovaries with drugs and tracking the development of follicles in the ovary using ultrasound (see page 455). The eggs are collected using a fine needle, fertilised in the laboratory, and returned to the uterus two or three days later. Usually, two embryos are used, and success rates are around 20–30 per cent per cycle. A more specialised form of IVF, involving returning embryos to the Fallopian tubes, is known as gamete intra-fallopian transfer, or GIFT.

In men with very low sperm counts, a single sperm can be obtained, either from a semen sample, or drawn off directly from the testicle, and injected into the egg. This is called intra-cytoplasmic sperm injection (ICSI). Donor sperm, or eggs, are sometimes used where conventional methods have failed, or are not appropriate.

Hypnosis and relaxation to enhance fertility

It has long been recognised that stress can contribute to some types of infertility. Hypnotherapy, where a trance-like state is induced in a susceptible individual, has been around for more than 6,000 years. Practitioners feel that during this state of relaxation, or trance, the mind begins to heal itself, and the body.

Relaxation, in combination with visualisation, is a technique that can teach you to use your imagination to cope with stress, or even activate the body's self-healing process. Relaxation and visualisation can be a part of positive thinking, and relaxation therapists regard positive thinking as a useful tool in keeping us well.

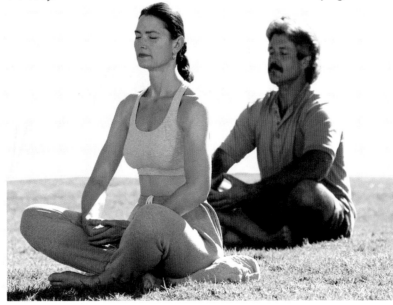

PREGNANCY

When an egg is fertilised by a sperm pregnancy begins, and complex changes take place within a woman's body to provide a protective and nourishing environment in which a baby can thrive. Pregnancy is conventionally divided into three stages, known as trimesters, which correspond to the phases in the development of the growing baby.

FIRST TRIMESTER

During the first thirteen weeks of pregnancy, the woman will notice the greatest changes in her body, although the majority are not visible. Most of these occur as a result of hormonal changes brought about by successful conception. In some women, these feelings can begin even before the first period is missed. Common symptoms include nausea and vomiting, tiredness, breast enlargement and tenderness, passing urine frequently, and emotional changes similar to premenstrual syndrome (see pages 420–21).

At conception, the future baby consists of a single cell, which, after dividing into two cells, implants into the lining of the uterus (womb). At this point, and for the next eight weeks, the developing baby is called an embryo. Some cells within the embryo develop, with cells from the mother, into an organ called the placenta, which allows exchange of nutrients and waste products between the blood of the embryo and the mother.

By the third week, the embryo is pear-shaped, with the head forming at the rounded end. Just one week later, the embryo, at only 0.75 cm (¼ in) long, already has many of the major organs present, such as the brain, the kidneys, the digestive system and the lungs. Ears begin to form as pits, eyes develop as stalks, and folds of tissue that will form the face appear.

Over the next four weeks, there is a rapid development of the major body systems, so that the 2.5 cm (1 in) long embryo is fully recognisable as a human, with a beating heart, jointed limbs and developing fingers and toes, facial features and muscles. During this period, the embryo is most at risk of developmental abnormalities. After eight weeks the embryo is known as a foetus, and by the end of the first trimester it is 5 cm (2 in) long and moving about.

SECOND TRIMESTER

During the middle third of pregnancy, the woman's abdomen begins to become noticeably swollen as the uterus expands to accommodate the foetus and the placenta. For many women this is the most pleasant trimester, as the irritating symptoms of early pregnancy have mostly

The developing foetus

By 12 weeks the foetus has all its major organs and limbs, and is recognisably human. Fingers and fingerprints develop by 16 weeks. At 28 weeks the foetus can suck its thumb. At 36 weeks the foetus is fully formed.

Face is now smooth

Hands are now fully formed

12 weeks   *16 weeks*   *28 weeks*   *36 weeks*

The baby in the womb

The growing foetus depends on its mother for a continuous supply of nutrients and oxygen. These are transferred from the mother's blood to the foetus's blood via the placenta, an organ attached to the uterus and connected to the foetus by the umbilical cord. At the same time, waste products pass from the foetus's blood into the mother's bloodstream.

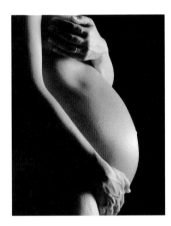

ABOVE *In the third trimester the mother's abdomen swells rapidly to accommodate the growing foetus.*

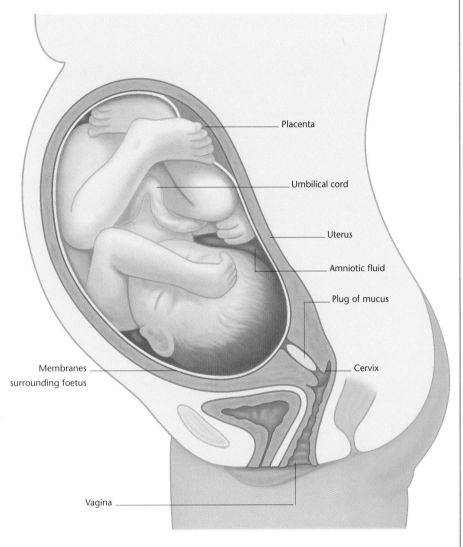

Placenta

Umbilical cord

Uterus

Amniotic fluid

Plug of mucus

Cervix

Membranes surrounding foetus

Vagina

disappeared to be replaced with a feeling of well-being.

The foetus continues to mature during the second trimester, so that by the end of the sixth month it has grown to about 25–30 cm (10–12 in). The bodily proportions change as the trunk and limbs expand. Around the fourth month, the mother can feel the foetus kicking, a sensation often described as a feeling of 'butterflies' in the stomach. In the fifth and sixth months, hair, eyebrows and eyelashes,

finger- and toe-nails develop. The ability to swallow, thumb-sucking and the grasp reflex, familiar in newborn babies, all are present by the end of the second trimester. The only organs not capable of functioning fully are the lungs, which remain immature until mid-way through the third trimester.

THIRD TRIMESTER

In the final third of pregnancy, the mother rapidly gains weight, and may experience a range of uncomfortable

symptoms once more as the uterus begins to fill the lower part of the abdomen. Heartburn, piles, varicose veins, constipation and a sensation of breathlessness may occur.

During this final stage of pregnancy, the foetus is capable of survival outside the uterus, although because of the immaturity of the lungs, most babies born before 36 weeks need to be in a special care unit. The average baby, born at 40 weeks, weighs about 3.3 kg (7 lb), and is about 50 cm (20 in) long.

PROBLEMS IN PREGNANCY

Most pregnancies are beset by minor problems and complications. Using simple remedies, or adjusting the diet, can deal with most of the common ailments, such as anaemia, constipation, swollen ankles, heartburn and piles. Nausea in early pregnancy is best dealt with by small, frequent meals, without resorting to medication. Sometimes, the vomiting is so severe, a condition known as hyperemesis, that there is a real risk of dehydration. In this situation, the use of anti-sickness medication along with a drip may be necessary.

ECTOPIC PREGNANCY

An ectopic pregnancy occurs when a fertilised egg implants outside the uterus. The most common site is in one of the Fallopian tubes, and it is possible for an affected woman to be unaware that she is pregnant until symptoms of ectopic pregnancy occur. For the majority of women, there is no underlying cause, but ectopic pregnancy can be associated with previous surgery on the Fallopian tubes, pelvic infection, pregnancy that occurs with a coil in place, IVF treatment (see page 269) and previous history of ectopic pregnancy.

As an ectopic pregnancy initially develops in the same way as a normal pregnancy, a late period, nausea and breast tenderness may be present.

However, many women are not aware they are pregnant, so the presence of increasingly severe, usually one-sided, abdominal pain may be the first symptom. Usually, this is accompanied by vaginal bleeding that may vary from a slight brown loss to torrential, bright red haemorrhage. An ectopic pregnancy should be regarded as potentially life-threatening, and medical help should be sought immediately.

PRE-ECLAMPSIA

This is a very common condition, particularly in late pregnancy, which may affect as many as 10 per cent of pregnancies in its mildest form, and about 1 in 50 in a moderately severe variety. In rare cases, the most severe type of pre-eclampsia, known as eclampsia, or toxaemia, can occur, although in the majority of women this life-threatening scenario can be avoided by careful monitoring of the pregnancy.

Pre-eclampsia is usually not seen until the sixth month of pregnancy. The syndrome comprises raised blood pressure (hypertension), protein in the urine (proteinuria), and retention of excessive amounts of fluid within the body. Certain factors may predispose a woman to pre-eclampsia, including: first pregnancy, diabetes,

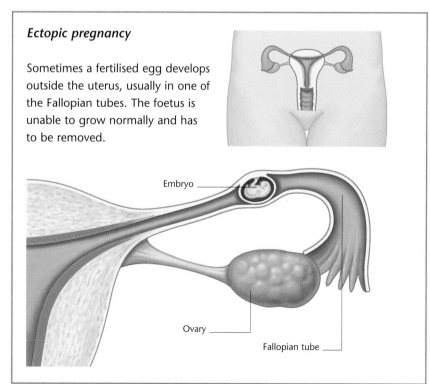

Ectopic pregnancy

Sometimes a fertilised egg develops outside the uterus, usually in one of the Fallopian tubes. The foetus is unable to grow normally and has to be removed.

Embryo

Ovary

Fallopian tube

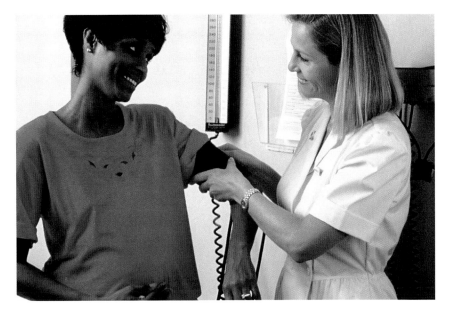

LEFT *Regular antenatal care is essential to monitor the progress of the foetus and the mother's health. Routine tests include blood pressure monitoring to detect the condition pre-eclampsia, which can be fatal if untreated.*

raised blood pressure, previous pre-eclampsia, chronic kidney disease or multiple pregnancy.

Regular monitoring during pregnancy should detect the condition before symptoms arise. Swelling of the ankles, fingers, or face, poor foetal growth, or rapid weight gain may indicate problems. In the latter stages of pregnancy, headache, blurred vision, confusion or abdominal pain can occur. Eclampsia can lead to convulsions or kidney failure, and may be fatal. In more than 40 per cent of cases, eclampsia occurs after the baby is delivered. Treatment may include drugs to lower blood pressure, or delivering the baby early. Some research has shown that aspirin given throughout pregnancy may reduce the rate of eclampsia in women who are at risk.

RHESUS INCOMPATIBILITY

This condition only occurs if the mother is Rhesus negative (see page 208), and has delivered a Rhesus-positive baby. During childbirth, blood from the foetus can enter the maternal bloodstream, causing the mother to develop antibodies against Rhesus factor. In subsequent pregnancies,

the Rhesus antibodies may enter the baby's bloodstream, damaging the red blood cells, and leading to a serious condition known as haemolytic disease of the newborn. Careful monitoring of antibody levels in the mother reduces the risk of the illness developing.

MISCARRIAGE

Miscarriage is the loss of a pregnancy before 24 weeks, but most miscarriages occur before 12 weeks. It is very

common, affecting 1 in 8 pregnancies, and half of all miscarriages are caused by an abnormality in the foetus. The risk of miscarriage is increased by smoking and rates also rise with maternal age. The usual symptoms of miscarriage are lower abdominal pain and vaginal bleeding. Some women have no symptoms, and the miscarriage is detected on a routine scan, when it is known as a missed abortion. Often, a small operation is required to remove the products of conception from the womb. Some women have recurrent problems and if a woman suffers three miscarriages, then she should be referred for investigation to determine the cause, if any.

BELOW *Ultrasound scanning is a safe and painless technique that uses sound waves to produce a picture of the internal organs. Ultrasound is routinely used in pregnancy to check the development of the foetus.*

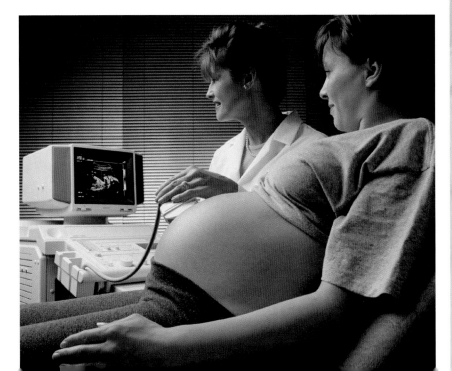

LABOUR AND BIRTH

Birth begins with the onset of labour, which is generally signalled by regular, rhythmic contractions of the muscles in the wall of the uterus (womb). Initially, these may be felt as tightenings across the abdomen, or in the lower part of the back. In some cases, the baby's waters breaking precede the contractions, felt as a gush of fluid from the vagina. More often, this occurs after labour is already established. Most women notice a 'show', a mucus-like discharge that may be blood-streaked, before labour occurs, but it is not a reliable indicator that labour is imminent.

STAGES OF LABOUR

The majority of women give birth without problems. Conventionally, labour is divided into three stages, and monitoring of the mother and baby takes place throughout. The baby's heartbeat is examined using a special foetal stethoscope applied to the mother's abdominal wall. If more continuous observation is necessary, then a cardiotocograph (CTG) is applied to the mother, held in place with a belt placed around the abdomen. Sometimes a special electrode is applied to the baby's scalp to record the baby's heartbeat during labour.

FIRST STAGE

This begins as the uterine contractions become regular and strong enough to cause the neck of the uterus (the cervix) to start opening. The position of the baby is checked by external examination of the abdomen. An internal (pelvic) examination is performed to assess the state of the cervix, which initially is long and closed. As the first stage of labour progresses, the cervix shortens (known as effacement), and opens, or dilates. The first stage is completed when the cervix is fully dilated – about 10 cm (4 in). It is very important that the

---

Delivering the baby

Labour usually begins around the 40th week of pregnancy, and is trouble-free for most women. There are three distinct phases: the first stage, with the initial strong contractions of the uterus and the dilation of the cervix; the second stage, when the baby travels from the uterus down the vagina and is born; and the third stage, when the placenta is expelled from the uterus. The length of each stage is different for every woman and may also be affected by whether or not she has given birth before.

1 *In the first stage of labour, strong, regular uterine contractions gradually push the baby's head against the cervix, causing it to become shorter and wider. During this stage the amniotic sac breaks.*

2 *In the second stage, uterine contractions push the baby along the birth canal. The baby's head presses on the pelvic floor, causing the mother to push down. When the head appears, birth is imminent.*

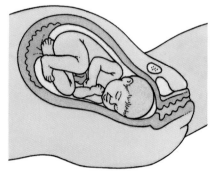

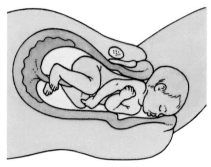

woman does not push before full dilation as the cervix can be damaged. The first stage of labour lasts, on average, about 12 hours.

SECOND STAGE

The second stage of labour starts when the cervix is fully dilated, and at this point the mother usually has a strong urge to push. By bearing down, the baby's head is eased through the cervix into the vagina. The second stage is concluded when the baby is delivered, and may last anything from 15 minutes to 2 hours.

THIRD STAGE

This is the delivery of the placenta (afterbirth), and is usually completed within 15 minutes. A drug is injected into the mother to stimulate uterine contractions as soon as the baby is born. This helps to expel the placenta and reduces the risk of bleeding (post-partum haemmorhage). Sometimes the placenta has to be removed medically, and this usually requires a short general anaesthetic.

3 In the third stage of labour, about 15 minutes after the delivery of the baby, the placenta detaches from the wall of the uterus and is pushed through the vagina by mild uterine contractions and expelled.

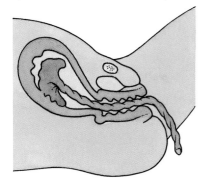

The role of raspberry leaf tea in pregnancy

Raspberry leaf tea is a commonly used herbal tonic for pregnancy. Its exact role is hotly debated, but generally it is accepted that it tones the uterine and pelvic muscles, and reduces constipation. Taken towards the end of the third trimester (after 36 weeks), it probably helps with the progress of labour, although it does not bring on labour. It is vital to check with your doctor before using this remedy.

Caesarean section

This accounts for between 10 and 20 per cent of births in the UK, a figure that is rising yearly. It may be planned (elective) or performed as an emergency. Common reasons for caesarean section include low-lying placenta, failure to progress during the first stage of labour, threats to the oxygen supply to the baby, previous caesarean section, and some breech deliveries. Caesarean section is usually performed under spinal anaesthesia (when the mother stays awake), or a short general anaesthetic, and the surgeon will make an incision about 20 cm (8 in) long across the lower abdomen through which to deliver the baby. The procedure takes about 20 to 30 minutes.

Pain relief

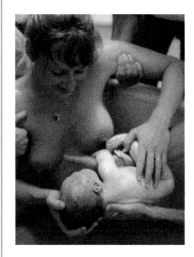

ABOVE *Using a birthing pool under supervision during labour can be relaxing and soothing. Lying in water renders you virtually weightless, which brings relief between contractions.*

Some mothers feel that they would rather not have pain relief (analgesia) during labour, wishing to keep the process as natural as possible. Analgesia, if requested, usually starts with entonox, known as gas and air, which is safe to use throughout the first stage. Pethidine, by injection, is often given in combination with entonox. Side-effects include nausea and drowsiness in the mother and, rarely, the baby may be slow to breathe after birth. Epidural anaesthesia, performed by an anaesthetist who inserts a needle into the lower part of the back, is a very effective, safe form of pain relief. Sometimes it makes the mother's efforts to push in the second stage less effective.

YOUR HEALTH AFTER BIRTH

In the days and weeks following the birth of a child, the parents may go through a confusing range of emotions. In most instances, because of the demands and obligations placed upon her by the new arrival, mothers take the brunt of the emotional turmoil. The exhilaration of the moments immediately after birth, cradling the newborn infant, and the banishment of the pain of labour, can sometimes rapidly be replaced by feelings of inadequacy, vulnerability and sadness. Moods can swing from elation to tearfulness in a matter of minutes.

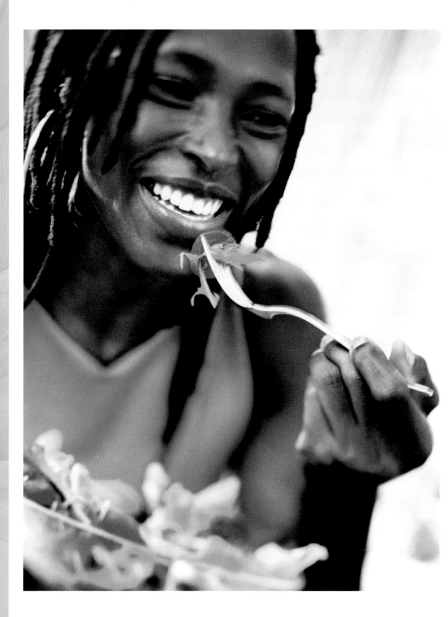

BABY BLUES

Maternal insecurity, combined with the fatigue that is naturally felt after childbirth, sudden changes in hormone levels and the responsibility of knowing that this small being is entirely dependent on its mother, often leads to a period of sadness called the 'baby blues'. This is a normal phenomenon, and usually occurs around the end of the first week after birth. Recognising the signs, and giving the mother the chance to gain some well-earned rest, almost always leads to the disappearance of symptoms.

POSTNATAL DEPRESSION

This should not be confused with the baby blues, which can almost be regarded as a normal event. Postnatal depression goes much deeper, with the usual symptoms of depression such as poor sleep, persistently low mood, loss of appetite and reduced levels of motivation often present. As many as 15 per cent of new mothers experience postnatal depression that lasts longer than two weeks. Half of these will require specific treatment such as

LEFT *A new mother needs to look after herself as well as the baby, and eating properly will help her stay healthy.*

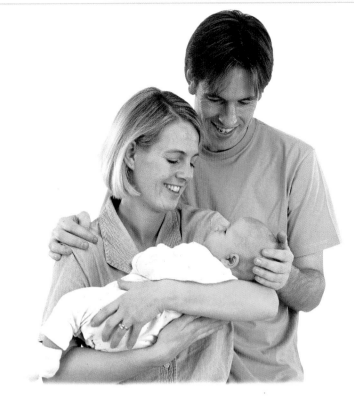

RIGHT *It usually takes new parents a while to get used to becoming new parents, but time spent together will help you all adjust.*

antidepressant tablets. Untreated, the condition may last for many months.

Two new mothers in every thousand will experience a severe form of mental illness known as puerperal psychosis. This usually occurs in the first two weeks after childbirth, and symptoms include confusion, irrational thoughts, hallucinations or delusions. Onset can be rapid, and urgent medical assessment is required, as the newborn baby may be at risk from the mother. Treatment may include medication, or electro-convulsive therapy (ECT).

LOSS OF SEXUAL DESIRE

For most women, the time immediately after childbirth is so busy and exhausting that the last thing they want to think about is resuming sexual relations with their partner. They may also have a genuine fear about becoming pregnant again. The majority of new mothers regain their desire after a couple of months.

Occasionally, new fathers feel they have been replaced in their partner's affections by the new baby, and may even feel jealous. Another barrier to resuming a sex life can be if a father, after witnessing the pain of childbirth, finds it difficult to consider love-making out of a sense of guilt. For these reasons, it is important for both partners to understand the other's point of view, and to be patient.

When sexual intimacy is being rekindled, it is probably wise to delay full intercourse until after the postnatal check-up has taken place at around six weeks. Try to find a time of day when you are not both worn out, and take advantage of any offers of baby-sitting to take time out to relax and enjoy each other's company.

Exercise after pregnancy

Generally, even if a new mother was exercising on a regular basis until the latter stages of pregnancy, it is usually sensible to wait until the all-clear at the postnatal examination before resuming any form of vigorous exercise.

However, this does not mean being idle during those first six or eight weeks. General fitness levels can be regained through exercise such as brisk walking or swimming. Gentle toning and stretching can improve abdominal muscle tone, and most importantly, pelvic floor exercises (details from your midwife) should be performed to reduce risks of urinary problems after birth, and to encourage the tissues in the perineum (the site of any stitches) to heal more quickly.

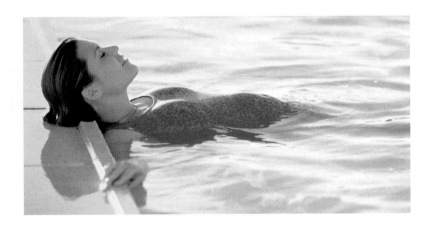

THE NEW BABY: BIRTH TO SIX WEEKS

For a new mother, the first weeks after childbirth seem to be a whirl of activity: feeding, bathing, changing nappies and snatching sleep. It is almost possible to miss the subtle changes that occur in the baby. By the end of the first six weeks, a baby might be following an object with her eyes, vocalising with sounds other than crying, be startled by loud noises and even be smiling at familiar faces. For the vast majority of people, this initial period of parenthood is relatively trouble-free, but unless they are very lucky, there are a few common problems that might be encountered.

COLIC

Around 10–15 per cent of babies suffer from colic, and although most medical staff accept that it exists, there is no agreement about the cause of colic, or what the best treatment is. All sorts of theories have been put forward, including spasm of the muscles in the intestines, and air in the intestines, causing wind.

The most common symptoms of colic include incessant crying, sometimes for several hours, where the baby is inconsolable. The crying occurs at the same time each day, usually in the early evening. The baby draws her knees up towards her chest, and clenches her hands into fists. There may be loud stomach rumbling and gurgling. Colic often begins at around two weeks of age, and may continue until the baby is three months old.

Coping with colic is difficult, and parents find it very distressing when their baby is so upset and they can do little to help. Some parents find that using gripe water helps, others use medication, such as Infacol, prescribed by their doctor, to good effect. However, many parents have to fall back on tried and tested routines such as walking around with the baby, often taking it in turns so that one can rest or eat. Singing, rocking, cuddling or taking the baby for a ride in a car often helps. Finally, crying may be a sign of illness, so if in doubt, it is important to have your baby checked by your GP.

Head is supported

Back is supported

LEFT *Your baby will feel secure in the crook of your elbow, her head and limbs well supported by your crossed arms. Rocking or cuddling your baby often helps stop her crying if she is suffering from colic.*

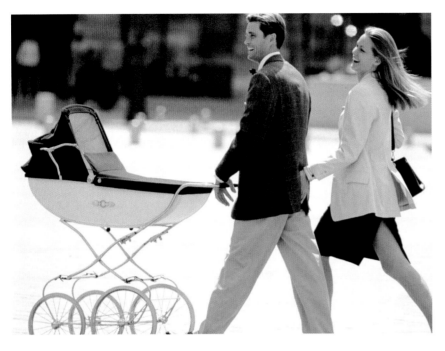

LEFT *For the first three months, your baby must be able to lie flat when being transported until she has head control. The pram you choose will depend on your budget and lifestyle.*

to sleep for an hour or so in the day, take it, and leave housework for another time.

Most parents would like to encourage their baby to sleep for the longest period at night. There are a few tips to aid this objective during night feeds. Close the curtains and keep lighting at low levels, and try to speak very quietly, if at all. Put your baby back to sleep as soon as the feed is finished, do not play with her and only change nappies if essential.

CRYING

All babies cry; it is a normal form of communication. Most times, the crying will be for an obvious reason such as hunger, thirst, a dirty nappy or colic, and that means an easy remedy is at hand. Sometimes, babies will cry constantly, and despite all that parents do to console the infant, nothing seems to work. This can be extremely difficult to cope with, but various methods, such as cuddling and gently rocking your baby, taking her for a walk in her pram or for a drive in the car may help. Gently stroking your baby while talking or singing often soothes a fractious child. It is important to remember that this phase will not last forever, and that many thousands of parents have been through the same experience, so do not be afraid to ask others for help.

SLEEP

Every baby has her own pattern of sleeping and waking, and this will change as the weeks go by. The one certainty is that your sleep requirements, and those of your baby, will rarely coincide. So if you get the chance

Cot death

Cot death (Sudden Infant Death Syndrome) occurs in infants up to the age of 12 months. The cause is unknown, but there are some important factors that can reduce the risk of cot death, including putting your baby to sleep on her back, avoiding smoking in the house, and making sure that your baby is not too hot. Do not let your baby fall asleep under a duvet as she may overheat.

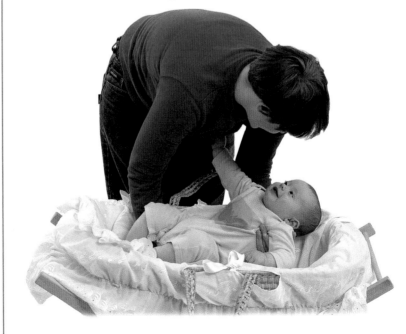

BASIC BABY CARE

During the first few months, new parents learn skills that they have never had to use before. Not all of these will come naturally, so it is important that you should not be afraid to seek advice and guidance from more experienced friends and family.

HOLDING YOUR BABY

Newborn babies are delicate, and it is essential that they are handled with care. Probably the most vital point to bear in mind when picking up your baby is the lack of head control. A baby's head is relatively heavy and the muscles in the neck are not strong enough to stop it flopping around, so placing one hand beneath the head to cradle it prevents injury.

Once the baby has been lifted safely, there are two positions in which to hold her to keep her safe, especially if walking around. The first is to cradle the baby with the head in the crook of your elbow, with your arms crossed beneath the baby's body. The second is to hold your baby so that she is facing backwards, resting her head on your shoulder. This position is often adopted when trying to encourage the baby to bring up wind. Make sure that young children do not attempt to hold the baby by themselves.

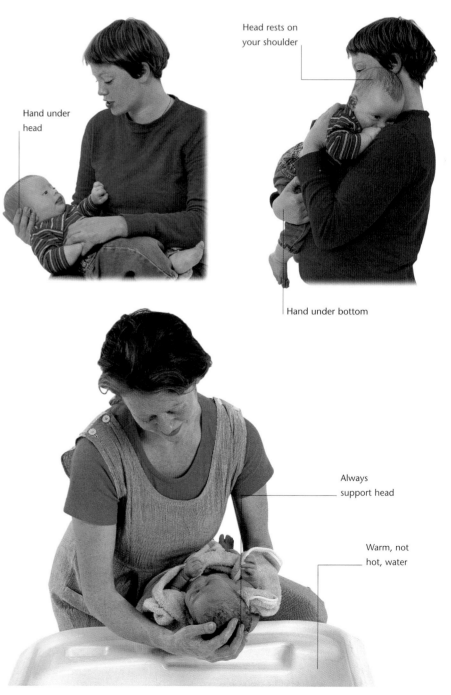

Hand under head

Head rests on your shoulder

Hand under bottom

Always support head

Warm, not hot, water

ABOVE LEFT *It is vital to support your baby's head during the first few weeks so that it doesn't loll and damage the neck muscles. Hold your baby firmly, with one hand under her head.*

ABOVE RIGHT *Your baby will feel secure when held upright against your shoulder. Take her weight with a hand under her bottom, and support her head. This is a good position to help your baby bring up wind after a feed.*

RIGHT *When bathing, support the baby's shoulders and neck on your forearm and cradle the bottom with the other. Slowly splash water over her body with your free hand.*

BATHING

Every day, you should carefully wash your baby's face, neck, hands and bottom. This is known as 'topping and tailing'. Topping and tailing is probably easiest to do on a changing mat. Bathing every other day is sufficient, but many babies enjoy bath time, so a bath could become part of your daily routine. Always make sure that you have everything you need to hand before you start bathing your baby – towels, a nappy and clean clothes. The water should be warm, but not hot: test it with your elbow or wrist.

When bathing, it is essential that you make sure that your baby's head is well supported at all times. Never leave your baby unattended in the bath, even for a second. When washing is completed, gently lift your baby out and pat the skin dry, paying particular attention to the skin creases. This is best done with the baby lying down, and is an ideal time to use moisturiser on your baby's skin.

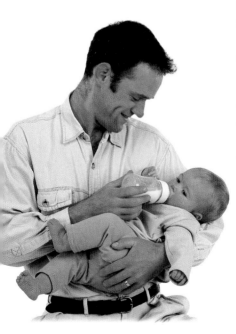

ABOVE *Encourage your partner to take equal responsibility for baby care – he can give breast milk in a bottle while you have a break.*

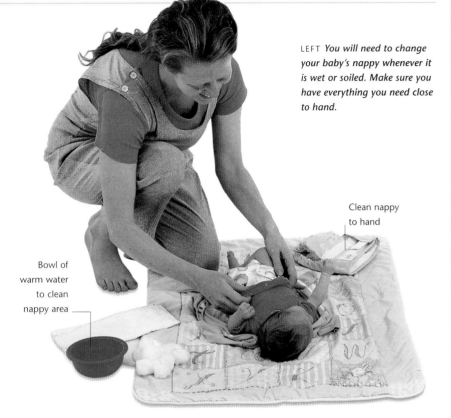

LEFT *You will need to change your baby's nappy whenever it is wet or soiled. Make sure you have everything you need close to hand.*

Clean nappy to hand

Bowl of warm water to clean nappy area

GIVING A BOTTLE

You will need about six bottles and teats to allow easy preparation of a full day's feeds. Sterilising equipment, usually in the form of a chemical sterilising unit, is essential to prevent infection. Teats come in all shapes and sizes, so you will probably have to experiment a little to find the most suitable one for your baby.

Although it is traditional to warm bottle feeds, this is not essential. If you have warmed the bottle, test the temperature by squirting a little on the back of your hand. Find a comfortable position that allows you to cuddle your baby while feeding. As you feed, keep the bottle tilted, and allow your baby to take her time. At the end of the feed, throw away any leftover milk. Never alter the concentration of the feeds you make up, and do not add solids because your baby may choke.

CHANGING A NAPPY

This is best done on a changing mat on the floor. Have a bowl of warm water, cotton wool or baby wipes, and a clean nappy to hand. If your baby is dirty, use the nappy to clean off most of the faeces. Changing nappies as soon as they are soiled helps prevent nappy rash. Clean the whole area thoroughly, wiping from front to back. It is a good idea to leave your baby without a nappy for a short time after changing to let some fresh air get to the skin. Use plenty of barrier cream before putting on a new nappy.

PUTTING DOWN TO SLEEP

Babies should always sleep on their backs to reduce the risk of cot death. The room should be smoke-free, and not too warm. Cover the baby with light bedding, making sure her head is left uncovered. Place the feet against the foot of the cot so the baby cannot wriggle down under the covers. Do not use pillows, quilts, baby nests or bedding rolls. Avoid plastic sheets or bumpers, or bits of string or ribbons from mobiles, because of the risk of your baby becoming entangled.

BREASTFEEDING

There is no doubt that breastfeeding your baby will give her the best start in life. Breast milk is a complete food, containing all of the nutrients your baby needs in the right proportions. If your baby is premature, then it is even more beneficial to breastfeed. In addition, breast milk contains vital hormones, growth factors and antibodies, and the advantages of breastfeeding, even if only carried out for a short time, can last for many years.

BEST FOR BABY

Breastfed babies are less likely to suffer from stomach upsets, constipation, ear infections and coughs and colds. The antibodies passed on from the mother in the milk protect against common childhood infections, and make babies less prone to developing allergic conditions such as asthma or eczema.

BENEFITS FOR MOTHERS

Breastfeeding has a number of advantages for mothers, in addition to the bonding that it promotes between mother and child. It helps the uterus to contract more quickly, and the extra fat that is laid down by pregnant women is used as an energy source to produce milk, allowing a speedier return to your pre-pregnancy figure. Breastfeeding for more than three months is thought to give some protection against breast and ovarian cancer later in life. It is also the most convenient baby food, allowing hungry infants to be fed instantly, wherever you are.

PRODUCING MILK

Breastfeeding can begin immediately after your baby is born, and in most maternity wards, babies are put to the breast as soon as they are delivered to promote milk production. For the first few days after birth, the breasts produce a liquid called colostrum that contains all the nutrients necessary for your baby. The change from colostrum to full breast milk begins around the third day, and is complete by four weeks.

Successful breastfeeding usually begins with finding the correct position for both mother and baby. Comfort is important, and as a suckling baby has to be held close to the breast for some time, make sure that your back and arms are well supported. It is best to bring the baby to the breast rather than vice versa, so placing your baby on a pillow on your lap may make feeding more comfortable.

FEEDING PATTERNS

Feeding patterns vary considerably in the first few weeks, and it is probably

Milk production

Each breast contains 15–20 groups of milk-producing glands (lobules), connected to the nipple by milk ducts. During pregnancy, increased hormone production stimulates the lobules to produce colostrum, a fluid rich in nutrients and antibodies. The production of colostrum stops and that of milk begins about 3–5 days after the baby is born.

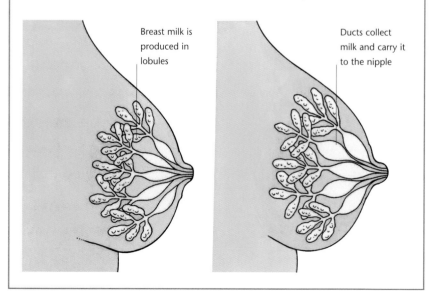

Breast milk is produced in lobules

Ducts collect milk and carry it to the nipple

best to feed on demand, taking as short or as long a time as your baby wishes. The more your baby feeds, the greater the amount of milk produced by the breasts. Sometimes, your baby will only feed at one breast, but most times, it will be necessary to switch breasts after ten or twenty minutes. Suckling is an automatic reflex for most babies, but sometimes encouragement is required, and stroking your baby's cheek or lips will promote the suckle reflex.

New mothers often worry that their baby is not getting enough breast milk, but if a number of wet nappies is being produced each day, and the baby is growing normally, then milk intake is more than adequate.

PROBLEMS WITH BREASTFEEDING

Common problems with breastfeeding include engorgement, where the breast becomes hard, swollen and painful. This is often a consequence of the start of breastfeeding having been delayed, or if the baby is being fed other than on demand. Bathing the breasts with warm water may help. Sometimes, a hard, painful lump appears, caused by a blocked duct in the breast, and can be alleviated by a good feed on that breast. If the area becomes hot and red, and flu-like symptoms develop, then this may be due to a condition known as mastitis. It is best to continue feeding, but sometimes the condition will only clear up with antibiotics, in which case your doctor may advise you to stop breastfeeding.

Ease sore nipples by checking that the baby is latching on properly, by swapping breasts frequently, and by wearing a comfortable bra. Check to make sure your baby does not have oral thrush (see page 425), because this can cause sore nipples. Herbal remedies for sore nipples include calendula, chamomile and comfrey.

Breastfeeding

The key to successful breastfeeding is getting your baby's mouth correctly latched on to your breast. When she is feeding correctly, her mouth will be wide open and you will see her ears and temples moving as her tongue and jaw muscles suck milk from your breast. Let your baby suck for as long as she likes on the first side so she gets the nourishing hindmilk as well as the thirst-quenching foremilk. The baby's jaws should be clamped on your breast tissue rather than on the nipple. This prevents the baby from sucking on the nipple and enables her to stimulate a good flow of milk.

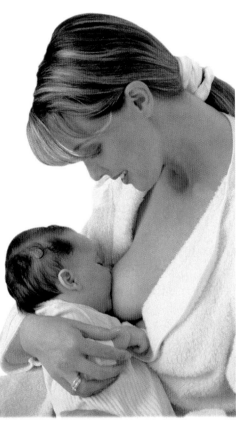

Cracked nipple

Breastfeeding sometimes causes raw areas and cracks on the nipple and surrounding skin, often because the baby has not been correctly positioned on the breast.

Chamomile flowers

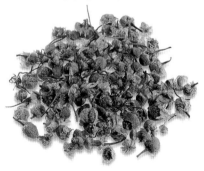

Marigold flower

Herbal remedies
Calendula (marigold) and chamomile oils are anti-inflammatory and can be applied to the breasts to ease nipple pain and inflammation – wash off before feeding.

THE GROWING BABY: SIX WEEKS TO THREE MONTHS

All babies are individuals, and throughout their childhood, rates of growth and speed of development will vary from child to child. It is important that parents view their child with this in mind and do not start to worry if their baby is not doing exactly the same as a friend's baby. Most children develop normally, but at different rates.

CHILD HEALTH RECORD

After their baby is born, all new parents are given a personal child health record, or parent-held record, for their baby, used to keep track of their child's development. Initially, height and weight measurements are recorded, but over time, immunisations, developmental milestones and information about childhood illnesses can be added.

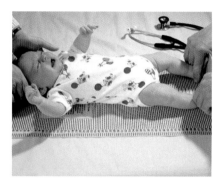

THE SIX-WEEK CHECK

Six weeks marks an important milestone in the life of your baby because it is at around this age that the first physical and developmental check-up takes place. This will usually involve

LEFT *Your baby will have her first medical check-up when she is six weeks old to see how she is developing and how you are coping.*

Height and weight charts

Your baby's growth is recorded during regular check-ups in the first two years of life. The range of normal heights or weights for a child at a given age is very wide, but if a growth curve falls outside the shaded area or follows an erratic pattern there may be a problem. To use the charts, draw a line from your baby's age and another from the measurement of height or weight and plot the point at which they cross. The 50th percentile is the average: 50 per cent of babies are bigger than this, 50 per cent are smaller.

Child's weight (0–2 years)

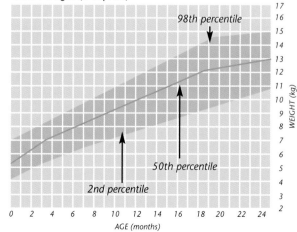

Child's length (0–2 years)

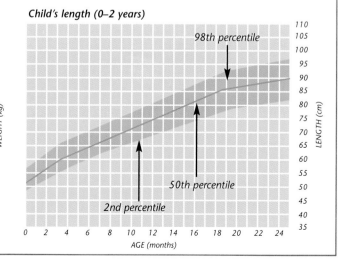

RIGHT *At three months your baby can now lie flat and support the weight of her shoulders and head on outstretched arms.*

both your health visitor and a doctor. Each time you attend a baby clinic, your baby will be weighed and measured, as this is a useful guide to the general progress of your baby. Even if you feel that all is well with your baby, it is important to attend the six-week check-up.

The review generally begins with some questions about how your baby is developing, and how well you are managing with looking after her. After weighing and measuring height, and sometimes head circumference, the doctor will examine your baby by looking at the eyes, mouth, palate (roof of the mouth), heart and lungs, genitalia, and include tests to ensure the hips are in place. The check-up is also an opportunity to ask any questions, or discuss any worries you might have regarding your baby. Advice is given about the immunisation programme, and concerns about vaccination issues can be discussed.

By the age of six weeks, most babies will be smiling, following objects with their eyes, responding to sounds, and communicating using sounds other than crying. Weight will normally have increased by around 30 per cent, and the majority of babies will have grown in length by 5 cm (2 in).

AT THREE MONTHS

In the six weeks following the first development check-up, your baby will begin to develop a character of her own as she starts to interact with the environment and the people involved in her life: parents, older siblings and grandparents. By the age of three months, a baby growing normally will have doubled her birth weight and be approximately 10–12 cm (4–5 in) taller.

The problems that were encountered in the period just after birth may still be present; in particular, colic may persist until the age of three months and sometimes beyond. Sleep patterns may be improved, and many babies will be sleeping through the night from six weeks onwards, giving their parents a well-earned rest. You should still place your baby on her back to sleep, as the risk of cot death does not lessen until the age of twelve months.

At three months, most babies will vocalise by gurgling or laughing, and will turn their heads towards familiar voices. A baby will look at her hands

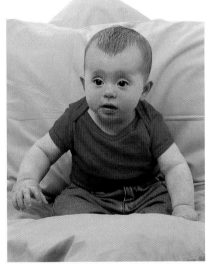

ABOVE *As coordination and muscle strength increase, you baby's body control continues to improve and at three months she should be able to sit up if supported by pillows.*

and move them. If put into a sitting position, a baby will be able to hold her head steady, and may be able to lift her head about 90 degrees while lying on her stomach. If held in a standing position, a baby may be able to bear her own weight. Finally, many babies will be able to grasp toys such as rattles if placed near an outstretched hand.

THE SETTLED BABY: THREE MONTHS TO ONE YEAR

This period, between three months and your baby's first birthday, is one of the most exciting as the pace of developmental changes is breathtaking. Your baby will learn to sit, then crawl, and later to walk, and will develop manipulative skills. She will observe and interact with the world and learn to communicate.

GROWTH AND DEVELOPMENT

At three months, your baby will be watching you, responding to your voice, and taking a lively interest in the surrounding environment. Your baby will listen to you talking, learning already about speech patterns, and will answer back with babbling or cooing sounds as early as the fourth month.

By six months, your baby will be trying to communicate with you using repetitive sounds such as 'ga-ga', or 'ba-ba', and vocalising with an increasing vocabulary of different sounds. Most babies will be reaching out for objects in months four and five, and may be passing things from hand to hand at six months. Your baby is likely to protest loudly if you try to take things from his grasp.

For many babies, the period between six months and one year represents the greatest change of all. You may be able to pull your baby up to a sitting position, and this will be followed shortly by sitting, without support, at around seven months. First teeth arrive about the same time, and you may find that your baby is babbling and dribbling continuously.

At around the same time, babies start to crawl, although some babies seem to miss out this stage completely, and begin to pull themselves up on furniture, trying to walk. This is known as 'cruising'. Sometimes babies who are good crawlers prefer to get around in this fashion for a considerable time, and may, therefore, be slow to walk.

By a year, the majority of babies will be able to walk alone. Most will be able to drink from a suitable cup, and feed

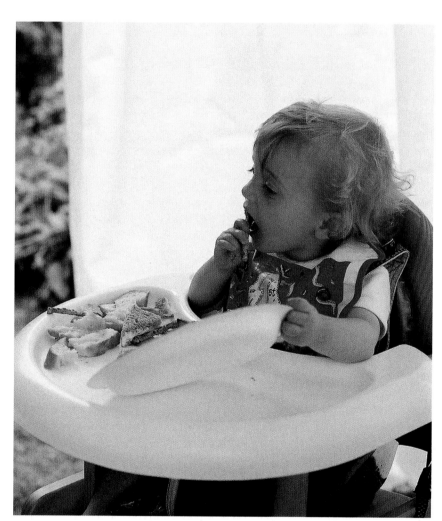

ABOVE *During your baby's first year she will be weaned onto solids. Mealtimes will become messier as she learns to feed herself. Once her neck and back muscles are strong enough to support her you can use a high chair. Always supervise your child when she is eating because she may gag on food.*

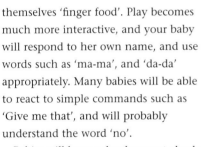

Think about introducing solid food if your baby is not satisfied after a normal feed, or wants feeding more often than usual. Hopefully, most babies will be eating the same food as the rest of the family by the age of one. Some babies enjoy the change of diet, but others take longer to adjust, so go at your baby's pace. Introduce your baby to a variety of tastes and textures.

Ideal first foods include puréed vegetables and fruit, or baby rice. If you use commercial baby foods, then make sure they are suitable for your baby's age, and that they contain no added salt or sugar. Always check that the seals are not broken, and follow the instructions for preparation. It is probably best to avoid wheat-based foods before six months, and it is important to continue breastfeeding alongside solid foods for as long as you both want to.

LEFT *As your baby sits unsupported for longer periods of time his coordination, sense of balance and desire to walk will increase.*

BELOW *By the age of one most babies are able to walk a few steps unaided. As a baby's independence increases, safety in his environment becomes increasingly important.*

themselves 'finger food'. Play becomes much more interactive, and your baby will respond to her own name, and use words such as 'ma-ma', and 'da-da' appropriately. Many babies will be able to react to simple commands such as 'Give me that', and will probably understand the word 'no'.

Babies will have a development check at seven or eight months, usually carried out by a health visitor. At the same time, your baby will have a hearing test. It is important to remember that all babies develop at different rates, and that if you have any concerns about your baby, you should discuss these with your health visitor or GP.

FEEDING

Babies are unable to digest anything other than breast milk or formula milk until they are at least four months old. Between four and six months is the best time to start introducing some solid foods (weaning). By then, babies will require more nutrients than milk alone can provide, and if weaning is delayed past six months, some babies have difficulty accepting 'lumpy' foods, and would rather eat purées.

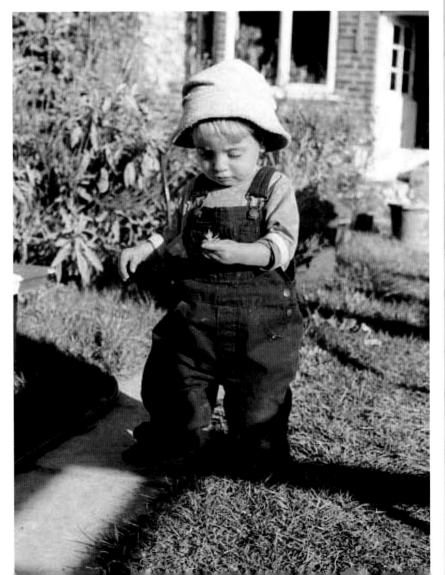

THE SETTLED BABY:
THREE MONTHS TO ONE YEAR

IMMUNISATIONS

Although babies are born with some natural immunity, and gain more through breastfeeding, it is important to have your child immunised to protect against potentially fatal illness that might be encountered in the future. The immunisation programme in the UK starts at eight weeks, and you will be invited to attend by your health visitor or GP.

The first immunisations are given at two, three and four months, and comprise diphtheria, pertussis (whooping cough), tetanus and Hib (bacterial) meningitis in one injection, and meningitis C in a second injection. Vaccination against polio is given orally (by mouth). Some of the illnesses that immunisation protects against are now very rare, but it is still necessary to vaccinate as many children as possible so that the illness may disappear altogether.

Your baby should be in good health when she is vaccinated. Immunisation should be postponed if your baby is feverish, or if she has had a severe reaction to a previous vaccine (a specialist may have to advise if it safe to continue the immunisation programme).

Side-effects of immunisation include prolonged crying, fever and redness at the vaccination site and, rarely, convulsions. If you feel that your baby had a bad reaction to an immunisation, you must discuss it when you attend for the next injection. Polio is a live vaccine that is excreted in the faeces for up to six weeks, and it is possible for an unvaccinated person to contract polio after changing a nappy. It is therefore essential to wash your hands thoroughly after changing the baby.

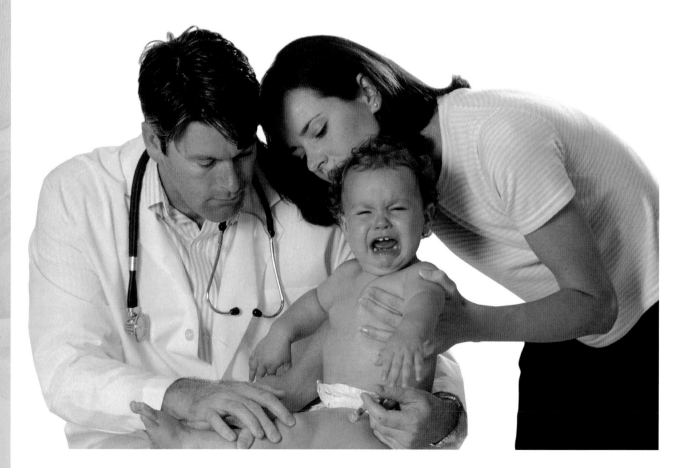

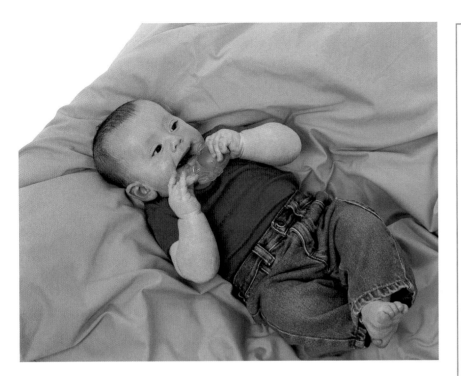

ABOVE *Giving your baby something to chew, such as a teething ring, can help relieve swollen gums caused by teething.*

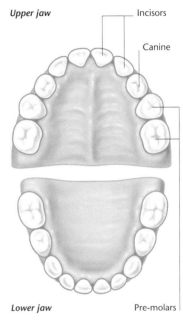

First milk teeth

The lower front two teeth are usually the first to erupt, then the upper front teeth.

Upper jaw   Incisors

                                               Canine

Lower jaw   Pre-molars

EARLY ILLNESSES

From time to time, all children are unwell. However, babies brought up in homes where there are smokers are more likely to suffer from coughs and colds, chest infections, ear infections and glue ear, and asthma. Most times, there will be obvious symptoms of illness such as a cough, fever, vomiting or diarrhoea. Sometimes, though, it is difficult to know if your baby is ill, and you may have to depend on your instincts in determining whether your child's listlessness or crying is unusual.

Illness is always more worrying in very young babies, and if parents are concerned then it is always better to seek help from their GP. Urgent symptoms include high fever, especially

LEFT *The incidence of potentially fatal childhood diseases such as polio has declined dramatically since the introduction of vaccination programmes, which protect your baby.*

if your baby feels cold or clammy, difficulty breathing, extreme drowsiness or fits (convulsions). A purple-red rash that does not disappear when pressure is applied may be a sign of meningitis and always merits urgent medical attention (see Meningitis, pages 414–15). If you cannot contact your GP, then go immediately to a hospital accident and emergency department.

Many illnesses in early childhood are short-lived, including coughs and colds, stomach upsets and diarrhoea. More serious conditions include croup, a viral infection of the voice box (larynx) that leads to a hard, barking cough, and sometimes difficulty breathing. Putting your child in a steamy atmosphere may help, but if the condition does not improve, medical help should be sought. Another viral infection, called bronchiolitis, may also cause breathing difficulties and require hospital treatment.

SLEEP PATTERNS

As the number of night feeds diminishes, it becomes easier to

establish a pattern of sleep for your baby. Having a simple routine for bedtime that is enjoyed by both you and your baby can often prevent problems in the future. This might include a period of relaxation such as bathing and feeding, followed by changing into nightclothes, along with a cuddle and a bedtime story. Putting your baby down awake will allow her to learn to fall asleep in her cot.

TEETHING

The first teeth come through at around six months and usually erupt without problems. There may be some redness or swelling of the gums. Often there is dribbling, and your baby might chew a lot. Using paracetamol or teething gels eases symptoms. Teething rarely makes babies ill, so beware of attributing more serious symptoms to teething.

TODDLER HEALTH

By the end of the first year of life, many children are already walking, talking in a basic manner, and joining in with the family at mealtimes and playtime. Probably the most dramatic changes that occur in the toddler years are linked to communication and behaviour. Speech develops, along with your child's ability to understand what is said to her. Around this time your child's individualism and character really begin to make themselves apparent.

GROWTH AND DEVELOPMENT
Vocabulary increases from the rudimentary 'ma-ma' and 'da-da' at 12 months, to around 20 words by the age of 18 months. At two years, most toddlers will be able to put two words together with a definite meaning. Meaningful play develops within the second year, and fine motor skills improve, allowing precise use of the hands to pick up small objects and build with bricks.

Soon, your baby is a miniature adult, walking up and down stairs, drawing with crayons, kicking a ball and pedalling a tricycle. Your child recognises different colours, can eat without making too much mess, and may even help to dress herself. This is a time to allow your child to explore and to discover things on her own. Parents should be doing things with their child, rather than just doing things for her.

IMMUNISATIONS
The only immunisation that your child will be offered as a toddler is the MMR vaccination at between twelve and fifteen months. This provides immunity

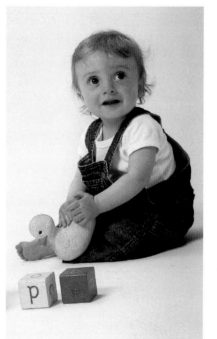

ABOVE *Bright, colourful toys of different shapes stimulate a child's perception of form and space as well as a sense of colour, and building blocks help improve manual dexterity.*

Common childhood illnesses

Many childhood infectious diseases have similar characteristics, such as a rash, fever, cold symptoms and a general feeling of being unwell. Diseases such as measles can lead to complications such as convulsions.

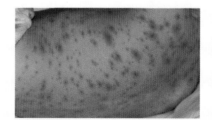

Chickenpox

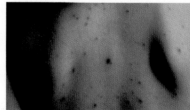

Measles

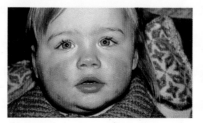

Mumps

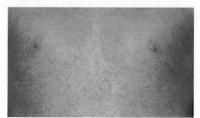

Rubella (German measles)

against measles, mumps and rubella (German measles). There is a second, booster dose of MMR at school entry between the ages of four and five.

Although rubella and mumps are usually regarded as mild illnesses, they can cause problems. If a pregnant woman contracts rubella it may damage the unborn baby. Mumps can cause deafness and can affect fertility in boys. Measles is an unpleasant illness, and may cause complications such as chest infections, convulsions and brain damage. In rare cases, it can be fatal.

Side-effects after MMR include a mild rash and fever about ten days after vaccination. A mild form of mumps sometimes occurs in the third week after immunisation. About one child in a thousand suffers a fit after the MMR jab, but this is about one-tenth the rate of convulsions after measles is contracted. For more information, see MMR, pages 412–13; Measles, page 413; and Mumps, page 414.

COMMON ILLNESSES

The increased social contact that your baby has as she begins to attend nurseries and toddler groups means that the risk of contracting the normal childhood infectious diseases rises. These include chickenpox (see page 415), with its widespread itchy, blistery rash and hand, foot and mouth disease, with greyish blisters on the hands, feet, tongue and sometimes on the buttocks. Scarlet fever, consisting of a sore throat and a widespread red rash that eventually peels, is also common.

Asthma is a chronic condition that affects the lungs, making children cough or wheeze, especially with colds, or on exertion. Sometimes it can be triggered by allergies to house dust, or to animal hair. It often runs in families, and is difficult to diagnose if it appears under the age of two. It appears to be on the increase, and may be provoked

by pollution, or the presence of smokers in the home. For further information, see Asthma, pages 366–67.

Another common illness at this age is 'toddler diarrhoea', manifested in frequent, sometimes offensive-smelling stools in a child who is otherwise well. No obvious cause is found and generally the condition clears up after a few months. Finally, this is a time when frequent ear infections associated with respiratory tract infections can culminate in glue ear, which can affect hearing, and consequently, speech.

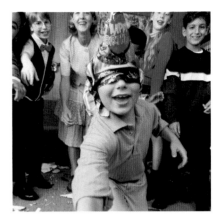

ABOVE *As your child becomes older he will have increased social contact, and his likelihood of contracting an infectious disease rises.*

LEFT *A young child will quickly become accustomed to taking medicine, and will need a spacer to enable asthma medication to reach the lungs.*

TODDLER TAMING

By the time your baby has developed into a toddler, he will have realised that he wields an uncanny and disproportionate amount of ability to completely disrupt the day-to-day goings-on in the house, and beyond. This power may be expressed in a number of ways, and although not every child will go through the 'terrible twos', it is best to be prepared.

BAD BEHAVIOUR

Everybody has their own ideas about what constitutes bad behaviour, and this may be based on your own experiences as a child, and how strict, or otherwise, the family discipline was. It is better to set your own rules depending on you, and your child, and how you wish your family to live. Remember, the behaviour problem may only be a problem in other people's eyes, and made worse by their comments.

TEMPER TANTRUMS

Tantrums usually begin at around 18 months, hit their zenith in the twos, and are rare after four. It is estimated that 20 per cent of two-year-olds have temper tantrums twice daily. Often they are born out of tiredness or hunger, or the frustration of being unable to express feelings adequately because speech is not fully developed.

If there is no obvious trigger for the outburst, then try to distract your toddler, or stay as calm as possible, and if circumstances allow, just sit it out without giving in to demands if you have already said 'no'. Changing your mind to end the tantrum sends the wrong messages to your toddler.

Tantrums often occur in shops, so it is a wise move to keep shopping trips short. Some parents find it helps to hold their child firmly until the tantrum passes, but this requires complete calmness on the part of the

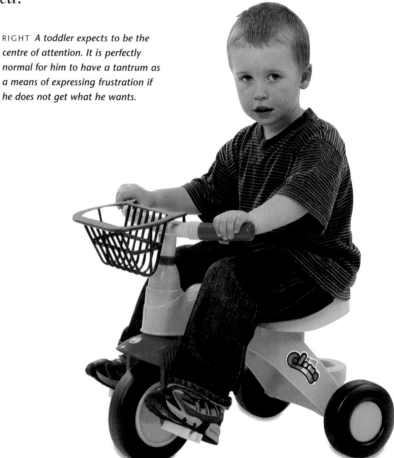

RIGHT *A toddler expects to be the centre of attention. It is perfectly normal for him to have a tantrum as a means of expressing frustration if he does not get what he wants.*

adult and is not always appropriate. Smacking should be avoided because it teaches your toddler that hitting is acceptable behaviour.

Similarly, if your toddler is aggressive, and kicks, bites, or fights with other children, or attacks you during a tantrum, it is essential not to respond in kind. This just reinforces aggression. Try to be firm, remove your child from the environment if other children are

involved, and talk to your toddler, explaining that, although you love him, the behaviour is wrong.

SLEEP PROBLEMS

During the toddler years all your carefully orchestrated bedtime routines may flounder. While in the newborn, the problem is usually coordinating sleep patterns, in the toddler, refusing to go to sleep may cause conflict.

Difficulties in settling down to sleep and waking in the night are common in the under-fives. How much a problem this is depends on whether, as a parent, you are bothered about what time your child goes to sleep. Some parents are happy for their toddler to go to bed at the same time as they do.

Some techniques for encouraging a sleep routine include setting a bedtime and starting a winding down regime about 20 minutes beforehand. Set a limit to how long you will spend in the room story-telling and putting your child down. Make sure that a favourite toy or comforter is nearby. Leave a crying child for about ten minutes before going into the room, and do not take your toddler out of bed to resettle him. Do not keep checking to see whether he has fallen asleep.

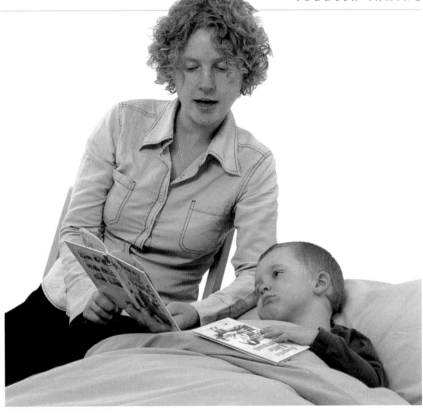

ABOVE *Try to follow a regular routine in the lead-up to bed – reading your child a story will help to calm him down.*

Cranial osteopathy and behaviour

Cranial osteopathy is a type of osteopathic treatment that encourages the release of stresses and tensions throughout the body, including the head. Practitioners feel that they can help with a range of problems in children, including hyperactivity, poor concentration, fidgeting, and problems arising from cerebral palsy and Down's syndrome.

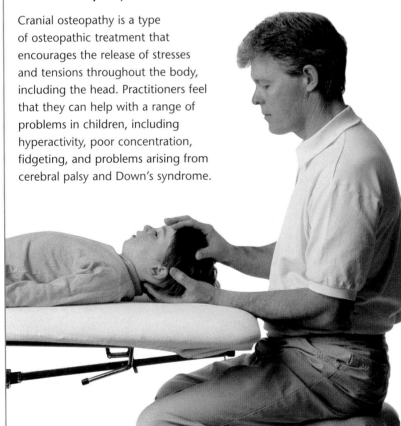

EATING PROBLEMS

Mealtimes can be a battleground as toddlers often become very fussy about what they will eat. Parents worry that their child is not getting enough nutrients, but children eat enough to keep themselves going, and rarely starve themselves to death. What an adult regards as a healthy diet might not appeal to a toddler, so unless your child seems ill, or is not gaining weight, there probably is not a problem.

Try not to force your child to eat, and arrange mealtimes at suitable times so that your child is not too tired to eat. Praise your toddler, and be patient if he doesn't eat very quickly as some children are slow eaters. If a mealtime is dragging on, calmly call a halt. Limit snacks between meals, and remember that children's tastes and appetite change from day to day.

THE GROWING CHILD: TO AGE TWELVE

By the time your child has reached the age of three, most of her movement (motor) skills will be fully developed, allowing a wide range of activities. Your child will be able to recognise the difference between male and female, know several different colours, and speak in sentences clearly enough to be understood by strangers. In play with other children, she will share toys without prompting, and take turns during games. Over the next nine years, most of the changes in your child, apart from the physical alterations in height and weight, will occur in language and social interaction.

EARLY YEARS

Many children start attending reception-type classes at between the ages of three and four as a preparation for starting school at four or five years of age. During these early years in the education system, children begin to develop reading and writing skills, as

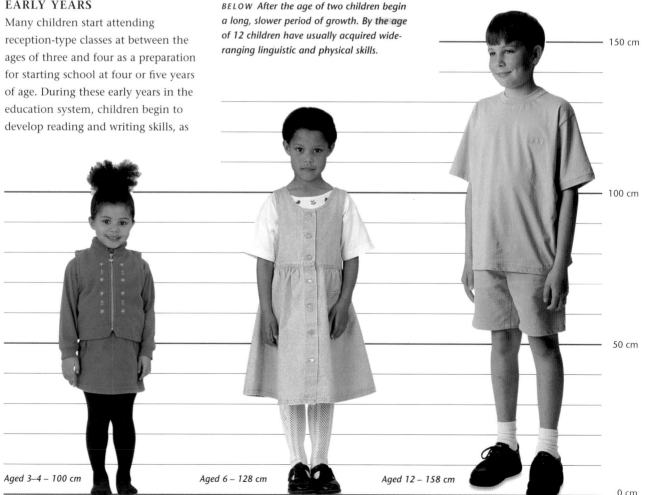

BELOW After the age of two children begin a long, slower period of growth. By the age of 12 children have usually acquired wide-ranging linguistic and physical skills.

150 cm

100 cm

50 cm

Aged 3–4 – 100 cm   *Aged 6 – 128 cm*   *Aged 12 – 158 cm*

0 cm

Adult teeth

As the jaw grows, a set of 32 secondary (adult) teeth erupts between the ages of 6 and 21, replacing primary (milk) teeth.

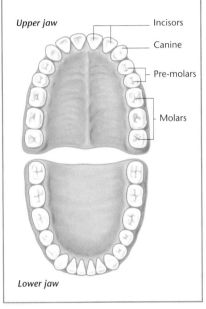

Upper jaw

Incisors

Canine

Pre-molars

Molars

Lower jaw

colds, it might indicate underlying asthma, and it would be worthwhile consulting your GP.

Sometimes, if your child has numerous ear infections, she can develop a condition called glue ear, whereby fluid is trapped behind the eardrum, interfering with hearing. This may be treated by careful monitoring over several months, or by inserting a grommet (a small plastic tube) to improve drainage in the ear.

Failure to thrive is not common, but is a serious condition of infancy and early childhood. Growth is a good indicator of general health, so any child that is not growing as expected may have some underlying illness such as a chronic bowel, heart or lung abnormality. Sometimes, it can be due to inadequate or unsuitable diet. It may also be a pointer for emotional problems and should always be investigated further by a specialist.

Abdominal pain is common in childhood, and can be divided into acute (sudden) and recurrent pain.

Acute pain might be due to gastroenteritis, colic, urine infection, appendicitis, or torsion (twisting) of a testicle. Stomach pain often accompanies infections such as tonsillitis and ear infections, and is thought to be due to the swelling of glands in the abdomen. Recurrent pain, for which there is no obvious cause, may be a form of migraine, or reflect emotional problems such as school avoidance. Most recurrent pain clears up by itself.

IMMUNISATIONS

The only vaccination offered up to the age of twelve is a booster at age four to coincide with school entry. It consists of diphtheria and tetanus in one injection, with MMR (see pages 412–13) given at the same time at a different site, and a booster dose of polio vaccine administered orally.

BELOW *By the time your child reaches the age of four he should enjoy playing with other children in an imaginative and interactive way.*

well as learning to play, interact and communicate with other children. By now, many children will enjoy doing most things independently, and will begin to understand concepts such as size and time.

From six onwards, your child will blossom into a miniature adult, thinking for herself, solving everyday problems, making permanent friends and learning to play team sports. The final link with babyhood is broken as the milk teeth are gradually lost, to be replaced by the eruption of the permanent teeth.

COMMON ILLNESSES

Many children, especially after they start to mix with others in playgroups and reception classes, are prone to viral coughs and colds. These are usually nothing to worry about, although if your child seems to have excessive

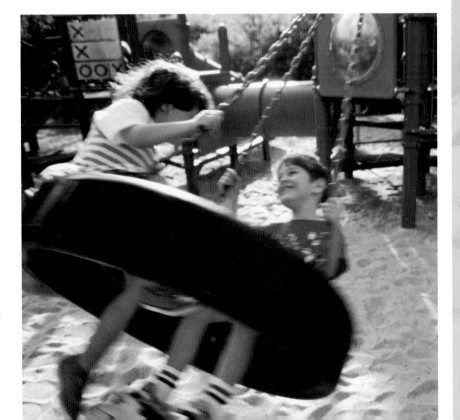

THE GROWING CHILD'S EMOTIONAL LIFE

Raising a child is often said to be one of the most difficult things any human being can do. Undoubtedly, it is a satisfying task, with huge responsibilities, and one for which most people are unprepared. However, there is usually a host of friends, relatives and 'experts' on hand to offer advice on successful parenting. For most parents, the potential minefield of coping with the demands of a new baby, an errant toddler or a difficult schoolchild is negotiated more or less successfully. But difficulties can arise when the problems are of a more emotional nature, where there may not be a perfect answer, and when the advice from various sources is conflicting.

BED-WETTING

Bed-wetting, or enuresis, is usually defined as frequent wetting of the bed in children over the age of five. Enuresis is common, affecting 10 per cent of five-year-olds, 5 per cent of ten-year-olds, and 1 per cent of fifteen-year-olds. Occasionally, it can persist into adult life.

The reasons why some children seem unable to gain bladder control during sleep is not known, although a number of children may start to wet the bed, after being previously dry at night, following a traumatic life event. This might be bereavement, a change of school, or even moving house, with subsequent loss of friends.

Treatment is aimed at controlling the problem, and may be undertaken by your GP, a special enuresis clinic, or a hospital doctor. In younger children,

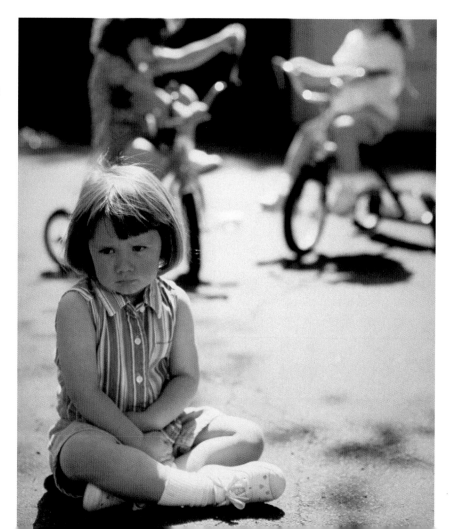

RIGHT *Some children find it difficult to build friendships and lack the confidence to be able to play readily with others, but you can help your child join in by teaching her how to approach others, or create your own opportunities for socialisation.*

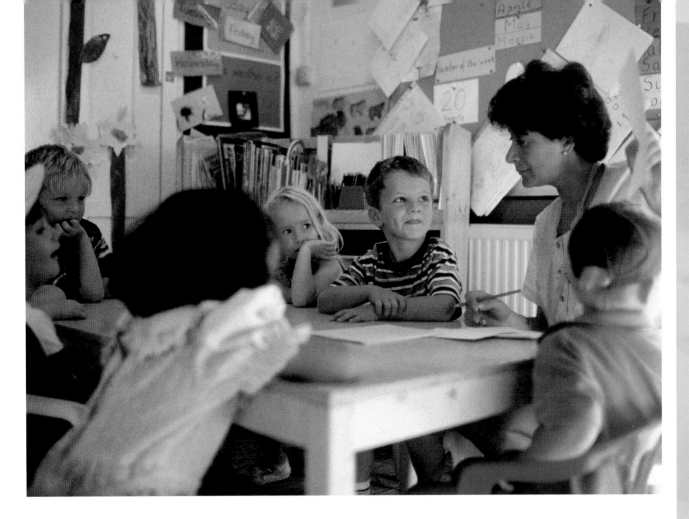

encouragement, lifting from sleep and taking to the toilet when parents go to bed, and a record of successful dry nights using a star chart may be all that is needed.

Sometimes, a buzzer alarm that wakes the child as wetting starts, helps to train the child to wake as the bladder becomes full. This can be very helpful, but relapse after the alarm is removed is quite common. Usually as a last resort, drugs are used. The most successful is desmopressin, a hormone produced by the body that reduces urine production overnight, and is usually very effective.

STARTING SCHOOL

Traditionally, the first day at school has been faced with dread by parents, as their offspring deal with the reality of being out of reach for the first time. Despite the growth of nurseries and reception classes, a child confronted with the scale of a 'proper' school, with its larger buildings, masses of strangers

and its formality, may panic.

For most children, this is a period of relative calm and stability, and the majority seize the opportunities presented to make friends, gain knowledge and develop as individuals. Problems in reading are common, affecting one in ten children, so it is important to spot if your child is struggling, or falling behind her peers, so that action can be taken. Whenever problems are suspected, then close liaison with the school is essential.

BULLYING

Bullying comes in many forms, and it is thought that 25 per cent of primary school children and 10 per cent of secondary school children are the victims of bullying at some time. Bullying may be physical (violence, or intimidating behaviour), verbal (name-calling, sarcasm), emotional (exclusion from the gang), racist or sexual.

Verbal and emotional bullying are on the increase, and are hard to prove,

ABOVE *Specific learning weaknesses, in reading, language and attention, are strongly hereditary. Be quick to ask a teacher for help if you think your child is falling behind.*

often wearing the victim down. Bullying is not restricted to the school environment, and may happen to anybody without an obvious reason. Over time, the effects of bullying can lead to depression, loneliness, poor academic achievement and even attempts at suicide.

If you suspect that your child is the victim of bullying, then it is best to ask her outright, and although she may deny it at first, hopefully she will open up about the problem. Discuss how your child wants to handle the bullying, as it is likely that the last thing that she wants you to do is storm into school, demanding to see the head and threatening retribution against the bully. Keeping a diary of incidents may be helpful, as may contacting the school in a low-key way.

A CHANGING BODY

For the vast majority of children, the first ten years or so of life are spent in a rather idyllic state of play, education and social interaction, which does not prepare them for their first and most significant life change. Puberty, the period in a young person's life when the changes in body and mind can lead to turmoil, then shows its ugly face.

WHAT IS PUBERTY?

Puberty is usually defined as the time in a child's life where sexual maturity begins. It is often preceded by changes in bodily appearance with a spurt of growth, and in emotional thoughts and responses. As a parent, you will notice the changes, although your child may not be fully aware of the bewildering array of physical and hormonal alterations that occur. These changes tend to start earlier in girls, and are known as secondary sexual characteristics.

PUBERTY IN BOYS

In boys, the physical side of puberty includes alteration in the voice, so that it becomes deeper in character, known as 'breaking', the development of pubic hair and a change in the size and appearance of the penis and scrotum as sexual maturity is reached. The testicles begin to produce sperm. The distribution of muscle tissue can change, causing the shoulders and limbs to become broader, while fat deposited around the abdomen may disappear, making the waist narrower.

There may also be the beginnings of facial and body hair growth.

PUBERTY IN GIRLS

The first sign of puberty in girls might be the appearance of the first period. This is usually an indication that the ovaries have started to produce sex hormones. These hormones will have far-reaching effects on the appearance of the female body. Secondary sexual changes in girls include a change in body proportions, with narrowing of the waist and widening of the hips.

Puberty in boys

Testosterone levels rise sharply during puberty, causing physical changes and, later, sperm production and increased sex drive.

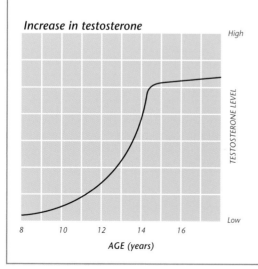

Increase in testosterone

High

TESTOSTERONE LEVEL

Low

8   10   12   14   16

AGE (years)

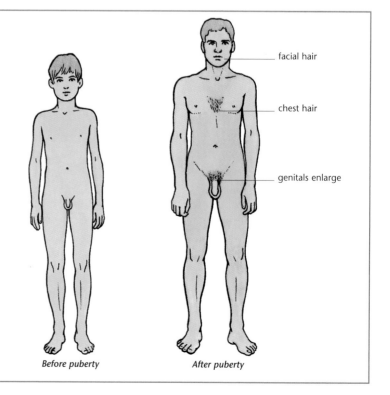

facial hair

chest hair

genitals enlarge

Before puberty   *After puberty*

Breast development begins, and pubic and underarm hair grows. The external sexual organs change in appearance as they mature in preparation for future sexual intercourse.

Most girls experience their first menstrual period between the ages of 10 and 16. It has the potential to be a frightening experience, so it is important to discuss what to expect with your daughter before the event, allowing her to be prepared. If you do not feel comfortable doing this, it would be helpful if another female relative or friend could discuss menstruation with her.

A TIME OF TRANSITION

In addition to the physical changes, puberty represents a period of limbo between childhood and adulthood. Conflict with parents is commonplace, and can almost be regarded as normal. Adolescents are seen as cheeky, moody, irritable know-alls by parents, and conversely, teenagers generally regard

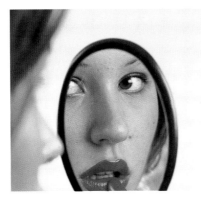

parents as old-fashioned, embarrassing and useless.

Many young people find the changes in their bodies hard to cope with, particularly if they stand out as early or late developers compared with their peers. They can feel shy, insecure and lack confidence. They may not be satisfied with their body image. It is important that parents offer support at this time, but beware of being over-protective as this can lead to problems establishing relationships with other people later in life.

LEFT *Girls become sexually mature earlier than boys and will often look much older than their age, particularly if they wear makeup.*

Sometimes, the final insult for many teenagers going through puberty is the appearance of a common skin condition called acne (see pages 370–71). At puberty, both boys and girls start to produce androgens, male sex hormones that increase the production of sebum (the skin's natural lubricant) by glands just below the surface of the skin. The long-term consequence of this, in some young people, is the typical appearance of acne.

Although for many youngsters acne is a mild, transient disorder that can be tackled by attention to skin care, for others, it requires treatment either with antibiotic lotions or tablets. The aim of the treatment is to improve the appearance of the skin and to reduce the risk of scarring in the future. Treatment may need to continue for months, or even years.

Puberty in girls

Oestrogen levels rise sharply in girls, prompting physical changes and then stimulating ovulation and menstruation.

Increase in oestrogen

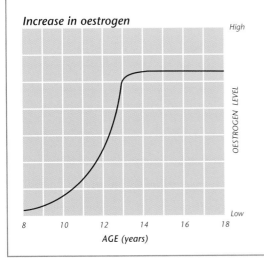

AGE (years)

OESTROGEN LEVEL

High

Low

8   10   12   14   16   18

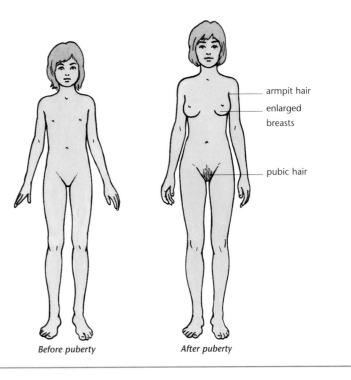

armpit hair

enlarged breasts

pubic hair

Before puberty   *After puberty*

THE EMOTIONAL ADOLESCENT

Bringing up a child is a difficult and demanding job, and most parents draw on their own upbringing and the role that their parents played. Parents who show their children patience, understanding, respect, honesty, unconditional love and kindness are much more likely to see these qualities reflected in their child's behaviour. Support during periods of difficulty, time spent together as a family, consistency with regard to discipline and setting acceptable limits of behaviour are likely to produce confident, self-assured teenagers who can communicate with both peers and parents.

EATING DISORDERS

For many young women there is a constant battle, usually because of peer and media pressure, to pursue the ideal body shape and weight. However, the vast majority look upon this battle as a minor irritation in life, and regard the occasional indulgence in chocolate or fast food as normal. For a small minority, the obsession with body image and calorie counting not only threatens to invade their whole life, but can also literally kill them.

Nobody is really certain what triggers an eating disorder such as bulimia or anorexia nervosa. Most probably environmental factors, and a genetic predisposition in an individual with low self-esteem combine to trigger the illness. Trigger factors include puberty, bereavement, and stress provoked by bullying and ridicule from friends. Although eating disorders mainly affect females, boys and young men can also develop problems.

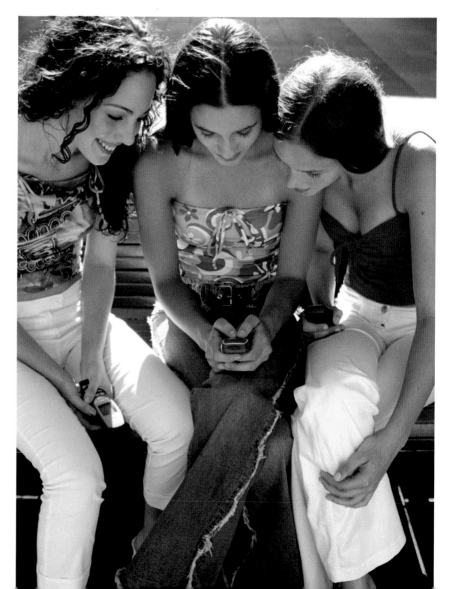

RIGHT *Teenagers are very concerned with looking good and will be subjected to constant pressure to attain the ideal weight and body shape, but most will take this in their stride.*

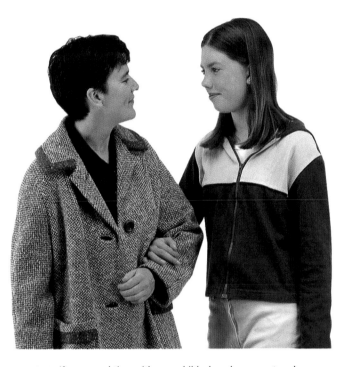

ABOVE *If you spend time with your child, show her respect and understanding, and give her unconditional love, her behaviour is likely to reflect these qualities.*

ABOVE *Teenagers are often moody but be alert if your child withdraws from friends and interests – he may be depressed, and if symptoms continue, you should seek professional help.*

ANOREXIA NERVOSA

Thought to affect around 1 per cent of teenage girls, anorexia nervosa may share some of the features of bulimia such as vomiting, use of laxatives and a fixation with body shape and weight, although binge eating is rare. Body weight, however, is usually at least 15 per cent below normal and sufferers live in fear of putting on weight. They become expert calorie counters and often have rules about how much they are allowed to eat.

Physical signs, other than being underweight, include dental problems, absence of periods, low blood pressure and low pulse rate. There may be symptoms of depression such as low mood and poor motivation.

If an eating disorder is suspected, it is vital that help is sought as soon as possible, but this may be hindered by the sufferer's lack of acknowledgement of her illness. There is no single therapy that guarantees success, but cognitive behavioural therapy, family therapy and antidepressants are used, usually under the care of a psychiatrist. For more information, see Anorexia, pages 352–53.

BULIMIA

Although less well known than anorexia, bulimia is far more common, affecting between 1–2 per cent of women aged 15 to 40. In bulimia, although there is often an obsession with body shape and weight, there are not the same efforts to lose weight as there are with anorexia. For this reason, a near normal weight may be maintained for many years without the diagnosis of bulimia being made.

Features of bulimia include binge eating, usually followed by self-induced vomiting or excessive exercise. Sometimes, shop-bought laxatives are used to promote weight loss. Excessive vomiting may lead to kidney damage, as well as eroding teeth enamel. For more information, see Bulimia, page 353.

DEPRESSION

Probably one in five teenagers has an episode of depression at some time. Usually these occur in response to the traumas and stresses of normal teenage life – relationships, exams and sexual maturation are just a few. It may show itself with low mood, irritability, anger, loss of appetite, weight changes, poor sleep and loss of interest in sport or hobbies.

It is often difficult to decide whether this sort of change in your child is due to depression, or just the typical ups and downs of a normal teenager. However, if symptoms persist for more than a couple of weeks, it is best to seek professional help, particularly if you have personal experience of depression, as it may be hereditary. For more information, see pages 348–50.

THE WELL WOMAN

In the UK, women, on average, live about five years longer than men. Part of this is due to the fact that there are some routine screening programmes available to women, whereas, as yet, no population screening programmes are aimed at men. Also, women come into contact with the health service much more frequently than men. They attend for contraception, are seen regularly in pregnancy and have dealings with midwives, health visitors and GPs when they have young children. There is ample opportunity to discuss health issues and worries.

HEALTHY LIVING

There is no doubt that good health is more likely to be maintained if your lifestyle encompasses a well-balanced diet, regular exercise, alcohol intake within the recommended limits and abstinence from smoking. Heart disease is the top cause of death for women in the UK, so addressing risk factors such as obesity and smoking should be a priority for all women.

Find out if you are overweight by calculating your BMI (Body Mass Index; see page 241). This is worked out by finding your weight in kilograms and dividing it by your height in metres squared. A normal result lies between 20 and 25, with obesity being present if the BMI is above 30. Look out for other risk factors such as raised blood pressure (hypertension), raised cholesterol and diabetes. If you have a family history of heart disease, then make sure that you have your blood pressure taken every year, and ask your doctor to screen you for diabetes (by testing a urine sample for sugar) and have a blood test for cholesterol.

You can protect your bones for the future by making sure your diet contains adequate amounts of calcium. Peak bone mass is reached in the thirties, and can be maintained by regular weight-bearing exercise, not smoking and avoiding excessive amounts of alcohol.

SCREENING FOR WOMEN

In the UK, screening for cancer of the cervix is offered from the age of 20 and ceases at around the age of 65. A cervical smear is taken every three years to detect early changes in the cells of the cervix. Sometimes, if abnormalities are detected, smears are carried out more frequently. Abnormal vaginal bleeding or a change in the amount, or character, of your normal vaginal discharge could indicate early problems and should always be reported to your doctor.

LEFT *Eating a healthy diet is essential for good health, and choosing fresh foods will help you obtain the maximum amount of nutrients.*

Similarly, women over the age of 50 are invited to attend for a breast X-ray, or mammogram, every three years. Although this national screening programme detects many breast cancers, more than 90 per cent of breast cancers are picked up by women themselves. Make sure you know what is normal for you, and examine your breasts on a regular basis. Report any changes to your doctor immediately, and do not wait to be screened.

Women who have a family history of cancer should find out about who was affected, the type of cancer, and discuss with their doctor the availability of screening tests. Common cancers where there may be a family link include breast cancer, cancer of the ovary and bowel cancer. Some larger hospitals now have family cancer clinics, where your risk of developing the disease can be estimated and the various screening tests discussed.

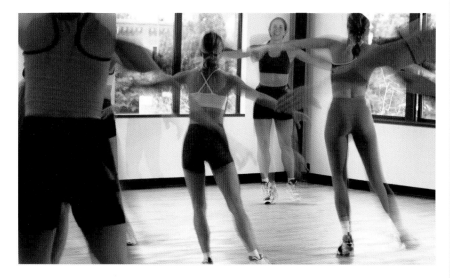

ABOVE *Aerobic exercise gives the heart and the lungs a good workout, making you feel more energetic and reducing your risk of developing heart disease and stroke.*

BELOW *Weight-bearing exercise such as walking helps keep bones healthy and slows down the loss of bone mass associated with declining oestrogen levels after the menopause.*

When to see a doctor

Some symptoms that might be a sign of a serious problem include:

• *Rapid weight loss, or loss of appetite lasting for more than a few days.*
• *Persistent tiredness, which could indicate anaemia, diabetes or an underactive thyroid gland.*
• *Irregular, prolonged or heavy vaginal bleeding.*
• *Change in bowel habits such as diarrhoea or constipation. This may be accompanied by other symptoms, including abdominal pain or bleeding from the rectum, and should always prompt a visit to the doctor.*
• *Vomiting or coughing up blood – this is always serious and should not be ignored.*
• *Blood in the urine – although this is fairly often a feature of cystitis, it should be reported to your doctor.*

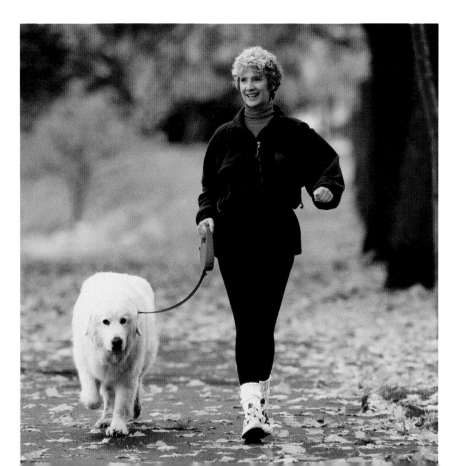

BREAST HEALTH

Breast development is one of the most obvious female secondary sexual characteristics, and can begin in girls from the age of ten onwards. Breast tissue is made up of about 85 per cent fat, interspersed with glandular tissue, and supported by a network of fibres known as connective tissue. Contrary to popular belief, breasts contain no muscles. Breast development is, to a degree, influenced by genetic factors that determine the final size and shape of the breasts.

SIZE AND SHAPE

Not only do breasts develop differently from woman to woman, they also change size and shape throughout each woman's life. Even the size of each breast can differ, often to a significant degree. In the early years after puberty, the breasts increase in size, sometimes at an alarming rate. The breast tissue tends to be much firmer, needing less in the way of support than later in life.

During pregnancy, the breasts usually enlarge in preparation for breastfeeding. The nipples change in size and colour under the influence of hormones produced by the body during pregnancy. Increased pigmentation makes the nipples look much darker, and this is a permanent change that will not go away after childbirth.

The breast enlargement seen during pregnancy may or may not be permanent, with many women returning to near their pre-pregnancy shape and size after they have finished breastfeeding. As women approach the menopause, some will notice that their breasts increase in size a little. As the effects of falling hormone levels become apparent, the supporting tissue can lose some of its elasticity, leading to sagging of the breasts that becomes more apparent with advancing age.

BREAST AWARENESS

Recent changes in the advice given to the medical and nursing professions has meant that the days of having breast checks routinely when attending for contraceptive advice and when taking HRT are gone. There is no evidence to show that a nurse or doctor examining the breasts in the absence of specific symptoms is of any benefit.

Instead, doctors and nurses are promoting breast awareness. The most vital aspect of breast awareness is for a woman to understand how the shape, size and consistency of her breasts vary, and to learn what is normal for her. The breasts change considerably throughout life, but more importantly, they change even from day to day during the menstrual cycle. These changes may involve discomfort or pain, a sensation of fullness before a period, lumpiness, or tenderness in a cyclical pattern. The ability to recognise changes from the normal pattern is the basis of breast awareness.

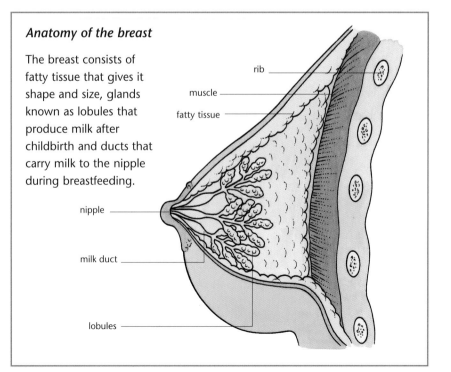

Anatomy of the breast

The breast consists of fatty tissue that gives it shape and size, glands known as lobules that produce milk after childbirth and ducts that carry milk to the nipple during breastfeeding.

rib

muscle

fatty tissue

nipple

milk duct

lobules

SELF-EXAMINATION OF THE BREASTS

Regular self-examination should be part
of every woman's monthly routine, and
is relatively simple to carry out.

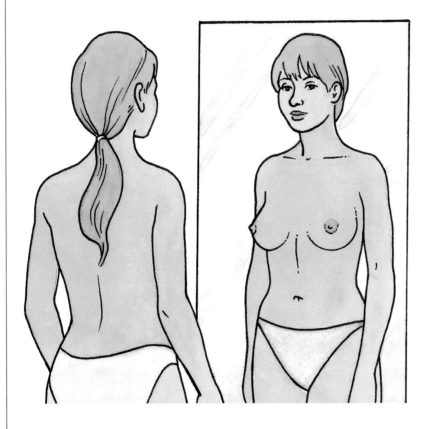

*1 The first part of the examination is to
observe the breasts, best done standing in
front of a mirror with the arms hanging loosely
down. Look for changes in the size or shape of
the breasts, and changes in the nipples,
particularly any bleeding or discharge.
Puckering of the skin is a significant symptom.*

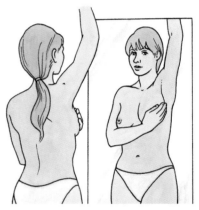

*2 By raising the arms above the head, and
moving from side to side, the breasts can
be viewed from all angles.*

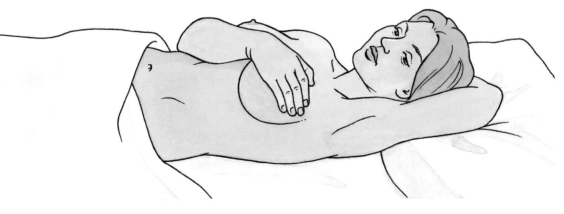

*3 The second part of the examination is
to feel both breasts for changes. Lying
on your back, extend one arm and place
the hand under your head. With your other*
*hand flat and fingers together, use the flats
of your fingers to feel around the breast
in small, circular movements, in an
anticlockwise direction. Cover the whole of*
*the breast, including the nipple. Examine the
armpit on that side for lumps. Examine the
other breast in the same fashion. If you find
anything that worries you, visit your doctor.*

MENSTRUATION: THE MENSTRUAL CYCLE

Menstruation, also known as having a period, refers to that part of the menstrual cycle where a woman loses blood from the uterus via the vagina. The onset of the first period indicates that sexual maturation is complete. The majority of girls have their first period between the ages of 10 and 16, and will continue to menstruate until the age of 45 to 55. The average woman will have around 500 periods in a lifetime. Periods usually occur about once every 28 days, and last for between three and seven days.

HOW THE MENSTRUAL CYCLE WORKS

The female reproductive system consists of a pair of ovaries, the Fallopian tubes, the uterus (or womb) and the vagina (see Female Reproductive System, pages 204–5). The menstrual cycle is a complex interplay between these female sexual organs and chemical messengers known as hormones, produced in the ovaries and by a structure in the brain called the hypothalamus, and by a nearby organ known as the pituitary gland.

PRE-OVULATION

The ovaries contain eggs (ova) from birth, but these eggs become available for fertilisation only with the onset of the first period. In the first part of the menstrual cycle, the hypothalamus releases a hormone called follicle-stimulating hormone (FSH) that causes a number of eggs within the ovaries to mature. As these eggs develop, the ovaries produce an increased level of the female hormone oestrogen.

This increased production of oestrogen has a direct effect on the lining of the uterus (the endometrium), causing it to thicken and to benefit from an improved blood supply. These changes in the endometrium prepare the uterus to receive a fertilised egg. Over the two weeks following the first day of a period, eggs continue to mature within the ovaries until the pituitary gland releases a hormone called luteinising hormone (LH) into the bloodstream.

OVULATION

This surge of luteinising hormone causes one of the maturing eggs to be released from the ovary, a process known as ovulation, which precedes the next period by 14 days. Some women know when they are ovulating because they feel a pain in the lower part of the abdomen, or they may experience some mid-cycle spotting of blood. Women who have no symptoms of ovulation can check when they ovulate by measuring their temperature daily, using the same site and taking the temperature before getting out of bed in the morning. A change in temperature of 0.5° Celsius indicates ovulation. The egg survives for 24 hours after ovulation and can be fertilised only during this time.

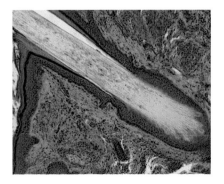

LEFT *In the first half of the menstrual cycle, about 20 eggs ripen in fluid-filled sacs (follicles). One of these follicles outgrows the others and matures and ruptures, releasing the egg.*

RIGHT *After ovulation, the hormones oestrogen and progesterone cause the endometrium to become thicker and spongy so that it is ready to receive the fertilised egg.*

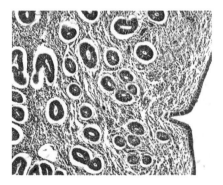

The menstrual cycle

During a woman's reproductive life, between puberty and the menopause, her ovaries release eggs in cycles in preparation for conception and pregnancy. Each menstrual cycle lasts about 28 days on average but varies from woman to woman. The menstrual cycle is controlled by complex interactions between four sex hormones: follicle-stimulating hormone (FSH) and luteinising hormone (LH), produced by the pituitary gland, and oestrogen and progesterone, produced by the ovaries. The development and release of an egg for fertilisation is known as ovulation, and the ovaries ovulate alternately.

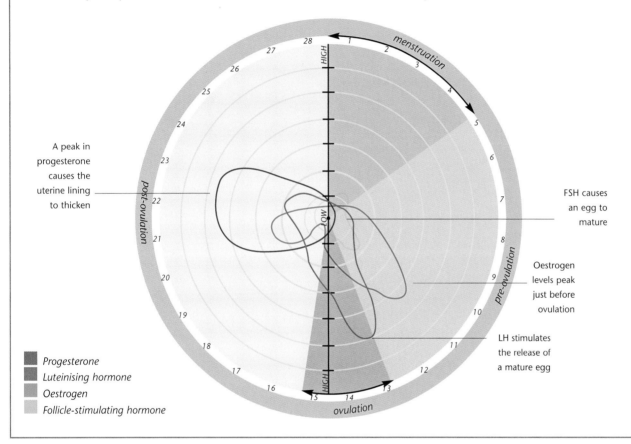

A peak in progesterone causes the uterine lining to thicken

FSH causes an egg to mature

Oestrogen levels peak just before ovulation

LH stimulates the release of a mature egg

menstruation

post-ovulation

pre-ovulation

ovulation

■ Progesterone
■ Luteinising hormone
■ Oestrogen
■ Follicle-stimulating hormone

POST-OVULATION

If fertilisation by a sperm occurs, then the egg implants into the thickened endometrium (see The Beginning of Life, pages 266–67). However, if the egg is not fertilised, then the levels of the two female hormones (oestrogen and progesterone) in the bloodstream begin to fall. This, in turn, leads to the death of the endometrium which, along with some fresh blood from the disrupted blood vessels, is shed as the menstrual flow. On average, about 80 ml (3 fl oz) of fluid is lost with each period.

FACTORS AFFECTING THE MENSTRUAL CYCLE

There is a number of factors that influence the menstrual cycle. The most important of these are the various hormones involved in the stimulation of the ovaries, and those produced by the ovaries themselves. Hormonal imbalance is a common cause of menstrual problems, but as each individual's normal levels are different, blood tests to check them often are not very helpful. Fluctuations in hormone levels are common in puberty, after childbirth and in the run up to the menopause, causing wide variations in a woman's normal pattern of bleeding.

Periods are also influenced by weight, with underweight women sometimes finding that periods cease. Obesity may also make the menstrual cycle erratic, leading to difficulties in conceiving. Regular exercise may be helpful in normalising the menstrual cycle, but too much exercise can stop periods completely, something seen in professional athletes, particularly long-distance runners.

MENSTRUAL PROBLEMS

With the complex interaction between the female sexual organs, hormones and the brain, it is hardly surprising that almost all women will, at some point in their lives, suffer from period problems. In fact, because painful periods are so common, it seems almost acceptable to regard the problem as a variation of normality, rather than an illness.

PAINFUL PERIODS (DYSMENORRHOEA)

It is estimated that around 70 per cent of young women use painkillers regularly for period pains, and for 50 per cent, painful periods disrupt daily living for at least a day or two each month. Period pains are often only one part of a collection of other unpleasant symptoms that happen as menstruation takes place each month, which can include headache, abdominal pain, nausea, sweating and pain in the vagina. Add to these the symptoms of premenstrual syndrome (see page 420), and it is easy to appreciate why so many women feel wretched during menstruation.

Painful periods are almost certainly caused by contractions of the muscles in the wall of the uterus, similar to those felt during labour. These occur all the time, but become much more intense during a period as the lining of the uterus is shed. At the same time, the body produces chemicals called prostaglandins in an effort to strengthen the contractions of the uterus during a period, but this can make the pain even worse.

Period pains, especially if present from the time that periods began, are rarely a sign that anything serious is going on. Pain is often at its worst in teenagers and in women nearing the menopause. However, because period pains are often accepted as being part of a woman's lot in life, more serious underlying causes may be ignored, or the diagnosis delayed.

If the pattern of dysmenorrhoea changes, or if the pain becomes much

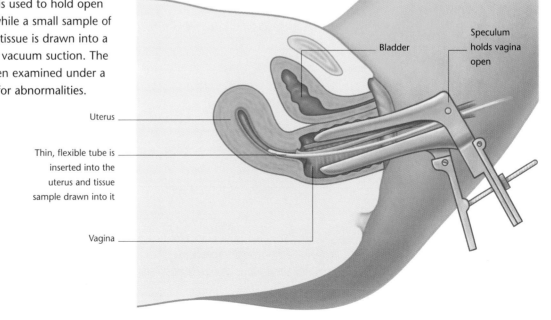

Endometrial sampling

A speculum is used to hold open the vagina while a small sample of endometrial tissue is drawn into a thin tube by vacuum suction. The sample is then examined under a microscope for abnormalities.

Bladder

Speculum holds vagina open

Uterus

Thin, flexible tube is inserted into the uterus and tissue sample drawn into it

Vagina

worse in the twenties or thirties, then it is much more likely that there may be a specific cause. If simple measures to deal with the pain are not enough to make it bearable, then medical help should be sought. A common cause of period pain in these circumstances is a condition called endometriosis (see page 423), where deposits of tissue similar to the lining of the womb are found outside the uterus.

If period pain is accompanied by other symptoms, such as pain during sexual intercourse, heavier bleeding during the period, or an irregular cycle, it is even more likely that there is a definite medical cause for the pain. Other conditions associated with painful periods include pelvic infection or inflammation and benign tumours in the uterus called fibroids (see page 424).

For many women, simple measures to reduce period pain will be successful. Painkillers, such as paracetamol, or anti-inflammatory drugs, including aspirin and ibuprofen, taken regularly throughout menstruation are helpful. Other remedies include:

- *Exercise*
- *Avoiding caffeinated drinks*
- *Relaxation or meditation to reduce stress*
- *Keeping the abdomen warm, for example by using a hot water bottle*
- *Complementary therapies, including oil of evening primrose and raspberry leaf tea (see page 275)*

If these measures fail to improve the pain, then your doctor may prescribe a drug called mefenamic acid, which reduces pain and blood loss by lowering the levels of prostaglandins. If endometriosis is suspected, further tests may be necessary, with the prescription of specific drugs. Rarely, hysterectomy might be required if dysmenorrhoea does not respond to medication.

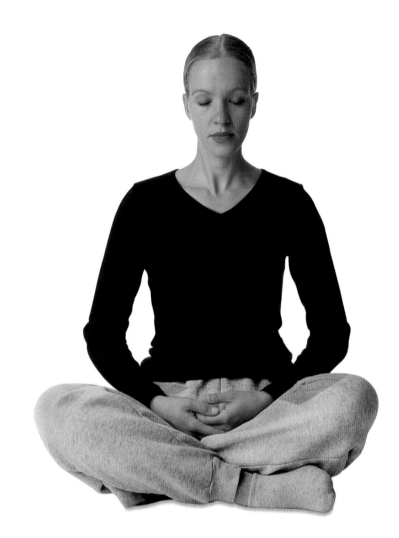

ABOVE *Meditation can be an effective way of reducing period pains because it alters the pattern of brain waves to those linked with deep relaxation, countering muscle pain.*

HEAVY PERIODS (MENORRHAGIA)

Heavy periods are more common as you grow older, and can be particularly troublesome in the years leading up to the menopause. Often caused by hormonal imbalance, especially if accompanied by an irregular cycle, female hormones might be prescribed to reduce blood loss. Other causes include fibroids and polyps in the uterus. Surgical treatments include techniques to destroy the lining of the uterus, or hysterectomy.

IRREGULAR OR ABSENT PERIODS

Lack of periods, or amenorrhoea, can be primary (never had a period) or secondary. Most girls will have had a period by the age of seventeen, so if this age is passed without any sign of bleeding, investigation into the cause is necessary. Conditions that lead to primary amenorrhoea include absent sexual organs or polycystic ovary syndrome (see page 422).

The most common cause of secondary amenorrhoea is pregnancy. Other reasons include early menopause, certain types of contraception, severe weight loss or an underactive thyroid gland. Irregular periods are frequently caused by hormonal imbalance, polycystic ovaries or the menopause.

CONTRACEPTION

Preventing unplanned pregnancies is preferable to the traumas of abortion, and for this reason contraception is freely available in the UK from GP's surgeries, family planning clinics, and, in the case of the morning-after pill, from some pharmacies without prescription. Over the past few years there has been an increase in the number of contraceptive methods available. In choosing which contraceptive is best for you, it is important to remember that the different types of contraception have varying success rates, and that a contraceptive will only work if the instructions for use are strictly followed.

TYPES OF CONTRACEPTION

Essentially, there are four groups of contraceptive methods: natural family planning, barrier methods, medication and operative techniques. The first of these, natural family planning, works well for some couples, but has to be strictly adhered to. It depends upon working out the part of the woman's cycle when it is safe to have sex: that is, avoiding mid-cycle. Some couples practise the withdrawal technique (coitus interruptus), but this is both risky and unsatisfying.

Barrier methods include the sheath, or condom, the only contraceptive to provide a degree of protection against sexually transmitted diseases; the female condom; the diaphragm and the cervical cap, which are generally used with spermicidal gel; and coils (intra-uterine devices). Coils, especially the newer, hormone-coated Mirena coil, are almost 100 per cent effective. The other methods' effectiveness depends on following the instructions fully.

Drugs used for contraception include the combined contraceptive pill, the progesterone-only pill, also called the mini-pill, and progesterone given by injection, or as an implant inserted under the skin. The combined pill is

Barrier methods

Male condom
Before unrolling a condom onto the penis, squeeze the air out of the end of the condom so that it does not split.

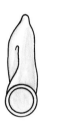
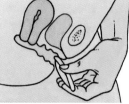

Female condom
The closed end of the condom is inserted into the cervix, and the open end extends beyond the vaginal opening.

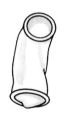
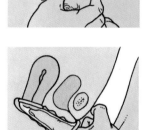

Diaphragm
Both sides are coated with spermicide. The concave side is placed over the cervix and left in place for at least 6 hours.

Cervical cap
The cap is filled with spermicide and pushed over the cervix. It must be left in place for at least 6 hours after sex.

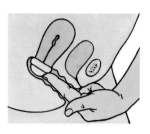

probably the most widely used contraceptive, and is almost 100 per cent effective. The mini-pill is used as an alternative to the combined pill, and is useful in older women, smokers and women who are breastfeeding.

The progesterone implant gives contraceptive cover for a year, and has to be fitted by a trained doctor or nurse. The contraceptive injection is given every three months. Both methods are probably 100 per cent effective. The final group of methods, female sterilisation and male vasectomy, should also be regarded as both completely effective and permanent.

Emergency contraception is available in two different forms. The morning-after pill, based on a progesterone preparation, can be taken up to 72 hours after unprotected sex, and consists of two tablets taken 12 hours apart. Alternatively, a coil can be inserted within five days of unprotected intercourse.

ABORTION

Terminating an unwanted pregnancy is probably one of the most difficult decisions a woman can make, and it is important that the process is not rushed. In the UK, abortion is legal up to the 24th week of pregnancy, although it would be more commonplace for a termination to be performed before 20 weeks if possible.

A woman considering termination should consult her GP as soon as possible, and if after discussion with her doctor she wishes to continue with that option, she will usually be referred to a clinic. At the clinic, she should be counselled fully about the procedure, the possible complications, and then examined by two doctors who have to agree that the abortion can be carried out.

There are two methods of abortion that are used. Surgical termination,

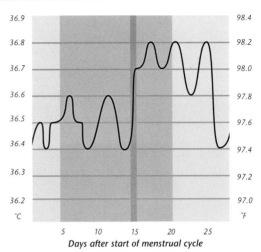

The rhythm method

A temperature chart can be used to identify days when you are fertile and days when you are less likely to conceive. Ovulation is followed by a rise in temperature for at least three days; a time of infertility follows.

◻ Infertile days, safe for sex
▨ Fertile days, unsafe for sex
▪ Ovulation, unsafe for sex

Days after start of menstrual cycle

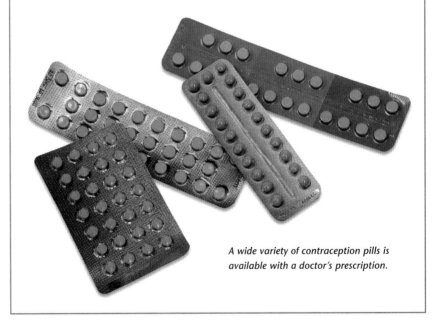

Hormonal methods

Hormones that prevent conception are usually given by pill, injection or as an implant inserted under the skin. These methods are almost 100 per cent effective.

A wide variety of contraception pills is available with a doctor's prescription.

involving a general anaesthetic, is the most common procedure, but can only be performed up to the 13th week of pregnancy. Medical terminations, using drugs called prostaglandins, stimulate labour, and can be performed up to the 24-week limit.

Complications of termination include bleeding and pain in the immediate post-operative period. Pelvic infection can occur after both surgical and medical terminations, but giving antibiotics routinely after abortion reduces the risk.

THE MENOPAUSE

Although in the strictest sense the term 'menopause' signifies the cessation of menstruation, more commonly it is used to describe a whole gamut of changes that occur in association with a woman's last period. Many years ago, few women reached the menopause, but in modern times the menopause signifies the beginning of a new phase in a woman's life that will last for around thirty years on average.

EARLY MENOPAUSE

In the UK, the average age for the onset of the menopause is 51, but it can occur naturally anywhere between 40 and 60. If the menopause begins before the age of 40, it is regarded as being premature. Consequences of an early menopause include osteoporosis (reduced bone density; see page 389) and possibly increased risk of heart disease. Even if the ovaries are left in place at hysterectomy, the menopause can come a couple of years earlier than expected if the uterus is still present.

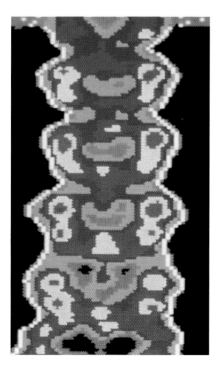

LEFT *Bone is a living tissue supplied with blood vessels and nerves that is constantly being broken down and rebuilt. As you become older, more bone is broken down than is replaced. Bone density can be measured by X-ray to screen for and diagnose osteoporosis. This colour-coded computerized image shows different densities of bone in the spine.*

HORMONE LEVELS

From the onset of the first period, the process whereby an egg (ovum) is brought to maturation each month releases the female hormone oestrogen. Although oestrogen is produced elsewhere in the body, the ovaries are responsible for the overwhelming majority of circulating oestrogen. As the ovaries begin to fail, and egg production dwindles, the level of oestrogen also falls. At the same time, the pituitary gland secretes more follicle-stimulating hormone (FSH) to stimulate the ovaries. Most symptoms associated with the menopause occur because of the reduced levels of oestrogen or increased amounts of FSH.

In addition to its role in preparing the lining of the uterus for a fertilised egg, oestrogen helps maintain the health of a number of the body's organs, including the breasts, vagina, skin and bladder. For many women, the menstrual cycle is rarely regular during menstruation. Usually periods become lighter, and the menstrual cycle

lengthens, making periods more sporadic. Paradoxically, some women find their periods are more frequent, or much heavier (menorrhagia). The time of life leading up to the menopause is known as the peri-menopause. Blood loss occurring more than a year after the last period should always be investigated by a gynaecologist. For some women, the menopause causes no symptoms whatsoever, and apart from the cessation of periods, there will be no evidence that oestrogen levels have fallen drastically. For most, however, the lack of female hormones may lead to numerous symptoms, many of which can be attributed to the fall in oestrogen levels. Other symptoms may not be directly linked to the menopause, but often seem to accompany it.

SIGNS AND SYMPTOMS OF THE MENOPAUSE

Common symptoms of the menopause, in addition to changes in the menstrual cycle, include hot flushes, night sweats and vaginal dryness that can lead to pain on sexual intercourse. Along with bladder problems, which often appear as cystitis-like symptoms, and dry skin, these symptoms are probably directly related to the drop in oestrogen levels.

Other symptoms that often appear at the menopause, but may not be

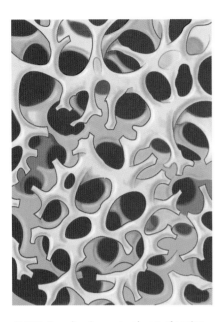

ABOVE *Bone loss is a natural part of ageing but the process speeds up in women after the menopause, because the ovaries stop producing oestrogen, a hormone that helps the body absorb calcium from the diet and deposit it in the bones. By the age of 70 a woman will have lost at least 30 per cent of her bone mass.*

directly due to lower oestrogen levels, include fatigue and loss of energy, headaches, and emotional changes such as mood swings, irritability and depression. Loss of libido may be a consequence of depression and vaginal problems making sex painful. Poor memory and concentration are frequently complained of, and sleep patterns may be disrupted. Weight gain is quite common.

Specific problems such as depression, sleeplessness and bladder infections can be treated and most of these disappear once the menopause is over. Eating a healthy diet will improve general health, and regular exercise will aid relaxation and reduce stress.

Finally, long-term consequences of the menopause include increased risk of both osteoporosis and heart disease. There might also be links with Alzheimer's disease (see page 345).

Parts of the body affected by the menopause

The drop in oestrogen levels increases health risks, such as osteoporosis and heart disease. The skin appears to be more wrinkled and there may be emotional problems associated with the loss of fertility.

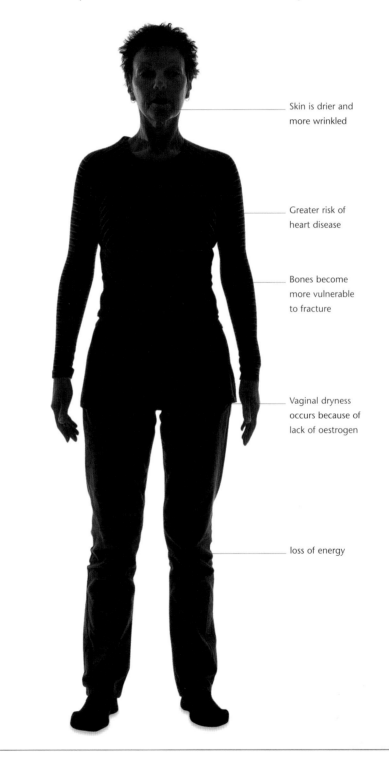

Skin is drier and more wrinkled

Greater risk of heart disease

Bones become more vulnerable to fracture

Vaginal dryness occurs because of lack of oestrogen

loss of energy

HORMONE REPLACEMENT THERAPY

A small minority of women pass through the menopause with few or no symptoms. Most women, however, experience a whole range of unpleasant, troublesome symptoms that can last for several years (see The Menopause, pages 312–13). Most of the symptoms experienced around the menopause are due to the fall in the level of the female hormone oestrogen circulating in the bloodstream. As the ovaries reach the end of their natural life, eggs are released sporadically, leading to an irregular bleeding pattern and a dwindling production of oestrogen. To combat the lack of oestrogen, and to try to maintain a healthy body, many women turn to hormone replacement therapy, or HRT.

HRT AND THE PERI-MENOPAUSE

The majority of women take HRT when they are sure they have reached the menopause. However, sometimes it is prescribed during the couple of years leading up to the change, during a period known as the peri-menopause, if a woman is experiencing frequent, heavy periods, often accompanied by hot flushes or night sweats. The use of HRT may relieve these symptoms. If you are not certain you have reached the menopause, your GP can arrange a blood test to determine hormone levels.

HRT is used to ease the short-term symptoms experienced during the menopause, and although not suitable for all women, most find it very effective. Long-term effects of the menopause include an increased risk of developing heart disease, stroke and a condition called osteoporosis. Osteoporosis is due to reduced levels of minerals, particularly calcium, in the bones, leading to an increased risk of suffering fractures of the spinal bones (vertebrae) or hips.

Slow-release method

Adhesive skin patches are a simple and effective way of releasing HRT into the body at a steady rate and over a period of time. The replacement hormones (usually oestrogen and synthetic progesterone) are absorbed through the skin directly into the bloodstream. Doctors recommend that HRT treatment continues for up to 10 years following the menopause.

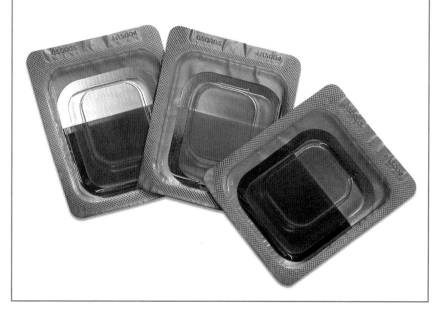

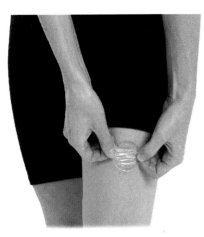

ABOVE *Adhesive skin patches are most effective when placed on the upper thigh or lower abdomen on dry, unbroken skin.*

RISK FACTORS FOR OSTEOPOROSIS

Risk factors for osteoporosis include early menopause, a family history of hip fracture, low body weight, smoking, excessive alcohol intake, poor diet and previous broken bones. Use of steroid tablets for conditions such as asthma can also increase the risk. HRT has been shown to reduce the long-term effects of the menopause for as long as medication is taken, although it is likely that therapy should be continued for at least five years to gain maximum benefit.

TYPES OF HRT

HRT comes in many forms, and if the first one tried causes problems, then it is worth persevering to find one that suits you. Preparations include tablets, patches applied to the skin once or twice weekly, a gel applied to the skin daily, creams to be inserted into the vagina and implants of pellets under the skin of the abdomen every six months.

Depending on your circumstances, you may be prescribed one of the three types of HRT available:

Unopposed HRT *This contains only oestrogen, and is suitable for women who have had a hysterectomy.*

Sequential HRT *In this form, another female hormone called progesterone is given for part of each month to prevent the lining of the womb becoming cancerous. Generally, there will be a light period each month.*

Combined, continuous HRT

This provides both oestrogen and progesterone throughout the month and can only be used in women at least a year past the menopause. The advantage is that it is bleed-free and after the first three to six months there is no period.

SIDE-EFFECTS OF HRT

Short-term side-effects of HRT include breast tenderness, leg cramps, emotional changes and possibly weight gain. More seriously, there is an increased risk of blood clots, and there is a small, but definite, increase in the rate of breast cancer among those women taking HRT for more than five years.

NATURAL HRT

Most conventional HRT contains oestrogen in the same natural form that appears in the female body before the menopause. For women who decide that HRT is not for them, there are some oestrogen-containing herbal remedies such as Dong Quai. Soya products such as tofu contain natural plant oestrogens.

Progesterone has no role in relieving menopausal symptoms, but is important in preventing build-up of the lining of the uterus. It may be appropriate to use 'natural' progesterone in these circumstances, available orally or as a skin cream, as an alternative component in conjunction with standard oestrogen preparations. There is no convincing evidence that natural progesterone prevents osteoporosis or heart disease.

BELOW *Drugs that act in a similar way to female hormones are used to reduce symptoms associated with the menopause, enabling you to live life to the full.*

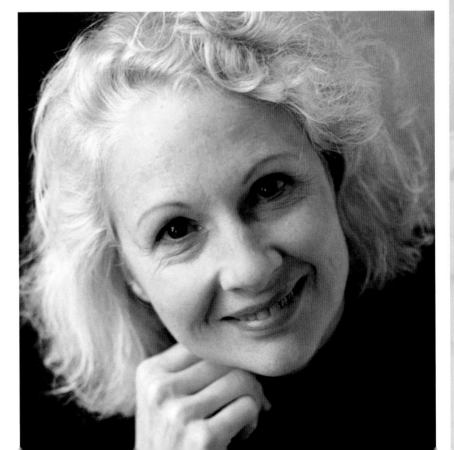

THE WELL MAN

All the evidence points to the fact that men take more chances with their health than women. They are more likely to smoke, drink alcohol and be overweight. They are less likely to attend their GP for acute illnesses and, more importantly, to ask for screening check-ups. The end result of this is that men in the UK live about five years less, on average, than women.

MALE HEALTH PROBLEMS

The main cause of male death is coronary heart disease, with around 20 per cent of men dying prematurely from heart attacks, angina and heart failure. Men are more likely than women to die from cancer of the lung and other smoking-related lung diseases such as chronic bronchitis and emphysema. To improve the lot of the UK male population is a challenge currently facing the medical profession. Greater awareness of male-related health problems through media campaigns is one answer. Encouraging men to live a healthier lifestyle with regard to diet, exercise, smoking and drinking will help reduce male premature deaths.

SELF-HELP

Most problems that affect men's health can be detected earlier if a few simple self-examination check-ups are carried out. The sooner a condition is picked up, the greater the likelihood that something can be done about it. Keeping an eye on your body is simple, and will take up only a tiny amount of your time.

A simple place to start is to measure your body mass index (BMI; see page 241) by dividing your weight in

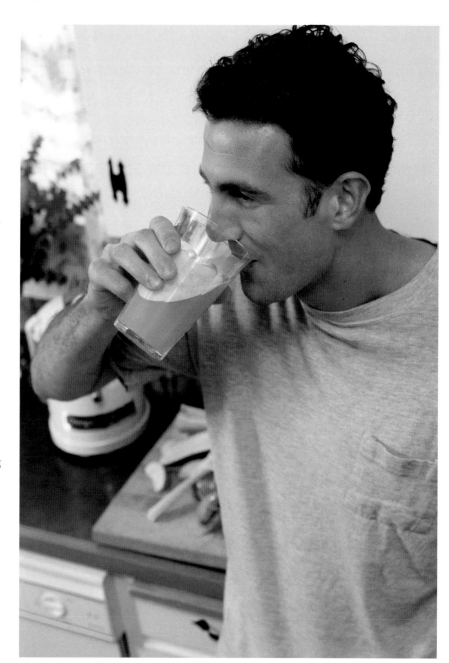

LEFT *Men are more likely to neglect their health than women. For most, a change of diet and lifestyle will increase their life expectancy.*

RIGHT *Regular exercise will benefit your heart and lungs, improve mobility and strength and help keep your weight under control.*

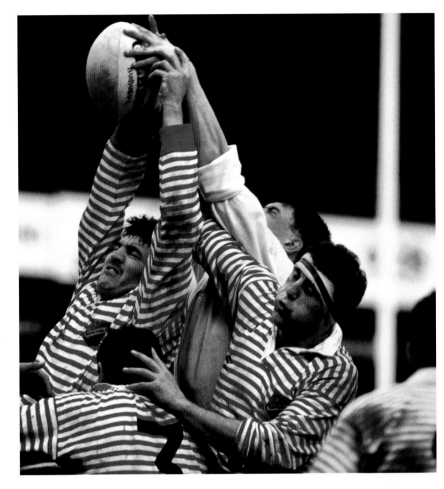

kilograms by the square of your height in metres. A BMI between 20 and 25 is healthy; above 30 indicates obesity, associated with higher rates of heart disease, diabetes and osteoarthritis. Weight loss not associated with change of diet can indicate problems such as diabetes or cancer. Weight gain might be due to hormonal imbalance, such as an underactive thyroid gland.

Raised blood pressure (hypertension) is a factor in heart attacks and stroke. The problem is that for almost everybody suffering from hypertension, the condition is symptomless, and it can only be detected if checked by your doctor. Blood pressure measurement is also performed as part of fitness checks at a gym, and home BP machines are becoming less expensive. If attending your doctor for a check-up, ask about a blood test for cholesterol, another risk factor for heart disease.

WARNING SIGNS

Keeping an eye on your bowel movements can allow early detection of problems such as bowel cancer, stomach ulcers or inflammation of the bowel. Any change from your usual frequency, whether diarrhoea or constipation, should be reported to your GP, especially if you notice any blood being passed in the stools.

Watch out for blood in the urine, as this may indicate bladder or kidney cancer. It can also be associated with prostate problems. Changes in the frequency of passing urine, particularly if you have to get up several times at night, can be due to prostate gland disease, or may sometimes be an early indicator of diabetes. Ask your doctor to check your urine for protein, sugar and blood if you are worried.

Testicular self-examination

Testicular cancer affects 14,000 men every year, many in the 25–35 age group. If detected early enough, this type of cancer is curable, so checking testicles should be encouraged from an early age. This is best done after a bath or shower, so that the scrotum is relaxed. Get to know what your testicles feel like normally by checking about once a month. Hold the scrotum in the palms of your hands, and gently squeeze the testicles, looking for firm lumps, or evidence of change in size. Do not worry if the testicles are not identical, or if one hangs lower than the other, because this

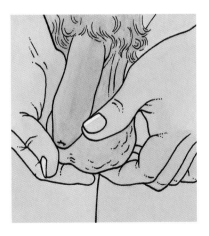

is normal. Report any testicular lumps or pain immediately, as any delay in diagnosis reduces the chance of cure.

THE PROSTATE AND PROSTATE PROBLEMS

The prostate gland is present only in males, and is about the size of a walnut. Lying near the base of the bladder, it envelops the first part of the urethra, the tube through which urine passes as the bladder empties. The prostate gland has a number of functions, including moisturising part of the lining of the urethra, and providing some of the secretions that go to make up semen. For further information, see The Male Reproductive System, pages 206–207.

PROSTATE GLAND GROWTH

From around the age of 40, the prostate gland slowly increases in size. The effect of this varies from man to man, with some having no symptoms at all, while others are seriously inconvenienced by the obstructive effects of the enlarging gland on the urinary flow. It is estimated that about 50 per cent of men over the age of 60 will be affected by symptoms of prostate gland growth.

BENIGN PROSTATIC HYPERPLASIA

Benign prostatic hyperplasia (BPH) is the most common cause of prostate symptoms, and occurs under the action of a derivative of the male hormone, testosterone, which stimulates growth of the gland. The symptoms experienced by sufferers are divided into two distinct categories. Firstly, irritation of the bladder leads to symptoms of passing urine frequently, having to get up more than once at night (nocturia), having to dash to the toilet (urgency), and sometimes a degree of incontinence. Secondly, symptoms caused by obstruction of the bladder outlet include poor stream, difficulty starting to pass urine (hesitancy) and incomplete emptying of the bladder with dribbling. Men who experience these symptoms may require surgery.

Sometimes, the symptoms can be so severe that the whole of a man's day-to-day existence is disrupted. Poor sleep, often also affecting his partner, leads to daytime drowsiness. Car journeys are interrupted, business meetings are faced with dread, and simple social pleasures cannot be enjoyed without careful planning of trips around the local public

---

The prostate gland

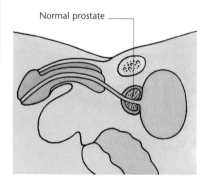

Normal prostate

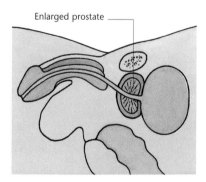

Enlarged prostate

NORMAL *The prostate is a small gland about 2.5 cm (1 in) round which lies under the bladder in front of the rectum. It surrounds the first part of the urethra, the tube leading from the bladder through which urine and semen are transported out of the body. The outer part of the prostate gland produces secretions that form part of semen, and the inner part manufactures fluid that keeps the urethra moist.*

ENLARGED *Enlargement of the prostate gland is seen as a natural part of ageing. From the age of about 40 the prostate gland slowly begins to get bigger. It may constrict the urethra, making it difficult to urinate and to empty the bladder completely. Urine may collect in the bladder and stagnate and, if the condition is not treated, the urinary tract and kidneys may become infected.*

conveniences. Many men accept this as normal, but if you suspect you have BPH, see your doctor.

Diagnosis depends on going through the symptoms and examining the prostate gland by rectal examination. Usually, a urine sample is analysed to rule out infection, and a blood test is performed to check the function of the kidneys and to detect a chemical produced by the prostate gland called prostatic specific antigen (PSA), used to screen for prostate cancer.

If the symptoms are mild, then no treatment may be necessary. However, medication can help either by relaxing the muscular part of the prostate gland and allowing better flow rates and reducing obstruction, or by reducing the size of the gland by blocking the effect of testosterone derivatives. More rarely nowadays, with the advent of more effective drug therapy, an operation might be necessary to remove part of the prostate gland.

PROSTATE CANCER

Prostate cancer affects about 20,000 men each year in the UK, and is the second most common cause of death from cancer after cancer of the lung. Symptoms of prostate cancer can be identical to those seen in BPH, and initial diagnostic tests are the same. Prostate cancer may be indicated if the prostate gland feels hard on rectal examination, or if the PSA levels are elevated.

Referral to a prostate specialist (urologist) for further tests is essential for accurate diagnosis. An ultrasound scan of the prostate gland, along with a biopsy to obtain a sample of tissue (see page 455) are the next steps. A bone scan might be necessary if the cancer is thought to have spread outside the prostate gland. Treatment, especially in younger men when the disease tends to be more aggressive,

Radical prostatectomy

If cancer is confined to the prostate your doctor may recommend removal of the entire prostate gland, along with the seminal vesicles and the neck of the bladder.

In a less radical operation, pictured below, you can see that the bladder wall, or neck, has been reconstructed and rejoined to the urethra and the seminal vesicle has been left intact.

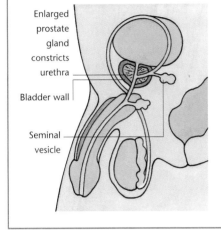

Enlarged prostate gland constricts urethra

Bladder wall

Seminal vesicle

Bladder neck remains

RIGHT *In a prostate gland biopsy, a small sample of prostate tissue is removed for examination under the microscope. The cells shown here are cancerous.*

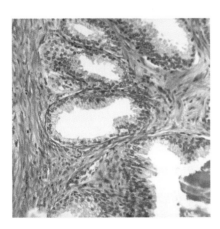

BOTTOM RIGHT *This sample of prostate gland cells shows non-cancerous, normal cells.*

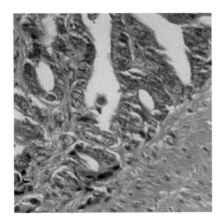

involves surgery to remove the prostate gland if the cancer is confined to the gland. In many patients, if the disease is more widespread, tablets or injections to lower the testosterone level is the usual treatment.

However, a diagnosis of prostate cancer does not always mean that the cancer will cause symptoms or be life-threatening. Especially in elderly men, the best policy may sometimes be to monitor the disease rather than to treat it. If a tumour is small, the patient is likely to live for a number of years. For further information on prostate cancer, see page 430.

SEXUAL HEALTH

There is evidence to demonstrate that men who are single and have no lasting relationships tend to die at an earlier age than to their married counterparts. Although this statistic cannot wholly be explained by the beneficial effect of a healthy sex life, it seems likely that it does play some part in improved levels of health for men.

BENEFITS OF LONG-TERM RELATIONSHIPS

Although predictions indicate that, in the next decade, the number of people marrying or remaining in long-term relationships may decline, stable relationships offer most people a much more satisfying sex life. When the novelty and excitement have worn off in a new relationship, there are lots of advantages from remaining with one partner rather than looking for the next one.

When you share a bed with somebody long term, there is greater intimacy, with less pressure to perform. Sex becomes more relaxed, less hurried and frenetic, and as time goes by, there is greater opportunity to vary sex, and to find out exactly what your partner enjoys. Often people in long-term relationships have better levels of communication generally, leading to a less stressful life outside the bedroom. Happy, relaxed people live longer. Importantly, sexual health is more

likely in a stable relationship with a faithful partner.

Finally, one of the great advantages of enjoying a long-standing sexual relationship is that sex is likely to continue into old age. Most older people find sex just as desirable and exciting as they did in their younger days. Usually the sex is less frequent, but more relaxed and less hurried. Women may even find it more enjoyable because there is no possibility of becoming pregnant.

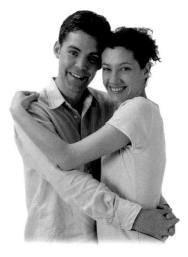

ABOVE *A satisfying physical relationship is an important part of life. With age and experience, most people become able to establish and fully enjoy sexual relationships.*

RIGHT *People who are involved in long-term sexual relationships tend to live longer than those without partners. Age should not be a barrier to sex, although it may be less frequent.*

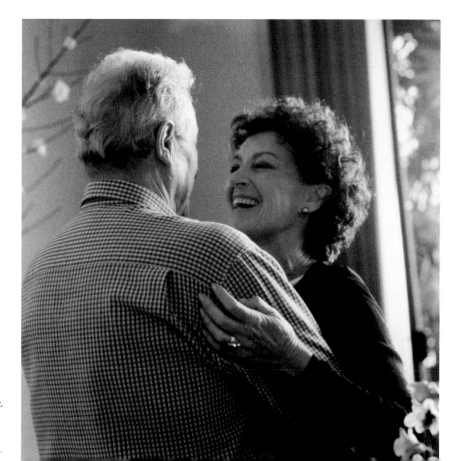

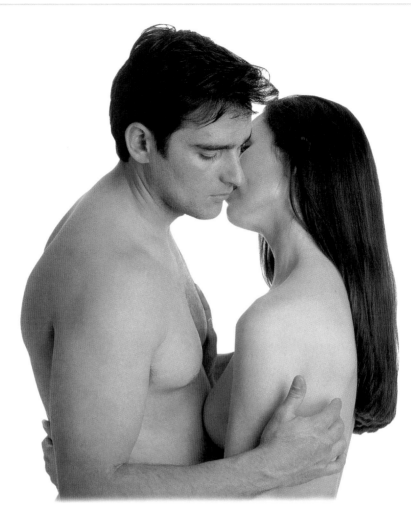

RIGHT *A loss of interest in sex may have physical or psychological causes. Sex therapy may help if the cause is psychological. The sensate focus technique involves experiencing pleasure through touch rather than sexual intercourse.*

COMMON SEXUAL PROBLEMS

Loss of desire is often confused with having a low sex drive (libido), but many women who complain of loss of desire still have a normal sex drive. Common causes include stress and anxiety, tiredness, particularly after childbirth, depression and hormonal imbalance, for example around the time of the menopause, or after hysterectomy.

Sometimes, medication such as antidepressants, or drug or alcohol abuse may reduce desire. A bad experience, such as previous sexual abuse or painful intercourse, even if this occurred many years ago, can lead to problems. Finally, trouble within a relationship may promote loss of desire.

Physical causes should be ruled out if possible, and this might involve seeing a gynaecologist. If the problem is thought to be psychological, then counselling can be very beneficial.

FAILURE TO REACH ORGASM

About one in ten women have never had an orgasm. Of those that have, three-quarters need stimulation other than penetration to achieve a satisfactory orgasm. Reaching orgasm is dependent on several factors, including feeling relaxed and comfortable with your partner, being able to feel sexually aroused and receiving appropriate sexual stimulation.

There can be several reasons why a woman fails to reach orgasm. Stress, anxiety and depression or previous sexual abuse are all possible causes. Sometimes, loss of the ability to reach orgasm can be a consequence of pelvic surgery, or may point to problems within a relationship. Once again, counselling after excluding physical problems is the mainstay of treatment.

IMPOTENCE

Impotence, or erectile dysfunction, affects most men at some time during their life. For the majority, this is a temporary phenomenon caused by stress or tiredness. For about 10 per cent, the problem persists, and causes upset and disappointment for both partners. The causes are broadly split into physical and psychological factors, but the two groups often occur together. Physical causes include poor circulation, diabetes, smoking, excessive alcohol intake and side-effects from anti-depressants or drugs to treat raised blood pressure. Impotence can occur after operations for prostate problems, or pelvic surgery. If a man has spontaneous morning erections, then the cause is more likely to be psychological and due to anxiety or depression, or 'performance anxiety' due to previous unsuccessful attempts at intercourse.

More and more treatments are becoming available, including tablets taken before intercourse, injections into the shaft of the penis to induce an erection, or a pellet introduced into the urethra, the tube leading from the bladder through which urine and semen are transported. Vacuum pump devices may also be used to produce an erection. Lifestyle changes such as giving up smoking or alcohol or a change in medication can also help.

SEXUALLY TRANSMITTED DISEASES

Sexually transmitted diseases (STDs) remain one of the biggest public health issues in the UK. The incidence of STDs continues to rise, with chlamydia (see page 419) set to become the next global epidemic, following hot on the heels of herpes and HIV. For many STDs, the initial symptoms may be so negligible that they are not noticed. Infection is spread during intercourse before the carrier of the STD even realises that he or she is infected.

SAFE SEX

The move away from monogamy to multiple sexual partners looks likely to make STDs even more widespread. The use of condoms is still the only way to try to protect yourself from catching a STD, and it is essential to practise safe sex with any new partner. If you suspect you may be suffering from a STD, then confidential advice, investigation and treatment can be obtained from your local STD clinics. For some STDs, the clinics will need to contact previous partners if test results are positive.

There is a number of infections that, although transmitted sexually, are not regarded as STDs in the true sense. These are summarised in the table below.

DISEASE	SYMPTOMS	DIAGNOSIS	MANAGEMENT
Candida (thrush; see also page 425)	*In women, vaginal irritation and itching, a thick white vaginal discharge, pain on passing urine and, rarely, vaginal bleeding. In men, there may be irritation or a rash on the end of the penis, but often there are no symptoms.*	*Often diagnosed by the typical signs on examination, and diagnosis can be confirmed by a high vaginal swab.*	*Simultaneous treatment of both partners with anti-fungal drugs. These can be taken by mouth, or applied to the genitalia as creams and pessaries. Natural yoghurt is often used instead of anti-fungal medication.*
Bacterial vaginosis	*In 50 per cent of women, there are no symptoms. There may be a fishy-smelling vaginal discharge. Slight irritation may be the only symptom in men.*	*Vaginal swab.*	*Oral antibiotics such as metronidazole for both partners. Intra-vaginal antibiotic creams are also effective.*
Trichomonas vaginalis (TV)	*In women, a heavy greenish-yellow discharge, pain on intercourse, genital irritation and, sometimes, abdominal pain. Men are almost always free of symptoms. Rarely, there can be pain on passing urine or a whitish discharge from the penis.*	*Vaginal swab or urethral swab in men.*	*Oral antibiotics for both partners, usually metronidazole.*

More serious STDs are listed in the next table.

DISEASE	SYMPTOMS	DIAGNOSIS	MANAGEMENT
Chlamydia (see also page 419)	Often no symptoms in either sex. Women may have discharge, lower abdominal pain, vaginal bleeding and pain on intercourse or when passing urine. Men may have discharge, pain on passing urine or testicular swelling.	By swab in both sexes, or by urine or blood sample.	Oral antibiotics. Previous sexual partners need to be traced. This is a major cause of female infertility, and it is routinely checked for during infertility investigations.
Gonorrhoea (see also page 418)	In females, symptoms are similar to chlamydia. There are often no symptoms. In men, a yellow discharge from the penis, pain on passing urine, blood in the urine or swollen glands in the groin.	By swab in both sexes.	Oral antibiotics. Previous sexual partners need to be traced.
Genital herpes	Painful genital blisters that may form ulcers. Can be accompanied by flu-like symptoms.	Swabs taken from the base of the blisters.	Oral anti-viral medication.
Syphilis	Painless red genital sores (chancres) initially, followed by rash and flu-like illness. Long-term consequences include damage to the heart and nervous system.	Detection of antibodies from a blood sample.	Antibiotic medication at a specialist treatment centre. It is essential to trace previous sexual partners.
Hepatitis B and C (see also page 405)	Often no symptoms, but may be initial flu-like illness.	Antibody blood test.	Specialist treatment essential, as is tracing previous sexual partners.
HIV (see also page 416–17)	Often symptom-free, but may be initial flu-like illness.	Antibody blood test 2–3 months after suspected infection.	Specialist treatment essential, as is tracing previous sexual partners.

WELL OVER SIXTY

The processes involved in ageing are the subject of considerable research as scientists strive to discover the secrets of an extended life span as well as attempting to slow the onset of medical conditions associated with old age. Already, we are living longer than ever, and are in better health. The current life expectancy for women is 75 to 80, with men living about five years less on average.

LIFE EXPECTANCY

It seems likely that the human body is not pre-programmed to die after a certain timespan. Problems begin to appear in a few of the billions of cells within the body, and despite the body's attempts to repair the damage, eventually the changes in DNA, cell structure and organs catch up with us. It is difficult to say why one person lives to a ripe old age and another dies early. Sometimes this is due to genetics, and sometimes it depends on our lifestyle and the dangers we expose ourselves to.

LIFESTYLE AND LONG LIFE

Many people stay fit and healthy into old age. Although some of the factors involved in determining how long we live may be outside our control, there are precautions and actions a person can take to improve the chances of longevity. Lifestyle is important in reaching a ripe old age as, unless you are very lucky, poor choices in the way you live will have a detrimental effect on your health. For detailed information on healthy living, see pages 220–61.

The single most important lifestyle change anybody can make to improve general health is to give up smoking, and it is never too late. Stopping smoking will slow down the deterioration of many organs, such as the heart and lungs, and will reduce the chance of developing heart disease and some types of cancer. If you have always blamed the stress of work for your bad habit, then retirement is the ideal time to stop smoking.

DIET AND EXERCISE

Eating healthily is important at any time of life, but as we age the body has a tendency to burn up calories more slowly. As a result it is easy to put on weight, even if the amount of food eaten is the same. There is less lean muscle in the older body, and since an older person is unlikely to perform as much vigorous exercise as a younger person, the chances are that any excess calories will end up as fat.

Sensible eating means plenty of fruit and vegetables, main meals of pasta or rice, with fish, lean red meat or poultry. Switch to low-fat dairy products, and try to avoid food with too much fat

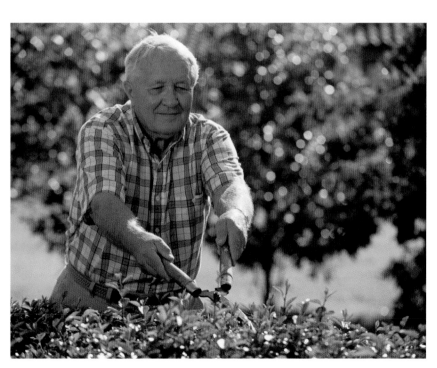

LEFT *It is important to stay active throughout life because it keeps you fit, and light activity such as gardening will keep you mobile and independent.*

Drop in calorie requirements

Your basal metabolic rate (BMR) slows down as you age and you will find that you need to eat less as you get older. Keeping active will help you avoid

Decline in BMR with age

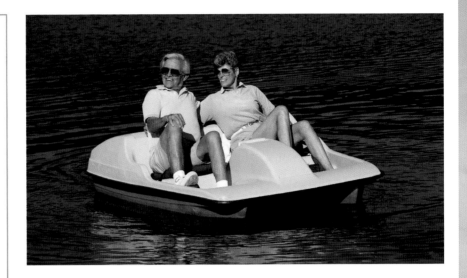

gaining weight. A person's BMR is measured in the number of kilojoules (1 kilojoule = 4 kilocalories) used per square metre of body surface per hour.

or sugar. This does not mean you should make yourself miserable by dieting too strictly – the occasional treat is important.

Regular exercise should be a part of any older person's routine to improve strength, muscle tone and coordination. This does not mean that you have to take up jogging or run marathons – there are plenty of sensible, sociable activities to improve levels of fitness without giving you a heart attack. Try tennis or badminton, or join an over-sixties' exercise class. Swimming, brisk walking, dancing, cycling, golf, bowling or gardening are all guaranteed to improve your levels of fitness, keep joints supple and improve your circulation. Improving your social life will also benefit your mental health.

STRESS

Stress may be something that you hoped had been left behind when retirement beckoned, but it can be a factor in health at all ages. For many people, stress is something they thrive on, and life without any stress would seem terribly boring. However, if stress is making you unhappy, it will be having a detrimental effect on your health.

ABOVE *Taking part in a sporting activity that both you and your partner enjoy will keep you flexible and mobile for longer, improving your quality of life.*

Learn to recognise stress and try to do something to combat it. Talk to your partner, or to friends. Try to have some time in the day to yourself that is just for you. Some herbal and homeopathic remedies can help alleviate stress. Depression, often caused by bereavement, is another problem that frequently affects the elderly, and you should visit your doctor if you are worried that you might be depressed.

LEFT *Staying active as you get older helps keep you fit and reduces problems associated with ageing. Regular exercise improves stamina, mobility and coordination.*

ILLNESSES OF AGEING

As the body ages, physical changes take place that can affect your health in old age. Failing eyesight and loss of hearing, a degree of urinary incontinence and a less efficient memory are common concerns among the elderly. More serious health illnesses include osteoporosis, rheumatism and arthritis, and heart disease.

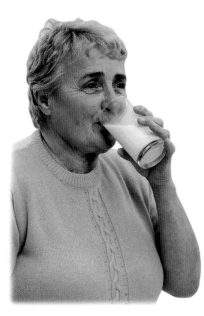

ABOVE *Calcium is essential for building and maintaining bones. Dairy products and oily fish are excellent sources of calcium and vitamin D, needed for calcium absorption.*

OSTEOPOROSIS

As with all medical problems, prevention is better than cure, and there can be few better examples than osteoporosis. Looking after your bones and reducing the risk of osteoporosis is one of the most vital aspects of remaining well in old age. The weakened bone structure caused by osteoporosis means that one woman in three will suffer a broken bone in their lifetime, usually after the menopause. Osteoporosis also affects men, with one in 12 experiencing a broken bone.

The consequences of osteoporosis are often underestimated, but half of all elderly people suffering a broken hip will never regain full mobility, and one in five will die within six months of the fracture. Other problems include loss of mobility, chronic pain, spontaneous fractures and spinal deformity, leading to breathing difficulties.

If you suspect you may be at risk of developing osteoporosis, consult your doctor to discuss your worries. Bone strength can be improved by regular weight-bearing exercise, reducing alcohol intake, making sure you have sufficient calcium in your diet and stopping smoking. Medication such as HRT can increase bone density, but its benefits last only as long as the hormones are taken. For more information, see HRT, pages 314–15 and Osteoporosis, page 389.

Hip replacement

If a joint has been severely damaged by arthritis it may be surgically replaced with an artificial one made of plastic or metal. The most commonly replaced joint is the hip. Both the pelvic socket and the head of the thigh bone are replaced during hip replacement.

RIGHT *An artificial hip joint has a pelvic socket and a femoral component which fits into the thigh bone*

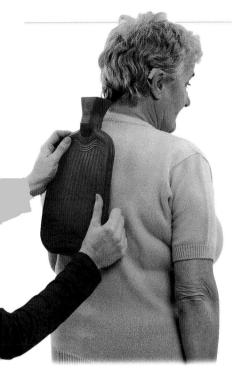

ABOVE *Applying a hot water bottle to an aching back helps to relieve pain and stiffness because the heat increases blood flow to the area and relaxes the muscles.*

RHEUMATISM AND ARTHRITIS

It is almost an accepted fact that old age and joint aches and pain go hand in hand, and that rheumatism and arthritis are inevitable. Rheumatism is really a term used by many people to describe the aches and pains felt in the joints, bones and muscles, often caused by overuse, or unaccustomed exercise, or even by changes in the weather. The discomfort and pain may last for days, and be made more unbearable if you are tired or anxious.

There is a number of ways to ease the aches and pains of rheumatism. Applying heat to the affected area using heated pads, heat lamps or hot water bottles can relieve symptoms. A hot bath can have the same effect, especially if combined with relaxing

RIGHT *It is important to exercise regularly throughout life in order to increase bone strength, remain mobile and flexible, and improve heart and lung function.*

bath oils. Changing your sleeping position can alleviate many aches and pains. Massage with anti-inflammatory creams or aromatherapy oils is a great way to ease muscle spasm and tension.

Arthritis is a term that means inflammation of the joints and, broadly speaking, can be divided into osteoarthritis and inflammatory arthritis (usually affecting younger people, causing hot, swollen joints). Osteoarthritis is often referred to as a problem with wear and tear in the joint and is usually associated with ageing. The exact cause of osteoarthritis is not known, but it tends to affect the weight-bearing joints, such as the knees and hips. For some people, it may be related to obesity, and losing weight will help the symptoms. For others, it might have occurred as the result of an injury in their younger years. Treatment often consists of adequate pain relief through medication. Physiotherapy might help some, but many people will need a joint replacement.

HEART DISEASE

This is an umbrella term covering angina, heart attack and heart failure.

The most common form is ischaemic heart disease, where the blood vessels supplying the heart muscle with oxygen begin to fur up and become narrow. At this stage you might experience chest pain on exertion, or angina. If an artery blocks off completely, part of the heart muscle is starved of oxygen, leading to death of the muscle cells. This is a heart attack. See also Heart Problems, pages 48–49 and Heart Attack, pages 392–93.

Ischaemic heart disease is the most common cause of death in men and women, and although there are genetic factors involved, lifestyle plays an important role in developing the disease. Smoking, obesity, lack of regular exercise, raised blood pressure and raised cholesterol are all contributing factors.

Stopping smoking and having your blood pressure and cholesterol levels routinely monitored by your doctor will go a long way to reducing heart disease. In addition, regular exercise, eating a low-fat diet and losing weight if necessary will not only help your heart stay healthy, but will also improve your sense of well-being.

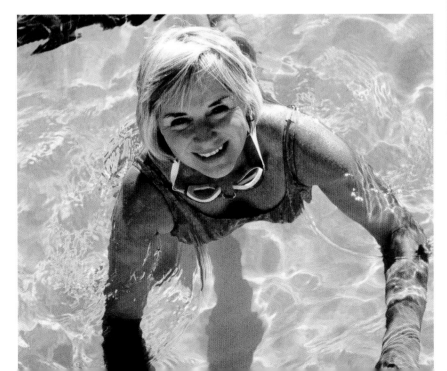

ILLNESSES

CONTENTS

INTRODUCTION

Good health is something we take for granted until we become ill ourselves, or become closely involved with those whose health is impaired. The human body is often compared to a machine, and both the physical body that carries out the day-to-day functions and the mental machinery that keeps us thinking clearly are important for well-being. Most ill health is a result of the failure of one or more parts of the body's machinery to work as we would like it to. However, sometimes the body is poisoned or damaged, making the parts work inefficiently or fail.

We rely on genes that we are born with and sensible feeding for our energy requirements to keep our bodies running well throughout life. You inherit your physical characteristics and susceptibility to certain diseases from your parents. You cannot change your genes but medicine may help prevent diseases to which you are prone and you may reduce your risk of disease by adapting your lifestyle.

Some risk factors are present before birth. Genetic defects may be transmitted through the generations. Sometimes genetic combinations from both parents produce an abnormality. Geneticists can assess the risk of inheriting a faulty gene, and you may want to take this into consideration before starting a family.

The first months of our lives, while we are growing in the uterus, are governed by our mothers. If pregnant women subject their bodies to dangers such as alcohol, smoking and other drugs, then there is a risk that the baby may be damaged. Sometimes, through no fault of the mother, there are problems while the baby is in the uterus. The placenta, which carries food and oxygen to the baby, may not function efficiently and the baby may suffer and be born unwell. The mother may suffer specific pregnancy health problems such as pre-eclampsia that endanger the baby. The process of being born is not without risk and serious birth problems still occur with lifelong consequences.

There are many external causes of physical and mental ill health: injury, infections, poisons and infestations being some of the most important. Internal causes may be due to failure of one of the body's systems involving the heart and blood vessels, the nerves, the hormones, breathing, reproduction, digestion, the skin and the mind. Rarely do problems occur exclusively in one part of the body. Usually problems in one area produce or go hand-in-hand with malfunction in another area of the body.

We are aware of how we normally look and feel and any departure from this makes us aware that we may have an illness. Sometimes the signs are obvious, as when someone collapses and becomes unrousable. Sometimes the signs are more subtle and in children it may be a mother's 'sixth sense' that recognises illness in a child.

The importance of preventing illness, as well as identifying and treating conditions, cannot be underestimated. Body and mind are intimately linked and keeping them healthy and free from external poisons and injuries as much as possible is very important.

It would be impossible to cover all possible areas of illness in one book but the aim is to give an overview of common illnesses, consider the symptoms, signs, possible causes, treatment and the likely outcome. The information here is not intended to replace conventional medical advice or treatment.

HEADACHES AND MIGRAINE

Headaches are an extremely common complaint, experienced by most people at some time in their lives. Headaches are mainly caused by muscular tension in the head, neck or shoulders, but can also result from factors such as stress, food allergies, poor posture or injury. There are many different types of headache and the degree of pain felt varies enormously. Migraine is a severe headache often associated with nausea or vomiting and visual disturbances.

THE DEGREE OF PAIN

More than 90 per cent of people admit to having had a headache at some point in their lives, and headaches are also common in children. Pain is a sensation carried in nerve fibres. When stimulated by chemicals, heavy pressure or extreme heat, nerves transmit messages to the brain, where they are interpreted as pain. The head has a rich nerve supply, and the skin of the head, the muscles, especially the scalp and jaw muscles, and the blood vessels are the commonest areas to produce pain. There are many different types of headache, and the degree of pain felt ranges from a dull thudding in the temples to intense, throbbing pain.

Why do headaches occur?

Most headaches are triggered by muscular tension, stress and anxiety, fever, head injury or local trauma, such as a sports injury. Overuse of medication may cause the headache to persist. Some pains in the head arise from the teeth, sinuses, ears, eyes and nasal passages. Rare causes include meningitis, brain tumours and brain haemorrhages or clots. The greatest worry for people with persistent headaches is that they have a brain tumour, but only 2 per cent of brain tumours first present as a headache – other signs such as weakness of a limb, slurred speech or memory loss usually occur long before tumours are large enough to cause pressure sufficient to cause a headache.

CLUSTER HEADACHES

These occur primarily in men. They are very severe indeed and are usually centred around one eye. They occur in

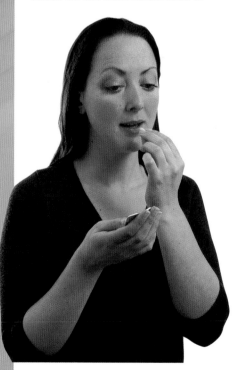

LEFT *Painkillers are frequently taken to treat headaches but if taken too often they may actually be the cause of them.*

Symptoms of tension headaches

• *Sensation of a band tightening around the skull*
• *Pain ranges in intensity*
• *A throbbing sensation that pulses in time with the heartbeat*
• *May be accompanied by eye or neck pain*

Sources of headaches

Muscular tension in the sinuses, ears, eyes and nasal passages can cause headaches.

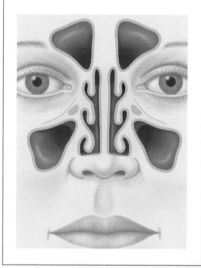

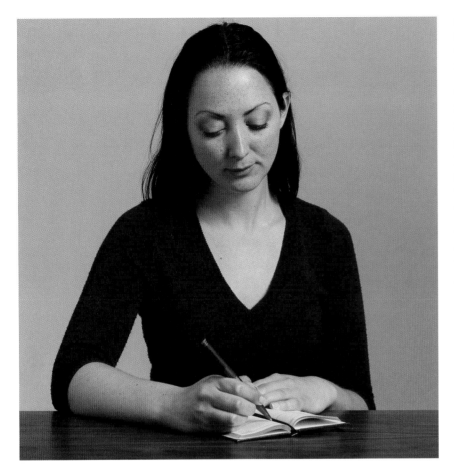

LEFT *A headache diary will help you keep track of the amount of medication you are taking and the frequency with which headaches occur.*

clusters often over several weeks or even months but then disappear. Unlike with migraine where people usually want to lie down and keep still, those with cluster headaches throw themselves around and may even bang their heads on the wall because the pain is so bad. There may be redness and excess watering of the affected eye, and a blocked nose on that side. The attacks last from ten minutes to a few hours and there may be several episodes in a day. There is specific medication for acute attacks, especially the triptan tablets used for migraines (see page 334), and oxygen therapy to relieve symptoms. However, because the clusters may last over many weeks, medication to prevent attacks may be required.

When a headache is a warning

Headaches frighten people, in spite of the fact that they are rarely a sign of something sinister in the brain. Sometimes they may be an indication of a much more serious condition. Seek urgent medical attention for the following cases:

- *The first ever or worst ever headache*
- *Sudden onset of very severe headache*
- *Recent head injury*
- *Headache starting in people over 50 years old*
- *Headache in the temple associated with tenderness*
- *Headache associated with fever and stiff neck*

Treatment for headaches

- *Standard painkillers are used in the short term to treat headaches. It is not uncommon to suffer from chronic daily headache, and although this may be severe, people with this condition manage to function in spite of their headaches. Headaches that have been troublesome most days over a period of months or years, with no other symptoms, are very rarely serious.*

- *Keeping a headache diary may be useful, especially to document the amount of medication taken, because very often it is the medication itself that keeps the headache going. Stopping the tablets, usually the sort bought over the counter, and often containing codeine, may stop the headaches.*

- *Your doctor may prescribe an antidepressant drug such as amitriptyline, which can help enormously in cases of chronic daily headache. The non-pharmaceutical therapies listed for migraine in the complementary remedies and therapies box (see page 335) may also be useful.*

HEADACHES AND MIGRAINE

MIGRAINE

Many people with recurrent headaches describe their headaches as migraine. However, migraine has a fairly strict definition, and the classic feature is a throbbing, often one-sided headache. Between attacks, people are perfectly well. During attacks sufferers cannot carry on with day-to-day activities and usually want to lie down in bed in a darkened room and, ideally, sleep (which may be prevented until the headache has subsided). The frequency of attacks varies: there may be a group of headaches over a few months and then none for another period of time. On average, people with migraine have between one to six attacks a month.

Only about 15 per cent of people with migraine experience what is

Symptoms of migraine

- *Well between attacks*
- *Incapacitating headache*
- *Made worse by activity*
- *Headache lasts 2–72 hours*
- *Pain often one-sided*
- *Pulsating, throbbing in character*
- *Nausea, sensitivity to light, sound and smells*
- *An aura of unusual sensations, including visual disturbances*

termed an aura, a forewarning of an attack that may consist of visual disturbances, speech problems, temperature changes or, occasionally, weakness of a part of the body, lasting

from a few minutes up to an hour. They are then frequently, though not always, followed by the headache.

Why do migraines occur?

Migraine is caused by spasm and dilation of the blood vessels overlying the brain. There are sometimes triggers but if you are unaware of these, keep a diary for a month or so, making note of foods, social events, stress and sleep patterns. Common triggers include foods such as chocolate, cheese and garlic, coffee and alcohol, which are thought to contain an amino acid that affects blood vessels. Others such as stress, too much sleep, too little sleep, perfumes, solvents and computer screens may affect certain individuals. Migraine in women may be triggered by hormonal changes.

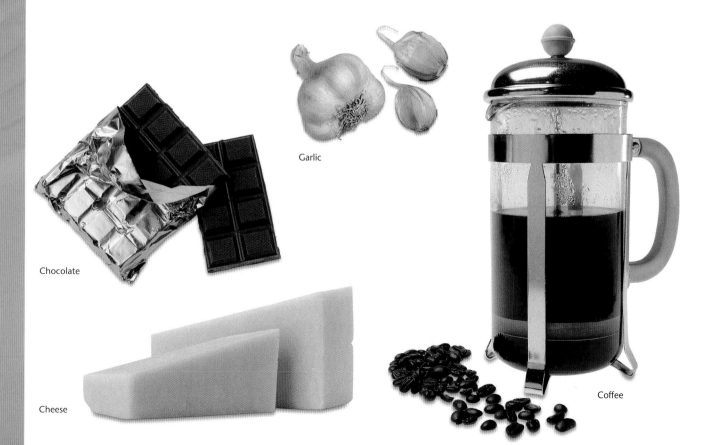

Garlic

Chocolate

Cheese

Coffee

Complementary remedies and therapies

If your migraine is not totally incapacitating, or you prefer not to take pharmaceutical preparations, you could try some of the following therapies and remedies:

- Feverfew (fresh leaves or in tablet form)
- Acupuncture
- Hypnotherapy
- Aromatherapy
- Relaxation therapy
- Exclusion diets
- Yoga
- Homeopathy
- Massage
- Botox injections

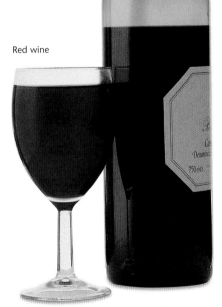

Red wine

Treatment for migraine

- Treatment is usually very successful but can require a battery of medicines to deal with the problem, because each attack may be different. Most people will have tried painkillers such as aspirin or paracetamol but sometimes, just for one dose, three tablets, rather than the usual two, may make all the difference.

- One of the main problems is that during a migraine attack the stomach contents are static. This means that tablets taken are not well absorbed and therefore don't work efficiently. Sometimes a doctor will prescribe medication to stop sickness and nausea and help empty the stomach, which will enable the painkiller to be more effective.

- Tablets containing codeine are not recommended because they can create dependence and a rebound headache once they are stopped. Anti-inflammatory tablets, such as ibuprofen, work for some people.

- New migraine-specific drugs called triptans, which control the changes in blood vessels that cause the migraine, have recently become available. These need to be prescribed by a doctor and come in the form of tablets, rapidly melting tablets, nasal sprays and injections for those whose migraine starts with vomiting.

- About three times more women than men are affected by migraine, and this is probably hormone related. Women with migraine react individually to extra hormones. About a third benefit from taking the contraceptive pill, in a third it makes little difference and in a third the migraine gets worse and the pill should be stopped. In that very rare group of women who have a numbness or weakness of part of the body when they have a migraine attack, the pill should definitely not be taken. During pregnancy, many women have fewer attacks and they may even disappear. A few have a really difficult time.

- For those troubled with very frequent attacks of migraine who find that painkillers don't work, daily preventive medicines such as beta-blockers (which help regulate heart rhythm) may reduce the severity and frequency of the attacks, but these may also have side-effects.

LEFT Certain foods such as red wine, coffee, chocolate and cheese are thought to contain the amino acid tyrosine, which affects the blood vessels. Try an elimination diet to detect culprit foods.

EPILEPSY

Epilepsy is an indication of an abnormality of brain function, often characterised by sudden seizures or loss of consciousness. This condition may start at any age, and can take many forms. The most important person to help a doctor make the diagnosis is an eyewitness, because the sufferer may have little or no idea what goes on before, during or directly after an attack. Investigation by electroencephalography, a technique that records brain waves, should confirm the diagnosis.

GRAND MAL EPILEPSY

This is what most people recognise as having a fit. In this form of epilepsy, there appears to be a massive electrical storm in the brain, and as the attack starts, the person usually collapses and makes regular, shaking movements that affect one or more limbs and sometimes the whole body.

During an attack, unless the person appears to be vomiting or going blue, the best help an onlooker can give may be to put something soft under the head to avoid head injury, keep others away and ensure that he is not in danger from traffic or other hazards. Once the jerking has stopped, turning the person on to his side will help prevent inhalation of vomit. Following the attack, the person who has had the fit usually just wants to sleep, and, ideally, should be left to do so.

The first grand mal attack should always be investigated by a doctor but subsequent ones will not generally require hospital treatment.

PETIT MAL EPILEPSY

These attacks usually show themselves first in childhood. Often a teacher or parent will recognise that the child has 'absences', which may take the form of stopping for a few seconds mid-sentence, or missing out while listening to information. When the condition affects children it is important that it is recognised, as children with epilepsy tend to under-achieve in school.

TEMPORAL LOBE EPILEPSY

This is less common than petit or grand mal epilepsy and may involve all sorts of strange patterns of stereotypical behaviour. Each time the person has an attack he tends to do exactly the same type of thing, though he will know nothing about it after the attack. For

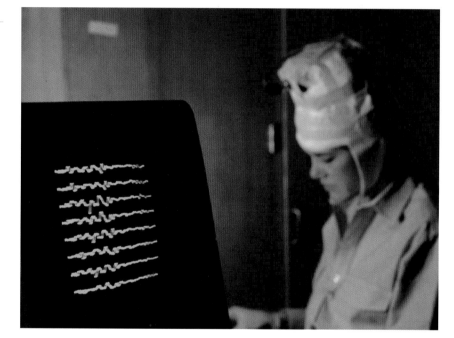

ABOVE *Electroencephalograghy (EEG) is a painless procedure used to diagnose abnormal electrical activity in the brain. Electrodes are attached to the scalp and recordings of the brain's activity are made.*

instance, he may look blank and lick his lips for several minutes and then carry on as if nothing has happened. He may go outside and walk to a shop, pick up a newspaper and walk out without paying. This type of repetitive, unusual behaviour does requires medical investigation and medication.

Symptoms

Grand Mal

• *May have warning signs of headache, yawning, odd tingles, dizziness and feelings of unreality*
• *Loss of consciousness*
• *Muscles, especially of the jaw, contract strongly then convulse*
• *Sometimes frothing at the mouth*
• *Person may vomit or lose control of bowel or bladder function*

Petit Mal

• *Brief losses of conscious awareness that may pass unnoticed by others*
• *Person feels he's lost a few moments daydreaming, or may appear vacant for seconds at a time*
• *Sometimes there are facial twitches*

Temporal Lobe Epilepsy

• *Sufferer unknowingly performs simple or complex tasks (automatism)*
• *Sufferer is usually unaware that an attack has occurred*

What causes epilepsy?

Birth injuries, high fevers and serious head injuries are recognised causes of epilepsy, particularly in young children. In older people, drugs, alcohol, serious head injury or brain tumours may be causes of late onset epilepsy. Frequently there are no obvious causes of epilepsy, particularly when the condition starts in childhood.

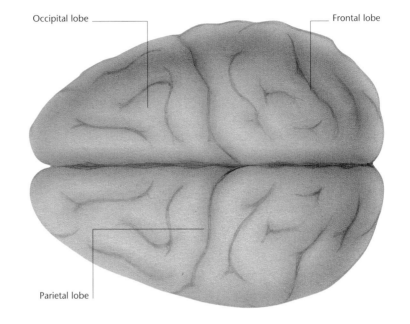

Occipital lobe — Frontal lobe — Parietal lobe

ABOVE *During an epileptic fit electrical impulses begin in one area of the brain and spread out. either over a particular part or all of the brain.*

Treatment

We can all be made to have a fit by being plugged directly into an electrical socket. Most people with epilepsy just have a lower threshold for having a fit. During a fit, the brain may be deprived of oxygen for a while, and if this happens frequently, then areas of the brain become damaged. The different forms of epilepsy can all be controlled by anti-epileptic drugs so that fewer fits occur. Not only are the short-term embarrassment and inconvenience helped, but the long-term brain damage is limited. Newer medications, giving better control and fewer side-effects, have recently become available.

Outlook

Medication taken continuously to prevent attacks is the mainstay of treatment, but when a person has been attack-free for a while it is often difficult to persuade him to continue medication. If you have not had seizures for 2–3 years it may be possible to reduce the drug treatment. Those who suffer from grand mal epilepsy should avoid known triggers such as flashing lights, loud music, fatigue, stress and hot, smoky rooms.

There are very strict laws regarding driving if you are an epileptic, and a person who has had an epileptic attack is legally bound to report it to the authorities. After a seizure-free period of time, driving licences may be reinstated.

STROKE

A stroke results from an interruption of the blood supply to the brain. Most people are aware that the effects of a stroke can vary widely, depending on its cause and the part of the brain affected. Damage to the brain results in damage to the body, which may be brief and trivial or massive and eventually fatal.

Why do strokes happen?

Essentially, a stroke is due to either a clot in a blood vessel supplying an area of brain or bleeding (haemorrhage) from a cerebral blood vessel into the brain tissue. Risk factors include smoking, high blood pressure, diabetes, high cholesterol levels and some oral contraceptives. Recognised causes of strokes are as follows:

- *weakness of blood vessels*
- *blood clots either in the brain vessels or carried there from elsewhere in the body*
- *very high blood pressure*
- *congenital weaknesses*
- *direct damage to the brain*
- *infection causing brain damage*

Symptoms

These can range from minor numbness to profound paralysis:

- *Sudden loss of speech or movement on one side of the body*
- *Headache*
- *Numbness or tingling in limbs*
- *Blurred vision*
- *Dizziness or confusion*
- *Seizures*
- *Incontinence*

TRANSIENT ISCHAEMIC ATTACKS (TIA)

These are common events, especially in older people, but they are important because they indicate a significant risk of developing a more serious full-blown stroke. TIAs are of brief duration and symptoms may be so minor that people ignore them. There may only be numbing sensations affecting a part of the body and they may even occur while the person is asleep.

In order to minimise the risk of larger strokes, TIAs need proper medical investigation and treatment. High blood pressure, over-active thyroid, irregular heartbeat, diabetes, high cholesterol levels and other blood

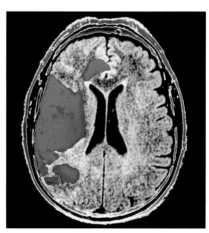

ABOVE *The red area in this brain scan shows a pool of blood (a cerebral haemorrhage), which occurs when an artery supplying the brain ruptures and blood seeps out into the surrounding tissue.*

vessel diseases may be diagnosed, which will need treatment in their own right. If you smoke, you should stop, and you will be advised to reduce the amount of fat in your diet if high cholesterol is a problem.

After medical investigation, the usual treatment, once any additional problems have been dealt with, is medication to stop clotting. Aspirin thins the blood and helps to prevent harmful blood clots forming. Initially, at the time of the attack, a dose of 300 mg (just one ordinary aspirin) is taken, but over time this dose may be reduced to just 75 mg daily. For those who are sensitive to aspirin, other drugs are available which help to prevent clotting.

MAJOR STROKES

If the blood supply to part of the brain is interrupted, a condition that is termed a stroke, the affected region fails to function properly. Sometimes the area of damaged brain from either a haemorrhage or a clot is so large, or in such a sensitive area (such as the area controlling breathing), that the outlook for any recovery is very limited. Many people thus affected develop pneumonia and die, but if they do survive they have a time of severe incapacity ahead of them. A lot of thought should be given to how to deal with the frustration and boredom frequently experienced by these individuals.

Areas of the brain affected by stroke

The brain processes information from different sense organs throughout the body and coordinates appropriate responses. Different types of stroke may affect functions such as speech, movement or mental processing, depending on the area of brain affected. If the area of damage is extensive or in a particularly sensitive place, such as that controlling breathing, full recovery is very unlikely.

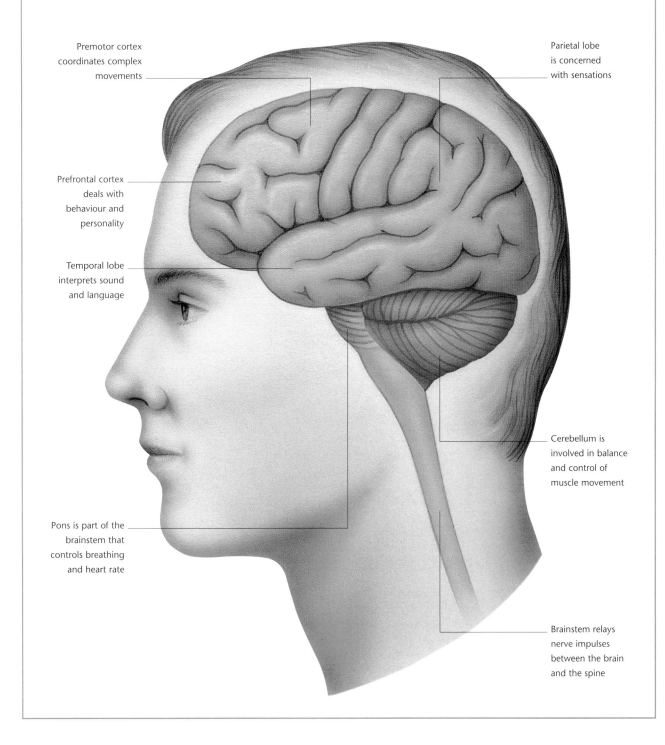

Premotor cortex coordinates complex movements

Prefrontal cortex deals with behaviour and personality

Temporal lobe interprets sound and language

Pons is part of the brainstem that controls breathing and heart rate

Parietal lobe is concerned with sensations

Cerebellum is involved in balance and control of muscle movement

Brainstem relays nerve impulses between the brain and the spine

STROKE

ABOVE AND LEFT *You can keep an eye on your blood pressure with a blood pressure monitoring kit, readily available from most chemists, and easy to use at home. Blood pressure kits record the systolic pressure, when the heart contracts, and the diastolic pressure, when the heart relaxes. Lifestyle changes such as cutting down on salt and fat will help reduce high blood pressure.*

Prevention of further strokes

• *It is essential to stop smoking to reduce the risk of further strokes and also to reduce the risk of clots forming in other parts of the body.*

• *Careful nutritional planning is essential as it is easy to gain weight when inactive and sufferers may seek consolation in sugary and fatty foods. The added weight not only makes it more difficult to get around but also makes it more difficult for carers. Fats should be cut back in an effort to reduce cholesterol levels.*

• *Regular blood pressure checks are important, and home blood pressure monitoring equipment is now readily available from most good chemists. The equipment is relatively cheap and accurate.*

• *Prevention of stiffness and contortion of limbs is possible with regular physiotherapy*

exercises. People often find it easy to do exercises initially, but see little benefit and give up on them. The exercises are there not just to gain some improvement but also to help prevent deterioration. Relatives can really help by encouraging exercise sessions several times a day.

Outcome

When we consider the size of the stroke we are concerned with the amount of functional loss that the body has suffered as a result of the brain damage. People who have had TIAs usually make a complete recovery. If there is permanent damage, in an ideal world all patients would firstly be admitted to hospital. This is to identify the brain damage accurately and ensure that everything possible has been done

to prevent a further episode or brain damage, and to be sure of the diagnosis; secondly, to ensure maximum early rehabilitation, which seems to be the key to minimising the final disability. Sometimes specialised stroke teams in the home may do even better work than hospital based teams, as the family can be involved in carrying on with rehabilitation when the professionals are not there.

Rehabilitation of stroke victims

Speech therapy and physiotherapy, provided at hospital or at home, are essential for stroke victims. If a person has a commonly recognized stroke, with weakness of the arm and leg on one side and sometimes associated speech disturbances, the sooner that physiotherapy starts, the less likely he is to end up with tight, spastic muscles. Early speech therapy, occupational therapy, psychological support and social workers, as well as nurses and doctors, are all important.

A person who suffers a major stroke has been used to a healthy, normal life and the change for him may be devastating. The sufferer may often be

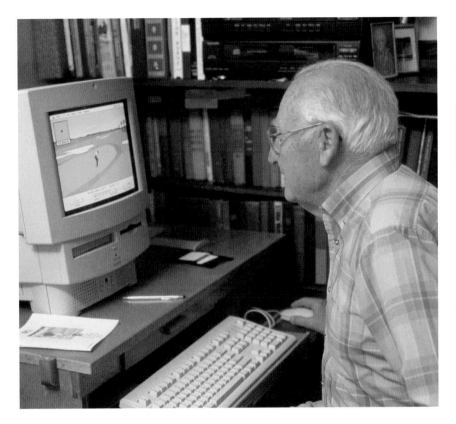

LEFT *Using a computer may help to improve reflex actions and fine muscle control, which may help you regain dexterity and coordination.*

totally dependent on others to do even the simplest task, which makes him feel humiliated and useless. His mind may well be very active and possibly functioning normally, but if speech is impaired then the frustration is immense. It is not surprising that so many of these people become depressed. They may neglect exercise and become even more severely disabled.

Sometimes antidepressants may be beneficial but they are only a part of the helping process. If visitors and friends can talk normally to the person, as they did before the stroke, this may help considerably.

Ways of communicating with someone who has had a stroke need to be inventive and individual. Reading may be a problem as eyesight may be affected, holding papers and books and

RIGHT *Discovering new ways of communicating with someone after a stroke may do more than anything else to help the person.*

turning pages may be difficult and sometimes the written word may be hard to understand because of the area of brain affected. Talking books and newspapers may be the answer.

It is important for both patient and carer to lead as normal a life as possible after a stroke.

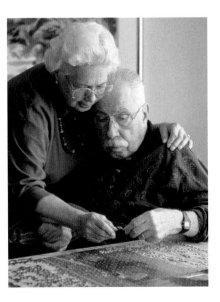

Treatment

• *If the stroke was caused by a clot (or an embolism, where a piece of blood clot breaks off from a clot in the heart), then medication to thin the blood is required. Aspirin is the most commonly used but in cases of sensitivity to aspirin there are alternatives; the anticoagulant warfarin may be prescribed in cases of irregular, fast heartbeats.*

• *If diabetes, high blood pressure (hypertension) or high cholesterol levels are identified, medical treatment for these conditions may prevent further, even more devastating, strokes.*

• *Muscle relaxant drugs relieve stiffness in the limbs, and physiotherapy is essential.*

• *For bladder problems, there are drugs to help loss of control caused by nervous system impairment, and regular catheterisation (the introduction of a tube to empty the bladder) may be required.*

• *Depression often accompanies a stroke, particularly if the sufferer is left disabled, and antidepressants may be appropriate.*

THINKING DISORDERS

It is not uncommon to joke about memory loss, saying it's all to do with getting older. Some people worry enormously about perfectly normal memory loss such as forgetting what they went upstairs for. Others have major memory impairment but show little anxiety about what they have forgotten. Major thinking disorders are usually noticed by family or friends. If there is concern about a a family member it is important to seek early medical help.

CONFUSION

This is a state of mental dysfunction when a person lacks either knowledge or confidence as to his identity or the current time and place. Often there is an awareness that he is not as alert as he has been. It may seem to onlookers that sufferers are indifferent to their lack of orientation but this may not be so, and panic may set in when a person understands how unsure he is of reality. There is little doubt that putting a confused person under stress raises his level of distress and lowers his level of functioning.

What causes confusion?

The condition occurs more commonly in the elderly but may come on suddenly or very gradually; it may be temporary if due to illness but can also be permanent. Causes include the following:

- *ageing*
- *dehydration*
- *infection*
- *fever*
- *hypothermia*
- *underactive thyroid gland (hypothyroidism)*
- *inebriation*
- *low blood sugar (hypoglycaemia)*
- *high blood sugar (hyperglycaemia)*

- *head injury*
- *low blood oxygen due to chronic lung disease or carbon monoxide poisoning*
- *numerous medications, including antidepressants and tablets for high blood pressure (hypertension)*
- *poor nutrition and vitamin deficiencies*

BELOW *As you grow older your memory may become less efficient but you can stimulate your mind with activities such as playing cards.*

Symptoms of confusion

- *Lack of orientation*
- *Forgetfulness*
- *Bewilderment*
- *Self-neglect*

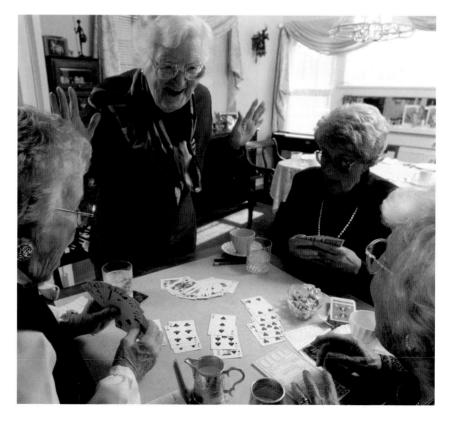

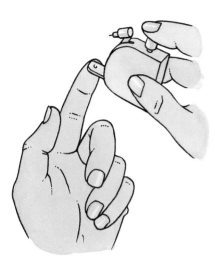

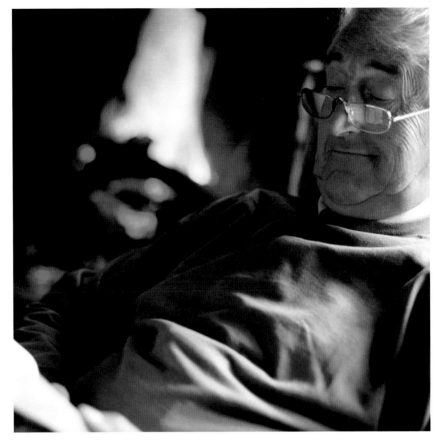

ABOVE *A simple finger-prick test can ascertain the presence of diabetes which may well be the underlying cause of confusion in an elderly person.*

RIGHT *Make sure your body temperature doesn't fall below the normal range. Inadequate heating can result in hypothermia which is a common cause of confusion.*

Treatment for confusion

• *It is essential that a full physical and mental examination is done to try to exclude any remediable cause of confusion.*

• *Some of the commonest causes of sudden onset of confusion are urinary infections or chest infections, and these are readily curable once they have been identified. A course of antibiotics will often enable a confused person to become lucid quite rapidly.*

• *Hypothermia is a common cause of confusion, especially in the winter when the elderly on low budgets fight to keep their heating bills down. As their body temperature cools they become very confused. Warming the person over many hours is necessary and as the temperature rises, so the confusion goes. It may take several weeks until an ill person returns to complete normality.*

• *Those who live in houses with old boilers may be exposed to chronic carbon monoxide poisoning, and those with chronic lung disease may become confused through lack of oxygen and may look blue. Giving oxygen from a cylinder, at the correct dosage, may cure the associated confusion.*

• *Diabetes should be looked for in all older people as it is often missed. The sugar level of the blood may rise over many months, making it appear that the confusion has come on slowly. A quick finger-prick blood test will confirm the blood sugar level very readily.*

• *In some people there seems to be no obvious reason for their confusion but if this is the case they will need constant care and attention as they can easily wander off and get lost or do other things that may endanger their lives and those of others.*

THINKING DISORDERS

DELIRIUM

This is a type of major confusion, which may be due to physical or mental illness. It is usually treatable and reversible. There are rapid swings of mental state, energy levels, thinking ability and paranoia, and the patient may not be aware of his condition.

Why does delirium happen?

There are many causes of delirium and some of them are an extension of those that cause confusion. There is no clear cut-off point when confusion becomes delirium except to say that confusion doesn't seem to fluctuate as wildly.

Investigations

As with confusion, a doctor will search for a physical cause of delirium to try to identify and treat any obvious cause. Tests are as follows:

• *blood tests to examine thyroid, liver and kidney function, and presence of anaemia, drugs or alcohol*
• *urine analysis*
• *eye tests*
• *hearing tests*
• *ECG to check the heart's electrical activity*
• *EEG to investigate patterns of activity in the brain*
• *head scans*
• *chest X-ray*

Symptoms of delirium

• *mumbling and continuous incoherent speech*
• *complete disorientation in space and time*
• *memory both past and recent may be seriously impaired and the person may lose any ability to concentrate*
• *hallucinations and paranoia, which makes it difficult to distinguish between physical and mental causes*
• *constant drowsiness or wakefulness*
• *abnormal movements, which may be wild and jerky*
• *wild fluctuations in activity, from total inactivity to rapid running around*
• *mood changes may be rapid and very marked, with a variation from happy to sad, angry to anxious and depressive to manic that may happen over very short periods of time*

Treatment for delirium

If no obvious cause is found, or if the delirium continues while specific treatment is being given for physical reasons, then various medicines to control the delirium may be needed. If the agitation is marked, the mood swings severe or the behaviour is violent and aggressive, then sedation or antidepressants may be very helpful. Psychotherapy may be appropriate to try to change behaviour patterns.

If the delirium seems to have no physical illness as its basis, then it may turn into a chronic mental illness and progress to dementia. If this happens, then appropriate help may be required in the form of medication and practical care.

BELOW *It is very important for people with major thinking disorders to have a strong support network.*

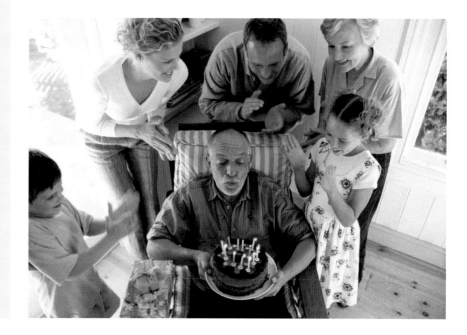

ALZHEIMER'S DISEASE

This is a progressive form of dementia. There is loss of memory, judgement, ability to make decisions, word finding and use of language, and inability to pay attention or retain new information. It is almost as if the brain is full and nothing new can be put into it, while other bits keep slowly slipping out. Usually the progression of the dementia happens over many years but for some the rate of deterioration is rapid.

Why does it happen?

Unfortunately we really do not know. It is not part of the normal ageing process and the only way to make a definite diagnosis is after death, when changes within the brain tissue can be found. Alzheimer's becomes more prevalent in old age and a family history of the disease tends to increase the likelihood it developing. It seems that women develop the disease more frequently than men but that may be because, on average, they live longer, and so more cases become prominent. A few forms of Alzheimer's occur before the age of 60, and these forms seem to have a much stronger genetic link. As yet, there is no form of prevention available, although scientists are working on various vaccines.

Outlook

The average life expectancy from diagnosis to death is about 14 years. This is a very distressing disease for the relatives of sufferers and they need much support from family, social workers and support groups.

The person with Alzheimer's will become unable to make decisions or deal with day-to-day money matters, and a family member should seek a power of attorney so that difficulties are avoided.

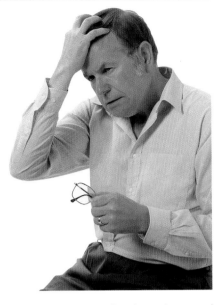

ABOVE *Some memory impairment is a natural part of ageing and minor forgetfulness should not be a cause for concern.*

Treatment for Alzheimer's

At present, the only drugs available seem to delay the rate of progress of the disease but it is likely that more effective drugs will soon be available that may stop the progression completely. Mood-controlling drugs may be necessary to control anger or agitation. These drugs can cause sedation and lethargy but this may be preferable to people putting themselves and others at risk.

Symptoms of Alzheimer's

These are early signs and often manageable by relatives and friends:

- *Difficulty remembering names*
- *Constantly repeating sentences*
- *Loss of memory, especially in relation to new information*
- *Forgetting where she is when outside in familiar places*
- *Change of personality, often becoming grumpy*
- *Loss of interest in previously enjoyable activities*
- *Inability to do everyday tasks*

However, as the disease progresses there may be more serious loss of brain function:

- *Loss of immediate and long-term memory*
- *Inability to dress independently*
- *Choosing inappropriate clothes and food*
- *Inability to remember who she is, her past and even her close family*
- *Violent and aggressive behaviour*
- *Hallucinations and sometimes hearing constant voices*
- *Severe depression*
- *Extreme agitation and inability to stay still*
- *Delusions and paranoia*

Often at this stage the family cannot cope and admission to a home for the mentally ill is necessary.

DEGENERATIVE CONDITIONS

Within this group of conditions lies a large number of tragic, progressive malfunctioning diseases of the nervous system. Fifty years ago, nearly all were untreatable and the outlook was one of a distressing, hopeless, downhill course with progressive loss of bodily and often mental function. Since then, new medicines have been developed that have helped delay the relentless deterioration and sometimes even allowed for improvement. Advances in physiotherapy and help in dealing with the psychological consequences of these diseases have enabled both patients and doctors to have a more positive attitude.

MULTIPLE SCLEROSIS (MS)

This is a condition confined entirely to the nervous system, thought to be due to auto-immunity, where the body fights against bits of itself, causing damage and inflammation. In this case, the body fights the white matter of the central nervous system. The most common form of the disease is a slow, general deterioration with periods of remission and then another attack. Eventually some of the weaknesses become permanent, and a few patients have a steadily progressive downhill course. The disease is twice as common in men as women, and has a peak age of onset at around 30 years of age.

What causes MS?
MS is caused by inflammation in the nervous system. The protective myelin sheaths that cover nerves become inflamed and scarred (a process termed demyelination), resulting in loss of nerve function. Some hold that the disease occurs following exposure to a virus in early life. However, there is a genetic factor – there is a one in twenty risk of developing the disease if a sibling has the condition.

Symptoms of MS

• *Sudden onset blurred vision or fairly sudden loss of vision in one eye*
• *Numbness, tingling and patchy areas of altered sensation*
• *Sudden weakness in limbs or the face*
• *Attack often short-lived and within a few days there may be nothing evident*
• *Dizziness, clumsiness or lack of coordination*

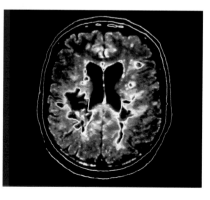

ABOVE *This brain scan shows tissue damaged by destruction of the myelin sheaths.*

Treatment for MS

Plaques of demyelination can be readily identified on an MRI (magnetic resolution imaging) scan, and this is essential for diagnosis of the disease. There is no cure for MS and treatment is aimed at alleviating symptoms. Steroids may shorten the length of an acute bad relapse. In a specific sort of person with a specific type of MS, drugs known as beta interferons may help prevent some relapses. There are also medicines available to help to deal with the symptoms of spasticity, muscle spasms, bladder dysfunction and erectile dysfunction. The efficacy of cannabis in helping MS patients with spasms and spasticity is still hotly debated. Physiotherapy, occupational therapy and psychotherapy all have an important part to play in managing this condition.

PARKINSON'S DISEASE

This is a slowly progressive brain disease associated with difficulty in walking, coordination and movement that occurs in approximately two in a thousand people. Most commonly it develops in those over the age of 50 but it can affect younger people, and it affects both sexes equally.

RIGHT *Physiotherapy aims to improve mobility, relieve pain and maintain normal body function through the use of physical techniques such as exercise and massage. Here, a person with Parkinson's disease is having his hand manipulated to extend the range of movement.*

Symptoms of Parkinson's

• *Stiffness and muscle rigidity*
• *Difficulty bending arms and legs*
• *Change of walking style and posture to shuffling and stooped gait*
• *Unsteadiness*
• *Poor balance*
• *Problems with starting movements which may improve once action has commenced*
• *Muscular aches and pains*
• *Shaking and trembling which tends to be worst at rest but may interfere with activities such as eating and drinking*
• *Mask-like expression where little emotion is shown*
• *Slow, monotonous speech tone*
• *Spider-like handwriting which goes up the page*
• *Loss of mental ability and depression*
• *Constipation*

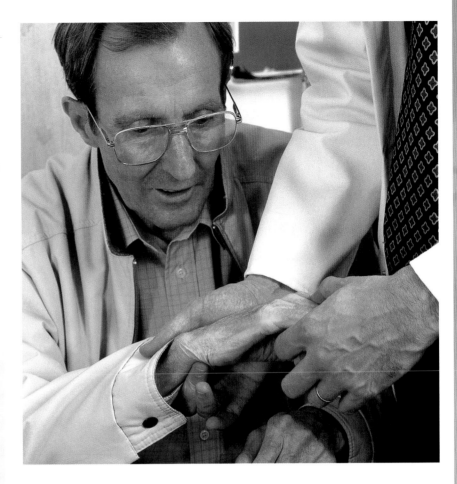

Treatment for Parkinson's

• *The aim of treatment at present is to slow down the progression of the disease. Parkinson's disease is thought to be caused by a lack of the chemical dopamine and drug management is geared towards trying to build up dopamine levels in the brain. Physiotherapy, education for the sufferer and relatives, and occupational therapy can help with physical and mental needs and diet. Nutrition may become badly impaired and weight can be lost easily if eating is difficult because of shaking or stiffness, and it is vital to provide a high-calorie intake in a form with which the sufferer can cope.*

• *Surgery is occasionally an option for shaking as this may occur as a result of areas of the brain being destroyed. Foetal tissue transplant aims to replenish the supplies of dopamine but this procedure is not well established.*

This is a very depressing condition for everyone as it involves progressive deterioration, but there is every reason to expect that medical advances will yield better and better results.

DEPRESSIVE ILLNESSES

When we are physically ill few of us hesitate to seek treatment but the case is very different if we become mentally ill. Most people find it very hard to accept that they have a mental health problem. However, disorders such as depression, anxiety and phobias are commonplace and in most cases readily treatable. It is important not to suffer alone and to seek medical help if you are suffering from a depressive illness.

DEPRESSION

Depression in some form is a common experience, but there are many grades and depths of this condition. Most people have days when they feel a bit fed up or not as happy as on other days but for some, depression is a very serious, sometimes life-threatening condition. Depression after childbirth is common.

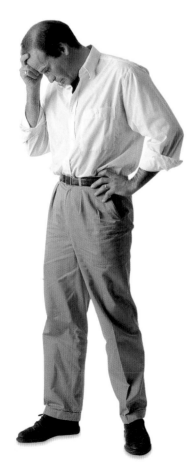

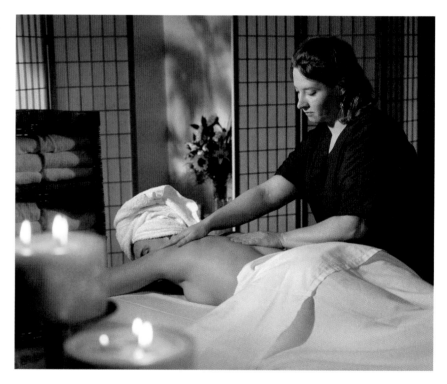

LEFT *A person with depression often feels very lonely. Talking things over with a sympathetic listener can be the first step to recovery.*

ABOVE *Combined with other forms of treatment, aromatherapy may be recommended as a therapy for depression.*

What causes depression?

There may be an obvious reason for depression (reactive depression) such as loss of a loved one, or the break-up of a relationship. In many cases it may be due to a chemical imbalance within the brain. Quite often there is no very obvious cause. It may even be that everything seems perfect: good health, secure job, no financial stress and loved ones around. Depression often comes from inside (endogenous depression) and is often inexplicable and difficult for non-sufferers to understand. With a depressive illness the sad mood may go on for long periods of time and may be severe enough to make life seem not worth living.

Historically, depression has been seen as a weakness, something not to

RIGHT *In group therapy small groups meet regularly to share experiences and feelings. It is often used to treat addictions such as alcoholism.*

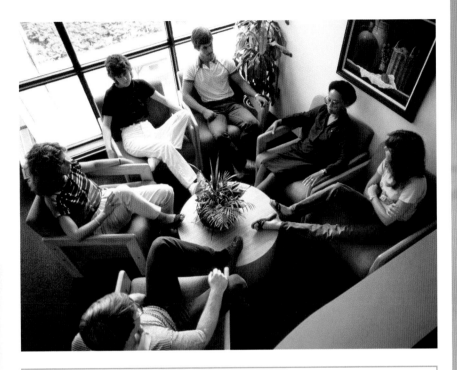

give in to. Nowadays we have much more understanding but many people with depression are still afraid to complain about it and feel that others will not understand. Others with depression may express it physically, complaining of constant headaches or stomach aches.

Symptoms of depression

One or several of the symptoms listed below is usually present in depression. The severity and constancy of the symptoms make the illness diagnosable as depression. Often other people recognise depression before the person suffering.

- *Constant tiredness*
- *Wanting to be in bed for long periods*
- *Long periods of sleep or poor sleeping*
- *Early morning wakening*
- *Feeling worse in the mornings*
- *Over-eating*
- *Loss of appetite*
- *Frequent weeping*
- *Anxiety and restlessness*
- *Lack of interest in things and people*
- *Lack of interest in sex*
- *Loss of self-esteem and self-worth*
- *Becoming isolated from others*
- *Feelings and thoughts of suicide*
- *Worries that you are going mad*

Treatment for depression

The most important part of treatment is recognising and accepting that you have an illness and need help. Friends and relatives may be aware of your depression but may be anxious not to upset you further by discussing it, or you may not be prepared to listen either to yourself or your friends. As in diabetes, treatment may need to be continued for life. Most people will require a minimum of six months' medication.

One or a combination of the following suggestions may be of help:

- *Talking things over with a doctor, family, friends, employers or the Samaritans*
- *Extra daylight (special daylight bulbs and light boxes are available)*
- *Relaxation therapy*
- *Homeopathy*
- *Herbal medicine*
- *Psychotherapy and counselling*
- *Change of diet*
- *Antidepressant medication*
- *ECT (electroconvulsive therapy, whereby an electric current is passed through the brain to alter patterns of thinking)*
- *Self-help groups*
- *Aromatherapy*
- *Exercise and fresh air*
- *Changing job*
- *Abstaining from alcohol*

DEPRESSIVE ILLNESSES

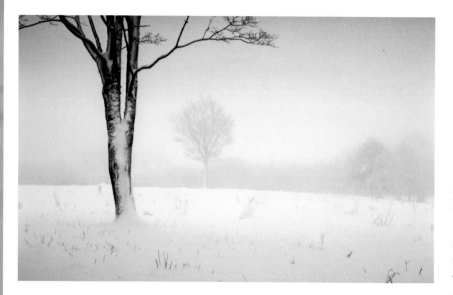

LEFT *Light plays an important role in regulating the body's biological clock and a lack of sunlight in winter is thought to cause seasonal affective disorder.*

SAD (SEASONAL AFFECTIVE DISORDER)

This form of depression always occurs during the winter months, which is why it is termed seasonal affective disorder. It is thought to occur because the daylight hours are so short in our winter. The condition affects about half a million Britons quite severely and others have it to a lesser degree. In the summer a lot of light enters the eye and then travels to the brain. Here it probably acts in two ways: it reduces the production of melatonin, which causes sleepiness and apathy; it also increases the production of serotonin, the feel-good chemical (low levels of serotonin are thought to be the basis of depression). Therefore when there is little daylight in the winter we have more melatonin, making us sleepy and also increasing apathy, and lower levels of serotonin, making depression more likely.

People who become depressed and apathetic in the winter often benefit from extra light exposure. Ideally this would mean migrating to a sunny climate, but a special light box (see www.outsidein.co.uk), may completely prevent the symptoms of depression.

ALCOHOL

Many people with depression find temporary relief from drinking more and more heavily, using alcohol to blot out feelings of sadness. It is very easy to become dependent on alcohol, which is itself a depressant, and drinking alcohol alone nearly always results in a downward spiral. If depressed, avoiding alcohol altogether is safest.

ANTIDEPRESSANTS

Many people suffering from depression are reluctant to acknowledge the disease or to take proven effective medication. This is because of the stigma of acknowledging they have what is widely perceived to be an unacceptable illness (a mental disorder) and fear of the possible side-effects of the medication, such as character changes, addiction and agitation. Some side-effects do occur with drug treatments, but it is worth bearing in mind that codeine/paracetamol medicines, readily available without prescription, may cause sleepiness, constipation, addiction, chronic headaches and liver and kidney poisoning, yet few people hesitate to take them.

Antidepressants are drugs specifically designed to overcome the problems in brain chemistry that cause depression. They are much more specific than painkillers. The SSRI drugs (marketed as Prozac, Seroxat, Lustral and many more) work specifically to raise the levels of serotonin in the brain. Others raise the levels of noradrenalin. Lack of these mood-enhancing substances can cause depression. Raising their levels, a process that usually takes about ten days, is usually very helpful.

There are side-effects but they are often mild, short-lived and pale into insignificance as the depression improves. Slight nausea, sleepiness, agitation, and a certain amount of dependency are common. Dependency probably occurs because depression can be a chronic disease. Like Type I diabetes, where insulin injections are necessary every day, depression is a disease that may be present all the time unless medication is taken to relieve it. Therefore a person who becomes reliant on his medicine does so because that is what is needed to keep him feeling well.

Anyone who has diagnosed themselves or seen a doctor who has diagnosed depression should think positively about taking antidepressants. For most people they work very well and relieve the depression.

Symptoms of anxiety and phobias

- *Sweating*
- *Palpitations (when the heart is felt to thud quickly)*
- *Fainting*
- *Diarrhoea and other bowel symptoms*
- *Hyperventilation (abnormally rapid breathing)*

Treatment

- *Talking about the problems*
- *Trying, with support, to work through them*
- *Psychotherapy*
- *Relaxation therapy*
- *Meditation*
- *Yoga*
- *Emergency medication (such as diazepam)*
- *Longer-term medication (such as risperidone)*
- *Support from self-help groups and friends*
- *The Samaritans*

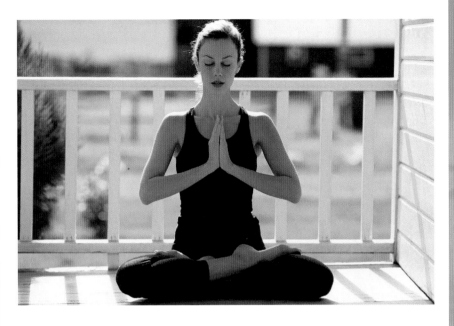

ABOVE *Focusing on breathing or meditating may calm you down and prevent panic.*

ANXIETIES AND PHOBIAS

These are normal reactions to stress, which may be obvious or unidentified. All of us worry and become distressed under different circumstances but when fears and anxieties are abnormal and prevent a person from carrying out everyday activities help is needed.

Excessive anxieties may be associated with obsessive thoughts and actions. Often there is a compulsion to check things and repeat things over and over again. One of the most common rituals is hand washing, and some people feel so anxious that they feel it is essential to wash their hands many, many times a day. They may become obsessed with dirt and germs. Other people worry excessively about noises or the wind or heights.

Anxieties, panic attacks and phobias can be paralysing, but the earlier help is sought, the more likely that the condition will be alleviated or even cured.

Why do anxieties and phobias occur?

Sometimes these disorders occur as a result of a severe, real stress such as a road traffic accident. Sometimes they occur because people set themselves unrealistic goals.

RIGHT *Yoga is a combination of physical exercises and controlled breathing techniques designed to harmonise the mind and body, helping you to relax and feel more serene.*

EATING DISORDERS

This term embraces the whole range of abnormal eating patterns. The most commonly recognised are anorexia, bulimia and obesity, and there is a whole range of eating styles and habits that span and include these. Eating patterns become abnormal when they either cause problems with lifestyle, such that a person cannot eat with others and eats far more or less than others, or when the resultant weight changes put health at risk.

ANOREXIA NERVOSA

Usually referred to as anorexia, this condition commonly occurs in adolescent females. However it is becoming more common in males, and can occur in very young children or in older people at times of great mental stress. The disease, usually associated with stress and distress in the first instance, involves eating less and less and dropping body weight. The sufferer is always thin; sometimes in extreme cases they can appear to be just skin and bone. There is nearly always a distorted body image, so however thin a person looks to others she considers herself to be fat. A person with anorexia is obsessed by body size and weight. Anorexics often take up cooking and make wonderful meals for others but always plead that they are too full to eat it themselves.

What causes anorexia?

Anorexia has become more common in recent years where there is a media pressure to be thin. Nearly all film stars are thin and the media messages are always that you need to be thin to look good. If your work involves your appearance, there is enormous pressure to be thin.

Frequently, a teenager starts off on a diet and enjoys the encouraging remarks made by others. She feels good as she loses weight but unfortunately she also loses her sense of proportion and becomes thinner. The sensation of hunger disappears rapidly and excuses for not eating with others trip off the tongue.

Health risks

Few anorexics are happy after the initial euphoria of becoming thin. They live in constant dread of gaining weight and also of others finding out that they hardly eat. As the weight falls, periods stop in girls (fertility may take years to recover even if the illness is brought to an end) and the body becomes covered with fine, downy hair. Depression, tearfulness and lack of concentration are frequent problems. In the longer term, thinning bones, where fractures can occur with the slightest fall, infection, heart failure, epileptic fits and kidney failure can all develop. Some patients are so obsessed with the fear of gaining weight that they literally starve themselves to death.

Symptoms of anorexia

- *Weight loss even after others have commented*
- *Reluctance to seek medical advice about the weight loss*
- *Using laxatives*
- *Over-exercising*
- *Feeling revolted by food*
- *Depression*
- *Lack of concentration*
- *Sleep disorders – most people with anorexia sleep little*

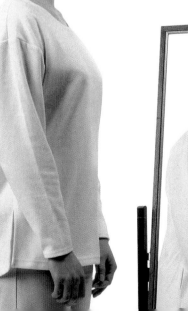
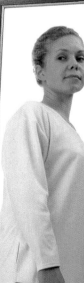

RIGHT *An obsession with body image can lead to anorexia, where the sufferer perceives herself to be fat even though she is actually underweight.*

Treatment for anorexia

• Treatment for anorexia is notoriously very difficult. If you or anyone in your family appears to be losing weight and has no other illness to explain it, then the sooner help is sought the more likely there is to be a happy outcome.

• Acknowledgement is the first step in dealing with the problem. Talking to family and friends and your doctor will help. However, there is no simple, quick cure. Setting goals to return to a normal style of eating is important. Eating with others may be a first step, even if initially it is just one meal a day. Try to eat half portions of what others are having. A target weight, which can be lower than others might think appropriate but still allows your body to be healthy, should be agreed by you. Depending upon your bone structure, aiming for a BMI (Body Mass Index, see page 241) of around 18 may be acceptable. It is important to understand the full health risks of this illness and if a target weight is agreed, any drop below this should alert you immediately to seek help.

• There is always a tendency to revert to anorexia, even many years after the illness appears to be resolved. Help and support from friends is vital. Being nagged to eat more and gain weight doesn't help and makes a person with anorexia even more determined to get thinner. Recognising triggers such as stress and anxiety may enable an attack to be curtailed before it takes hold again. In extreme cases specialised psychiatric help is essential.

Symptoms of bulimia

• Eating thousands of calories at a time: entire cakes, boxes of chocolates, biscuits and huge meals may all be consumed in a very short period
• Forcibly vomiting as soon as the binge is over
• Taking huge amounts of laxatives to ensure that none of the binged food is absorbed

Treatment for bulimia

A bulimic is aware that binge eating is abnormal and is more likely than an anorexic to go to her doctor for treatment. Keeping a diary may help spread food intake more evenly. Families can help by ensuring the house is not full of readily consumable, high-calorie foods, not leaving the sufferer alone for long, eating with her on a regular basis and ensuring that she has no access to laxatives. Frequently psychological support and counselling may be useful.

BULIMIA

This condition has some similarities with anorexia. A person feels she is overweight; eats little or nothing for a period of time and then binges. Bulimics tend to be on the thin side of normal but not always so. Even when a person is binge eating she is aware that she is going to try to bring it all back up, but she is unable to stop the binge at the time. The person wants to be thin but cannot maintain a low food intake for long. She then overeats, knowing she has the fallback mechanism of vomiting and laxatives.

What causes bulimia?

Most bulimia sufferers have had adverse comments made about their weight. They have better body image recognition than anorexics, and know when they are over- or undersized.

Health risks

There are several areas of risk, especially in the mental distress that this condition causes and the reasons for which it has arisen. Bulimia can cause major damage to the teeth through vomiting, and generalised weakness following the vomiting and diarrhoea. Depression and poor concentration may occur as a result of bulimia and there is the possibility of relapse many years after the condition appears to be cured.

RIGHT *Eating meals with others is often a first step in treating anorexia, even if the sufferer is consuming smaller portions than is normal.*

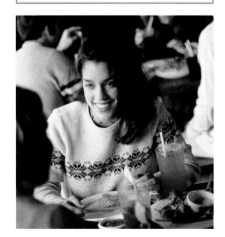

EATING DISORDERS

OBESITY

This is probably the major health problem in the West, with both mental and physical effects. Although there are a few medical conditions that do result in being overweight, the vast majority of people are obese because they eat more than their body needs. We all need different amounts of food to maintain a

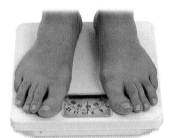

ABOVE *Weighing yourself at regular intervals – once a week, first thing in the morning, is best – enables you to keep track of your weight.*

'normal' body weight, and anyone who exceeds his individual need will become fat. The only way to lose weight is to eat less.

Health risks

Obesity causes many health risks. The chances of suffering from heart disease and stroke are considerably increased because of the extra pressure put on the heart and blood vessels. Strain is put on the respiratory system and a person becomes progressively breathless. The whole of the skeleton and its joints are put under pressure the more the weight rises. Arthritis, back pain and aching muscles and joints are also common. There is a general slowing down, which compounds the problem, since exercise becomes limited or even non-existent. Digestive disorders such as indigestion, ulcers and irritable bowel syndrome (IBS) are more likely to occur. Obesity also increases the chances of developing Type II (non-insulin-dependent) diabetes. Obesity can affect fertility and increase the risk of developing certain types of cancer.

The risks to mental health cannot be overestimated. We live in a society that values thinness, viewing those who are overweight as unattractive and, because they are physically slower, unintelligent.

What causes obesity?

There are a few medical conditions that can cause someone to gain weight and with correction of the condition the weight will return to normal.

• *An underactive thyroid gland can cause increasing weight but is nearly always associated with other features such as sleepiness, coarsening of facial features, loss of the outer third of the eyebrows, slow pulse and deepening of the voice. If this is diagnosed and corrected with thyroid replacement therapy, the weight may slowly drop off. Taking thyroid tablets if your thyroid works normally will not cause weight loss and is extremely dangerous.*

• *Taking steroid tablets for arthritic diseases, asthma and various other medical conditions may cause the weight to rise as appetite is increased and fat distribution alters. However, most people taking long-term steroids need them and cannot stop them abruptly. Cushing's disease, a rare disorder caused when the body makes too much of its own steroid hormone, causes central obesity with thin arms and legs.*

• *Certain genetic causes associated with mental retardation have an association with obesity, but these are few and far between and are usually readily recognised in infants or children.*

• *If one particular area appears to have put on weight while the rest of the body stays relatively slim, this needs medical investigation. For instance, in a non-pregnant woman with slim arms and legs but a very protuberant stomach, the possibility of ovarian cysts and other gynaecological tumours must be excluded.*

• *In both sexes, a condition called ascites, where fluid fills the abdomen, is uncommon but needs to be excluded if this is the only area affected. Women frequently worry that they are retaining water and this can explain their obesity. Occasionally, women may retain some fluid at certain times of their menstrual cycle but the quantities rarely amount to more than a few pounds and what is gained will be lost during other parts of the cycle. It is rare for much fluid to be retained except in cases of renal or heart failure where other signs will be uppermost.*

Treatment for obesity

• *The only solution to being overweight is to eat fewer calories or to maintain the same calorie intake and burn up more calories through exercise, but if obesity is severe then exercise capabilities will be very limited. To lose weight, most sedentary people need to eat about 1,000 calories a day; those with heavy manual jobs will need 1,500 calories. Slimming clubs have different ways of disguising this fact and use points and various diets but the truth remains that one way or another fewer calories need to be taken in than previously to lose weight. However, slimming clubs do help many people as the community spirit and encouragement from others increases the willpower and the determination to continue dieting.*

• *Various drugs have been used in the past to treat obesity. One group produced to speed up metabolism proved to increase the risk of developing heart disease and had side-effects such as palpitations, insomnia and general anxiety. These are now rarely prescribed. Another group of medicines based on cellulose aimed to trick the brain into thinking the stomach was full. The idea was that the person felt full and the appetite decreased, but these drugs were not very successful because the problem of eating patterns was not addressed.*

• *Currently two drugs are used for people who have severe obesity. One stops the absorption of fat, a highly calorific substance. This in turn reduces calorie intake and so induces weight loss. The major side-effect is diarrhoea. The problem is that overweight people quickly learn to substitute fatty foods with others and so, after initial success, there is a return to the previous body weight and the drug is then deemed unsuccessful. Another new drug aims to reduce food intake by up to 20 per cent by reducing feelings of hunger, but it is far from a miraculous answer to the problem because it doesn't change eating habits.*

• *All sorts of diets have been in and out of fashion: different food combinations, food timings, special one-food diets and many other individual programmes. Some of these have good short-term results but almost inevitably the weight returns.*

• *The only way to control your weight and maintain it within a healthy range for your height is a lifetime of re-educating the body to make do with less food. Avoiding specific high-calorie foods such as cakes, crisps, biscuits and chocolates is essential. One of the biggest culprits when people estimate their food intake is underestimating how many calories are contained in drinks. Milk, fresh orange juice, apple juice, fizzy drinks and especially alcohol contain far more calories than anyone suspects. Cutting out this source of calorie intake often helps dieters enormously.*

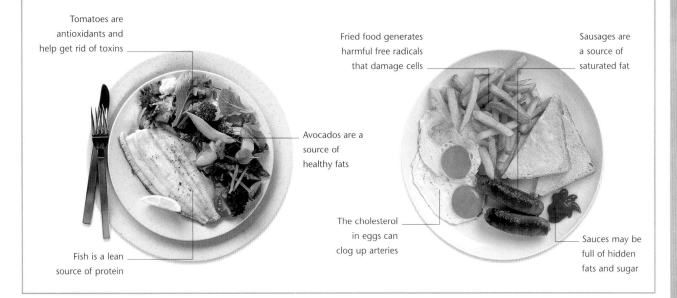

Tomatoes are antioxidants and help get rid of toxins

Avocados are a source of healthy fats

Fish is a lean source of protein

Fried food generates harmful free radicals that damage cells

The cholesterol in eggs can clog up arteries

Sausages are a source of saturated fat

Sauces may be full of hidden fats and sugar

SCHIZOPHRENIA

Schizophrenia is a serious mental illness that encompasses a group of mental disorders where there are disturbances of thought, behaviour, communication, mood and action. There is frequently lack of insight that anything is wrong. There can be many symptoms of varying severity between individuals and within each individual. Depression be closely interrelated: people with schizophrenia have a high rate of suicide and experts debate whether this is part of the actual illness or whether the accompanying depression causes this.

WHAT CAUSES SCHIZOPHRENIA?

No one knows for certain what causes schizophrenia, but there is undoubtedly a predisposition to it, particularly if there is a family member with the illness. Just as with migraine and asthma, the disease may be triggered by different life situations. Job loss, bereavement, break-up of a relationship, examinations, alcohol abuse, misuse of drugs, and inability to cope with financial pressures may all be triggers.

This is a much more common illness than most people realise. At some point in their lives one in a hundred people will be diagnosed as suffering from schizophrenia. It is equally common in men and women and usually starts between the ages of 25 and 30. A small group of the over-65s will develop the condition for the first time. The disease

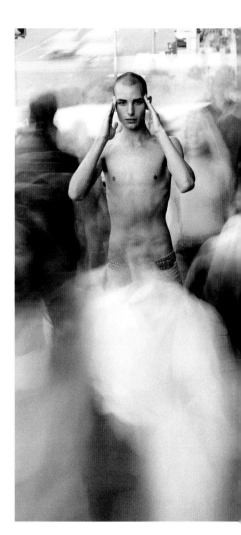

ABOVE *Schizophrenia is a severe mental illness whereby sufferers have an impaired sense of reality, which leads to irrational behaviour and disturbed emotional reactions.*

Symptoms

People with a schizophrenic illness may have just a few or many of the following symptoms:

• *Hallucinations*
• *A feeling of being watched*
• *Being constantly afraid*
• *Becoming withdrawn*
• *Belief that others can hear their thoughts*
• *Belief that they are someone famous*
• *Disjointed or disorientated speech*
• *Apathy*
• *Laziness*

• *Under- or over-emotional reactions*
• *Refusing or feeling unable to communicate*
• *Unusual, sometimes child-like, behaviour*
• *Self-harm*
• *Attempted suicide*
• *Strange movements and rapid changes of pace*
• *Fear for others*
• *Bizarre anxieties and acting as they believe they are being instructed*
• *Very strong religious feelings*

Treatment

• Schizophrenia is a disease that is managed rather than cured. Although it may be effectively treated with medication and help from many quarters, it is usually a chronic disorder and the risk of a relapse is always present. After a first bout of a schizophrenic illness, many people will be unable to pursue the job they were doing at a high level and many are at risk of becoming less functionally able than they were.

• Although family and friends are the first to realise that the person has a mental problem, the sufferer is often relieved to get medical assistance. If the person has sought help early, then medication may be enough, with family support, to restore a good level of normal functioning. Frequently, however, the first time the problem is faced head-on is when a crisis has occurred. The person may refuse to talk, or eat, or is constantly in fear, or is hearing voices. Under these circumstances, a doctor may feel that the person with schizophrenia requires hospitalisation. The sufferer may have to be committed to hospital involuntarily under the Mental Health Act, after assessment by a consultant psychiatrist and approved social worker. In these circumstances, the safety of the sufferer and those around him is of paramount importance. During the early days in hospital strong sedation may be necessary to prevent dangerous situations arising and to enable the sufferer to sleep. Quite quickly people with schizophrenia view hospital as a safe place and agree to stay there voluntarily while receiving treatment.

• On discharge a sufferer will need support from friends, relatives and often community psychiatric nurses. Talking to others with the illness and with community psychiatric nurses may be of great help. Doctors and psychiatrists will be available if relatives need assistance. Rehabilitation and adjusting to life back in the community take varying lengths of time, which is true of any illness.

• Exercise is a very good relaxant and a way of helping restore normality. Relaxation therapies, especially tapes and music, yoga, aromatherapy, reflexology, and Indian head massage may also be of great benefit.

BELOW *Massage aids relaxation by directly affecting the body systems that govern blood pressure, breathing and digestion, inducing a sense of profound well-being and alleviating feelings of distress.*

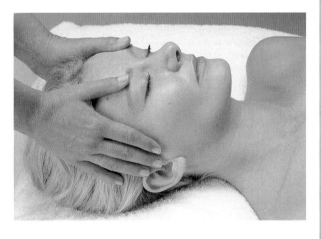

may occur as an isolated episode or as a progression of slow or rapid deterioration.

MEDICATION

Tranquillisers are generally used to treat schizophrenia. In some patients a great deal of sedation may be helpful for some time, but there may be side-effects of abnormal movements, twitching and clouded thinking. Most patients with schizophrenia do not like taking medication and unless closely supervised most will stop quickly, long before they are well. If there is a relapse, it seems to become more and more difficult to regain control and heavier drugs in larger doses need to be used. An injection of medication which acts over a period of time is often a good option for those who prefer not to take daily tablets or for those who forget.

OUTLOOK

Unfortunately, relapses are common with schizophrenia, particularly if it develops while the person is young.

Warning signs of a relapse include:

- *slow withdrawal from society*
- *failure to take medication*
- *missing meetings with professionals*
- *apprehension*
- *lack of personal hygiene*
- *poor sleeping pattern*
- *depression*
- *impaired concentration*
- *inactivity*
- *inability to recognise the symptoms of the illness*

EYE DISORDERS

Signals received through our eyes bombard us with pictures of the world around us, and many people fear losing sight more than any other faculty. We rely on sight for work and leisure, we gather information from studying people's faces and by looking at their eyes to assess emotion and reaction. Any disease that threatens to mar the appearance of the eyes or impair their function usually causes people to seek medical advice. Early intervention can often prevent sight loss.

GLAUCOMA

This is an eye disease that can affect one or both eyes, either at the same time or many years apart. Normally, the eye is filled with a clear, watery fluid, which is constantly being manufactured within the eye and which escapes through small channels. If these channels become blocked, they cause the pressure to rise. The rise in pressure over time squashes the optic nerve at the back of the eye, causing blindness.

In acute glaucoma, there is a sudden rise in pressure, pain and rapid loss of sight. If a sufferer is seen quickly by an eye specialist, then surgery may save some or all of the eyesight.

Chronic or open-angle glaucoma is the more common form of glaucoma and is slowly progressive. The pressure in the eye rises so slowly that the small day-to-day changes pass unnoticed and it is only when severe, irreversible changes have occurred that the problem is identified. By this time treatment is too late.

Why does glaucoma happen?

This very serious condition tends to run in families and is also a result of ageing, usually affecting people over 40. The

Symptoms of glaucoma

Gradual loss of vision at the outside of the field is the first sign of glaucoma. It is not usually noticed unless specifically looked for by an optician. Gradually the field of vision becomes narrower and narrower until only a blurred central area, known as tunnel vision, remains.

• *Blurring of vision, especially at the edges*
• *Failing sight in dim light*
• *Bumping into things when in unknown places*
• *Eye pain or headaches, especially if on one side*
• *Haloes around bright lights*

What happens with glaucoma

Fluid continually moves in and out of the eye to maintain its shape and nourish the tissues. With glaucoma, the eye's drainage system becomes blocked, causing a rise in pressure and a build-up of fluid. The high pressure may damage the optic nerve and, if untreated, lead to blindness.

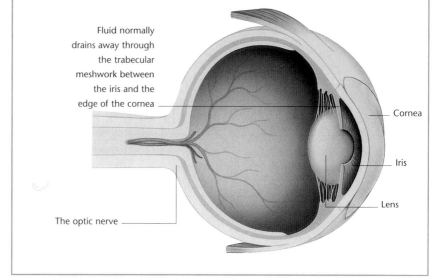

Fluid normally drains away through the trabecular meshwork between the iris and the edge of the cornea

Cornea

Iris

Lens

The optic nerve

main worry about glaucoma is that it may lead to irreversible blindness.

Prevention

This is a condition where special care should be taken to identify the problem early. Regular eye testing will pick up this condition before it does any damage. If there is a family history of glaucoma, then it is essential that everyone over the age of 40 should be tested every two years. Currently, testing is free for those with close relatives who have or have had glaucoma.

Treatment for glaucoma

• If the optician or your doctor suspects glaucoma you will be referred to hospital. If, after thorough examination, the condition is confirmed, then eyedrops to reduce pressure by aiding drainage of fluid from the eye are usually the first line of treatment. The drops sometimes sting to start with but they quickly become easy to tolerate. Sometimes tablets are needed to reduce the eye pressure. Occasionally surgery to widen the drainage tube from the eye will be necessary. Often this is done by laser therapy and literally takes minutes.

• If there is considerable eyesight loss you may be eligible to claim benefits for partial sightedness. The consultant at the hospital can help with this.

STYE

A stye is a painful lump that forms along the edge of the eyelid, caused by bacterial infection in the hair follicle of the lashes. Pus may be seen at the tip of the lump. Warm flannels may be applied to try to draw out the infection. Applying an antibiotic ointment (available from a doctor) will make the stye disappear more quickly. Some styes rupture, drain and heal without treatment.

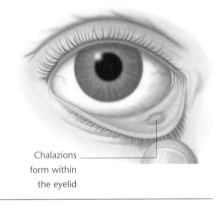

Styes form on the edge of the eyelid

FOREIGN BODIES

Most of us experience a foreign body in the eye at some time. Often it is a speck of dust and with much watering the eye gets rid of it itself. Sometimes an eyelash can be the culprit, and if this is obvious it can be wiped off by using very clean cotton wool. If you feel that a lash may be trapped under the upper lid, you could try to pull it down over the lower one and this may wipe it out. If there is pain and watering, filling a bowl with cool water and opening the eye under the water may wash it out. Any suggestion of metal in the eye, for example, after using a hammer and nails, requires immediate medical attention. The concern about foreign bodies is that they may cause permanent damage or scarring to the clear cornea covering the eye.

CHALAZION

This is a lump that forms within the eyelid, top or bottom. It looks like a pea and if in the upper lid, it sticks out when the eye is closed. It probably occurs as a result of a blocked duct, and secretions mount up as a cyst behind the obstruction. A chalazion is not serious, although it may irritate and be cosmetically unacceptable. It can be removed under local anaesthetic. This is usually done by an ophthalmologist at an eye hospital.

Chalazions form within the eyelid

Unless the foreign body is easy to remove, or very obvious, it is important to seek medical advice sooner rather than later. Pain, redness and constant watering are warning signs.

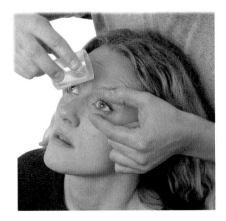

ABOVE *If a foreign body is proving difficult to remove you may need assistance. Flushing the affected eye carefully with cool, clean water may help to wash it out.*

SORE THROATS, COLDS AND COUGHS

Ninety per cent of people who get sore throats, colds and coughs recover after a week, irrespective of any treatment. Most of the symptoms are caused by a virus, which cannot be cured by antibiotics. Anyone who is young and fit will probably cope with all the symptoms without the need to see a doctor, and it is usually only the elderly or very young, or those with other serious illnesses, who may be at risk. Antibiotics are not useful in cases of viral infection and can cause diarrhoea, vomiting, allergy and thrush. Another major concern is that bacteria may develop resistance to antibiotics and so create a global problem with fighting germs in the future.

SORE THROAT

A sore throat usually lasts two or three days and often indicates that a cold is on its way. Most people who have a sore throat do not have tonsillitis but sometimes it is the first sign of an infection of the tonsils, the almond-shaped glands at the back of the throat.

What causes a sore throat?

A sore throat is usually caused by infection, generally viral in origin, but it can also be caused by smoking, heavy drinking and food allergy.

Symptoms of sore throat

- *Back of the throat may be red or pink; sometimes shiny and swollen*
- *Tonsils may be pink*
- *Tonsillitis produces red tonsils and often yellow spots of pus*
- *Quinsy is a collection of pus on the soft palate*

Treatment for a sore throat

- *There is no rapid way to get rid of a common sore throat. Sucking lozenges, using antiseptic sprays, regular painkillers and very frequent cool drinks or ice cubes are the only answers. The sufferer may find it be too painful to eat, but provided fluid intake is maintained there is little need to worry as the illness is short-lived.*

- *Older people or tiny babies may need medical advice but it is rare for these groups of people to get sore throats. Antibiotics are rarely necessary but a doctor may give parents of tiny babies a prescription to use if the throat hasn't improved after three days.*

- *If the throat continues to be very painful or there is an extremely high temperature then it may be appropriate to send a throat swab to the laboratory to see what bugs are causing the illness.*

- *If prone to sore throats or tonsillitis, strengthen your immune system by increasing your intake of garlic and vitamin C, and follow a diet rich in fruit and vegetables. Reducing stress levels may also help.*

COLDS

The common cold results from an infection that causes inflammation of the membranes that line the nose, sinuses and throat. Often people with colds start with a sore throat and the rest develops. However, the symptoms can come in any order. There is rarely loss of appetite, except if the throat is sore, making swallowing painful.

What causes a cold?

Like sore throats, these too are nearly always caused by a virus. There are more than 200 viruses that can cause a cold, and these are spread by breathing in tiny droplets coughed or sneezed into the air by an infected person.

Nose and throat

The upper respiratory system comprises the nose and throat and associated structures such as the sinuses (the air-filled spaces in the front of the skull) and the larynx, or voice box. The throat or pharynx connects the mouth and the nose to the voice box. The tonsils are the almond-shaped glands that lie at the back of the throat and form part of the body's defence system. The nose and throat can be affected by a variety of disorders, from nosebleeds to snoring and coughs and colds, caused by infection or obstruction in the nasal passages.

Symptoms of colds

- *Fever*
- *Sore throat*
- *Cough*
- *Blocked nose*
- *Sinus pain*
- *Thick, sticky mucus*
- *Earache*
- *Generally feeling unwell*

Treatment for colds

- *The blocked nose, cough and facial pain are often most helped by steam inhalations. Add a teaspoon of menthol or eucalyptus oil to boiling water then inhale the steam, under a towel, for at least ten minutes, three times a day. Make sure you drink plenty of fluids to avoid becoming dehydrated. Take regular warm drinks and painkillers such as paracetamol or aspirin. There are scores of over-the-counter cold remedies and your pharmacist will advise you about which is best for your particular symptoms.*

- *Nasal sprays that relieve congestion should not be used for more than a few days as they can lead to problems which cause the nasal blockage to persist.*

Nasal cavity
Sinus
Soft palate
Pharynx
Tonsil
Vocal cords
Larynx

QUINSY

This happens when an area of the soft palate, the part of the roof of the mouth that is just in front of the tonsils, swells up and fills with pus. This is a very serious disease. The sufferer is very ill with fever and can hardly swallow his own saliva. There may be dribbling from the sides of the mouth. The condition is really an abscess formation and will often require emergency surgery to relieve the swelling and pain. Antibiotics may be needed and sometimes the person will have to stay in hospital.

SORE THROATS, COLDS AND COUGHS

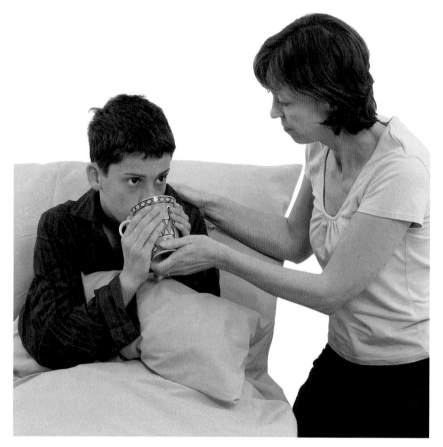

EARACHE

This condition seems to affect some people more than others. In children especially there is a great variation, which is probably due to the size of the Eustachian tube, which drains the ear into the back of the throat (those with small tubes tend to suffer from earache more frequently).

What causes earache?

Most recent studies show that, like colds, 90 per cent of earaches are due to viral infections.

Treatment for earache

Although when a child has earache it is also very distressing for parents, who feel helpless, regular fluids, with painkillers, steam inhalation and ensuring that the head is kept as upright as possible are the best courses of action. Antibiotics are rarely needed, but sometimes antibiotic drops may be used in the affected ear to reduce inflammation and kill any local bacteria.

COUGHS

People cough for many reasons. If there is a cough as well as the symptoms of a cold, most coughs should be treated as little as possible because the purpose of coughing is to get rid of the mucus and bugs travelling down the windpipe (trachea). If the cough is suppressed then nature cannot do its job.

If nighttime coughing is disturbing sleep, a cough syrup may help. Lying on several pillows at night will help to control the cough, particularly in small children.

If the cough becomes a chest infection, it is not unusual to cough up tiny streaks of blood. Within the

ABOVE *Drinking plenty of fluids will help to ease a sore throat and clear congestion of the nasal passages. Lying propped up on several pillows will help to control nighttime coughing.*

context of a severe cold, it is not an alarming sign, but if it continues after the cold is better it does need medical investigation. If you think that the infection has spread into the chest and the phlegm is green and the person feels unwell, seek medical advice. Antibiotics may or may not be needed.

Those who have asthma may need to increase the amount of inhaled medicine taken when suffering from a cold. This should be discussed with your doctor, perhaps just over the telephone.

SINUSITIS

This is a painful condition usually felt just below the eyes or above the nose. The membrane that lines the sinuses, the air-filled cavities in the bones around the nose, becomes inflamed and swollen. A build-up of mucus results, causing intense pressure.

RIGHT *Air-filled cavities known as sinuses are found in the skull bones around the nose and eyes. The mucus-secreting membrane that lines them can become blocked due to infection.*

There may be terrible pain and a feeling of being blocked up, and the face may be painful when touched.

What causes sinusitis?

Sinusitus usually develops following a cold or as a result of allergy, but can be triggered by pollution and tobacco smoke.

Symptoms of sinusitis

- *Nasal congestion*
- *Thick mucus discharge*
- *Severe pain around the eyes and cheekbones*
- *Headache*
- *Loss of sense of smell*
- *Sometimes swollen eyelids*
- *Nosebleeds and sneezing*

Treatment for sinusitis

Painkillers and steam inhalations should alleviate the condition. Often antibiotics are necessary but there is much debate as to how long the course should be – your own experience, if you have had the condition before, may serve as a good guide. Occasionally surgery or sinus wash-outs may be needed.

RIGHT *To help relieve a blocked nose, try a steam inhalation of a teaspoon of peppermint or menthol oil added to a bowl of hot water for at least ten minutes three times a day.*

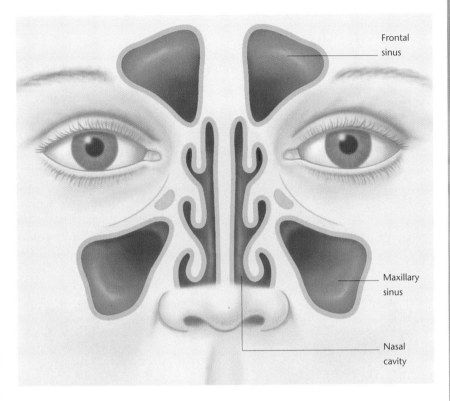

Frontal sinus

Maxillary sinus

Nasal cavity

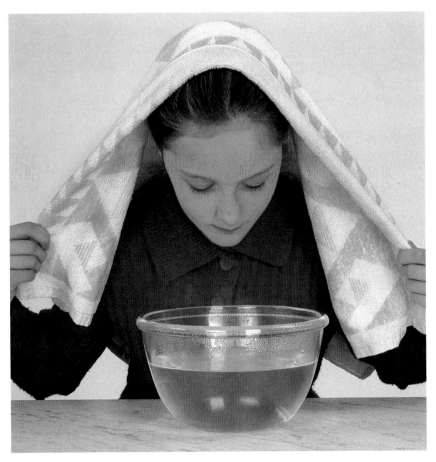

INFLUENZA

It is very true to say that lots of people with colds diagnose themselves as having flu (influenza) but nobody with flu would ever declare themselves to have a cold. Influenza is a serious disease which kills thousands of people (currently around 12,500) every year in the UK.

WHAT CAUSES FLU?

Influenza is a highly contagious viral disease. There are three main strains, which means that even if you have had flu once, you could catch it again. Like the common cold, flu is contracted by breathing in contaminated droplets coughed or sneezed into the air by an infected person. Particularly virulent strains can cause millions of deaths worldwide in what are known as pandemics, which occurred several times in the twentieth century.

COMPLICATIONS

The most common and worrying complication of flu is pneumonia, which can be life-threatening for those in high-risk groups, such as the elderly, those with bronchitis or other serious chest infections, children and those with lowered immunity such as occurs after chemotherapy or if a person is HIV positive. Very occasionally the heart muscle becomes inflamed and a condition called myocarditis develops, which is potentially fatal. Inflammation of the brain (encephalitis) is another rare complication.

PREVENTION

This is one condition where prevention is very effective, readily available and very rarely causes side-effects. Influenza vaccine will protect the majority of people who receive it from developing

Symptoms

The symptoms are usually severe for one to three days and require bed rest. Sufferers rarely want to eat much and usually just fluids are required in copious amounts. Once a sufferer feels able to get out of bed he will still be very weak and it may be ten days before he is strong enough to return to work. Depression is common in the weeks after an attack because the body has been put under a lot of stress in fighting the infection.

*   • Sudden onset of feeling very unwell
*   • Fever
*   • Headache
*   • Shivers
*   • Muscle pain
*   • Backache
*   • Sore throat
*   • Cough
*   • Sweating
*   • Insomnia

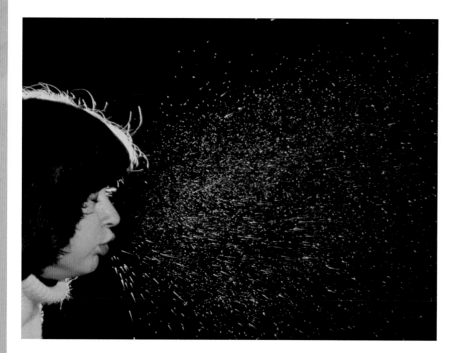

LEFT *Tiny airborne droplets rapidly spread viral infections if an infected person coughs or sneezes and another person breathes these in. This photograph shows how far droplets are sprayed by a sneeze.*

RIGHT *Immunisation prevents flu infection in about two-thirds of people who are vaccinated. It can never be 100 percent effective because the virus mutates and different strains are responsible for outbreaks. Recommendations for types of vaccine are issued by the World Health Organization depending on which strains of virus are expected to be prevalent. Vaccination is advised for those in high risk groups (except babies) such as the elderly or those whose immune systems are depleted.*

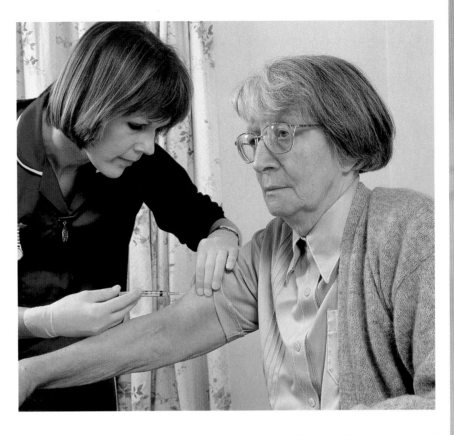

flu. The vaccine is different each year because the viruses that cause the flu vary, and scientists incorporate those that are most likely to cause problems. The virus is inactivated by one of several processes and, when injected, the body will make specialised cells known as antibodies to neutralise it. This means that when the body meets the real virus, it has already formed its own defensive army against it, and so avoids falling prey to the illness.

Some people are reluctant to have the injection. One reason people give is that it may give them flu but this is impossible as the virus in the injection is inactive. Very occasionally people who are particularly sensitive may react to the solvent in which the virus is suspended (a red lump may develop or a person may collapse). Sometimes flu may develop at a similar time to receiving the injection but this is probably because it was given just a bit too late and the flu was already developing.

New drugs are being developed to try to treat flu at the first sign but, as yet, these anti-viral drugs are not readily available unless a person has other serious illnesses and is seen within 48 hours of developing influenza.

If everyone who can do so has their influenza injection, it would not only save the individual from suffering but also prevent the spread of the disease to others. The injection is freely available to those over 65 and those considered to be in a high-risk group.

Treatment

The only treatments for influenza that are readily available are rest, aspirin or paracetamol and lots of fluids. Many over-the-counter remedies alleviate the symptoms. Some people feel that large quantities of vitamin C may help and this is certainly worth trying. Antibiotics have no part to play unless pneumonia sets in, but this usually happens long after the initial symptoms have passed.

RESPIRATORY DISEASES

Respiratory diseases are the main cause of death in the UK, accounting for nearly a quarter of all fatalities (deaths from heart disease account for a fifth). Of these deaths, around 40 per cent are due to pneumonia and influenza, 23 per cent are due to cancers of the respiratory tract and 20 per cent are caused by long-term obstructive lung disease. Many of these respiratory diseases are directly related to smoking.

ASTHMA

This condition still kills more than 1,200 people every year in the UK. Asthma can start at any age, but it often begins in childhood. It is the most common long-term (chronic) childhood disease and is thought to affect about 15 per cent of all children. However, not all children who have attacks of wheezing go on to develop chronic asthma.

What causes asthma?

Asthma is a result of the airways become inflamed and narrower, making it a struggle to breathe out. This causes wheezing, which is the noise air makes as it is breathed out over narrowed tubes. Many factors may contribute to asthma:

- *family history*
- *exposure to cigarette smoke*
- *allergy*
- *reaction to stress*
- *infection*
- *reaction to certain foods*
- *immune system problems*

Metered-dose inhaler

Prevention

Avoiding known allergens, increasing lung capacity by regular aerobic exercise such as swimming and avoiding tobacco smoke should help to control the disorder.

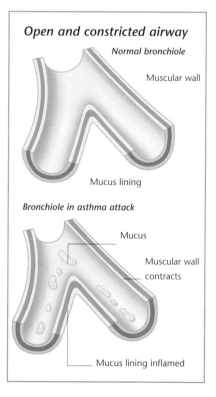

Open and constricted airway

Normal bronchiole

Muscular wall

Mucus lining

Bronchiole in asthma attack

Mucus

Muscular wall contracts

Mucus lining inflamed

Symptoms of asthma

- *Wheezing, especially on breathing out, which is typically at its worst at 2 am*
- *Dry cough*
- *Feeling of fighting for breath*

A person's airways may be so tight that he cannot get enough oxygen into the blood and he may turn blue. A severe attack is very frightening: if it does not respond quickly to self-administered remedies, seek urgent medical attention.

Treatment for asthma

As the problem lies in the airways that carry air into and out of the lungs, treatment usually consists of medication inhaled directly into the lungs. Corticosteroids prevent the airways from contracting, and drugs known as bronchodilators dilate the airways. Current medical opinion is that it may not be necessary or wise, particularly in children, to use too much of these medicines.

The lungs

Air is breathed into the lungs through the nose or mouth and enters the windpipe in the throat. The windpipe divides into two branching airways (bronchi), each leading to a lung. Within each lung, these airways branch and subdivide into thousands of tiny air passages. The very smallest passages (bronchioles) carry air into balloon-like sacs called alveoli. Oxygen passes through the thin alveoli walls into the bloodstream.

Blood vessel

Bronchiole

Windpipe (trachea)

Bronchus

Alveolus

LEFT AND RIGHT *Drugs to treat or prevent asthma are often inhaled because they reach the lungs quickly. An inhaler delivers a measured dose of a drug. A nebuliser, which delivers a much larger dose, can be used to treat a severe attack.*

Drugs inhaled through a face mask

Press the inhaler while breathing in

Nebuliser

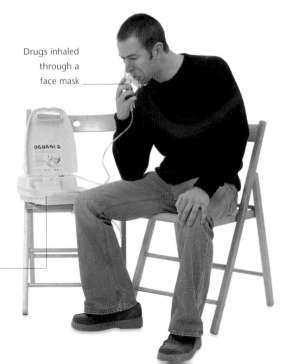

RESPIRATORY DISEASES

PNEUMONIA

This is the name given to an infection deep within the lung tissue, which can be life-threatening. It may affect one or both lungs (when it is known as double pneumonia).

What causes pneumonia?

Many types of bacteria may cause pneumonia but the most common bacterium is called *Streptococcus pneumoniae*. Occasionally it is caused by a virus. This disease will often follow a flu-like illness. It particularly strikes

Symptoms of pneumonia

- *May follow viral illness*
- *High fever*
- *Dry cough*
- *Pain on deep breathing*

Later:
- *Coughing up of rust-coloured mucus*
- *Cold sores around the mouth*
- *Rapid, shallow breathing*

Treatment for pneumonia

- *Appropriate antibiotics will be prescribed, depending on the type of bacterium causing the infection. Sometimes those who are extremely ill may need an injection of antibiotics or have them administered into the bloodstream by intravenous drip.*

- *Physiotherapy is a very important part of the treatment, to get the sufferer to cough up the infected sputum (a mixture of saliva, mucus and/or pus). The physiotherapist will also encourage ways of coughing and deep breathing. If the disease is recognised and treated early most people will recover. However in those who are very vulnerable there is a considerable death toll.*

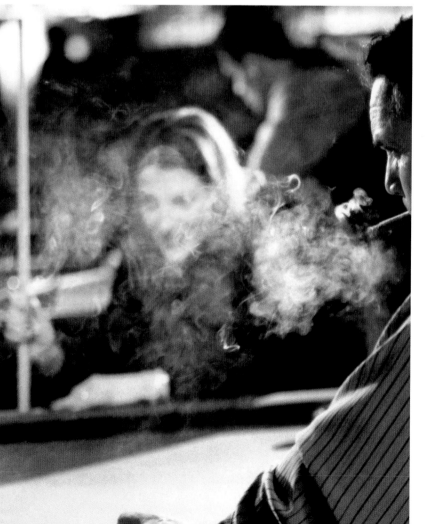

those whose resistance is low, including the elderly, those who have had their spleen removed, young babies, people with AIDS, those with cancer (especially of the lung), those with long-term lung disease, cigarette smokers and alcoholics.

Tests

Often a person with pneumonia is so ill that hospitalisation is necessary.

LEFT *Substances in tobacco smoke damage the lungs because they irritate and inflame the mucus membranes and reduce the oxygen-carrying capacity of red blood cells.*

A chest X-ray will confirm that the disease is pneumonia, as a shadow will be seen where the infection is. A sputum sample (whereby the material coughed up from the lungs is analysed) is essential to confirm which particular bacterium is causing the pneumonia. Blood tests for anaemia and to measure inflammation within the body will also be carried out. Several X-rays may be needed to ensure that the infection is responding to treatment.

Prevention

All those who are over 65, or at risk, may qualify for a free vaccination against the major bacterium that causes pneumonia. This same group should also receive a flu jab to prevent the flu that may lead to pneumonia.

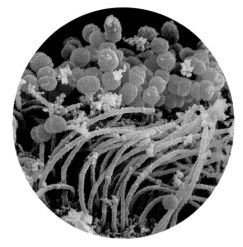

RIGHT *This highly magnified image shows the bacteria that cause pneumonia blocking up the fine hair-like strands that line the airways.*

Chest X-ray

A chest X-ray is a harmless and quick test used to investigate lung conditions. You will be positioned against a special surface so that your chest lies between a drawer containing a film cassette and the X-ray machine. You will be asked to raise your arms to move shoulder blades away from your body, to take a deep breath, and to remain still while the X-ray is being taken, usually from behind. To create an image, X-rays are passed through your chest on to photographic film. Dense tissues (i.e. bones) appear white, soft tissues grey, and air black.

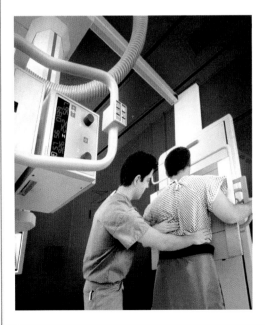

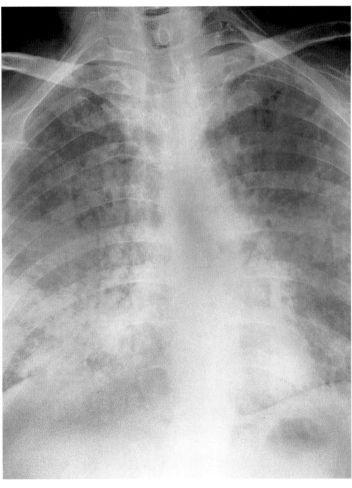

ABOVE *Damaged or abnormal tissue shows up as a white area on an X-ray because it does not contain air as healthy tissue. This X-ray shows abnormal shadowing on both lungs.*

SKIN DISORDERS

The skin is the largest organ in the body. It is constantly on display to a greater or lesser extent. Anything out of the ordinary can cause upset not merely for its own sake but because the disease and disfigurement is obvious to others. The port-wine stains that some people are born with, where an area of skin (often the face) is purple, are harmless but can cause a lifelong loss of self-esteem. Most skin diseases are made worse by stress but the diseases themselves lead to stress.

Acne spots

Acne spots are caused by the blockage and infection of the hair follicle in the skin. When the sebaceous glands surrounding the hair follicle produce too much of the skin's natural oil, sebum, a plug forms and darkens to become a blackhead. Bacteria multiply in the trapped sebum, causing infection, a pus-filled pimple to form, and inflammation of the surrounding tissues.

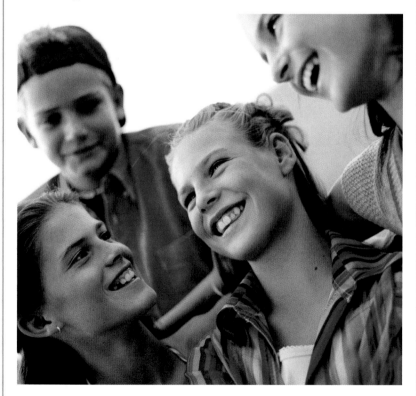

ABOVE *Acne is common among teenagers and is thought to be mainly due to the hormonal changes at puberty triggering the increased production of sebum in the skin glands, but it may also be hereditary.*

ACNE

This is a very common disease affecting the skin, usually on the face but it may also occur on the chest and back. Acne happens when skin pores become blocked by an overproduction of sebum, the skin's natural oil, which is made to lubricate the skin. If the top of the pore is open, then a black plug is visible, known as a blackhead. If the sebum becomes infected (often by a bacterium), a pus-filled pimple forms.

What causes acne?

Acne is not caused by being unclean, or by eating too much chocolate or cheese. There is a tendency for acne to be hereditary but this may be either because some families produce thicker sebum than others do or because bacteria is passed between members of the family. Hormones play a part: changes at puberty may stimulate the overproduction of the oil-producing glands.

Nearly 80 per cent of adolescents are affected by some form of acne and it can also occur in later life. Acne may cause considerable mental distress and self-consciousness at the time it is most active and result in scarring or changes in skin colour.

Managing acne

This should be aimed at trying to ensure that the sebum can escape more freely, and there is some evidence that drinking lots of fluids can help. Wash the skin twice daily with hot water and medicated cleanser to try to kill the bugs that live on the skin so they don't infect the spots. Facial steaming may help soothe spots and draw out infection.

It is important to try to improve the condition as soon and as thoroughly as possible. This may help to prevent scarring and depression.

Treatment for acne

• It is sometimes surprisingly difficult to get teenagers to the doctor for treatment, and some young people will not use prescribed medicines or, if they do, they will not persist with them. Many people with mild acne feel very embarrassed by it and want assistance. Others, with quite disfiguring acne, say they have no problem and don't want to be bothered with creams or tablets.

• For mild acne, usually a cream or lotion applied directly to the spots will help greatly. Benzoyl peroxide kills bacteria and helps reduce inflammation. It usually comes in a cream or gel and needs daily application. Topical retinoids, drugs derived from vitamin A that are applied directly to the spots, cause skin peeling and help expose the blocked pores. Both of these preparations may cause redness and may appear to make matters worse before any improvement is seen.

• Antibiotic lotions or liquids, applied to the spots once or twice a day, appear to be useful when there is a lot of infection and pus.

• Moderate and severe acne may require a course of antibiotics taken by mouth. These have an anti-inflammatory action and are successful in most people after the first month. They can be used in combination with a skin preparation such as benzoyl peroxide. Some female acne sufferers seem to have an excess of the male hormone androgen and a contraceptive pill such as Dianette may prove very useful.

• For the very bad cases, those that don't respond to usual treatments or those that are creating great mental distress, referral to a skin specialist (dermatologist) may be appropriate. If scarring is very bad then the dermatologist might arrange dermabrasion, where the skin is literally filed down to become level.

• Some people think of acne as something trivial. For others it is extremely depressing and distressing. Treatment is usually very successful for most people, although it may be prolonged. Early treatment helps to avoid all the problems associated with scarring and mental distress.

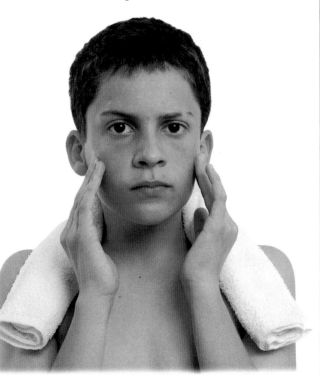

RIGHT *Washing the skin twice daily with warm water and a mild cleanser may help clear up acne and prevent further outbreaks.*

SKIN DISORDERS

ECZEMA

This is a condition of the skin that usually occurs on the insides of joints but in severe cases can break out all over the body, including the face. The skin reacts to a wide range of irritants and allergies and breaks out in a red, itchy, dry and inflamed rash, usually in patches. The intense scratching eczema provokes can cause bleeding and weeping sores. The word 'dermatitis' means skin inflammation and is often used to describe eczema.

What causes eczema?

Eczema is very common, affects up to one in five people and can start at any age. External factors may be a trigger, and people often become well aware of what sets off their eczema, such as a soap or fibre or plant, for example. One common substance is latex rubber: because eczema and dermatitis are dry-skin conditions, many people try to keep their hands dry by using rubber gloves, but this could make matters worse as the gloves may be irritant. Wearing creams covered by cotton gloves underneath the gloves is ideal.

Symptoms of eczema

- *dry skin*
- *intense itching*
- *red, scaly patches of skin*
- *blisters*
- *weeping areas*

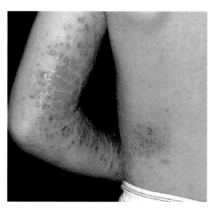

ABOVE *The itchy, dry, inflamed rash of atopic eczema is the most common form of eczema and usually first appears in childhood. Those who have a tendency to allergies are much more susceptible to it.*

BELOW *In nummular or discoid eczema, which is much more common in men than in women, itchy, coin-shaped patches develop, generally on the arms or legs. The affected areas may ooze and blister.*

Some foodstuffs may cause outbreaks of eczema. In children, in particular, it may be worthwhile trying to exclude dairy products from the diet for at least two months to see whether there is any improvement. Various perfumes, lanolin and metals may also trigger an outbreak of eczema. Often there may be no obvious cause. Sometimes eczema appears to be made worse by stress, but being itchy and sore is stressful in itself, so it is difficult to be sure which comes first.

Are there different types of eczema?

There are several types of eczema, and the most common one is atopic eczema, which seems to run in families. This usually starts in childhood and may be associated with asthma and other allergies. Atopic eczema may be constantly present and can be extremely severe. It can have a devastating physical and emotional effect on the whole family, because of the constant need for treatment. Brothers and sisters who do not have eczema may become jealous, as the affected child seems to have more attention. The affected child feels 'different', may think that she looks diseased and that others are constantly staring at her skin. Her sleep pattern is also badly affected, as unless appropriate medicine is given the itching can keep her awake.

Unfortunately, a quick and permanent cure is not available. However, atopic eczema generally improves with age.

Some people have patches of eczema that irritate but are less life-affecting. Often, eczema can be treated successfully and the condition cured when the triggers are avoided.

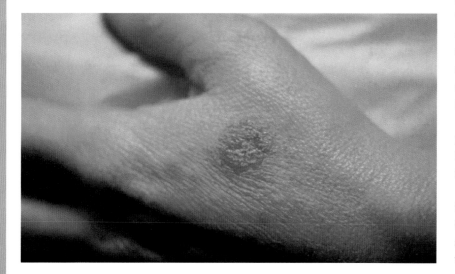

Treatment for eczema

• The worst part of eczema is usually the itching, which always causes scratching. Scratching causes a release of chemicals, one of which is called histamine, which in itself causes itching. Once the itch–scratch cycle has been set up it must be broken, which is achieved through the use of antihistamine tablets or medicines. There are some very powerful modern antihistamines that work without causing drowsiness.

• Three other major problems exist in eczema. The fundamental problem is very dry, easy to crack skin. To treat this, masses of skin softeners should be used. Ointments are ideal as they trap moisture into the skin and stop water leaking out, but because they are greasy these may be best applied at night. Moisturising creams should be liberally applied during the day. Add moisturising oils to bathwater to counteract skin dryness. It is essential not to feel limited by the amounts supplied by your doctor or the cost of over-the-counter preparations. For children all prescriptions are free, and it may well be that your doctor doesn't realise just how much moisturiser you need in a month – if you are using them regularly and liberally you may need to ask for more.

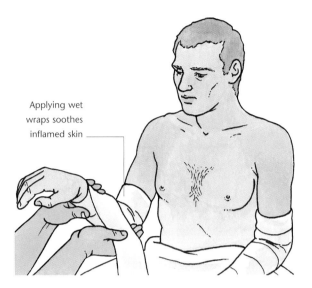

Applying wet wraps soothes inflamed skin

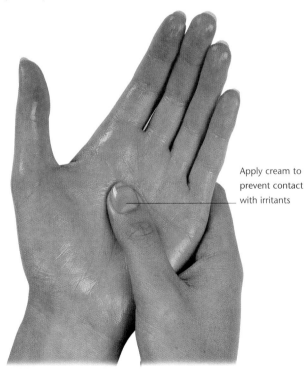

Apply cream to prevent contact with irritants

• Inflammation of the skin, causing redness and itching, is an important part of the eczema story. The best treatments to suppress inflammation are steroid creams, but many people dislike using them. Undoubtedly strong steroids used over years can cause skin thinning and possibly growth retardation in children, but this must be balanced by the relief that they give to sufferers. For a very bad flare-up a short course of strong steroid creams for a period of a week or so will have no long-lasting effect, provided it isn't repeated too often. Once the condition has come under control, reduction to a much weaker steroid is very safe and will help to prevent recurrences.

• The final important factor in eczema is infection. A bacterium called staphylococcus lives on the skin and when itching begins it can be scratched into the deeper layers. This sets up infection which can spread rapidly over the skin in a person with eczema. Antibiotic ointments and sometimes antibiotics by mouth are needed if there has been a bad flare-up.

• Very occasionally, when the whole skin is red, hot, constantly itching and the person is deeply distressed, a course of steroids for a week by mouth and sometimes even a short stay in hospital with soothing bandages applied frequently may be required. Though laborious, covering hot, itchy limbs in wet wrappings may help severe eczema tremendously.

SKIN DISORDERS

PSORIASIS

Psoriasis is a red, itchy, scaly skin condition that occurs in patches of varying size. It is usually found on the front of the knees and elbows or the edge of the scalp, but any part of the skin may be affected. The area is frequently very itchy and there may be tremendous amounts of flaking skin, which can look almost like a snowstorm. Psoriasis can be very distressing, because it is so itchy and because it may be disfiguring, especially if it is widespread on the areas of skin generally on display.

This very common skin complaint affects about two people in every hundred. Men and women seem to suffer equally and it can start for the first time at any age. Its severity may vary within the individual, so that sometimes it is hardly noticeable and at others it is extensive and red, itchy and scaly.

What causes psoriasis?

Psoriasis occurs because the skin cells tend to renew themselves too quickly and so they flake off easily, leaving reddened skin showing through. It is not really known why it occurs in some people rather than others but it tends to run in families – often a parent or grandparent will have the condition in some form. Stress, anxiety and exposure to some medicines or chemicals may play a part in worsening the condition.

Self-help

As this condition affects so many, there are lots of people who can offer advice based on their own experience and knowledge. The Psoriasis Association is particularly useful for those who want to know more about their illness and how they can help both the physical disability and mental distress this condition may cause.

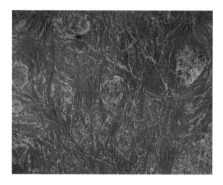

ABOVE *Psoriasis happens when new skin cells are produced faster than old ones are shed, and the excess skin forms thick red scaly patches.*

Symptoms of psoriasis

• *Pink or red patches of skin*
• *Areas covered with silvery-grey scales*
• *Itching*
• *Skin is dry and may crack easily*
• *Sometimes pitting of the nails*

Treatment for psoriasis

• *Psoriasis cannot be cured but it can be managed. Often, once the condition has been diagnosed properly, the best person to manage the problem is the sufferer, because he will become aware of what treatment to use according to how bad the condition is. Sometimes there may be long periods of time when the skin looks completely normal but then, for some reason, the psoriasis will suddenly appear again.*

• *Skin softeners, especially ointments that trap moisture, have an important part to play. Steroids are sometimes useful in a bad flare-up. Creams and ointments containing derivatives of vitamin D seem to be very safe and effective. Sometimes because the skin becomes cracked infection can set in and then antibiotics may be useful.*

• *Sunlight often improves psoriasis. If the condition becomes very severe and widespread, various forms of light treatment have been found to be helpful but these are usually only available via the hospital. Occasionally sufferers of psoriasis develop arthritis in various joints and the back, and if this happens then specialist medical care is required.*

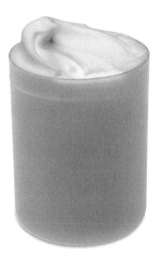

WARTS

These are small, solid growths in the top layer of the skin that can occur anywhere on the body. They are particularly common on the hands and on the feet (where they are called verrucas). When they occur on the bottom of the foot, because they are constantly being squashed by the body's weight, they are not raised. On the feet they can occur on all parts but often the heel, the ball and the toes are most

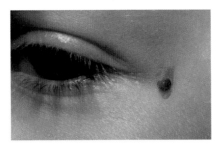

commonly affected. Warts last from a few weeks to many years but on average, without any treatment, they will disappear in about two and a half years.

RIGHT *Warts are small skin growths caused by a viral infection and are generally harmless.*

What causes warts?

Warts are caused by one of the many strains of the human papilloma virus. They are spread by contact either within the individual or passed to others by direct contact. They spread most readily if there are any cuts or grazes that are exposed to the wart.

Symptoms of warts

• *Thickened, raised areas of skin that can vary enormously in size*
• *Verrucas: areas of skin with tiny black pinpricks on them (these are blood vessels showing through)*

GENITAL WARTS

These occur on the vulva, vagina and cervix in women and on the penis in men. In women the virus may be detected by a cervical smear as it changes the appearance of cervical cells. Genital warts require medical treatment as they are linked to cervical cancer.

Treatment for warts

There are three basic treatments:

• *Do nothing. This is ideal and eventually all warts do go. However some warts are so large, extensive or cosmetically disfiguring that people feel they would like to do something about them.*

• *Cryotherapy. This involves freezing the area of the wart or verruca by spraying it with liquid nitrogen. This causes the cells holding the virus to crack open and release the virus particles. The body then has a rush of wart virus, makes antibodies and hopefully dissuades the wart from staying. The procedure is painful and is unsuitable for small children. After spraying the wart with liquid nitrogen the area may be sore for many days and may blister.*

• *Paint the area with salicylic or lactic acid, which works by burning out the wart. The cream, paint or ointment containing the acid can cause damage to the surrounding skin, so Vaseline or paraffin ointment needs to be spread around the wart before the acid is applied. The area where the wart was may become badly infected, blistered and burned after using this method.*

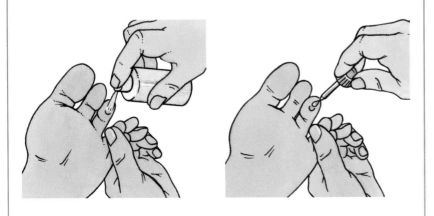

Treatment for genital warts

Genital warts are treated by using cryotherapy, laser therapy or painting with an acid, as for other types of wart. Genital warts may be spread by sexual contact, so condoms should be used to try to prevent this. Once genital warts have been diagnosed it is advisable to use condoms always as they do sometimes recur.

HAIR AND SCALP PROBLEMS

Hair and scalp problems may occur separately or together. The most common concerns are hair loss and scaly, itchy scalps. These conditions are generally harmless but may be unsightly. There are as yet no guaranteed cures for either of these conditions but management can help.

HAIR LOSS

Alopecia is the medical name for this condition, which may take many forms. It may even be total, where all head and body hair is lost, a condition called *alopecia universalis*. Total hair loss doesn't usually respond to treatment. Occasionally hair regrows as a soft down, often white or blonde for no obvious reason. Alopecia may occur in small patches, often due to stress or fungal infection. Males in particular may show hair loss from quite an early age, which is usually noticed as a receding hairline over both temples and the crown. It may occur in women, too. Usually this type of hair loss runs in families.

Loss of hair in patches may occur in those who pull out their own hair, a condition usually associated with extreme stress and anxiety but does sometimes happen in children. It is particularly difficult to treat without curing the underlying mental illness.

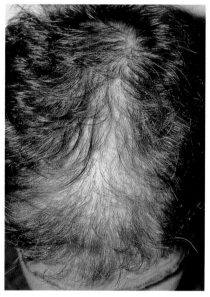

RIGHT *Alopecia or hair loss has many causes and can occur on any part of the body but is most noticeable on the scalp. Hair loss may be temporary or permanent, and may occur in patches or all over the scalp.*

What causes hair loss?

There are many reasons for hair loss, but the following tend to cause generalised hair thinning rather than patches of baldness:

• *Genetics*
• *Iron deficiency and other forms of anaemia*
• *Thyroid gland disorders*
• *Immune system problems*
• *Pregnancy*
• *Rapid weight loss*
• *Certain drugs*
• *Hormonal imbalance*
• *Lichen planus (a type of wart)*
• *Shock*
• *Stress*
• *Down's syndrome*

Treatment for hair loss

• *If there is an obvious cause for hair loss then treatment may help, particularly in the cases of anaemia and thyroid abnormalities. Treatment for stress and anxiety may help those with patchy alopecia or those who pull their hair out.*

• *The only medicines known to work are steroids, which cannot be taken long-term because of side-effects, and the substance minoxidil, which is expensive and only works while being used.*

• *Finesteride (a medicine used in men with enlarged prostate glands) is effective in male pattern baldness but is obviously unsuitable for women. Most men with this type of baldness accept it and it is currently fashionable to have closely shaven heads, so it is not the disaster it once was. In women with severe hair loss, the only answer may be a wig.*

• *If fungal infection is the cause of baldness then three months of anti-fungal tablets will almost certainly cure the condition.*

Male-pattern baldness

Male-pattern baldness is the progressive loss of scalp hair, usually in a characteristic pattern. Hair is lost over several years, beginning at the temples and spreading to the crown until it leaves a ring of hair like a monk's tonsure around the scalp. Male-pattern baldness affects most men to some extent after the age of 30. It is thought to be hereditary and caused by an imbalance in the hormone testosterone, which is why it mainly affects men.

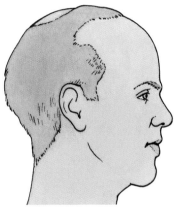 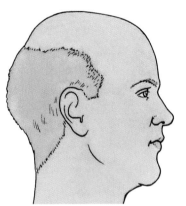

1 *Hair loss in men is common after the age of 30 but may start at an even earlier age, and begins with a receding at the temples or forehead.*

2 *Over the next few years, probably due to an imbalance in hormones, hair continues to be lost from the sides of the head and the crown.*

3 *The condition rarely ends in total baldness but seems to arrest when the top of the head is hairless. The only permanent solution is a wig or transplant.*

Hair transplant

The only way to permanently treat hair loss is to have a hair transplant, a surgical process performed under local anaesthetic that takes about an hour. In a transplant, baldness is treated by removing a strip of skin and hair from another part of the body, usually behind your ears or at the back of your scalp. Tiny incisions are then made in the area that is to receive the transplanted hair.

The removed hairs and their attached hair follicles are then inserted into the incisions using tweezers. The transplanted hairs fall out in few days but new hair starts to grow from the transplanted hair follicles.

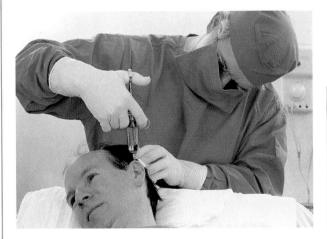

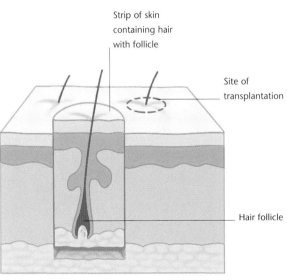

Strip of skin containing hair with follicle

Site of transplantation

Hair follicle

HAIR AND SCALP PROBLEMS

SCALP DISEASE

This usually shows itself as one or all of the following:

- *redness*
- *itchiness*
- *scaling or flaking of the scalp*

Psoriasis tends to occur around the hair margins, often over the forehead and at the back of the neck. The area is usually demarcated by a red edge and the top will be covered with scale of varying thickness. Often there will be signs of psoriasis elsewhere, particularly over the front of the knees and back of the elbows.

Seborrhoeic dermatitis is a fungal infection, occasionally linked to AIDS. It tends to cause great flakiness of the scalp and the snow-like fallout can be very distressing.

Lichen planus can lead to a build-up of scale and scarring of the scalp.

Dandruff is the name we give to excess scaling and skin flaking from the scalp.

Some people create scalp conditions by constantly picking at spots or slight build-up of scale on the scalp. Use of a barrier cream on top of spots, so that the area cannot be scratched, may help.

What causes scalp disease?

- *Psoriasis*
- *Seborrhoeic dermatitis*
- *Lichen planus (a type of wart)*
- *Fungal infections*
- *Dandruff*
- *Spot picking*

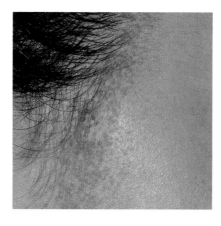

ABOVE *Seborrhoeic dermatitis is a red, scaly, itchy rash that commonly occurs on the face and the scalp, where it causes flaking of the skin. It is a fungal infection and outbreaks may also be triggered by stress or illness.*

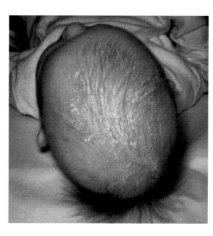

ABOVE *The red skin and thick patches of yellowish scales on top of a baby's head are typical of cradle cap. The condition is harmless and usually disappears of its own accord without any treatment but you can prevent build-up of scale by washing the hair and scalp regularly.*

RIGHT *There are many over-the-counter preparations available to treat scalp conditions. Coconut oil will help to remove dandruff and improve the condition of the scalp. Rosemary, cedarwood or tea tree oil can be massaged into the scalp or used in the final rinse when washing your hair to treat fungal infections and flaking.*

Treatment for scalp disease

By and large, the treatments for scalp conditions are steroid creams and scalp applications. There is thought to be little absorption from the scalp into the body and so extended courses may be followed. Anti-fungal shampoos are available to treat seborrhoeic dermatitis. Removing scale with oils, such as coconut oil, and then using a coal tar shampoo may prove successful. Treatment of psoriasis is very specific, including treatments with vitamin D-derived creams and ointments and sometimes steroid creams. A coal tar shampoo may help.

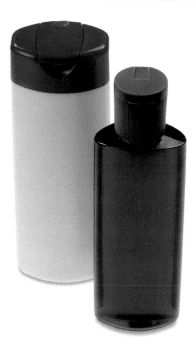

HEAD LICE

These are small, blood-sucking parasites that live in the hair. Head lice live for most of the time on the scalp, gripping tightly with special claws. They are small, grey or brown in colour and look like tiny beetles. The females lay about eight eggs (nits) a night and glue each one to the base of a hair. After seven days a new white louse hatches and leaves the egg case attached to the hair. The attached empty egg-case is often a good pointer that the cause of head itching is due to lice. Often the lice themselves, unless very plentiful, may move so quickly they can be difficult to see. The newly hatched white louse (nymph) starts to feed on blood from the scalp or the skin just below the hairline or behind the ears. Within ten days of hatching it is fertile and able to produce more eggs.

The creatures are rarely seen unless searched for but may be most apparent around the edges of the hairline or behind the ears. Scratch marks in these areas will also give warning of the likely diagnosis. Combing the hair with a nit comb over white paper may indicate head lice if they can be combed out and if they have been present longer than a week; the egg-cases may be seen still attached to the hair.

Symptoms of head lice

• Itching on the scalp and the area behind the ears
• Shirt collars may appear dirty more quickly than usual, because the black faeces are shed from the head and discolour collars

What causes head lice?

Head lice cannot fly, hop or jump and so the only way they can travel from head to head is by walking. This is why they occur so frequently in young children, who constantly put their heads close together. They cannot be passed on by sharing hats, combs or towels.

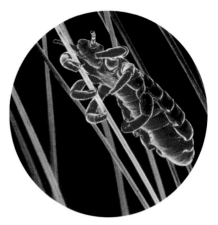

RIGHT *This magnification of a head louse shows how it attaches to the hair. Head lice live on the scalp and suck blood from the skin.*

Treatment

• *This can be very troublesome, because unless everyone who has them within a group acknowledges the fact and everyone is treated, they can be passed around again and again. Ideally everyone in a family with one affected child and all friends should be treated. Check hair at least once a week. Regular vigilance is the key to success. There is no shame in having head lice, but it is vital to acknowledge the condition.*

• *If lice are found, then several methods may work: twice-daily combing with a special nit comb after conditioner has been applied; application of a special lice killer to the scalp and all the hair followed by the requisite wait and then further combing (different products require different lengths of application to ensure all lice are killed). If medication is used, it must be repeated within a week to ensure that all newly hatched nymphs are killed.*

• *Various homeopathic treatments such as tea tree oil may be beneficial, especially if regular combing is done as well. There are some electric combs that electrocute the insects but these are not that successful and need very careful handling.*

• *Studies have shown that having head lice over long periods of time may lead to anaemia and can sometimes cause the child to under-perform at school.*

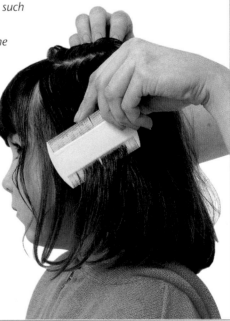

FOOT AND TOE PROBLEMS

Feet are the site of many maladies, from athlete's foot, a fungal infection, to osteoarthritis, where wear and tear on the many joints in the feet causes constant pain even at rest. As more and more people become overweight, feet are subjected to increasing pressure and damage.

INGROWING TOE-NAILS

These are painful and can occur on any toe but usually affect the big toe. They affect the edge of the nail, which grows into the soft skin surrounding the toe-nail. The nail can cut in at the side or the edge.

What causes ingrowing toe-nails?

They are usually caused by pressure on the toe-nail, from wearing shoes that are too tight. They may also occur when the toe-nail is cut too short and

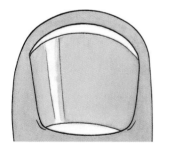

ABOVE *If you cut toe-nails too short and in a curve the nail may cut into the surrounding skin, causing inflammation and possibly infection.*

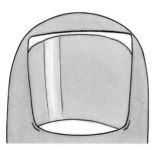

ABOVE *Cut the toe-nail straight across at the level of the skin to prevent the sides from curving under and cutting into the skin.*

curves down at the sides. Ideally, it should be cut at the level of the skin and straight across.

Symptoms of ingrowing toe-nails

- *Pain and inflammation at the edge of the nail*
- *If infected, pus, redness and swollen red tissue alongside the nail*

Treatment for ingrowing toe-nails

- *If the nail becomes infected then antibiotics may be necessary. If this settles the nail down it is important to keep the nails longish and avoid tight-fitting shoes. If the problem becomes recurrent, then either a part or the whole toe-nail may have to be removed under local anaesthetic. This is usually done in hospital.*

- *If the toe-nail regrows after this and still causes problems, then the base of the nail bed may have to be destroyed, leaving the toe-nail unable to grow. This leaves the toe with a soft skin covering rather than a proper toe-nail.*

GOUT

Gout is a form of arthritis in which a chemical called uric acid, a waste product made in the body, builds up in the joints and the kidneys, where it can form stones. Usually this disease will show itself as a sudden pain, redness and swelling at the base of one of the big toes. It can start in any joint but it is excruciatingly painful.

What causes gout?

Gout happens either because too much uric acid is made by the body or the kidneys fail to get rid of it properly. It may run in families or develop in people with diabetes, kidney disease or polycythaemia (too many red blood cells). Certain drugs may also cause the disease. Water tablets (diuretics) are particularly liable to cause this condition.

Symptoms of acute gout

- *Sudden, severe joint pain in one or more joints (typically big toe, ankle, wrist or elbow)*
- *Joint may be stiff, red, swollen and hot*
- *Sometimes white chalky matter leaks from joint*
- *Fever*

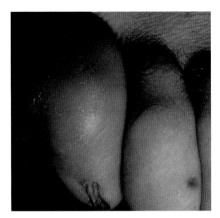

ABOVE *Gout is a type of arthritis in which uric acid crystalline deposits form in the joints, causing them to become painful and swollen. The base of the big toe is the site most commonly affected. The symptoms of gout usually flare up quite quickly.*

Stages

There are four stages:

1 *No symptoms, but raised uric acid levels in the blood*
2 *Acute gout, affecting one or more joints suddenly*
3 *Recurrent gout, when bouts are frequent*
4 *Chronic (long-term) gout, with joint deformity and deposits of uric acid outside the joints*

Tests

As the joint pain is sudden and there is redness and swelling, it is vital to ensure that it is not an infected joint, where symptoms may be very similar. Blood tests should be taken as soon as possible and if it is gout these will reveal a high level of uric acid in the blood. If there is fluid in the joint, it may be withdrawn and sent to the laboratory for analysis. In the case of gout, crystals of uric acid may be seen in the fluid. In suspected

RIGHT *Foods high in substances called purines increase levels of uric acid in the blood, and foods to be avoided include poultry, strawberries, shellfish, game, caffeine and alcohol.*

cases of infection the laboratory will look for bacteria. If it is the first attack the joint will usually be X-rayed.

Chronic gout

The aim of treating the high level of uric acid in the blood is to stop the development of chronic gout. In this condition, uric acid crystals are laid down as gouty lumps. A common site is on the edge of the outer ear. Chronic gout can lead to gross joint deformity and may be bad enough to confine a sufferer to bed. The development of kidney stones, caused by too much uric acid in the kidneys, is serious. Small stones may be passed down the tube to the bladder (the ureter) but this causes terrible pain and surgery may be required to remove the stone if it becomes stuck. If the stones cause blockage from the kidney, they may lead to total kidney (renal) failure and death.

Prevention

Modify the diet to exclude foods rich in purines, such as strawberries, shellfish and game, which increase levels of uric acid in the blood. Losing weight will be beneficial. It used to be thought that gout was caused by drinking too much port, which is not the case, but excess alcohol should be avoided. Drink

plenty of water in order to avoid concentrating uric acid and ensure that it is washed through the kidneys before it has time to crystallise. Aspirin and diuretics will make the condition worse, and should be avoided.

Treatment for gout

• *The aim of treatment is to stop the pain and then prevent future attacks. Colchicine works quickly and effectively against the pain and swelling. Often non-steroidal anti-inflammatory drugs (NSAIDs), such as ibuprofen, are given at the same time. Ordinary painkillers (except aspirin) may be useful.*

• *If the uric acid levels are high it is likely there will be further attacks in joints and there is a possibility of kidney stones developing. If a person has raised uric acid levels he may well need daily medicine to keep the levels down.*

Bunions

Bunions are swellings on toes that arise because the toe bone sticks out at the joint and pressure from shoes causes inflammation and pain. Bunions can be prevented by wearing well-fitting shoes, and by putting cotton wool between the toes to separate them. If bunions have formed, reduce pressure on the joint by wearing wide, flat shoes.

MUSCLES, BONES AND JOINTS

We generally take muscles and joints for granted but even a small amount of damage can cause severe pain and inconvenience, whereas damage to large joints can cause immobility. Older people tend to have the most problems because the muscles and joints have been subjected to years of mistreatment and hard work.

BACK PAIN

Eighty per cent of the adult population in the West will experience back pain of varying severity, disability and length at some point in their lives. Most back pain will get better within a month, with or without treatment.

What causes back pain?

Most back pain is caused by muscle spasm. The muscles and ligaments support the back; when there is injury the muscles respond by tightening, twisting the back and causing pain. The most common place to experience back pain is in the lower backbone (the lumbar vertebrae).

Only about one in ten people with a painful back will have a more serious disorder. Slipped or prolapsed disc is a condition where the soft, spongy pad between the hard back bones is squashed out of shape because of abnormal pressures. This causes pain, and if the disc bulges out of the line of the spine it may exert pressure on

a passing nerve. As the disc problem is usually in the lower part of the spine, the squashed nerve will cause shooting pain that goes into the bottom or thigh or travels down the leg. The pain may feel like an electric shock and can be excruciating. In extreme cases the nerves that supply the bowels and bladder may be affected, and when this happens hospital treatment and surgery to remove the disc may be required.

Occasionally, tumours of the spine or collapse of back bones from conditions such as osteoporosis (see page 389) or cancer can cause terrible back pain. Certain rheumatic disorders such as psoriatic arthritis or ankylosing spondylitis may also cause severe pain.

Tests

Tests are very rarely necessary, and X-rays are hardly ever appropriate, except when osteoporosis is suspected. X-rays expose people to unnecessary radiation and seldom show any abnormality. Finding a little wear and tear or degeneration in the back bones doesn't explain the back pain.

If back pain continues for longer than six weeks or there are signs of nerve damage then you will be referred to a specialist for appropriate tests.

Symptoms of back pain

- *Muscle spasms*
- *Back pain, ranging from mild to excruciating*
- *Stiffness*
- *Twisted body tilting to one side*

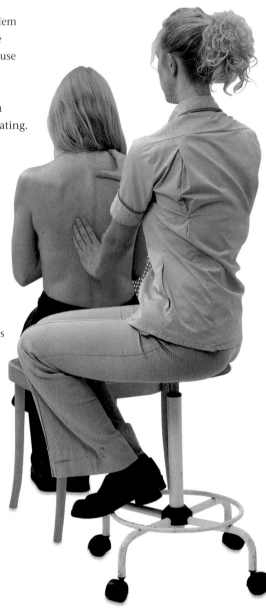

ABOVE *Chiropractic treatment is particularly successful at relieving back pain. Special manipulative techniques bring the back and neck vertebrae into alignment.*

Muscles and movement

Skeletal muscles make up the majority of the body's muscles. They are formed of long, strong fibres which can contract powerfully and quickly to produce movement. Muscles are attached to the skeleton by tendons, flexible cords of fibrous tissue. Movement depends on the integration of muscles, bones and joints in response to signals from the brain. When a muscle contracts, it pulls on the bone to which it is attached and produces movement. Muscles are arranged in pairs because they can only pull, not push.

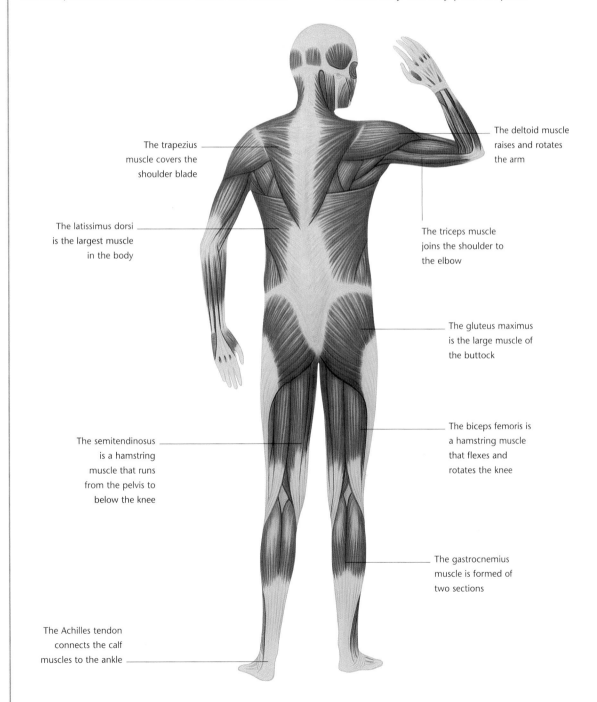

The trapezius muscle covers the shoulder blade

The latissimus dorsi is the largest muscle in the body

The semitendinosus is a hamstring muscle that runs from the pelvis to below the knee

The Achilles tendon connects the calf muscles to the ankle

The deltoid muscle raises and rotates the arm

The triceps muscle joins the shoulder to the elbow

The gluteus maximus is the large muscle of the buttock

The biceps femoris is a hamstring muscle that flexes and rotates the knee

The gastrocnemius muscle is formed of two sections

MUSCLES, BONES AND JOINTS

Prevention

Bad back pain can occur in anyone at any age, but it tends to occur most in those who drive, sit or have a heavy manual job. Posture is very important and movement therapies such as the Alexander technique and Pilates will help prevent many kinds of recurring back problems. Make sure your chair supports the small of your back, and buy a supportive mattress for your bed. If you have recurrent problems, a physiotherapist can teach you back-strengthening exercises.

When lifting heavy objects, bend the knees, keeping the back straight. Carry heavy weights in rucksacks. Exercise, particularly swimming, helps prevent and treat bad backs.

Treatment for back pain

• *Rest and painkillers are usually recommended for back pain. Bed rest may cause more harm than keeping going, and staying active is the key to getting better for most bad backs. For severe back pain ice, heat, massage and ultrasound may prove helpful. Treatment may include the use of muscle-relaxant drugs for pain and muscle spasm, which can cause drowsiness and constipation. Sometimes it will be necessary to have time off work because of the medication.*

• *Alternative therapies such as acupuncture, osteopathy and chiropractic have an excellent reputation for treating short-term back pain.*

• *If back pain is very severe and lasts longer than six weeks, physiotherapy may be helpful. Painkilling epidural anaesthetics may also be useful. Affected nerves will sometimes require surgery.*

How to lift

Back pain is often caused by sudden muscle strain, and learning how to lift heavy objects correctly can help you avoid putting undue stress on your spine. When lifting a heavy object, keep the object close to you so that you can use your full strength to lift it.

1 *Keeping your back straight, squat down to pick up the object. Balance your weight evenly on both feet with the object between your legs. Grasp the object.*

2 *Lean forwards slightly, still holding your back straight. Stand up in a single movement, pushing yourself up using your leg muscles and keeping the object close.*

3 *When you are upright, keep your head up, back straight and your weight distributed evenly on both feet to balance your body. Keep the object close to your body.*

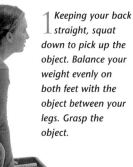

NECK PAIN

About a half of the population will have a pain in their neck at some point in their lives. Many of those who do will suffer discomfort for up to six months and it may be a condition that keeps coming back.

ACUTE TORTICOLLIS

This is the medical term for what is usually known as a stiff neck. The muscles in the neck, usually on one side only, go into spasm. This may be related to bad posture or doing a different activity but there is usually no obvious cause. Muscle relaxants, anti-inflammatory tablets and gels, and painkillers may be necessary. Keeping the neck warm may also help relieve the spasm. The stiffness usually fades away over a period of one to three weeks. Rarely, a condition where the neck keeps pulling the head to one side occurs. If this is persistent, injections of botulinum toxin, a powerful nerve poison, are required.

CERVICAL SPONDYLOSIS

This and other similar conditions are associated with wear and tear of and around the neck bones. They cause pain, especially on movement. Severe pain may be alleviated by wearing a soft, felt collar to support the neck. If the pain passes into the arms then this may indicate that the nerves from the neck are becoming trapped. Occasionally, very severe cases require surgery.

WHIPLASH

Sudden jerking of the head and neck may result in damage, and this is most commonly caused by being involved in a car crash. The pain may not appear at the time of the accident but hours or even days later. Neck movements may be painful and restricted and spread

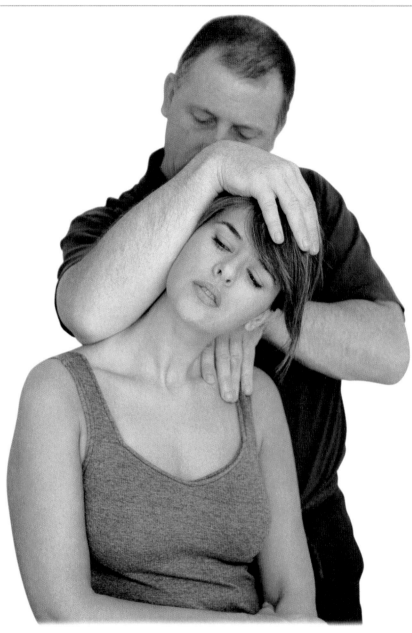

into the shoulders and arms. Treatment involves taking painkillers, anti-inflammatories and perhaps muscle relaxants. A collar should be avoided except in the most painful of necks, because the aim is to try to keep the neck moving gently. After a road traffic accident there is usually a lot of stress and upset, which can make the neck stiffness even worse.

Other causes of neck pain
- *Inflammation caused by rheumatic diseases, such as rheumatoid arthritis,*

ABOVE *Osteopathy uses massage and stretching techniques to reduce muscle tension and improve blood supply to the tissues to restore the full range of movement to the joints. Neck pain and whiplash injuries can be treated by having the neck vertebrae realigned.*

ankylosing spondylitis and polymyalgia rheumatica
- *Cancer*
- *Infection, including tuberculosis and other diseases*
- *Osteoporosis*

MUSCLES, BONES AND JOINTS

How to stand

The Alexander technique is a well-respected therapy that aims to improve posture so the body can function with minimum strain. By learning to stand correctly, your body is under less stress and conditions made worse by poor posture are relieved.

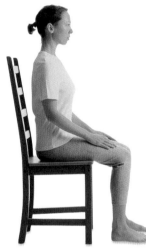

1 Let your neck go forwards and upwards and let your back lengthen and widen. Hold your back straight to avoid compressing the spinal vertebrae.

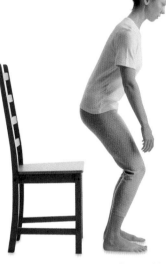

2 As you move into a standing position, lead with your head and try not to jerk it back. Concentrate on moving without strain and keep your spine long.

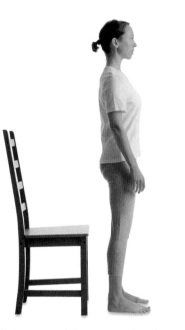

3 As you stand, keep your neck and your back free. Your shoulders should be relaxed. Backache and neck pain can be alleviated as you regain a natural posture.

Investigations

Neck X-rays are rarely of any use and expose the body to unnecessary irradiation. This is because pain usually comes from the joints and ligaments (tough bands of tissue that link bones) around the neck which do not show up on X-ray. Signs of wear and tear in the neck bones are common in many people over 40 and seeing these on X-ray doesn't mean they are the cause of the pain. If there are indications of

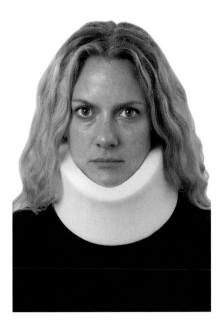

LEFT *A neck collar supports and protects vertebrae displaced by whiplash (caused by sudden extreme bending of the spine) but should only be used if pain is severe because the aim of treatment is to keep the neck moving.*

Treatment for neck pain

Only a very brief period of rest and inactivity for the neck is recommended for most painful necks. Getting the neck moving with gentle exercises and sometimes manipulation by a trained physiotherapist or osteopath may be the quickest way to get better. Posture is important and learning the Alexander technique can be beneficial when there is much neck tension.

trapped nerves and anything else worrying, you may be referred to a specialist for CT (computerised tomography) or MRI (magnetic resonance imaging) scanning, high-tech diagnostic techniques.

ELBOWS AND SHOULDERS

PAINFUL ELBOW

Apart from breaks on and around the elbow after falls or bangs, it is not uncommon for the area on either side of the elbow to become painful. This seems to arise for no particular reason but can be long-lasting and troublesome.

GOLFER'S ELBOW

This occurs on the inside of the elbow, i.e. when the arms are hanging down straight. The area near to the so-called 'funny bone', becomes tender and prevents people doing certain actions. Typing and anything that bends the wrist upwards may make it worse as may gripping and twisting. It has nothing to do with golf.

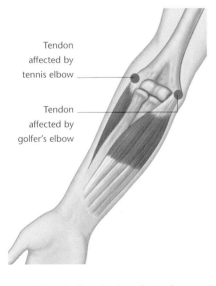

Tendon affected by tennis elbow

Tendon affected by golfer's elbow

ABOVE *Tennis elbow is where the tendon attached to the bone on the outer side of the elbow is injured; golfer's elbow is where the tendon on the inner side is affected.*

Treatment for golfer's and tennis elbow

This is similar for both conditions. Initially a period of rest and anti-inflammatory tablets or locally applied creams may help. Painkillers too may be necessary. If the pain is very severe, long-lasting or makes work impossible then one or two injections of steroids may be needed. These are not without risk and should only be undertaken when the pain is very bad indeed. Ultrasound treatment may help but in the most severe cases of golfer's elbow a surgical operation can be performed.

TENNIS ELBOW

Like golfer's elbow, this condition occurs in those who play tennis and those who have never held a racket. The pain in this case is situated over the top of the elbow when the arms are positioned held out and bent in. The pain may spread down the forearm.

SHOULDER PAIN

As the shoulder is the most mobile joint in the body, it depends on strong muscles and ligaments to keep it stable. The main supporter is the rotator cuff which is made up of muscles and tendons. Injury to this is the major cause of shoulder pain.

Causes

The commonest cause of injury in those under 40 is excessive use, weight-bearing or exercise and this leads to the so-called 'impingement syndrome'. Pain is felt in the upper arm and it may be impossible to sleep lying on the affected side. The main pain is felt

when the arm is moved outwards and upwards. An X-ray may show some calcification. In older people there may be outgrowths of bony tissue that actually tear the cuff and can result in severe pain. If pain occurs on the tip of the shoulder or above the shoulder blades then this may be coming from a joint between the clavicle and the shoulder or from the neck.

Other causes of shoulder pain and stiffness include:

Joint inflammation *rheumatoid or psoriatic arthritis or infection*

Capsulitis *caused by stickiness of the capsule around the joint. Sometimes occurs in diabetes or lung cancer*

Osteoarthritis *this may follow an accident, wear and tear or diabetes*

Lack of use *after a stroke, or after being bandaged for too long*

Polymyalgia rheumatica *a disease, usually of the elderly, alleviated by steroids*

Treatment for shoulder pain

Rest, anti-inflammatory tablets and possible steroid injection into the joint are the usual treatments. Painkillers may be necessary, too. After an initial period of rest, as the pain subsides, it is important to start exercising the shoulder gently until a full range of movement is established. Sometimes it will be necessary to use the unaffected arm to move the affected arm.

MUSCLES, BONES AND JOINTS

Healthy joints

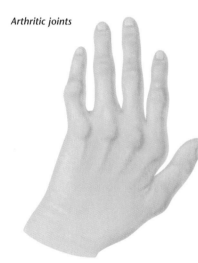

Arthritic joints

RHEUMATOID ARTHRITIS

This painful inflammatory disease is an auto-immune disorder, in which the body attacks itself. Rheumatoid arthritis usually starts in the small joints in the hands and feet and then spreads to affect other joints and parts of the body. The lining of the joint becomes inflamed and produces extra fluid, which causes swelling. The membrane overlying the bone surfaces in the joint becomes rough and eventually, often within a couple of years, the bone will start to be destroyed. The joints are painful and unstable and if the neck is involved then the collapse of the neck bones may, if left unchecked, result in paralysis. Rheumatoid arthritis may also affect the lungs, and lead to anaemia, skin ulceration, stomach ulcers, strokes, heart attacks and heart failure.

What causes rheumatoid arthritis?

There are thought to be many factors that may combine to produce rheumatoid disease. Hormones, genetics and infectious causes have been cited. This condition can occur at any age, with a peak between 25 and 55. There are two-and-a-half times more women affected by rheumatoid arthritis than men and there can be a great variation in the severity of the illness. Between 1 and 2 per cent of the UK population is affected. A similar but distinct condition can also develop in children.

Symptoms of rheumatoid arthritis

- *Tiredness and feeling unwell*
- *poor appetite*
- *Fever*
- *Joint pain and stiffness, usually on both sides of the body*
- *Stiffness in the morning*
- *Pale skin*
- *Small swellings under the skin*
- *Swollen glands*
- *Painful eyes, with burning and itching*
- *Restricted joint movement*
- *Hand and foot deformities*
- *Numbness and tingling*

Treatment for rheumatoid arthritis

- *Rheumatoid arthritis cannot be prevented but early diagnosis allows prompt treatment and raises awareness of complications. Diagnosis relies on blood tests to establish the presence of a substance called rheumatoid factor, found in about 70 per cent of sufferers, and to see whether inflammation is present in the body. X-rays may be taken to assess the extent of joint damage, with a view to surgery. If other organs are affected by rheumatoid disease then further tests for these may be required, such as chest X-rays to investigate the cause of breathlessness.*

- *With severe pain and other symptoms this disease may need to be managed initially in hospital. Use of steroid drugs may be necessary, as may gold injections and other strong drugs, to stop the body destroying itself. Many of these drugs have both short- and long-term side-effects and regular blood tests will be needed to ensure that more good is being done than harm.*

- *When the initial attack has died down, painkillers and anti-inflammatory drugs will probably be needed long-term. Many people with rheumatoid arthritis eventually see an end to the pain but may be left with seriously deformed joints.*

OSTEOPOROSIS

This is a condition in which the bones lose their mass and density, becoming weak and brittle. Loss of bone density is a natural part of ageing, and osteoporosis (meaning porous bones) is becoming more and more prevalent in our ageing society.

What causes osteoporosis?

Bone is a dynamic living structure that is constantly being built up and knocked down. It is composed of a protein framework strengthened with a 'brickwork' of calcium. In later life, particularly in women after the menopause, the framework is

Symptoms of osteoporosis

- Loss of height
- Easy fractures
- Humped back
- Bone pain
- Loose teeth

Treatment

Treatment concentrates on preventing further loss of bone density:

- Hormone replacement therapy for women
- Raloxetine, for women, has oestrogen-like effects
- Biphosphonates (drugs that prevent bone loss and increase bone density)
- A diet rich in vitamin D, calcium, magnesium, zinc and other minerals

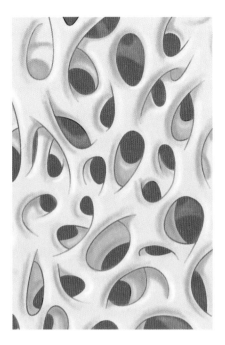

ABOVE *Bone is a living tissue that is constantly being broken down and replaced. Healthy bones have a layer of spongy bone underneath the hard shell that consists of a network of bony bars with many interconnecting spaces containing marrow.*

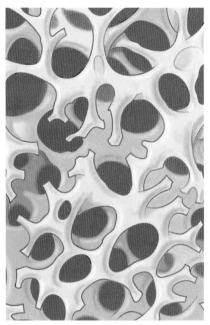

ABOVE *In osteoporosis, the network of bony bars breaks down, causing bones to lose their mass and density. It is a natural process of ageing but the severity of the condition varies from person to person. Here there is severe loss of bone density.*

constantly being broken down and not rebuilt. However many 'bricks' are available, the bone gradually becomes weaker because there is no firm structure to fix them to.

Prevention

As with all things, prevention is better than cure. Osteoporosis affects women more than men because after the menopause the ovaries stop producing oestrogen, a hormone that helps the body store calcium in the bones. After the menopause, unless the hormone oestrogen is replaced, the bones tend to become thinner. Therefore if hormone replacement therapy (HRT) is used early it is not a treatment but a preventative because it stops osteoporosis from developing. Likewise, in men who are found to have low testosterone levels, giving testosterone by implant or patches may prevent osteoporosis. Older men are often another, often

forgotten, group who may suffer badly from osteoporosis.

It is important to supply the body with materials to make the building bricks for bone, and your daily diet should include calcium (1000 mg daily until 50 and then 1500 mg daily), magnesium and zinc. Vitamin D is essential to help the absorption of these minerals. Enough calories are also needed,otherwise the body rebels and starts breaking down its own bones to get the chemicals it needs. People who suffer from anorexia are very prone to early osteoporosis. Other risk factors include smoking, excessive alcohol and caffeine intake.

People who are immobile, especially those who are bed-bound, are at great risk of developing osteoporosis. Exercise at all levels will help to prevent the condition. Twenty minutes' brisk walking each day will do wonders in terms of prevention.

HEART AND CIRCULATORY SYSTEM

Modern medicine has enabled diagnosis of heart disease even before birth and babies born with congenital heart defects are likely to have surgery that enables them to lead a normal, healthy life. The use of drugs, pacemakers, heart transplants and bypass surgery has revolutionised the management of heart disease. However, the risk of heart and circulatory diseases is increasing, mainly due to people becoming more overweight, smoking and taking less exercise.

HIGH BLOOD PRESSURE

Blood pressure describes the force with which the blood presses against the walls of the main arteries (vessels that carry blood away from the heart). It is recorded as the *systolic*, the pressure the heart has to use to push blood out of the heart, and the *diastolic*, the pressure the main artery (the aorta) uses to propel blood forward. Blood pressure constantly fluctuates, being low in the morning and rising in response to stress or physical exertion.

Between 20 to 30 per cent of the adult population of the UK suffers from high blood pressure. The figure varies

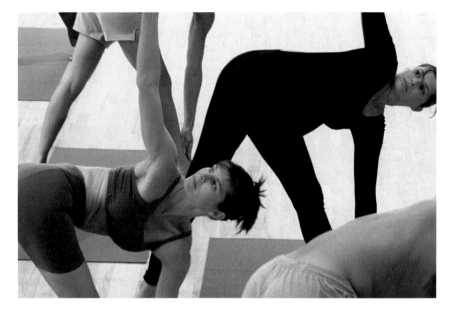

ABOVE *Aerobic exercises help protect you from heart disease as they make your heart stronger and more efficient, and able to pump more blood with every heartbeat.*

because doctors consider different levels as normal. The ideal levels of blood pressure are less than 140/80 (120/80 in the young or pregnant) but achieving these values is often impossible. It is scientifically proven that the higher the blood pressure, the greater the risk of heart disease, stroke and kidney damage, so it is important to treat this condition.

What causes high blood pressure?

High blood pressure often runs in families and, as yet, nothing can be done to change our genes. Only very

occasionally will a specific cause be found, such as kidney problems, heart defects or hormonal abnormalities. Many lifestyle factors can affect blood pressure, and losing weight, giving up smoking, reducing stress, reducing salt intake, and trying relaxation therapy, yoga and other forms of regular exercise may help reduce raised blood pressure.

Symptoms of high blood pressure

If blood pressure is very high, symptoms may include headaches, nosebleeds, dizziness, visual disturbances and breathlessness. High blood pressure is usually symptomless until damage to other parts of the body has occurred, and many people are unaware that they have the condition.

Treatment for high blood pressure

Avocado

• Blood tests are often performed to ensure that cholesterol levels are not high, the thyroid gland is not over-active and that the kidneys are working properly. If the cholesterol is raised then dietary advice will be given (but any change in diet has to be for life), and if these levels are unacceptably high then the only way to bring cholesterol down is by medication. The combination of high blood pressure and high cholesterol greatly increases the risks of stroke and heart disease.

Potatoes

• If a doctor feels that blood pressure is unacceptably high then the next step is to begin medication, which usually will be for life. Some people, particularly if they are young, feel unhappy doing this and want to put off taking tablets until they are older. It is easy to understand a reluctance to take tablets for a disease that is usually symptom-free, particularly as many of the medicines that lower blood pressure have side-effects. However, once high blood pressure starts, the damage to the heart, kidneys and blood vessels begins and it is better to begin treatment sooner rather than later.

There are four main groups of tablets:
• Diuretics (water pills): these aim to reduce blood pressure by ridding the body of excess water.
• Beta blockers, which reduce the activity of the heart. These may have side-effects of tiredness, cold hands and feet, and can make some asthmatics wheezy.
• Calcium channel blockers: these work with variable success. Side-effects include swollen ankles, headaches, flushing and constipation.
• Vasodilators, which widen the blood vessels and thus lower blood pressure. May induce a dry, irritating cough.

Current guidelines suggest that if blood pressure is difficult to control, it is better to have a small dose from two or more of the above groups than to have ever-increasing doses of one sort. However, from a people point of view, prescription charges may be difficult to afford and having four different tablets a month costs four times as much in charges.

Eating the following foods may help reduce raised blood pressure:

• celery
• garlic
• oily fish
• potatoes
• avocado
• salmon
• bananas
• Some people advise taking extra vitamin C, potassium and calcium

Bananas

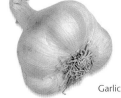

Celery   Garlic

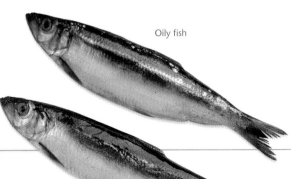

Oily fish

HEART AND CIRCULATORY SYSTEM

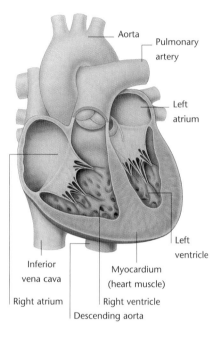

Aorta

Pulmonary artery

Left atrium

Left ventricle

Inferior vena cava

Right atrium

Myocardium (heart muscle)

Right ventricle

Descending aorta

HEART ATTACK

The classic heart attack, or myocardial infarction, occurs when a person feels a heavy pressure gripping across the front of the chest. The pain may spread up into the jaw and down the left or both arms. The person may look pale or even blue, start sweating, feel light-headed and may even vomit. Sometimes there will be shortness of breath and collapse.

LEFT *A heart attack is caused by loss of blood supply to part of the heart muscles. This usually happens because the arteries that supply the heart with oxygenated blood become narrowed by fatty deposits that build up on the artery walls.*

However, sometimes the pain may be very mild and occasionally can happen when sleeping, without even waking the person.

What causes a heart attack?

The pain and all the other signs and symptoms of a heart attack occur because the blood supply to a part of the heart has been cut off and an area of heart muscle damaged. Every year 5 people in 1,000 in the UK have a heart attack. Many factors make it more likely to be amongst those five. Some things we can do nothing about: age, being male, family history and ethnic origin (Asian people are more at risk). Some things we can identify as putting

Coronary heart disease

A number of factors can contribute to heart damage, and coronary heart disease is a prime cause. Atherosclerosis (narrowing of the arteries) and hypertension (high blood pressure) are conditions that can result in coronary heart disease. Both conditions usually develop over a number of years and tend to run in families, although diet and lifestyle also play a part in their development. As well as damaging the heart, narrowed arteries can result in stroke or poor circulation. Artherosclerosis occurs when fat deposits accumulate inside the arteries, eventually restricting the blood flow. Men are more likely to develop it than women, although by the age of 60 the risk is evenly shared. Hypertension affects about 16 per cent of adults in the UK and can also lead to coronary heart disease, stroke or heart attack. There is no obvious cause for hypertension but genetic factors and lifestyle may play a part in its development. Over time, the risk of damage to the arteries and to organs such as the heart, kidneys and eyes increases.

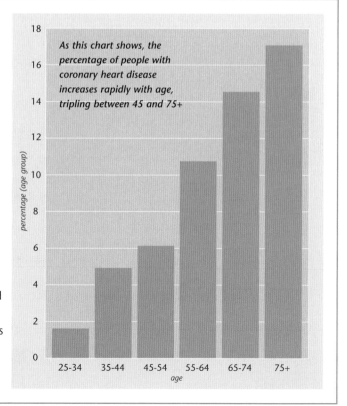

As this chart shows, the percentage of people with coronary heart disease increases rapidly with age, tripling between 45 and 75+

percentage (age group)

age

25-34　35-44　45-54　55-64　65-74　75+

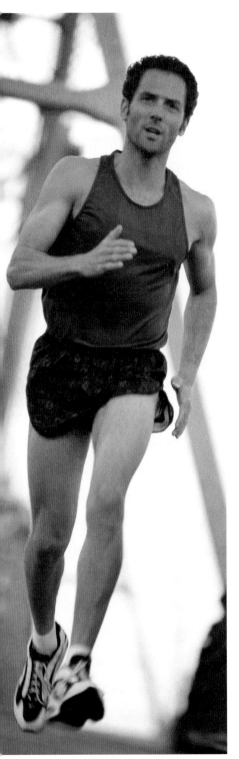

us more at risk and try and modify. These include high blood pressure, diabetes, smoking, high blood fats and being overweight.

Outlook

The size and position of the damage will determine the outlook for the patient. The damage done to the heart may be seen on an ECG (electrocardiogram: a recording of electrical activity in the heart), a chest X-ray may be helpful and measurement of the enzymes that the heart produces can confirm the diagnosis and may suggest how much muscle has been affected. In some hospitals, an angiogram, where dye is injected into the arteries supplying the heart, may show where the blockage to the blood supply has occurred and sometimes immediate removal or dissolving of the clot can be performed.

BELOW *This angiogram shows how a section of a coronary artery has become narrowed, restricting blood flow to the heart.*

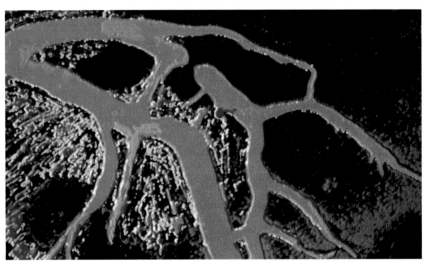

ABOVE *Regular exercise strengthens the heart and reduces blood cholesterol levels and blood pressure, both of which are factors in developing blockages in the arteries. Statistically, those who exercise regularly are more likely to survive a heart attack.*

Treatment

• *The immediate concern is whether the heart will stop, in which case first aid may be life-saving. The next most important worry is whether the heart rhythm will change to either very slow or very fast. Both of these may need immediate help.*

• *If available, oxygen, strong painkillers and drugs to dissolve the clot are ideal. An aspirin given at the time of a heart attack may make a considerable difference to how much the heart muscle is damaged. It may also prevent further clots.*

• *The first few hours after a heart attack are critical, and the sooner treatment is started, the better. If a heart attack is ever suspected then it is important to ask a doctor for advice and possibly transfer the person to hospital.*

HEART AND CIRCULATORY SYSTEM

ANAEMIA

This word literally means 'without blood', and is generally used to describe some form of blood abnormality. Anaemia may be either the cause or the result of ill health. The most common form is iron-deficiency anaemia, which happens either because the intake of iron is too low, the iron is not being absorbed or so much is being lost from the body that output exceeds input. Iron is an essential ingredient in making red blood cells.

What causes anaemia?

Women are particularly susceptible to iron-deficiency anaemia because of their monthly blood loss. If the periods are heavy and/or the intake of iron is low then anaemia results. Vegetarianism is common nowadays

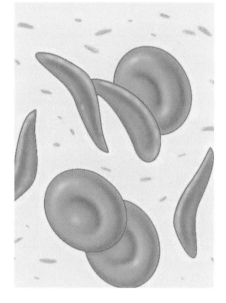

and although this diet is very healthy in many ways, its greatest weakness is that iron intake tends to be low. The incidence of anaemia in menstruating vegetarian women is high. Internal bleeding and various rheumatic diseases are common causes of anaemia that need investigation. Most causes of anaemia are treatable.

LEFT *Sickle cell anaemia is an inherited form of anaemia in which red blood cells become sickle-shaped because of an abnormality of the haemoglobin. These sickle-shaped cells are rigid and can block blood vessels, depriving the tissues of oxygen.*

Other types of anaemia

These are much less common but include:

- *pernicious anaemia: caused by vitamin B^{12} deficiency*
- *sickle-cell anaemia: an inherited disorder that occurs in black people*
- *thalassaemia: a genetic disorder that usually occurs in those of Mediterranean origin*
- *leukaemia: where the bone marrow makes too many white blood cells and not enough red blood cells*

There are dozens of other types of anaemia, which can be identified when a blood sample is taken. These need specialist diagnosis and treatment.

Symptoms of anaemia

- *Tiredness*
- *Breathlessness*
- *Headaches*
- *Irregular heartbeat (palpitations)*
- *Fainting*
- *Chest pain on effort (angina)*

Signs of anaemia include pale, grey or sallow skin; swollen ankles; fast heartbeat or heart failure; spoon-shaped or brittle nails; smooth tongue, brittle or thin hair and cracks at the side of the mouth.

Treatment for anaemia

- *Simple blood tests check levels of haemoglobin, the substance that binds with oxygen and carries it around the body in the blood, of which iron is an essential component. In pregnancy the levels are frequently lower than normal but rise after the birth of the baby. Further tests may be necessary to find out why the anaemia has occurred.*

- *The usual treatments include iron or vitamin B^{12} supplements along with dietary advice. To ensure adequate amounts of iron in your diet, the following foods are ideal: red meat, liver, spinach, breakfast cereals and green, leafy vegetables.*

VARICOSE VEINS

Varicose veins are swollen, twisted veins visible beneath the skin. They are most commonly found in the legs but can occur in other parts of the body, notably the rectum (where they are known as piles or haemorrhoids). They are a common problem, and in severe cases they sometimes lead to leg ulcers, open sores that are slow to heal.

What causes varicose veins?

Varicose veins develop when the valves in the vein (which control blood flow) become weak, preventing the blood from flowing efficiently and allowing it to stagnate. Many women first notice varicose veins during pregnancy, when they are caused by the pressure of the baby. Other contributing factors include standing for long periods of time, obesity, constipation, deep vein thrombosis and heredity.

Complications

The main worry is the development of leg ulcers. The first sign is often a patch of inflammation that becomes itchy, scaly, greasy and changes colour. The skin surface then breaks down to form the ulcer, typically on the inner ankle. Leg ulcers last for a long time – around 40 per cent will not have healed after one year and 10 per cent last for more than five years. The skin will change appearance when it heals to become red, shiny, thin and uneven.

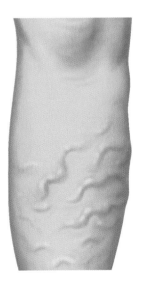

ABOVE *Visibly swollen, twisted veins that lie just beneath the skin are known as varicose veins. They are caused by an abnormal backflow of blood caused by weak valves in the veins.*

Symptoms of varicose veins

- *Sore, swollen and tender veins*
- *Aching legs*
- *Scaly patches of skin*

Treatment

- *Medical examination will establish the exact site of weakened valves and check the efficiency of blood flow in the legs to help determine treatment.*

- *The mainstay of conventional treatment is regular exercise, weight loss, wearing support stockings and avoidance of prolonged standing.*

- *The aim of support stockings is to compress the veins close to the skin's surface, thereby forcing blood to flow back to the heart. Graduated support stockings, where the pressure at ankle level is the highest, are classed 1, 2, 3 according to performance. There are several styles – thigh length, below knee, toe open (so foot length matters less) or toe closed – and different colours are available. Your doctor or pharmacist can assist you in measuring your legs so that you can choose from a wide range of sizes. Made-to-measure stockings are also available in all three classes.*

- *Putting on support stockings can be difficult. Wearing rubber gloves may help, or you could try putting on a nylon stocking first. If you want your stockings to last as long as possible wash them in warm, not hot, water and do not wring them out.*

- *Resting with the feet above chest level will help blood flow back to the heart. Painful inflammation may be treated with creams applied to the affected areas and anti-inflammatory tablets.*

- *Severe cases of swollen veins, especially below knee level, may be injected with a chemical that causes them to collapse. Up to two weeks after the injections a very tight bandage is applied to avoid losing the effect of the therapy. This clots the surface veins and sends the blood deeper down.*

- *Finally, depending on the exact site, the veins may be stripped out through incisions in the leg. The legs will then be tightly bandaged and early activity encouraged, including several walks every day.*

DIGESTIVE DISORDERS

In the West, many problems of the digestive system are caused by over-eating, obesity and the type of food we eat, including fast food, and the chemicals used in the manufacturing of foodstuffs. Operations and medications can ease many digestive disorders, and the use of acid-suppressing drugs has revolutionised the treatment of ulcers and indigestion.

INDIGESTION AND HEARTBURN

Indigestion is a general term used to describe abdominal discomfort, generally felt after eating. There can be few people over 40 who have never experienced heartburn. This is severe indigestion, caused when food flows back from the stomach into the oesophagus or gullet (the muscular tube that extends from the throat to the stomach). With the food come stomach acids and enzymes that irritate the lining of the oesophagus, causing pain right under the breastbone. The pain may be severe and frightening, particularly if it is recurrent.

Typically the pain occurs after meals and happens when food and acid travel upwards towards the mouth rather than downwards. The stomach may also be bloated. Symptoms may come on when bending forwards, lying down flat or after drinking hot liquids or alcohol. In severe cases, the reflux (backflow) at night may cause bouts of coughing or wheezing as food or acid spills over into the lungs. Repeated spills of stomach contents into the lungs may cause inflammation.

Symptoms of indigestion and heartburn

- *Nausea*
- *Burning sensation in the chest*
- *Belching*
- *Hiccups*
- *Flatulence*

What causes indigestion and heartburn?

Many factors can lead to increased production of gastric acid, which irritates the stomach. Eating too

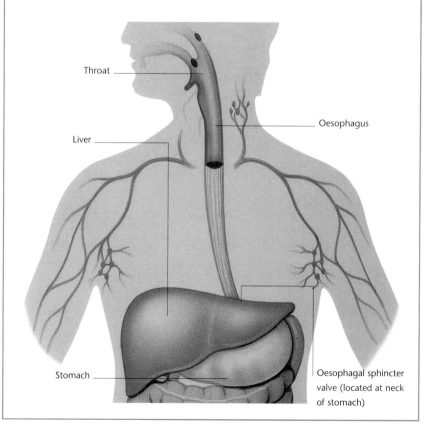

Causes of reflux

The pain of indigestion is due to the flow of acidic juices from the stomach back up into the gullet which irritate its lining. Stomach contents are kept from re-entering the oesophagus by a double-action valve, but this may leak, and certain foods may increase the production of stomach acid.

Throat

Liver

Oesophagus

Stomach

Oesophagal sphincter valve (located at neck of stomach)

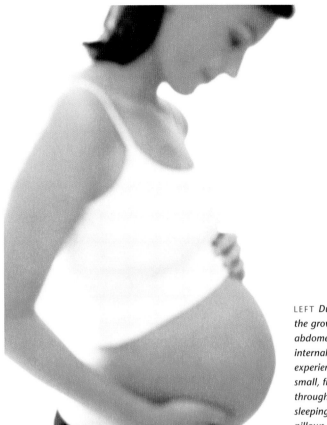

LEFT *During pregnancy, as the growing baby fills the abdomen and squashes the internal organs many women experience heartburn. Eating small, frequent meals throughout the day and sleeping propped up on pillows may ease symptoms.*

much rich, spicy or fatty food, eating too quickly, drinking too much alcohol or coffee, and excessive smoking are all causes of digestive discomfort, as are stress and anxiety. Pregnant women and those who are overweight are prone to reflux because their internal organs press on the digestive system. In some cases it may be a symptom of a peptic ulcer, gallstones or other disease.

Investigation

In severe and persistent cases of heartburn, medical investigation is desirable. Nowadays this usually involves endoscopy, where a tube containing fibre-optic filaments is swallowed (the patient is usually sedated). The doctor can then see any damage that has been done to the oesophagus, as it will appear red and will sometimes be bleeding. He will also see the reflux taking place. If there is a hiatus hernia,

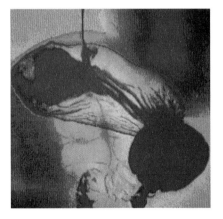

ABOVE *This X-ray shows a hiatus hernia, a cause of heartburn. Part of the stomach passes into the chest, and as a result stomach contents regurgitate into the oesophagus, causing pain.*

which occurs when a portion of the stomach, usually below the diaphragm, slips up above it, this too will be visible through the tube. Once the cause of the indigestion has been diagnosed a treatment plan can be formulated.

Treatment for indigestion and heartburn

- *Lose weight*
- *Eat less, and earlier in the evening*
- *Reduce alcohol intake*
- *Raise pillows to avoid lying flat*
- *Avoid bending after eating*
- *Eat bland foods*
- *Stop smoking*

- *All of these measures should help. However, sometimes medication is needed to neutralise the acid and stop the burning. Antacids are readily available from chemists. If these are not sufficient, drugs know as H_2 blockers reduce stomach acid. These are available in low dosages over the counter. Proton pump inhibitors may be prescribed by doctors and are very effective.*

- *In all but the most severe cases, this will be more than sufficient to control symptoms. In extreme cases, where, in spite of all the usual management measures, a person is waking at night coughing and wheezing, or there is anaemia caused by bleeding from the raw gullet, surgery may be performed. The surgery aims to stop the stomach contents flowing back, and it involves wrapping the top of the stomach round the oesophagus to act rather like a rubber band. It can be extremely successful but may create complications such as difficulty in swallowing solids. It is not undertaken lightly.*

DIGESTIVE DISORDERS

PEPTIC ULCERS

Peptic ulcers are breaks in the lining of the digestive tract caused by the action of gastric juices. There are two types of peptic ulcer: duodenal and gastric (stomach). They cause pain, bloating, wind, vomiting and other forms of abdominal upset and discomfort. Ulcers may be short- or long-term, single or multiple, deep or superficial. More effective remedies for reducing acid levels in the stomach have become available over recent years and peptic ulcers are now uncommon.

Symptoms of peptic ulcers

Pain is the most common symptom of early ulcer formation in the stomach or the short area of intestine below the stomach, known as the duodenum. Typically people with ulceration will point to an area just below the breastbone. The pain is said to be like having a hole burned into the inside. Frequently the pain has been smouldering away for some time and most people will have tried antacids from the pharmacy. Ulcers typically make people afraid to eat as food makes the stomach produce acid, and when this pours on to the ulcer it causes more pain.

Effects on the stomach and duodenum

Severe ulcers that form in the stomach or duodenum may be caused by certain bacteria. After carrying out tests to confirm this, treatment with drugs can begin.

RIGHT *This breath test will detect the presence of the bacterium Helicobacter pylori which can cause peptic ulcers.*

BELOW *This view through an endoscope shows a peptic ulcer (the yellow area) in the stomach lining.*

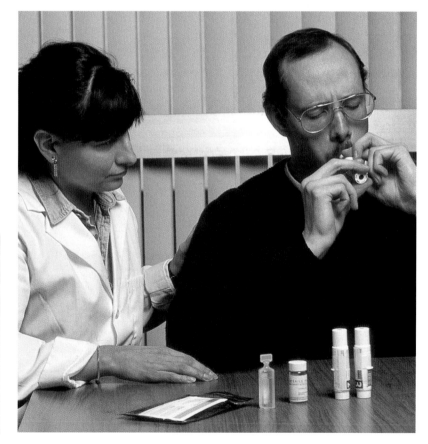

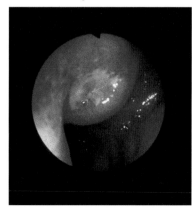

What causes peptic ulcers?

Gastritis, where the stomach may have many small ulcers, may be caused by anti-inflammatory tablets, especially aspirin and ibuprofen. Once these are stopped the ulcers may heal spontaneously.

Deeper, more severe ulcers are found in the stomach and duodenum, the first part of the small intestine. The bacterium *Helicobacter pylori* is often found in association with these ulcers, but it is not clear whether the ulcers are caused by the bacteria or whether these are present because there is an ulcer.

Other causes of peptic ulcers include poor diet, stress, hereditary factors, smoking and excessive alcohol consumption.

Management

In addition to drug treatment, lifestyle advice is vital in managing this condition. It is imperative to stop smoking. Weight loss may help, together with avoidance of acidic or spicy foods.

Regular weight checks are good to ensure that weight loss is not a problem. Blood tests to show that an ulcer is not bleeding chronically and causing anaemia should also be done.

Complications

These ulcers may go so deep that they perforate the wall of the stomach or duodenum. This is a surgical emergency as peritonitis (a form of severe abdominal infection) and death may follow. Constant bleeding may lead to anaemia. Ulcers may also become cancerous and require surgical removal.

Treatment for peptic ulcers

If a person under 45 has typical symptoms of an ulcer, he will probably be treated with H_2 blockers to reduce stomach acid production. Above this age, because there is an ever-increasing risk that the ulcer may be cancerous, sufferers will probably be investigated using an endoscopy (see page 397-98). People who have lost a lot of weight may also need this test. The doctor will then be able to see if and where any ulceration is. Through the instrument tests may be done to detect if the *Helicobacter pylori* bug is present. If it is, then two sorts of antibiotics may be given, together with the acid-suppressing drugs. If the ulcer looks worrying, biopsies (small samples) of tissue will be removed for examination. In older people, ulcers may be cancerous and surgery necessary.

LEFT *When ulcers start to form in the stomach or duodenum a burning pain will be felt just below the breastbone. Treatment of a peptic ulcer aims to heal the ulcer and to prevent it from recurring. Giving up smoking and cutting down on alcohol should ease symptoms.*

DIGESTIVE DISORDERS

IRRITABLE BOWEL SYNDROME (IBS)

This is a very upsetting and common condition. It is not linked to any serious disease but its symptoms are distressing and it is often difficult to accept that there is nothing dangerous going on. IBS occurs because the muscles that lie in the long tube of the bowel (also known as the gut or intestine) don't function well and become uncoordinated. This means that part of the bowel at the top might want to push the food onwards but because the bit below hasn't relaxed the top pushes harder and harder, becoming more and more blown up with food. The distended part of the bowel feels bloated while the tight bit below is in spasm and is very painful.

What causes IBS?

No one knows what actually causes IBS but both diet and stress are undoubtedly factors. Different diets can affect individuals in different ways, and although a particular diet can help one person with IBS it will not necessarily help another. Stress causes different symptoms in different people.

Muscle dysfunction

Irritable bowel syndrome often results from erratic contractions of the muscles in the walls of the intestines. Peristalsis, the wave-like action that propels food through the digestive system, becomes irregular, causing constipation, diarrhoea and pain.

Some people experience headaches, palpitations or panic attacks when they are stressed. IBS sufferers may have a bad, painful bout of their condition.

There is little doubt that IBS varies in its severity among sufferers, and there are good and bad spells. Sometimes there are no obvious triggers, or IBS itself may be a trigger. It is easy to become anxious that these bowel symptoms are suggestive of something sinister going on and so stress builds up and the condition may worsen.

Management

It is impossible to avoid stress in today's world but discovering different ways of dealing with it may be helpful. Avoid rushing by allowing plenty of time for a journey, or travel by train rather than driving. Putting aside half an hour a day for calm pursuits such as reading, painting, or doing crosswords or jigsaw puzzles is important.

Regular gentle exercise may help. A ten-minute stroll, rather than strenuous jogging, may be best.

Symptoms of IBS

• Pain in the abdomen which varies hourly and daily
• Alternating constipation and diarrhoea
• Bloating
• Feeling that the bowel isn't properly emptied
• Small, rabbit-like pellets of faeces
• Relief from pain after passing a stool or wind

Food

There are no right or wrong foods for people with IBS. It is a matter of tracking down the foods that suit best and eliminating others that cause upset. Leave time to eat meals slowly and enjoy them, ensuring that you consume foods that suit you. The amount of fibre we need in the diet varies between individuals. Most people find that a diet with a reasonable quantity of fibre, reduced amounts of refined sugars (such as biscuits and cakes) and small amounts of fatty foods works best. Peppermint tea is often useful and may be very soothing at stressful times.

Medicines

In IBS medicines may be needed if one aspect of the condition becomes disabling, such as profuse diarrhoea. Severe constipation may require the use of gentle laxatives – bulk-forming laxatives rather than irritative ones are best. Spasm and pain may both be treated by medication, of which there are many types. Peppermint oil, in the form of capsules, can be very soothing and help prevent spasm.

DIVERTICULAR DISEASE

Diverticular disease occurs when the lining of the colon, or large intestine, pushes out in pockets through the muscles of the colon. If the pockets become infected or inflamed they can cause pain and abscesses. This condition is often present without symptoms. Without symptoms it is known as diverticular disease, with symptoms it is known as diverticulitis. Only about a quarter of people with the condition develop symptoms.

ABOVE *Eating a high-fibre diet will keep your digestive system running smoothly. However, water-soluble fibre, found in leafy vegetables, fruit and oats, is easier to digest than the fibre in wheatbran, lentils and beans.*

Symptoms of diverticular disease

- No symptoms
- Occasional colicky pain
- Irregular bowel action

What causes diverticular disease?

Diverticular disease is thought to occur mainly because of a low-fibre diet, which is why it is so much more common in developed countries. It tends to increase in frequency with age and almost a third of those over the age of 65 suffer from this condition.

Investigations

Usually the only way to be sure of the diagnosis is admission to hospital for a colonoscopy, where a tube is passed into the anus and up through the bowel. The tube is filled with fibre-optic filaments that allow light to be passed into the bowel and permit the doctor to see the lining of the gut.

Another useful examination is the barium enema. Here barium, a chemical that can be seen, is passed into the bowel via a hollow tube. By twisting and turning and passing volumes of gas into the bowel as well, the lining of the bowel is clearly visible. Any fistulas (tiny passages between parts of the bowel) may be clearly seen as the barium trickles down them. Even more complex tests with large machinery such as the MRI scanner (see pages 456–57) may occasionally be needed.

Symptoms of diverticulitis

- Fever
- Constant central abdominal pain
- Nausea and vomiting
- Irregular bowel habits, especially constipation
- Bleeding
- Tenderness over the abdomen

Treatment for diverticular disease

- Often, if symptomless, no treatment is needed for diverticular disease. Ideally a diet high in fibre should be adhered to and if pain occurs from time to time a medicine to prevent muscle spasm may be useful. If constipation is a problem then regular use of laxatives is advisable.

- If inflammation or infection has set in with pain and bleeding, then the first line of treatment is rest, antibiotics and lots of fluids and painkillers.

- If the condition becomes worse, application of antibiotics to the affected area and intravenous antibiotics may settle the condition. Occasionally a badly affected area may have to be surgically removed. In the worst cases, a stoma may need to be performed, where the bowel is brought out of the skin at the side of the abdomen and into a bag that collects the faeces. This can be a temporary measure, which may be reversed when the bowel has had time to rest and recover.

DIGESTIVE DISORDERS

ULCERATIVE COLITIS

This in an inflammatory bowel disease that leads to ulceration of the lining of the intestine, the part of the alimentary (food) canal that extends from the stomach to the anus. This condition, though not very common, affecting about 6 people out of 10,000, can cause a lifetime of distress.

What causes ulcerative colitis?

Up to 10 per cent of people affected will have a family history of the condition. We are still unsure what causes the disease but milk allergy, autoimmune disease (where the body attacks itself) and unusual bowel bacteria may all play a part. It is one of the very few diseases where smoking may possibly do something to prevent the disease rather than cause it.

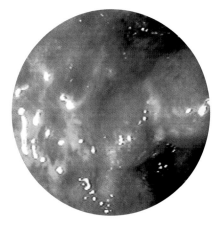

Symptoms of ulcerative colitis

- *Frequent passage of stools*
- *Blood and mucus in the faeces*
- *Lower abdominal pain*
- *Weight loss*

Area affected by ulcerative colitis

Ulcerative colitis is a form of inflammatory bowel disease that causes inflammation of the colon and/or rectum, leading to ulceration of the intestine lining. It varies in severity from month to month, and is usually treated by drugs. Complications include anaemia due to malabsorption and toxins from the intestines entering the bloodstream. Severe or extensive ulcerative colitis may be treated by surgery, particularly if the risk of colorectal cancer is high.

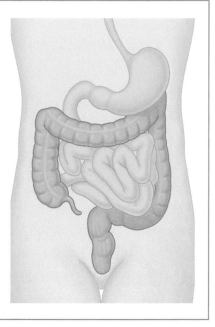

Diagnosis

Often the diagnosis is made from the history of passage of lots of blood and mucus. Sigmoidoscopy, where a tube is passed into the lower bowel, usually

This picture taken during sigmoidoscopy shows ulcerative colitis of the lining of the intestine, which causes long-term intermittent inflammation and ulceration.

confirms the condition as the bowel is seen to be red and bleeding and sometimes ulcers are visible. Tiny pieces of tissue (biopsies) are taken at the time of sigmoidoscopy for examination under the microscope. Colonoscopy (see page 401) will confirm the diagnosis and can be used for check-ups when required.

Treatment for ulcerative colitis

- *This condition can frequently be managed by medicines such as steroids. Sometimes, if the condition cannot be managed by medicines, surgery is required to remove the affected part of the bowel. Occasionally a stoma, where the bowel is brought out through the skin and drains into a bag, is necessary.*

- *Ulcerative colitis, particularly if it is extensive, has a tendency to become cancerous. For this reason, once it has been diagnosed, repeated colonoscopy will be necessary. Occasionally, if the condition has been troublesome for many years and the doctor feels the risk of cancer is high, the person will be offered surgery to remove the affected part of the bowel to prevent cancer developing.*

CROHN'S DISEASE

This serious condition affects about half as many people as ulcerative colitis, that is, 3 per 10,000 people. It may affect any part of the digestive tract throughout its length from mouth to anus, but is usually present in the last part of the small intestine, the ileum. Affected parts become inflamed, ulcerated and thickened.

What causes Crohn's disease?

Ten per cent of sufferers will have a family history of the condition. It seems that some form of infection may be responsible for the disease, and both measles and a type of tuberculosis bacterium have been cited as possible causes. It tends to affect young people, especially females, and there is a possible link to the MMR vaccine.

Outlook

This is a long-term disease with periods where the disease seems to be quiet and then suddenly flares up again. To all but the most stable of people, it is a very frightening condition, as no one knows what will happen next. Depression may be present and need treating.

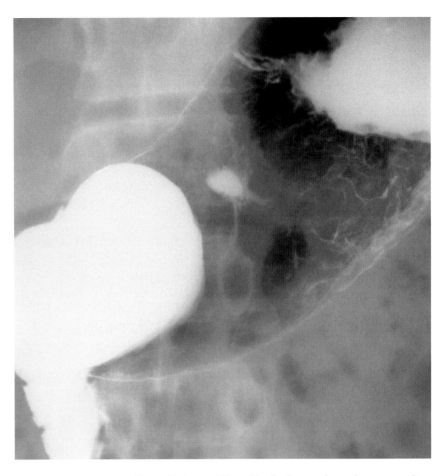

ABOVE *When a patient swallows a barium meal it enables the X-ray to detect the presence of Crohn's disease, whereby a part of the diegstive system has become inflamed and ulcerated. If it is present in the small intestine, it may interfere with the absorption of nutrients and anaemia may result. A sufferer may need dietary supplements to counteract malabsorption.*

Symptoms of Crohn's disease

- *Waves of abdominal pain*
- *Loud stomach rumbles after meals*
- *Bloated abdomen after eating*
- *Abnormal opening (fistula) on to the skin around the anus*
- *Blood and mucus in the faeces*
- *Occasionally the joints, eyes and skin may become inflamed, and there may be other unpleasant skin conditions*

Treatment for Crohn's disease

- *It is important to keep the person with Crohn's disease in as good general health as possible. A balanced diet and a constant weight are desirable. Sudden flare-ups may require steroid courses of high dosage, but alternatives are available if steroids are being used too frequently. Regular blood tests to check for inflammation and infection are advisable. Drugs that prevent the growth of bacteria may be useful to keep the disease under control.*

- *Over time, surgery becomes a progressively important part of management to remove damaged tissue.*

- *As the disease can be present throughout the bowel, regular checks of the small and large intestine are necessary, usually with a colonoscope (see page 401).*

DIGESTIVE DISORDERS

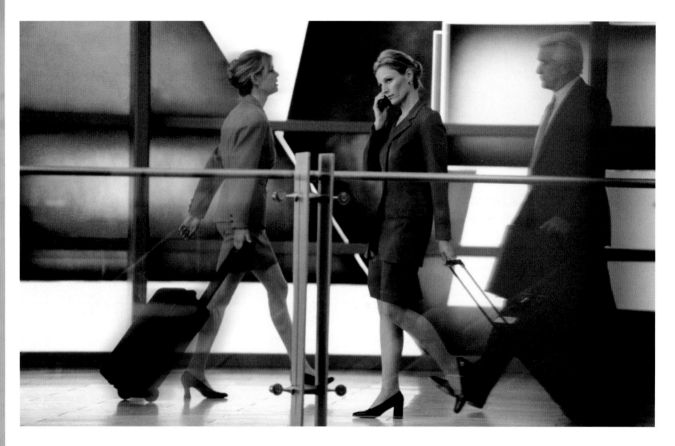

ABOVE *The most common cause of hepatitis is infection, and people at risk of hepatitis include travellers, drug users, homosexuals, those who work in institutions or day care centres and those who have regular blood transfusions, such as haemophiliacs.*

HEPATITIS

The term 'hepatitis' means inflammation of the liver. There are many different types, which are given alphabetical titles. Currently there are at least 13 separate groups, with Hepatitis M as the most recent, but undoubtedly there will be more to come. The most common are types A, B and C. Hepatitis can vary from very mild to very severe, life threatening or long-term. Cirrhosis, a liver disease, is a major complication and may need

hospital treatment. Occasionally a liver transplant is required to save life.

There are many different causes of hepatitis and a rapidly expanding number of treatments. Vaccination is available for Hepatitis A, B and C, and travellers to places where they are particularly at risk should always take the opportunity to protect themselves.

All types of hepatitis can be diagnosed by blood tests. Blood tests are readily available, either from your doctor or a local genito-urinary clinic. The tests are able to distinguish whether you have had the illness or whether you are currently suffering and infectious. A person who is very ill with hepatitis may need a liver biopsy, whereby a small sample of tissue is analysed to see how much damage has been done to the liver.

Most people with hepatitis will recover within three months, but will have to avoid alcohol during the illness and for a minimum of three months after they have recovered.

HEPATITIS A

This is a viral infection of the liver and is one of the most common diseases in the world. A person who has the disease passes the virus out with their faeces, and either through contact with that person or their excretions, someone else gets the infection. It can also be contracted through infected food or water.

Jaundice is the term used to describe yellowed skin. The first sign of jaundice is usually in the eyes, where the white of the eye becomes progressively more yellow. The person may become unwell

Symptoms of hepatitis A

- *Flu-like illness*
- *Fever*
- *Nausea and vomiting*
- *Fatigue*
- *Abdominal pain*
- *Loss of appetite*
- *Dark urine*
- *Jaundice*

The symptoms may be mild or even go unrecognised. A person may be infectious for two weeks after catching the infection and so can pass it on without even realising he has the disease.

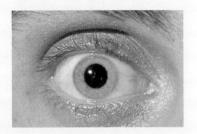

Jaundice (yellowing) of the skin and the white of the eye is often a sign of liver infection such as hepatitis. The yellowing results from excessive blood levels of the pigment bilirubin, a breakdown product of red blood cells, which is processed in the liver.

before the appearance of jaundice and get better while he is still very yellow. Generally, the darker the jaundice, the more severe the hepatitis.

Those at risk

- *Travellers, particularly in areas where sanitation is poor, such as South America*
- *Homosexual men*
- *People living where there is currently an outbreak*
- *Drug users*
- *Those with blood clotting disorders such as haemophilia*
- *Those who live or work in institutions*
- *Workers in child day care centres*

Treatment for hepatitis A

Treatment includes plenty of fluids, extra potassium and calcium and sugar. Sometimes, if clotting is a problem, a blood transfusion may be needed. Most people with symptoms recover from the worst of the disease in one or two months. In about 12 per cent of people the disease will keep recurring for up to six months.

HEPATITIS B AND C

These types can be short- or long-term. People with type B can recover from their symptoms but may still be infectious. Both are carried in the blood, and the virus may stay alive in dried blood for three months.

What causes hepatitis B and C?

- *Blood transfusion*
- *Sharing needles and drug paraphernalia*
- *Sharing razors and toothbrushes*
- *Unprotected sex*
- *Transmission at birth*
- *Unsterile piercings and tattoos*

Symptoms of hepatitis B and C

These are similar to type A.

Treatment for hepatitis B and C

For most people, treatment of the symptoms will be enough. This will involve rest, lots of fluids and very mild, bland, non-fatty foods. An antiviral drug such as interferon may be necessary, but treatment with this requires specialist medical care.

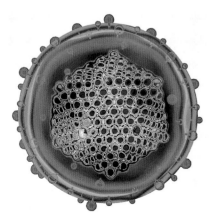

Hepatitis A virus

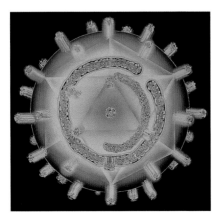

Hepatitis B virus

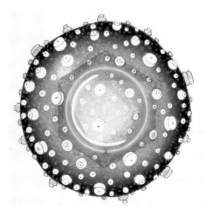

Hepatitis C virus

DIGESTIVE DISORDERS

APPENDICITIS

The appendix is a blind-ended sac that arises at the end of the colon, or large bowel. It normally does little in humans, but in rabbits it is very important in helping to digest the plant material cellulose. When the appendix becomes infected or obstructed by food pellets or swollen glands, then the symptoms of appendicitis arise. Appendicitis is one of the most common and best known causes of abdominal pain. It can occur at any age, although it is rare before the age of 2, and about 1 in 6 people undergoes an appendectomy to remove the affected organ.

Site of appendix

The appendix is a short, thin, blind-ended tube approximately 7–10 cm (3–4 in) long that is attached to the caecum, a pouch that forms the first section of the large intestine. It has no known function in humans. The appendix is liable to become infected, particularly amongst young people, and appendectomy is one of the most commonly performed emergency operations in the UK.

Appendix

Symptoms of appendicitis

- *Usually takes place over 24–48 hours*
- *Starts with central abdominal waves of pain*
- *Pain usually moves to the right side of lower abdomen*
- *Patient is flushed and feverish*
- *Fast heartbeat*
- *Unwillingness to eat*
- *After pressing over the site of the pain, the pain gets worse when pressure is released*

There are many conditions that can cause similar pains in the abdomen but appendicitis is the most common cause.

Treatment of appendicitis

- *If appendicitis is suspected then the person needs to be in hospital for further tests such as X-rays, blood tests and urine analysis.*

- *If the diagnosis is confirmed then removal of the appendix, as soon as possible, should be done. If left untreated, the appendix may form an abscess, which may burst and cause infection throughout the abdomen. For most, the operation is relatively straightforward and people often leave hospital two or three days after surgery.*

LEFT *Symptoms of appendicitis usually develop over 1–2 days. It starts with the sudden onset of waves of pain felt around the navel, then progresses to the lower right abdomen. If it is not treated the appendix may burst.*

BLADDER INFECTIONS

In most cases, disorders of the urinary system are simple to treat. Bacterial infection of the bladder is especially common in women and can be cured with an over-the-counter remedy or a course of antibiotics. The symptoms are easily recognised and early treatment will prevent infection spreading further to the kidneys. However, if you are at all worried or suffer recurrent infections, do not hesitate to talk to your doctor.

CYSTITIS

This is a common condition affecting the bladder, usually caused by an infection that causes pain on urination, sometimes pain at the base of the abdomen and an increased need to pass urine. Many cases of cystitis go on to cause kidney infection, which will result in fever, back pain and often sickness as well. For this reason it is important to try to avoid getting cystitis in the first place, but if the condition does start then early treatment is essential.

What causes cystitis?
Cystitis usually happens as a result of infection by bacteria that travel from the anus to the bladder. Women are more at risk than men because the urethra, the tube that empties the bladder, is shorter, and its opening is closer to the anus than it is in men. This means that germs have only a short journey to make before they get to the bladder.

Prevention
- *Drink lots of fluids, especially in hot weather*
- *Urinate before and after sex*
- *Wipe the bottom from back to front and never forwards*
- *Make sure all tampons used are newly unwrapped*
- *Urinate when you need to rather than holding on*
- *If you are past the menopause you may need hormonal help*
- *Avoid frequent, over-enthusiastic sex*
- *Avoid scented soaps, bubble baths and oils*
- *Drinking cranberry juice can help prevent bacteria remaining in the urinary system*
- *Avoid very acidic drinks, alcohol and caffeine*

Bladder infections in men
In men, bladder infections are less common due to the length of the urethra. An infection is likely to be related to an obstruction due to an enlarged prostate gland (see page 430).

Symptoms of cystitis

- *Frequent urge to urinate but often only tiny drops of urine are passed*
- *Urine may be very dark, cloudy or bloodstained*
- *Unpleasant-smelling urine*
- *Burning or scalding pain on urination*

Treatment for cystitis

At the onset of symptoms drinking alkaline mixtures to reduce the urine's acidity, so that it does not sting, may help. Dissolve a teaspoonful of bicarbonate of soda in a pint of water and drink freely. There are some over-the-counter remedies that a pharmacist should be able to recommend. If the symptoms are severe then antibiotics are usually required, and you will have to see a doctor. Take a specimen of urine in a freshly scalded container when you go. This will enable the doctor to check for signs of blood and infection. The specimen may be sent to the laboratory to identify the bacteria but sometimes this is not necessary and the doctor will prescribe an antibiotic that is likely to work (but only if you finish the course). Drinking lots of water will help dilute the acids and so ease the pain. Sometimes a painkiller such as paracetamol may be needed and a hot-water bottle (wrapped in a towel) held on the abdomen may be comforting.

HORMONAL DISORDERS

The endocrine glands are organs situated around the body that secrete hormones, chemical messengers that regulate important body processes and functions, such as growth, reproduction and metabolism. The major endocrine glands are the pituitary, thyroid, pancreas, adrenals, ovaries and testes. The bean-sized pituitary gland, situated at the bottom of the brain, just above the nose, has overall control of most hormone production. Hormonal disorders usually occur when there is under- or over-production of a particular hormone, either in a specific endocrine gland or in the pituitary gland, which affects output.

DIABETES

This is a condition that arises because the body cannot deal with the amount of sugar in the blood, which leads to permanently raised blood glucose levels. When sugar is absorbed into the blood from digested food in the intestines it is used by cells in the body as a source of energy. Normally a hormone called insulin, made in the pancreas, allows this process to occur. If this does not happen – either because

Symptoms of diabetes

• *Excessive thirst*
• *Frequent urination*
• *Recurrent thrush in women*
• *Boils*
• *General itching*
• *Weight loss*

Over a period of time, if the blood sugar level continues to rise, the person may become progressively tired and may eventually lose consciousness and fall into a coma.

The effects of diabetes

Diabetes is a metabolic disorder, which means that the chemical processes that take place in the body fail to work properly because of the body's inability to use glucose for energy production. Unused glucose builds up in the blood, eventually causing widespread damage to many parts of the body, including the blood vessels, the nerves and the kidneys. However, with proper management most diabetics are able to enjoy a normal life.

Type 1 diabetes is treated with daily insulin injections. Patients inject themselves with the correct dose from a pen-like insulin carrier the pancreas produces insufficient amounts of insulin or body cells become resistant to the hormone's effects – the level of blood sugar rises, and this in turn causes damage to the eyes, blood vessels, heart and kidneys. The immune system becomes weakened and there is increased susceptibility to infections such as cystitis.

There are two main forms of diabetes. Type I occurs when the body is unable to make any insulin. It usually happens in younger people and may even be present from birth. This sort of diabetes is known as insulin-dependent diabetes mellitus (IDDM). In Type II diabetes the pancreas can still make some insulin but either it cannot make enough or, for some reason, the insulin does not work as well as it should. This type usually occurs in older people and is known as non-insulin-dependent diabetes mellitus (NIDDM).

Complications

Diabetes is a common condition but the problem is controlling it well. If it is left untreated, life-threatening comas may result. If badly controlled, damage to the blood vessels, causing blockages and heart attacks, may occur. Damage to the kidneys and nerves (because of damage to the tiny blood vessels supplying the nerves) may also happen. The closer the blood sugar is kept to normal, the better the long-term outlook and the lower the risk of damage to other organs. This is why regular checking of blood sugar levels is essential in both types of diabetes.

Regular check-ups of eyes, feet, blood pressure, heart and kidneys are essential to keep on top of the disease. With good management and self-care, many diabetics live a normal life and enjoy generally good health. Special care should be taken to limit exposure to infection and to protect against influenza and other diseases by vaccination.

Treatment for diabetes

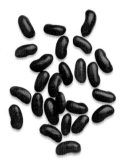

The aim of treatment in both types of diabetes is to try to maintain a near normal blood sugar level without wild fluctuations. If the blood sugar level is constantly too high then damage to the organs of the body occurs. If it falls too low then fainting and eventually coma and unconsciousness happen.

Treating Type I Diabetes

• *In patients with Type I diabetes, the only way to get insulin into the body is by injecting it. New types of insulin, where it can be absorbed rapidly when needed and slowly throughout the day, are constantly being produced. Most people who need it use a small cartridge of insulin that is concealed in a pen-like carrier with a small needle attached. A dial at the side of the pen permits different amounts of insulin to be injected.*

• *A person with IDDM has to check the level of blood sugar by pricking a finger and measuring a drop of blood with a small gadget. When the level is known, the correct amount of insulin required can be used. Many people with diabetes become expert at measuring their own blood sugar levels and working out the quantity of insulin they need. Others will require more assistance but there are many sources of information and help available from doctors, hospitals and diabetic societies.*

Treating Type II Diabetes

• *Type II diabetes is not any less serious than Type I, but it does require different management. A healthy diet and increased exercise are essential. Losing weight, in those who are overweight, will improve the condition. In people with Type II diabetes the first line of treatment is usually diet. Cutting out foods high in sugars and eating more starchy foods may help considerably. Advice from practice nurses and dieticians is essential.*

• *Some people with Type II diabetes will need tablets to help make the pancreas produce more insulin and also to make the cells less resistant to the insulin that is present. Recently, drugs called glitazones have been introduced in the UK to use in combination with some of the older medicines. These are especially useful in helping the cells make use of the available insulin.*

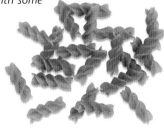

• *Eventually some Type II diabetics need to inject insulin either on its own or with their tablets.*

HORMONAL DISORDERS

THYROID DISEASE

The thyroid gland, situated at the front of the neck, produces the hormone thyroxine, which is essential for the conversion of food into energy within the body and for mental and physical development. Overproduction of thyroxine can cause major problems with overactivity of the body and its tissues. Under-production of thyroxine causes a general slowing down of all systems. The thyroid gland may also swell but produce no change in its hormonal output, so that the swelling seems to be the only problem.

HYPERTHYROIDISM

This describes the overproduction of the thyroid hormones, which causes

Symptoms of hyperthyroidism

- *Weight loss*
- *Irregular heartbeat (palpitations) and heart failure*
- *Sweating*
- *Swollen thyroid gland (a goitre)*
- *Eyes that appear large and swollen*
- *Eyelids may not shut fully*
- *Feeling hot even when others are cold*
- *Increased appetite*
- *Heavy periods*
- *Swollen shins*

Treatment for hyperthyroidism

- *There are two main reasons why an overactive thyroid needs to be treated. Firstly, the effect on the heart can produce very severe palpitations, abnormal rhythms that may cause clots, strokes and heart failure. Secondly, the effect of too much thyroxine on the eyes may cause them to bulge. This may result in damage to the surface of the eye (the cornea) or to the eye and eyesight by stretching it forward.*

- *The most commonly used medicine is carbimazole, which blocks the effect of the thyroxine and causes the metabolic rate of the body to slow down. Sometimes, even after stopping the carbimazole, the thyroid makes too little thyroxine and the symptoms of an underactive thyroid result. At this stage doses of thyroxine may need to be taken by mouth.*

- *Other treatments include surgery, especially if there is a large goitre (or swelling), or taking radioactive iodine. Swallowing radioactive iodine results in a gentle slowing down of the production of the thyroid hormone but eventually it may slow down too much and replacement thyroxine may be needed.*

Thyroid gland

The thyroid gland is situated in the neck, wrapped around the front of the windpipe (trachea). It produces the hormone thyroxine, which regulates the rate of many chemical processes in the body, including the use of energy. The pituitary gland in the brain produces thyroid stimulating hormone (TSH), which acts on the thyroid gland.

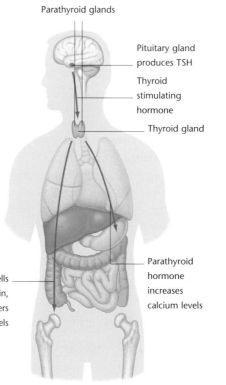

Parathyroid glands

Pituitary gland produces TSH

Thyroid stimulating hormone

Thyroid gland

Parathyroid hormone increases calcium levels

Some thyroid cells release calcitonin, which lowers calcium levels

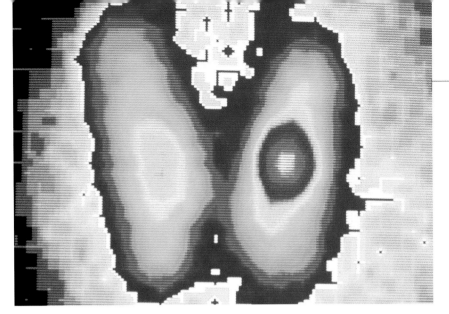

LEFT *This MRI scan shows an enlarged thyroid gland, which is known as a goitre when it becomes a visible swelling in the neck.*

many body functions to speed up. Hyperthyroidism affects about one person in a hundred. For some reason, this condition is ten times more common in women than in men, and it can occur at any age.

What causes hyperthyroidism?

Overactivity of the thyroid occurs commonly after childbirth. At this time, medication may calm down the effect of too much of the thyroid hormone. Eventually the problem may correct itself, which happens in other forms of overactive thyroid disease. Hyperthyroidism sometimes occurs because the body makes antibodies against its own thyroid and a condition known as Graves' disease, a particular type of hyperthyroidism that is thought to be hereditary, results. Blood tests to measure the level of thyroxine hormone in the blood are essential to diagnose the condition. Symptoms in most cases develop over several weeks.

HYPOTHYROIDISM

Hypothyroidism occurs in 1–2 per cent of the population and is ten times more common in women than in men. It tends to occur in older people but can be present even at birth, when treatment is urgent to prevent lifelong brain damage.

What causes hypothyroidism?

In the past, much hypothyroidism was related to iodine deficiency, but now that this chemical is added to bread and water, shortage of iodine is rare. The most common cause of hypothyroidism is when the body, over a number of years, makes antibodies against the thyroid (Hashimoto's disease).

Swollen thyroid gland

Sometimes the thyroid gland may be swollen but cause no symptoms of over- or under-activity. Most swellings of the thyroid are benign. However, they may cause problems if they swell behind the trachea, the tube that carries oxygen to the lungs. If the swelling becomes big, it may cause obstruction to breathing or swallowing, and it will need to be surgically removed.

Occasionally a swelling of the thyroid may be cancerous. Risk factors include:

- *a rapidly swelling lump*
- *being a male aged over 60 or under 20*
- *family history of cancer of the thyroid*
- *a hard lump on the thyroid*
- *painless lump*
- *surrounding swollen glands*
- *previous radiation therapy to the neck*

To find out whether a thyroid lump is benign or cancerous a biopsy will be carried out. Surgery to remove the whole gland is usually very successful but following it, thyroid replacement tablets will need to be taken.

Symptoms of hypothyroidism

- *Weight gain*
- *Sleepiness*
- *Lethargy*
- *Loss of outer third of eyebrow*
- *Dry skin that may be tinged yellowish*
- *Poor appetite*
- *Hair loss*
- *Dry hair*
- *Puffiness and swelling around the eyes*
- *Feeling cold all the time*
- *Constipation*
- *Aching, painful muscles*
- *Slowing of mental activity*
- *Heavy periods*
- *Pain in both wrists, especially at night (carpal tunnel syndrome)*

Treatment for hypothyroidism

Because the disease comes on slowly it is often missed. Only gradually does the body seem to slow down or the weight creep on. The disease is easy to diagnose, once it has been thought of, as a simple blood test to measure the levels of thyroid hormone will confirm it. Treatment is thyroxine hormone given by mouth. Blood tests are necessary every so often to ensure the dosage is correct.

COMMON VIRAL INFECTIONS

Infection was once the single largest cause of death. With the advent of antibiotics and anti-viral agents many infections, at one time fatal, are now entirely curable. Immunisation of children has revolutionised life expectancy in the West. There are worries about possible risks from all vaccines but these have to be balanced against the numbers of children saved from major complications or deaths from these infections.

MMR

In the UK, much publicity has recently been given to worries about the immunisation of young children with the measles, mumps and rubella (MMR) vaccine. This is offered routinely at around 14 months, with a booster dose at around four years. The government has put forward strong arguments in favour of immunisation but finds it hard to allay the emotional worries that parents are subjected to when making the choice of whether or not to have their child immunised. Parents must be able to make a choice, as undoubtedly there are risks and possible side-effects with any injection.

Against the MMR vaccine

- *These illnesses have been around for many years and in developed countries are rarely serious or have complications.*
- *There are grave concerns that a child might have a reaction at the time of the injection (anaphylaxis) and collapse shortly afterwards.*
- *The site of injection may be painful and sometimes there is fever and a mild rash or dose of one of the illnesses may follow.*
- *There is some evidence that the immunity gained from getting the disease naturally is better than that given artificially.*
- *There may be a risk of high fever and convulsions, which can possibly cause brain damage.*
- *Some scientists have suggested there is a link between the MMR immunisation and Crohn's disease and autism, a mental disorder in which children become self-absorbed and withdrawn. Other scientists dispute this.*

For the MMR vaccine

- *The MMR vaccine protects most children from measles, mumps and rubella. It appears to be very safe for the vast majority of children.*
- *Unless the vaccines are given together and early on, there is a window between*

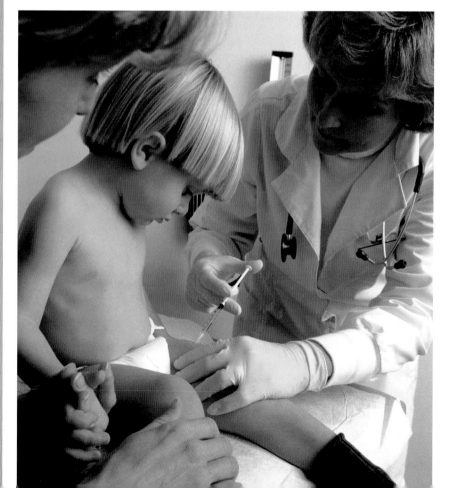

LEFT *Routine immunisation of babies against polio, diptheria and tetanus has made these diseases very rare in the Western world.*

the injections when the child is still susceptible to the infection. Giving a combined vaccine spares a child the trauma of three injections.

● *Measles can be a very serious illness, and the risk of brain disease from it is 1 in 5,000, which is much higher than the risk of getting it from the vaccine (1 in 1 million).*

● *Before the introduction of mumps vaccine, mumps meningitis was the major cause of viral meningitis in children. Since MMR was started it has rarely been seen.*

● *Protection of the child gives what is known as herd immunity, which protects whole communities and thus prevents mothers in early pregnancy from contracting rubella and having damaged babies.*

● *The apparent increased incidence of Crohn's disease and autism may well be accounted for by better and more accurate diagnosis in recent years.*

The balance would seem for most to be vastly in favour of taking the slight risk of danger from the vaccine against the tiny risks that may affect the individual. However, parents would hate to feel that they had been guilty of subjecting their child to unnecessary dangers to protect others. Those who feel that the risks of the injection are too high to accept should speak to a health professional before making a final decision.

MEASLES

This viral illness is highly infectious and can vary from being very mild to being a life-threatening disorder. The virus is carried in the nose, mouth and throat and it is usually passed on via direct contact or in airborne droplets before symptoms appear. It mostly affects children and it is preventable in most by immunisation in the form of the MMR vaccine.

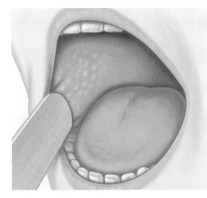

ABOVE *Measles is a highly contagious illness spread via direct contact or inhaling infected airborne droplets. Tiny white spots with a red base, known as Koplik spots, appear on the insides of the cheeks shortly before the onset of the rash on the head and the body.*

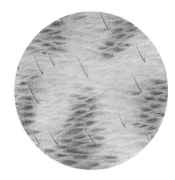

ABOVE *The measles rash consists of separate flat red spots which merge after a few days to form blotchy, raised skin.*

Treatment for measles

Usually little treatment is needed except for a few doses of children's paracetamol if there is fever or if there is pain from earache. If complications develop, such as chest infections or extreme sleepiness, dislike of bright lights or bleeding, then professional help should be sought immediately. A doctor can confirm the disease by taking blood samples or swabs from the mouth for analysis.

Symptoms of measles

There may be no symptoms of measles. Before the rash appears, an affected person may have a runny nose, cough, muscle pains, sore throat, fever, white spots inside the mouth (on the insides of the cheek) and red eyes. A rash then starts behind the ears and is red, slightly raised and may become purplish. The spots may merge to form a generally red, raised skin. The rash tends to occur five days into the illness and lasts about five days.

Serious symptoms

The main concern with measles is that the minor symptoms described above will progress to more serious complications. These include:

● *Sudden severe earache and pain*
● *Severe chest infections, including bronchitis and pneumonia*
● *Brain inflammation (encephalitis)*
● *Internal bleeding*

It is particularly important because of the risk of severe brain damage to try to protect children from measles by having them immunised early in life.

COMMON VIRAL INFECTIONS

MUMPS

This viral disease affects the salivary glands in front of the ears and those under the chin. It can be very painful and cause more serious problems if it affects older people. Mumps is spread by tiny droplets of saliva containing the virus passed on through coughing and sneezing. The incubation period, the interval between exposure to the virus and the appearance of the first symptoms, may be as long as three weeks, and people may easily pass the disease on without realising they are infectious. Mumps can be prevented by immunisation with the MMR vaccine.

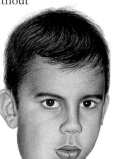

Treatment for mumps

There is no specific treatment for mumps, but the swollen glands are often quite painful. Paracetamol will help deal with pain and fever. Applying alternate hot and cold compresses (pieces of fabric soaked in water then wrung out) to the glands may relieve symptoms. It may be difficult to open the mouth because of pain and swelling, and using drinking straws may be necessary for a few days.

LEFT *In the viral infection mumps the salivary (parotid) glands situated below and in front of each ear may become swollen.*

Symptoms of mumps

• *Swelling of the salivary glands and pain, on one or both sides*
• *Sore throat*
• *Headache*
• *Fever*
• *Pain in and around the forehead and jaw*

These symptoms are typical of children with the illness, but when passed to male adults mumps may cause testicular pain, swelling and infertility. Mumps occasionally causes prostate problems, breast pain and swelling, and may spread to the pancreas and brain, where it causes a form of meningitis.

MENINGITIS

Meningitis is an inflammation of the tissues surrounding the brain and spinal cord due to bacterial or viral infection, and may be life threatening. Many types of bacteria can cause the illness, but immunisation introduced over recent years against the more common strains has been very effective in reducing the incidence of the disease. Viral meningitis is not usually such a serious condition, though the person affected may be very unwell.

The box (right) lists worrying warning signs of meningitis. Should anyone, of any age, show some of these signs and need to be seen by a doctor,

Symptoms of meningitis

• *Headache*
• *Fever*
• *Dislike of light*
• *Dislike of noise*
• *Vomiting*
• *Sleepiness*
• *Floppiness*
• *Stiff neck*

RIGHT *Because meningitis is a disease of the nervous system its effects are felt throughout the body, from fever and aches and pains to a haemorrhagic rash if the cause is bacterial.*

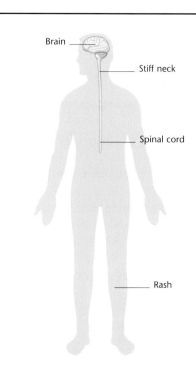

Brain
Stiff neck
Spinal cord
Rash

LEFT *The distinctive red rash of bacterial meningitis does not always appear and is usually a late sign of the disease.*

it may be quicker and better for the patient to take him directly to a surgery than to wait for a home visit.

Many people reading this list may be aware that meningitis can be associated with a reddish-purple rash that doesn't disappear when a a clear glass is pressed over it. The rash does not occur in every case of meningitis and when it does, it is usually a late sign. It is not necessary to have a rash to make the diagnosis.

Treatment for meningitis

• *There are many forms of meningitis. If diagnosed early enough, most people with meningitis make a complete recovery with the help of antibiotics. Sometimes, artificial ventilation using a machine that helps a person breathe normally is necessary for a while. If the disease is identified too late it may be fatal.*

• *Viral meningitis usually follows a viral illness such as chickenpox or mumps. Often general nursing care, rest and (occasionally) antiviral drugs may be needed.*

• *There is no doubt that in this illness prevention is better than cure, as the illness mimics many others. Delayed treatment can result in death or permanent brain damage.*

CHICKENPOX

Caused by the herpes zoster virus, which also causes shingles, this is usually a mild but highly infectious childhood disease. It tends to be much more severe in adults. Older people, those who have immune deficiency and even healthy adults may become very ill with chickenpox. They tend to feel quite restless, feverish and

Symptoms of chickenpox

• *General malaise, irritability and fever prior to the rash*
• *Small, reddish spots that fill with fluid to form blisters*
• *Variable outbursts of the rash, with sudden new patches*
• *Number of spots varies from very few to total body cover*
• *Itching, which may be severe*
• *Rash usually starts on trunk or limbs but can go to scalp*
• *Sometimes affects the inside of the mouth, the eyes, the genitals and the rectum*
• *Blisters form scabs after bursting and may remain for many days*

The appearance of the blisters usually confirms the diagnosis of chickenpox and blood tests are rarely necessary. If the blisters are not scratched, the skin may be left unmarked. However, usually a few will have been so itchy that scars will remain, often for life.

If there has been much scratching, the blisters may become infected and antibiotics are sometimes needed. The whole illness usually last about two weeks from the few days before the rash to the last scabs dropping off.

Treatment for chickenpox

Usually treatment is aimed at relieving the symptoms. Paracetamol will help if there is fever. Antihistamine tablets or syrups and soothing creams applied to the skin may relieve itching. In small children, cutting nails very short and wearing mittens overnight will help stop scratching. Those who have a depleted immune system, especially those with AIDS, may be given antiviral drugs.

lose their appetite. The chickenpox rash is often very severe, covering every bit of skin. In pregnant women, the danger period for the baby is in the middle three months: injections of immunoglobulins, which contain antibodies to the chickenpox, may be given.

What causes chickenpox?
Chickenpox is spread by a virus transmitted in droplets of fluid, which may be coughed or sneezed out. The blisters contain live virus. The person with chickenpox is infectious from two days before the rash starts until all the scabs have been shed. The incubation period is two to three weeks. Once a person has had chickenpox, the virus remains dormant in the nerve cells and may reactivate later in a condition known as shingles (herpes zoster).

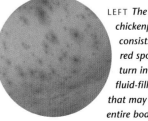

LEFT *The chickenpox rash consists of tiny red spots that turn into itchy, fluid-filled blisters that may cover the entire body.*

SEXUALLY TRANSMITTED DISEASES

Since records began, sexually transmitted diseases (STDs) have abounded. Each time a new disease has emerged, scientists have eventually found a way to treat it. Syphilis, once so prevalent, has become rare. Even AIDS, a huge problem in Africa and Asia, can be managed by drugs, though for most developing countries the cost is prohibitive. The key to control of STDs is safe sex. This means protecting the genital organs from direct contact with other people's. Widespread use of barrier methods and fewer sexual partners would reduce the risk of sexually transmitted diseases enormously.

HIV AND AIDS

HIV is the human immunodeficiency virus, which attacks and destroys the white blood cells, the body's infection-fighting cells. There are two strains, HIV-1 and HIV-2 (which is most common in Africa). HIV causes acquired immune deficiency syndrome (AIDS), which leaves the body open to a range of fatal diseases. About 40,000 people in the UK have the disease, a number that is growing rapidly.

What causes HIV?
The virus is most commonly contracted by sexual intercourse or blood transfusion. It usually takes three months until the body makes antibodies against the virus, so testing for HIV should be delayed for three months after possible exposure.

Prevention
This is the most important aspect when considering this condition. HIV is transmitted primarily by sexual intercourse, and condoms are excellent at protecting against the disease

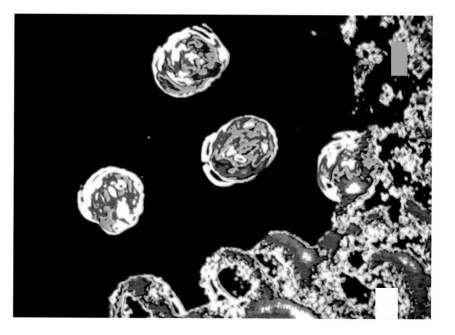

spreading. Many new cases are occurring in the heterosexual community and some cases are found for the first time in pregnancy. As the results of treatment are so good, many women who have the disease want to have children. If the baby is delivered by Caesarean section and not breast-fed, then the risk to the baby of contracting the infection is very small.

ABOVE *The HIV virus enters the bloodstream and infects the white blood cells, which are responsible for fighting infection. The virus reproduces within the cells, destroying them in the process, and leaving the person vulnerable to a range of diseases.*

The risk from blood transfusion is very low nowadays and rarely, with needle exchange programmes available, are drug users at risk.

RIGHT *HIV support groups help sufferers share experiences and methods of coping with the illness and exchange information on treatment.*

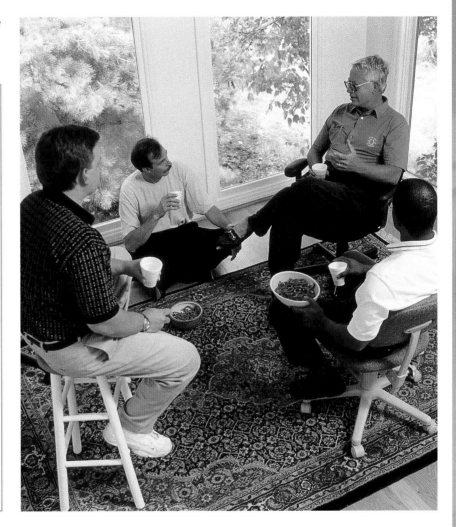

Treatment for HIV

HIV is no longer considered to be the death sentence it once was. New medicine regimes, usually involving using three special drugs at once, have reduced the terror of the disease and turned it into a long-term illness. Treatment is very expensive, currently being in the region of £10,000 a year, but those on treatment can live a relatively normal life. Specialist clinics are available throughout the country to deal with the need to keep up-to-the-minute with newly developed drugs. Drugs are not usually necessary until the number of white cells is very low or the amount of virus in the blood high.

Symptoms of HIV

Most people who carry the virus are initially symptom-free. Some appear to remain so for up to 15 years, or even longer. For some people, the first sign of being HIV-positive is when they have a flu-like illness, sometimes with a rash and swollen glands, lasting about two weeks. This usually occurs from two to six weeks after they have been exposed to the virus.

Once people become HIV-positive they may develop any of the following:
• *A red, greasy rash, usually affecting the face*
• *Oral thrush*
• *Shingles*
• *Runny nose*

• *Sinusitis*
• *Red and sometimes pus-filled pimples*
• *Mouth ulcers*
• *Tuberculosis*
• *Recurrent severe chest infections*
• *Genital herpes*
• *Abnormal cervical cells (shown on smear)*
• *Long-lasting shiny blisters with a central crater (a condition known as molluscum contagiosum, usually found in children)*
• *Diarrhoea*
• *Weight loss*
• *Cancerous tumours of the lymph nodes (lymphomas)*
• *Meningitis*

SEXUALLY TRANSMITTED DISEASES

GONORRHOEA

One of the most common sexually transmitted diseases, gonorrhoea is caused by a bacteria. It can affect the vagina, urethra (tube to the bladder), rectum, throat or eyes.

Anyone who suspects that they may have a sexually transmitted disease should either see their doctor or visit a genito-urinary clinic. Swabs (using cotton buds or similiar) will be taken from the vagina or penis. Gonorrhoea is sometimes not transmitted as the only infection and the doctor will ask if you would like to be checked for other sexually transmitted diseases at the same time. The others to be considered are hepatitis A, B and C, syphilis, thrush and HIV.

A woman who has gonorrhoea when she delivers her baby may,

inadvertently, spread the disease to the baby's eyes. Any eye infection in babies before the age of six weeks should be checked (using a swab) for gonorrhoea.

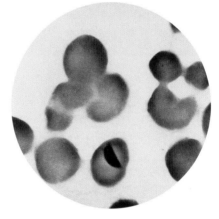

ABOVE *Gonorrhoea is a sexually transmitted infection caused by the Neisseria gonorrhoeae bacterium. It affects the cells in the genital mucous membranes, and can spread in the bloodstream to other parts of the body.*

LEFT *If you think you may have a sexually transmitted disease, seek medical advice to avoid spreading the illness.*

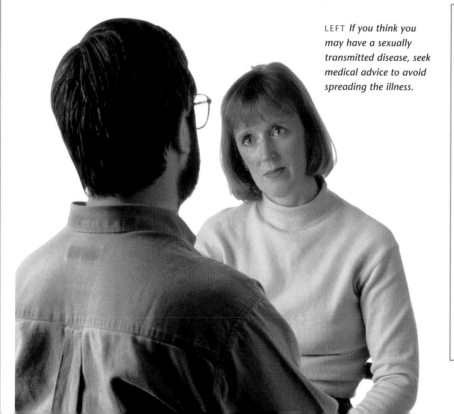

Symptoms of gonorrhoea

There may be none at all, but women may notice:

• *Vaginal discharge, which may be just more in volume, thin or green*
• *Pain on urination*
• *Sore throat*

Men may notice:

• *Yellowish discharge from the penis*
• *Pain on urination*
• *Anal itching*
• *Sore throat*

Treatment for gonorrhoea

Usually all that is required is a course of antibiotics to cure the disease. If the illness is left untreated because there are no signs or because people are too frightened to see a doctor, then it may lead to pelvic inflammatory disease and sterility in women. In men, the infection can spread to the testicles and prostate, causing pain, difficulty in passing urine and possible infertility. It is therefore essential to visit your doctor if you have any worries about your sexual health.

CHLAMYDIA

This is a bacterial infection caused by the bacterium *Chlamydia trachomatis* and it is thought to be the most common sexually transmitted disease in the UK. There has been a rapid increase in sufferers in recent years, which is probably because there may be no symptoms. Even though nothing may be obvious at the time of the infection, there can be very serious long-term health consequences.

What Causes Chlamydia?

Chlamydia is nearly always passed on by sexual intercourse. It can be transmitted from mother to baby at the

Symptoms of chlamydia

At least 50 per cent of men and maybe even more women have no symptoms. Chlamydia is often present with other sexually transmitted diseases and it is the symptoms of these that suggest chlamydia may be present. Occasionally there may be a discharge, lower abdominal pain, irregular periods or pain on urination. Symptoms of chlamydia may be similar in men and women.

time of birth. The newborn baby may show signs of having chlamydia in the first few days of life by developing an eye infection. Condoms, if used during every sexual occurrence, may help to prevent the spread of infection.

The Risks

Left untreated, chlamydial infection can lead to a number of serious health consequences, including infection of the reproductive organs and possible infertility. It is important that both partners are treated for the disease even if there are no symptoms.

- *pelvic inflammatory disease in women*
- *non-specific urethritis in men*
- *infection in babies, including eye disorders*
- *miscarriage*
- *infertility in women and possibly in men*
- *ectopic pregnancy, where the baby develops outside the womb; unlikely to result in a live birth*

Most common STDs

Sexually transmitted diseases, transmitted through sexual intercourse, are a major health issue and are on the increase owing to a switch away from monogamy to multiple sexual partners. The most common diseases include HIV, gonorrhoea, chlamydia, thrush and genital herpes. Different strains of hepatitis are also transmitted sexually. The symptoms may be so negligible that a carrier may not even realise he or she is infected.

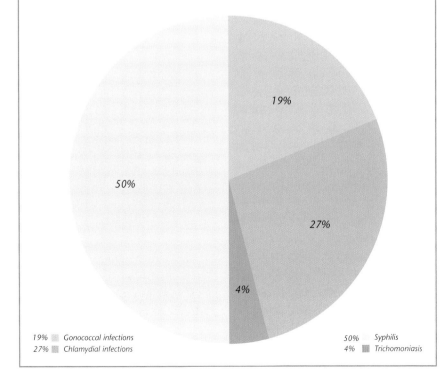

19%

50%

27%

4%

| 19% | Gonococcal infections | 50% | Syphilis |
| 27% | Chlamydial infections | 4% | Trichomoniasis |

Treatment for chlamydia

Treatment is available in the form of specific antibiotics but because chlamydia is often transmitted with other sexually transmitted diseases, it is best treated at a special clinic where tests for other infections can be done. The addresses of these clinics are available from your doctor or in the telephone book under NHS sexual health clinics.

FEMALE REPRODUCTIVE SYSTEM

The female reproductive system is the site of much distress and illness, from period pains to menopausal problems, but for many women the problems their female organs cause are outweighed by the joy of childbearing. Major landmarks include the contraceptive pill and improved procedures in childbirth. Cancer is still a major problem, some forms with a poor outlook.

PREMENSTRUAL SYNDROME (PMS)

This is the term used to describe the many forms of physical discomfort and emotional distress experienced by women in the runup to menstruation. By definition, this occurs only in women who have reached puberty, and usually happens in the 14 days before the period starts. Often it is a shorter time than this, sometimes lasting just a few days or a week before the period starts. To make this diagnosis, all the symptoms should disappear within a day of the period starting.

Symptoms of PMS

The following symptoms may occur:

• *Mood changes, especially anger and aggression*
• *Tension*
• *Depression*
• *Anxiety*
• *Sore breasts*
• *Headaches (often migrainous in character)*
• *Poor concentration*
• *Clumsiness*
• *Cravings for particular foods*
• *Fluid retention*

Self-Help

• *Keeping a diary and being aware of when your symptoms may occur is essential. Reducing activities and avoiding stress at this time can be especially beneficial.*
• *The diet needs to be well balanced, and rich in vegetables and fruit. Eat small, regular meals with good quantities of starches and proteins and try to consume as few sugary foods as possible (which can make the symptoms worse). Bananas, brown bread, rice and chicken are all beneficial foods. It is wise to avoid fatty foods and coffee, tea and cola.*
• *Anticipate your difficult days by minimising stress and travel and avoiding making vital decisions. Try resting or meditating for a period each day with a relaxation tape.*
• *Exercise can be helpful because it improves the circulation, relieves fluid retention and reduces stress levels but it is important to do regular and controlled exercise. It should be something you do regularly and easily each day, such as brisk walking or swimming.*
• *Extra vitamins and minerals may help with some of your symptoms but if your diet is sensible you should not need nutritional supplements.*
• *Take evening primrose oil every day for a minimum period of three months to assess whether it will help you. For some people the relief it brings is miraculous. For others the benefits are minimal.*

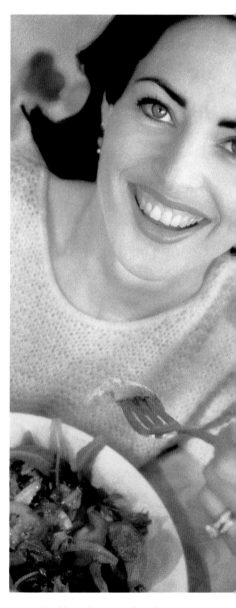

ABOVE *Healthy eating can reduce the symptoms of premenstrual syndrome, particularly if you avoid fatty, sugary foods and caffeine.*

Treatment for PMS

There is no one miracle medication that suits all. The following may be tried for a minimum of three months and frequently one of these will produce great improvements in symptoms.

- *the contraceptive pill*
- *oestrogen patches before the period*
- *progesterone, often in pessary form*
- *antidepressants for a week before the period*
- *particularly high doses of evening primrose oil*
- *some women respond well to vitamin B₆ supplements*

Evening primrose flowers

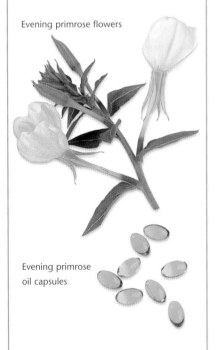

Evening primrose oil capsules

Evening primrose oil contains essential fatty acids that are thought to help reduce symptoms of bloating, water retention, stomach cramps, irritability and depression associated with PMS.

OVARIAN CYSTS

The ovaries are reproductive organs that produce female sex cells (known as eggs or ova). Many women develop growths or cysts on or within their ovaries. Ovarian cysts are sacs or cavities containing liquid or semi-solid matter, rather like a blister. Some cysts are completely harmless, others can be cancerous. There are two main types of ovarian cyst: functional (non disease-related) and abnormal.

What Causes Ovarian Cysts?

Ovarian cysts may happen at any time during childbearing years. Women usually have two ovaries that become active at the time of puberty. From then on, throughout a monthly cycle, the ovaries are bombarded by hormones from the pituitary gland. During the phases of the monthly cycle, eggs develop in sacs known as follicles, which ripen until they release

Symptoms of ovarian cysts
Warning signs include:

- *Sudden or intermittent abdominal pain (often to one side or other of the navel)*
- *Irregular periods*
- *Swollen abdomen*
- *Hirsutism (increased, masculine-type growth of body hair)*
- *Weight gain*
- *Acne*
- *Infertility*
- *Sudden, devastating pain on one side of the abdomen*

BELOW *A woman can suffer from various illnesses of the reproductive organs throughout her life and it is important to have regular health checks and screening for certain conditions to detect illnesses before they become serious.*

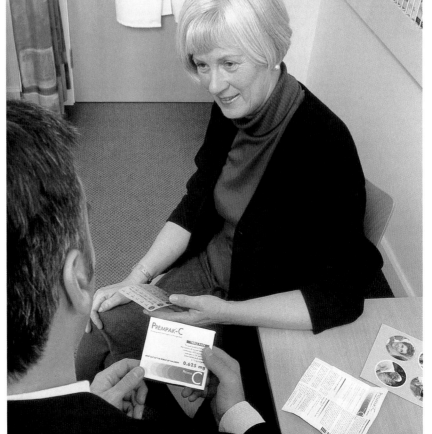

FEMALE REPRODUCTIVE SYSTEM

an egg. The majority of follicles do not mature and are reabsorbed by the body. Sometimes the follicle persists and forms a cyst instead. These are functional cysts, caused by a slight alteration in the normal function of the ovary, usually by hormonal imbalance.

Abnormal cysts result from abnormal cell growth, and it is not known why this happens.

Types of cyst

Many types of cyst grow in and on ovarian tissue. Some contain abnormal tissues such as teeth and hair and are known as dermoid cysts. Others secrete hormones and can cause serious illnesses. Some ovaries are covered with cysts and there may also be cysts on other organs such as the kidney and the pancreas. Almost every type of ovarian cyst needs to be investigated by a doctor.

In polycystic ovary syndrome (PCOS), the ova fail to mature and accumulate as cysts instead. This characteristically leads to increased weight gain, greasy hair, acne, hirsutism and infertility, though some women with polycystic ovaries have no symptoms.

The Problem with Cysts

An ovarian cyst may show up by chance when investigations are taking place for irregular periods or infertility. It may suddenly seem to grow and manifest as a rapidly swelling lump. Sometimes a cyst is discovered when there is sudden, severe abdominal pain, which may be caused by bleeding into the cyst, infection or rupture. A huge cyst may press on the bladder and cause symptoms there. Cancerous cysts are not uncommon and unless caught early the outlook is not good. They may be present for many months before showing any symptoms and therefore become difficult to treat.

Tests

Most ovarian cysts are benign or related to ovulation, but any irregular bleeding and pain should be reported to a doctor, who will carry out a pelvic examination. An ultrasound scan of the ovary to produce images of the interior of the body will almost certainly be needed. Specific blood tests can determine whether or not there are tumours in the ovary.

BELOW *In polycystic ovary syndrome, follicles in the ovaries fail to mature and remain as multiple cysts instead, usually because of slight hormonal imbalances. The first line of treatment is to administer appropriate hormones, in the form of oral contraceptives, patches, gels or capsules.*

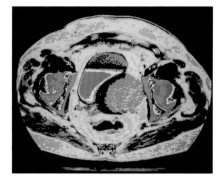

ABOVE *Ovarian cysts are fluid-filled swellings that grow in or on the ovaries. Most cysts are caused by hormonal imbalance and arise when follicles in which eggs mature continue to grow and fill with fluid.*

Treatment for ovarian cysts

• *This depends upon what sort of cyst is present. Most non-disease-related cysts clear up without treatment in a couple of months.*

• *Surgery for polycystic ovary syndrome is sometimes undertaken, but because this is a hormonal disorder, hormone manipulation in the form of oral contraception may be the first and best treatment.*

• *Many very large cysts require surgical removal, as do ovarian cysts that bleed or twist or cause pain. Cancerous cysts may need surgery to remove them, followed by drug treatment and sometimes radiotherapy.*

ENDOMETRIOSIS

The endometrium is the lining of the womb, or uterus. Sometimes it grows in other parts of a woman's body, especially inside the pelvic area. It can be found on the outside of the uterus, the bowel, the ovaries, the bladder, and on the membrane lining of the pelvis, where its presence is described as endometriosis. Typically this condition affects women in their early 20s and is not uncommon.

Symptoms of endometriosis

- *Painful periods*
- *Pain in the pelvis at non-period times*
- *Pain during sex*
- *Irregular bleeding*
- *Pain on defecation*
- *Infertility*

Not all women who suffer from endometriosis have symptoms. Some women will have severe pain with only small amounts of endometriosis.

The only way to be certain that endometriosis is the cause of the symptoms is for your doctor to send you to hospital for a laparoscopy. In this examination, while you are asleep, the surgeon will pass a fibre-optic tube into the cavity above the uterus to see if there are areas of endometrial tissue present. Once the condition is diagnosed treatment can start.

Sites of endometriosis

In endometriosis, tissue that normally lines the uterus spreads to other organs in the pelvic cavity, including the ovaries, Fallopian tubes, cervix, vagina and even the lower intestine. This tissue undergoes the same menstrual changes as the endometrium, causing painful periods and irregular bleeding. It may lead to fertility problems.

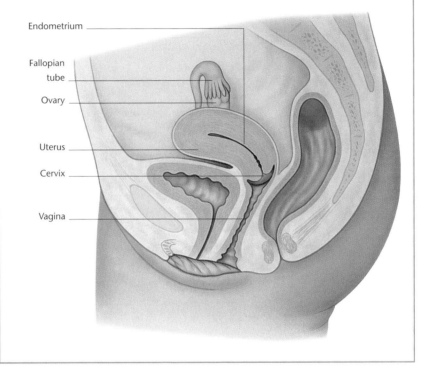

Endometrium

Fallopian tube

Ovary

Uterus

Cervix

Vagina

Treatment for endometriosis

- *This depends how bad the symptoms are, and whether or not infertility is a problem. If the main problem is pain, then painkillers may be appropriate to take as and when they are needed. The contraceptive pill will help most women with endometriosis but may take up to nine months to relieve the symptoms.*

- *Drugs may be prescribed to suppress the body's hormonal cycle but, depending on which ones are used, may have side-effects such as weight gain and excessive growth of facial and body hair.*

- *Surgery may be necessary for the most severe cases, particularly if infertility is a problem. Sometimes this can be done by laser treatment. Interestingly, some women's endometriosis will improve or even disappear after childbirth.*

FEMALE REPRODUCTIVE SYSTEM

UTERINE FIBROIDS

These are benign (non-cancerous) tumours that develop on the muscular wall of the uterus (womb). They can vary enormously in size, from smaller than a pea-sized lump to huge, heavy swellings that fill the whole of the uterus and weigh several pounds. It is estimated that 15–40 per cent of women have fibroids.

Symptoms of fibroids

- *heavy, long-lasting periods*
- *anaemia*
- *severe pain and pelvic cramps with periods*
- *swollen abdomen*
- *increased need to urinate*
- *infertility, if the fibroid is large and distorts the uterine cavity*

Treatment for fibroids

For heavy periods and cramps, anti-inflammatory tablets such as mefenamic acid may be extremely effective. These are taken two days before the period and for the first few days of bleeding. If heavy, painful periods persist and pregnancy is not an issue then intra-uterine contraceptive devices (IUCDs) may reduce the bleeding to little or nothing. Fibroids may be surgically shrunk or removed if they are particularly troublesome or thought to be interfering with fertility. If none of the above methods proves adequate then hysterectomy, when the whole uterus is removed, may be a last resort in older women whose families are complete, but this procedure is rarely necessary nowadays.

What causes fibroids?

It is not known what causes the tumour to appear in the first place but it does seem that the hormone oestrogen encourages their growth. Fibroids usually occur in women over 20 years old and can grow as long as the body produces oestrogen. Pregnancy, oral contraceptives and some forms of hormone replacement therapy may increase their size. Fibroids rarely occur singly, and often several are present. These uterine growths are much more common in women of Afro-Caribbean or Afro-American descent. If symptoms are a problem or are preventing conception fibroids can be removed surgically.

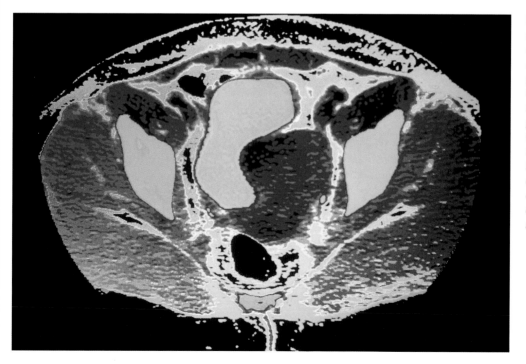

LEFT *This scan shows the presence of fibroids in the muscular wall of the uterus. Fibroids are non-malignant growths but if they are large they can cause heavy menstrual bleeding, pelvic pain and interfere with fertility. Fibroids appear to be linked to high oestrogen levels and may increase during times of pregnancy or when taking oral contraceptives or hormone replacement therapy.*

THRUSH

This is caused by a fungus called *Candida albicans*. Fungi, like mushrooms, like to grow in warm, dark, damp areas, which is why women commonly get the condition within the vagina. It also can occur in skin creases, especially under heavy breasts, in the groin, and in the crease between the bottom cheeks. Men can have the fungus on the tip of the penis.

Diagnosis and Treatment

Thrush is very common and usually easy to recognise. If there is any doubt then swabs can be sent to the laboratory where the condition can be confirmed. Treatment usually involves the use of an anti-fungal cream or pessary (to be inserted into the vagina) or capsule by mouth. Many of these are available over the counter directly from a pharmacy.

Some women have recurrent thrush and do not want to take medication all the time. Sometimes using live yogurt, especially if it is put on to a tampon and kept overnight in the vagina, may cure thrush. Taking frequent baths with vinegar in the water may also help. The condition may also get better on its own.

What Causes Thrush?

The fungus is present normally on most people's skin and in the mouth and gut. When the body is healthy, Candida is kept under control by the other organisms that live around it. However, if something happens to upset the balance of the bugs the body carries then Candida may take over and grow out of control. Overgrowth of Candida may be caused by one of the following:

- *Pregnancy*
- *Antibiotics*
- *Tight trousers or nylon underwear*
- *Cancer*
- *Chemotherapy or radiotherapy*
- *Diabetes*
- *Lowered immunity and generally being unwell*
- *Oral contraceptive pill*

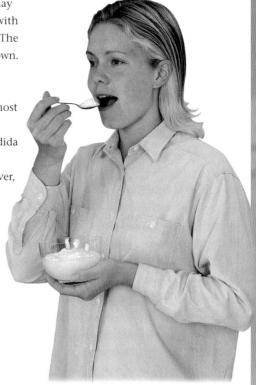

ABOVE *Live yoghurt contains healthy bacteria that will help prevent fungal infections and helps to restore the natural balance of micro-organisms in the digestive tract.*

- *Having sex with someone who has thrush*
- *Being very overweight with large skin creases*
- *Being breast-fed by a mother who has thrush*

Prevention

- *Women should wipe themselves from front to back*
- *Avoid tight, synthetic underwear*
- *Avoid using perfumes and strong soaps in the genital area*
- *Use sanitary towels rather than tampons*
- *Avoid intercourse if either you or your partner is sore*
- *Use condoms, especially if you have a new partner*
- *Do not take antibiotics unless you really need them*

Symptoms of thrush

In women the most common symptom is genital itching. There is often a thick white or creamy discharge. The area may become very swollen, sore and even bleed. Sexual intercourse may be painful, and there may be extreme pain on urination. Other symptoms include redness, itching and soreness in skin creases.

In men, when thrush attacks the penis, there may be no symptoms or the end of the penis may become red, sore and have white, scaly strips of skin which flake off. There may be a discharge, pain on urination and difficulty and soreness when the foreskin is retracted.

Women who are breast-feeding may get thrush around the nipples, making them very sore. Babies can contract oral thrush, manifested by white patches, typically around the inside of the mouth and on the tongue.

BREAST DISORDERS

The female breast consists of milk-producing glands (lobules) with ducts leading to the nipple. The glands are embedded in fatty tissue, which gives the breast its shape and size. The breasts undergo changes throughout life in response to varying levels of sex hormones, often accompanied by pain and lumpiness.

BREAST PAIN

This is very common and usually known as mastalgia. Only in about 5 per cent of cases of breast cancer is pain a feature. Unusually breast pain is harmless but it can cause great distress and interfere with everyday life. Most cases of breast pain happen within the monthly cycle, occurring in the week before the period is due. It may be associated with small pea-sized lumps in the breast.

Breast pain that occurs when breast-feeding may be due to infection, which will need antibiotics. This may occasionally occur at other times, often if there are cracked nipples. The breast becomes red and hot and a throbbing pain may be present.

Treatment for breast pain

• *Wearing a firm supportive bra, even at night*
• *Reassurance by a doctor or nurse who has done a proper and thorough examination*
• *Restricting caffeine intake*
• *A high-carbohydrate, low-fat diet may help*
• *Evening primrose oil in high doses over many months*
• *The combined contraceptive pill*
• *Prescription drugs and hormone injections*

BREAST LUMPS

These cause more distress in women than virtually any other condition. Every woman who feels a breast lump will immediately worry that she has breast cancer. Often lumps are benign (non-cancerous) but sometimes the anxiety that goes with the lump is very real and debilitating.

Variations within individuals

There is no doubt that women's breasts vary considerably in their consistency. Some breast tissue seems to be entirely made up of tiny lumps, while others have entirely smooth tissue. Some women have lumps that come and go with their monthly cycle and many doctors who think that a woman's breast lumps are harmless will ask for a return visit in two weeks' time to see if there is a variation within the monthly

LEFT *If you examine your breasts regularly you will notice if there is a change in the way they feel or look. It is important to detect potentially cancerous lumps, because the disease is more easily curable when found at an early stage. The best time to examine your breasts is just after a period.*

cycle. For some women, lumpy breasts are normal.

Isolated lumps, which are smooth, can be moved around and are not attached to surface skin or to deeper tissue are usually benign and are known as fibroadenomas.

Breast cysts are not uncommon, and can vary from tiny to the size of an orange. If a cyst is present, fluid is usually withdrawn from it so that cells can be examined in the laboratory. Very occasionally cysts are cancerous.

BREAST CANCER

The very thought of breast cancer strikes terror into most women. Any lump that is irregular in size, shape and consistency needs further investigation. Often a small piece of tissue will be removed under anaesthetic and the tissue analysed in the laboratory.

Prevention

In the UK the government has funded a national screening service, offered to all women between the ages of 50–64. Many women fail to be screened by mammography for many reasons: 'it hurts' (it is uncomfortable but a very small price to pay to pick up a cancer when it is curable); 'I don't want to know' (not knowing won't make it go away but knowing may put you in a position to save your life and lots of suffering); and 'I don't need to go as cancer doesn't run in the family' (you may be the first).

Self-examination of the breasts is very important. Your practice nurse or doctor will show you how to do this and helpful leaflets are available. Ideally, check your breasts once a month.

Treatment for breast cancer

• *The earlier a lump is found, in general, the more likely the treatment is to be successful. This is why it is essential to seek medical advice as soon as possible when any lump is found in the breast. Treatment may involve simply removing the lump with a small operation. Removing the breast (particularly if there is a large lump, or more than one, or if it is difficult to be sure that the whole lump has been removed) and sometimes removing the lymph nodes up into the armpit may be advised. Nowadays, in some cases, reconstruction of a new breast, using tissue from the back, is done at the same time as surgery or shortly after.*

• *Some patients will need the lump removed and/or radiotherapy. Radiotherapy is very carefully planned to do maximum damage to cancerous cells and minimal damage to surrounding tissue. This usually means daily visits over several weeks so that short, sharp bursts of radiation are given, and so that side-effects may be minimal. Sometimes there will be redness or nausea but generally radiotherapy is not too distressing.*

• *With some cancers of particular types, or if it has spread outside the breast, chemotherapy will be needed, usually with surgery and maybe radiotherapy, too. This is to enable the maximum chance of obliterating all the cancer cells from the body before they do damage elsewhere. Chemotherapy involves giving toxic medicines to try to kill the cancer cells. Almost inevitably there are some effects on the normal cells of the body. Side-effects may be minimal or very severe and distressing. Hair loss, nausea and generally feeling unwell are not uncommon. However, no doctor will suggest this treatment unless it is necessary and offers a considerable chance of helping beat the disease.*

• *Diet may be helpful with breast cancer and suggestions include eating lots of broccoli, cabbage, beans, soya, oily fish, wheat bran and tomatoes.*

• *Being of strong and determined mind has always been thought to increase the chances of recovering from breast cancer. The Cancer Clinic in Bristol pioneered this idea and has been very successful in helping many people.*

RIGHT *Fresh fruit and vegetables contain anti-oxidants that counteract free radicals, which damage cells. Pulses and wholegrains are high in fibre, helping to move food though the bowel so that toxins are not absorbed.*

FEMALE CANCERS

There is little doubt that cancer is an ever increasing cause of death. There are many possible causes for this: fewer deaths from infection so people live longer, better diagnosis of cancer, increasing numbers of smokers, the long-term effects of exposure to pollution and probably the ingestion of more carcinogens in our food.

OVARIAN CANCER

There are over 7,000 deaths from this disease each year in the UK. The survival rate five years after diagnosis is only 30 per cent.

What Causes Ovarian Cancer?

There are several factors that are thought to increase the risk of developing this disease. They include: having fewer babies or no children; bottle- rather than breast-feeding; and possibly infertility treatment and family history.

Factors that reduce the risk of developing ovarian cancer include: having children at an early age; having more babies; breast-feeding; and taking the contraceptive pill.

Diagnosis

Scanning of the ovaries using an ultrasound probe in the vagina to see the ovaries most clearly is essential. A blood test that measures the level of a protein called CA125 will also help to detect the disease. Using the two tests together will help to pick up even more cases earlier.

Symptoms of ovarian cancer

Often symptoms are late in showing themselves, which means the disease is diagnosed at an advanced stage and may be why treatment is not that successful. The usual symptoms are common in middle-aged women and include abdominal swelling, abdominal pain, nausea, bloating and weight loss.

Treatment for ovarian cancer

The earlier the diagnosis is made, the more successful the treatment. If the condition is confined to the ovaries then surgical removal can cure the illness. If the disease has spread, radiotherapy and chemotherapy may be used. The later the detection of the disease and the more widespread the condition, the less hopeful is the outlook.

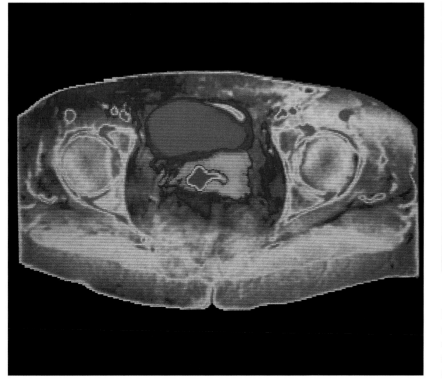

LEFT *This colour-enhanced MRI scan shows a large cancerous tumour (green) lying just beneath the bladder (purple). If cervical cancer is diagnosed and treated early, nearly all women recover completely.*

CERVICAL CANCER

Deaths from cervical cancer are declining due to nationwide screening. Most women affected by cervical cancer are between 40 and 70 but very young teenagers have been known to suffer from the condition.

If there is abnormal bleeding, then it is essential to report this to the doctor who, if you have not had a cervical smear, will examine you and send a smear off to the laboratory. Usually cervical cancer is slow growing and regular smears will pick it up at an early stage before it has time to become invasive and spread to other organs.

Prevention

The chances of getting cervical cancer are increased by:

- *Smoking*
- *Early sexual experiences*
- *Many partners*
- *Abnormal sexual practices*
- *Not having cervical smears*

Symptoms of cervical cancer

These are rare, which is why screening by cervical smear is essential. Sometimes there may be an abnormal discharge, or there may be irregular bleeding, especially after sex. After the menopause, bleeding is a very important symptom.

Diet may be important, and garlic, soya, vegetables, citrus fruit, fish, milk and tea are said to reduce the risk. cancers in general.

UTERINE CANCER

Most uterine cancers arise from the lining or endometrium. Very occasionally, a fibroid will give rise to uterine cancer. It causes about 3 per cent of female deaths each year and usually affects post-menopausal women.

Three-quarters of all women who get uterine cancer are over 50 when they are diagnosed. Earlier detection by examination when women start very abnormal bleeding in their 40s may help to reduce the death rate by catching the cancer earlier. Obesity is one of the known factors that increases the risk of developing uterine cancer.

Symptoms of uterine cancer

- *Post-menopausal bleeding*
- *Abnormal vaginal bleeding at any age*
- *Very heavy bleeding*
- *Constant bleeding*
- *Period-type pains*

Diagnosis and treatment for cervical cancer

- *If a smear is done and abnormal cells found, the next step is usually a visit to the hospital for a colposcopy. Colposcopy is where a speculum (the same as used for having a smear) is put in place to hold the vagina open. Then, using a powerful microscope, the cervix is stained and abnormal cells show up. Often treatment is performed there and then. The cervix is numbed using a small injection and the affected area will be burned or cut away, often with a laser. Other methods of getting rid of the cells are also used. After that the condition may well be cured, and apart from having more regular smears, that is the end of it.*

- *If the area of abnormality is large and long-standing (which usually only occurs in those who have not had regular smears), then surgery to remove diseased tissue or even a hysterectomy may be needed. If it has spread from outside of the cervix and womb, then radiotherapy and/or chemotherapy may be required and the outlook is much less certain.*

Treatment for uterine cancer

As with most of the other gynaecological cancers, once diagnosed the usual sequence of treatment is surgery to remove the uterus and ovaries. Chemotherapy and radiotherapy may be needed.

MALE CANCERS

Men are prey to three types of exclusive cancer: prostate, penile and testicular.
Prostate cancer typically attacks the older man; penile cancer is rare while
testicular cancer is increasingly common in the 20–45 years age group.
The sooner these illnesses are diagnosed, the more promising is the outlook.

The prostate gland

The prostate gland is an organ about the size of a walnut that surrounds and opens into the urethra, the tube that connects the bladder to the outside of the body. The prostate adds fluid to semen to help the sperm swim and to keep them healthy. Enlargement of the prostate is common with age. A doctor can check if the prostate is enlarged or lumpy by performing a digital rectal examination, inserting a gloved finger into the rectum to feel the prostate.

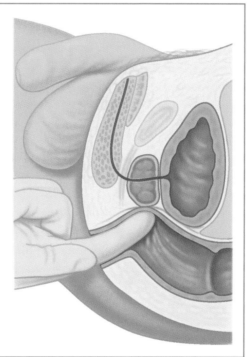

Tests and treatment

A doctor may perform a blood test to check the level of PSA (prostate specific antigen), which is raised in prostatic cancer. If the level is normal and the gland feels smooth but enlarged, tablets may be prescribed to help shrink the prostate. However, if the gland is lumpy and/or the PSA level is raised, you will undoubtedly need to see a urologist for expert advice and treatment. Treatment is usually a choice of surgery or radiotherapy. The urologist will guide you as to the best option for you. If the prostate cancer has been caught early then the outlook is extremely good. Many men live a full and normal life span after prostate cancer. Only if it has spread to the bones is it more difficult to treat.

PROSTATE CANCER

This typically affects men over 60 and may be heralded by symptoms of enlargement of the prostate gland. Often there is frequency, where you feel you have to pass urine many times but the stream is poor and only a little urine is produced. As soon as you've urinated you may feel as if you need to go again. Occasionally there may be blood in the urine. Similar problems occur at night with frequent wakening and passing of small dribbles of urine. This may be due to an enlarged prostate or due to prostate cancer. Either way, it is essential to visit your

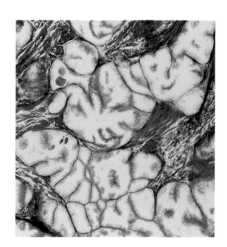

ABOVE *This tissue sample shows cancerous cells in the prostate gland. Symptoms arise when the tumour starts to constrict the urethra, and may include an increased need to urinate.*

doctor who will examine you by placing a gloved finger into the rectum. From here the doctor can feel the prostate gland, which may be enlarged and smooth, or lumpy, which tends to be more worrying.

Self-examination

• Examine the testicles after a warm bath or shower. This tends to relax the scrotum, in which the testicles sit.
• Look in the mirror first and see if you notice any difference from the last time you looked. Most men have one testicle that hangs lower than the other. Providing this is your normal appearance, all is fine.
• Feel the outline of the testicle through the scrotum. It should be smooth, soft and oval in shape.
• Across the top of the testicle and running down the back is the epididymis, the tube that carries the sperm from the testicles down to the penis. It feels a little like spaghetti but it should be soft.
• Consult your doctor immediately if there is any change in the appearance or texture of the scrotum or testes.

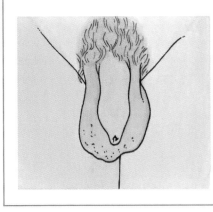 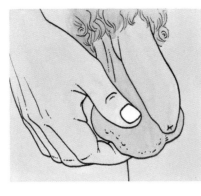

TESTICULAR CANCER

This form of cancer most often affects young men between the ages of 20 and 40, and it is vital to diagnose it early, as it is curable. You need to examine yourself, or ask your partner to do monthly examinations for you.

Symptoms of testicular cancer

• If the testicles do not appear to hang normally when you look in the mirror.
• If one testicle appears to be hanging in a different position.
• If there appears to be any change in testicle shape or size.
• If the testicle has any hard or firm patches in or around it.
• Pain in the testicles, groin or backache spreading to the scrotum.
• Any patches or sores on the penis that fail to heal.

Treatment for testicular cancer

If the doctor has any concerns, the next step may well be an ultrasound scan of the testes. This is painless and usually clearly highlights any tumours. Surgery may be necessary if cancer of the testes is diagnosed but if it is caught early it can be cured.

Any man who has the slightest worry should see his doctor or visit a sexual health (GUM) clinic as soon as possible. Generally it is the men who have held back because of embarrassment who end up with major problems, and it is better to be a little embarrassed than die from a curable condition.

PENILE CANCER

This is a rare illness. The first sign is a sore, often towards the end of the penis, which does not heal but continues to grow. The glands in the groin may also swell. Sores on the penis always need medical attention. Surgery or radiotherapy may be required but the earlier the treatment, the less likely there are to be long-term problems. If in doubt, see the doctor and get help before it becomes serious.

OTHER MALE CANCERS

Men are more at risk of developing cancer of the lung, stomach, skin, stomach, oesophagus and bowel. Smoking is thought to increase the risk of all cancers but particularly lung, voice box and oesophageal cancer. All of these are particularly difficult to treat. When the sun is shining, men are less likely than women to apply a lotion with a sun protection factor. This increases the risks of developing skin cancer, or malignant melanoma, which can rapidly be fatal. All suspect moles should be checked by your doctor.

PART FIVE

MEDICAL CARE, TESTS, TREATMENTS AND MEDICINES

CONTENTS

INTRODUCTION

This part of the book describes the basics of medical care, including various tests, methods of treatment and medicines that are routinely prescribed. It explains how common imaging techniques work and why they are used. There is also an article on examinations you can perform yourself, such as monitoring your weight, pulse and blood sugar levels.

The first part of this chapter explains what happens when you visit your doctor and the basic physical examination you may undergo.

A doctor will assess main body systems such as the heart, lungs and nervous system, and information on the techniques and equipment used is given. Sometimes all a doctor will need to reach a diagnosis is an assessment of your symptoms but in other cases further tests will be needed.

There are numerous tests routinely carried out to investigate disease, and this section explains the most common ones used to help a doctor reach a diagnosis. Blood tests are frequently used to look for disease and to assess general health. The various types of blood test include measuring the amounts of particular blood components and investigating their structure to help diagnose a wide range of disorders. Urine and stool tests are also useful diagnostic tools.

Different tests can be carried out at the doctor's surgery or may require investigation in a laboratory, where they are analysed by machines.

Laboratory analysis of fluid or tissue samples is one of the most important ways of confirming the diagnosis of an illness. A wide range of genetic conditions can also be identified by laboratory tests.

Various types of screening can pick up diseases before they become serious. Detecting a disease in its early stages can mean the difference between life and death. Articles on mammography and cervical screening explain the procedures and why they are so important for women's health. Heart disease is the major cause of death in the UK, and information is given on how it is diagnosed.

Imaging techniques are used to help arrive at a diagnosis if the results of other tests are unclear. X-rays are the oldest form of imaging technique. Computer-aided techniques include ultrasound, computerised tomography and magnetic resonance imaging. A particular technique may be more suitable for a specific part of the body. There are also different risks and levels of discomfort associated with various techniques.

Many disorders require more than medication to be cured, and there is a section that explains why surgery may be carried out, what happens and what the outlook is. Cosmetic surgery is becoming more and more commonplace, and the reasons why you may choose to have it done and what the disadvantages may be are discussed.

Finally, information is given on how to use and store medication safely. There is also an explanation of how common drugs work and their possible side-effects.

WHEN TO SEE THE DOCTOR

In the UK, the first point of contact when seeking health care is the family GP, or doctor, even if you wish to pursue private treatment. There are around 34,000 GPs, each responsible, on average, for about 1,800 patients. Most consultations last around seven to ten minutes, so it is important to have a clear reason in mind when attending.

REASONS FOR SEEING A DOCTOR

Generally, most people attend their GP for one of three reasons. The first of these is during an episode of sudden illness, to try to find out what the illness is, and whether treatment is required. Fortunately, many of these illnesses clear up on their own, and require only relief of symptoms. Examples include coughs and colds, flu, backache and gastroenteritis. Many people are happy to manage these illnesses at home, perhaps with the help of their local pharmacist, without visiting the doctor.

Secondly, a large number of consultations is now taken up with seeing people who have a long-standing (chronic) medical condition, which requires periodic monitoring. Illnesses in this group comprise ailments such as raised blood pressure (hypertension), asthma, diabetes and heart disease. With improved detection of these conditions, the numbers of sufferers have increased markedly, leading to a situation where trained nurses within special clinics in the surgery now carry out many of the consultations.

The final reason for attending the doctor's surgery is the one we will concentrate on, and concerns those patients who are generally well, but have noticed some change within their

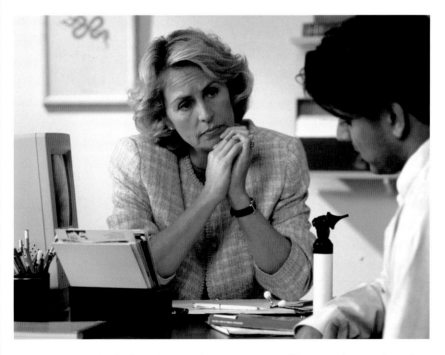

ABOVE *A person visits the doctor in times of sudden illness, if he has a long-standing condition that needs regular monitoring, or if he notices a change in the normal functioning of his body and is concerned by this.*

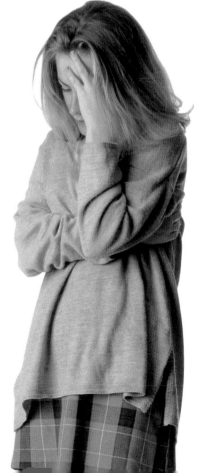

RIGHT *Many illnesses, such as coughs and colds, backache and stomach upsets, can be managed at home without needing to see a doctor, but if symptoms persist then you should seek medical advice.*

Checking blood pressure

Measuring blood pressure is a normal part of any medical examination. A cuff is wrapped around your arm and inflated by squeezing a bulb. The cuff is slowly deflated while the doctor listens to the bloodflow in an artery in your arm using a stethoscope. Arterial blood pressure rises as the heart pumps blood out (systolic pressure) but lowers when the heart fills with blood (diastolic pressure). Systolic and diastolic pressure are expressed in units of millimetres of mercury (mmHg), recorded by a measuring device (sphygmomanometer). Blood pressure rises with activity but in a healthy young adult at rest is usually 120/80 mmHg. It also increases with age and weight.

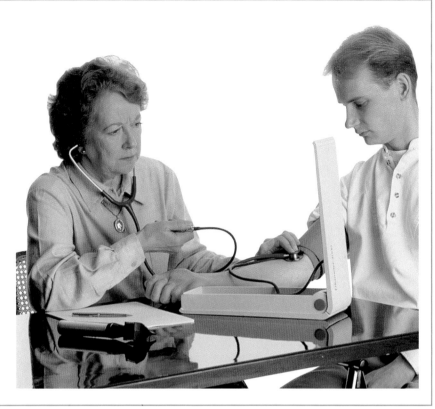

normal pattern of body rhythms or functions. The following paragraphs deal with symptoms and signs, which may indicate some form of serious illness, although the presence of such changes does not necessarily imply that a sinister cause is responsible.

WEIGHT CHANGES

Most people experience fluctuations in weight, but changes that happen in a reasonably short period of time, in the absence of dieting or increased calorie intake, should be reported to your doctor. Weight loss is sometimes the earliest symptom of disorders of the digestive system, for example, cancer, or inflammation of the bowel lining. Even without other symptoms being present, this is an important pointer. Weight gain can occasionally signal hormonal problems, although it is more often due to increasing age and loss of fitness levels.

PAIN

Persistent pain of any sort that is not easily explained by a specific injury should not be ignored. Sudden chest pain, in particular, should be regarded as an emergency and, generally, an ambulance should be called. Pain in the abdomen, headache or back pain, if sudden in onset or severe in nature, requires medical attention.

BOWEL MOVEMENTS

Diarrhoea or constipation that lasts for more than a week or two, and is not due to an obvious infection or change in diet, should trigger a check-up with your doctor. This is particularly important if there is any evidence of bleeding from the intestines. Bleeding may be obvious, with bright red blood on the toilet paper, or in the lavatory bowl. Often, however, the bleeding is hidden (occult), being mixed with the faeces high up in the digestive tract,

leading to a dark brown, or black, tarry stool known as malaena. This should never be ignored. When bleeding from other body openings, such as blood in the urine, coughing up blood, or vomiting blood, it is always vital to consult with your doctor.

TIREDNESS

Unexplained fatigue, or general malaise without an obvious cause such as a viral infection, can be due to a number of potentially serious causes, and should be investigated by a doctor if it does not go away on its own.

LUMPS

Finally, the discovery of a lump, in particular in the breast in women or in the testes in men, is potentially a tumour, and must be checked out as soon as possible. Similarly, pain in the breast or testes should also be investigated.

SELF-EXAMINATIONS

At most consultations with your doctor, a number of instruments and pieces of equipment will be used to measure many of your body's functions. The various types of apparatus used during a consultation are not generally available, and even if they were, they would be completely useless in the hands of the average person. However, there are some examinations that you can perform in the comfort of your own home, with the minimum of effort, which can help you see if there are problems with your health.

MEASURING BODY WEIGHT

Body weight is probably the simplest thing to determine. Although this is a very basic measurement, there are a few easy steps that should be followed to ensure that an accurate and meaningful result is obtained. This is particularly important if you wish to monitor your weight as part of a healthy eating and exercise regime.

An accurate set of scales is essential, and a set routine makes comparison from reading to reading more valuable. It is best to pick a particular time of day – first thing in the morning may be most convenient – and stick to the same day each week. As weight can vary considerably from day to day, checking your weight each day can be demoralising. Wear the same clothes, or better still, weigh yourself in a bathrobe or nothing at all.

A more helpful measurement of whether you are maintaining a healthy body weight is body mass index (BMI), which is an internationally recognised measurement determined by dividing your weight in kilograms by the square of your height in metres. As frame sizes vary, and there is no way of accurately working out a person's frame, then the BMI gives a range of weights to aim for. A healthy body weight is defined as a

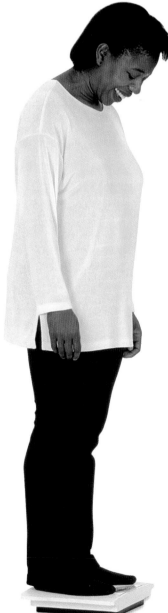

BMI of between 20 and 25. For more information, see *Finding the Right Weight*, pages 240–41.

PULSE RATE

The resting pulse rate can be used as a measure of fitness and cardiovascular (heart and blood vessels) health (see *Aerobic Activities*, pages 248–49). The pulse is best felt at the wrist, on the palm side of the forearm, about a centimetre (½ inch) below the base of the thumb. Using the second hand of a watch, the number of beats in a 15-second interval is recorded, and this figure is multiplied by four to obtain the number of beats per minute.

Generally, the normal pulse rate is between 60 and 70. Rates as low as 50 can be normal in trained athletes, but if the pulse is lower than 50, it may indicate a problem with the electrical conduction system of the heart. A rapid resting pulse sometimes indicates an overactive thyroid gland (the organ responsible for controlling the body's metabolic rate, see pages 202–3). Different types of rapid heart rate can

LEFT *You can monitor your weight at home with a set of scales. Weigh yourself once a week at the same time of day to see whether you are maintaining, gaining or losing weight.*

Checking blood glucose levels

If you have diabetes you need to maintain the level of glucose in the blood within the normal range, and you will have to take responsibility for monitoring your glucose levels and adjusting your diet and medication as needed. You can monitor your blood glucose levels at home by applying a drop of blood to a chemically impregnated strip and then using a digital meter to check the reaction. Monitor your levels at least once a day.

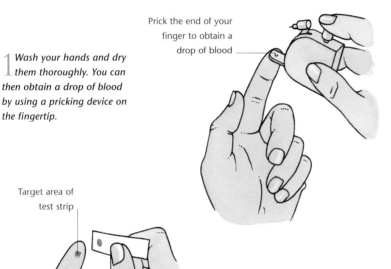

Prick the end of your finger to obtain a drop of blood

1 *Wash your hands and dry them thoroughly. You can then obtain a drop of blood by using a pricking device on the fingertip.*

Target area of test strip

2 *Cover the drop of blood with the target area of the chemically impregnated test strip. Wait for as long as is recommended by the instructions that come with the meter (generally about 60 seconds).*

Digital display gives a reading of the blood glucose level

3 *Insert the test strip into the digital meter. The meter analyses the blood sample and gives an almost instantaneous reading of the glucose level.*

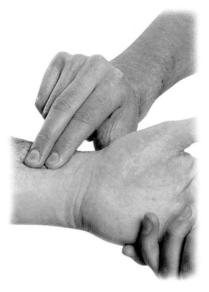

ABOVE *To check the pulse rate, place two fingers about 1 cm (½ in) below the wrist joint and count the number of beats felt in 15 seconds. Multiply this number by four.*

be detected by this method, which is particularly helpful for your doctor if you suffer from intermittent palpitations.

With the advent of less expensive automatic machines for testing blood pressure, many people can monitor their own readings at home. This may be of benefit if the diagnosis of raised blood pressure is uncertain. However, although the newer machines are easy to use, their accuracy is sometimes debatable. For this reason, if a reading is obtained that is particularly high, it is important to sit quietly for a few minutes and then repeat the measurement. If results are consistently high, advice should be sought from your doctor.

BLOOD SUGAR

It is also possible for patients suffering from diabetes to check blood sugar levels using simple monitoring machines, and for most diabetics this is part of their daily routine. It is particularly helpful if patients are taking different amounts of insulin throughout the day.

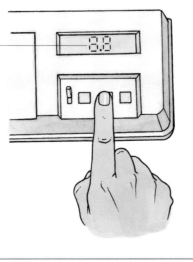

THE ROUTINE PHYSICAL

If you are visiting your doctor with a specific problem, the extent of the physical examination that takes place will be determined by what you have discussed during the consultation. For some illnesses, your doctor will need to look at a number of the body's systems, whereas for others, no examination of any kind is necessary.

BASIC OBSERVATIONS

If a full examination does take place, then it is likely that some basic observations will have been made before the doctor starts. For example, the doctor will have observed whether you look pale, suggesting anaemia, or yellow, signifying jaundice, or whether there is any sign of poor circulation, visible in blueish or white discoloration of the hands, or a blue tinge to the lips, known as cyanosis.

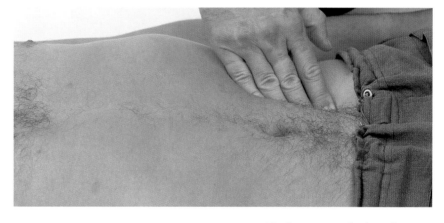

ABOVE *The doctor presses firmly on the abdomen with one or two hands to detect tender or enlarged internal organs or swellings.*

LEFT *By pressing his fingers across the patient's back the doctor can determine if there is any fluid around the lungs.*

Fingers are used to produce sounds that indicate the state of the lungs

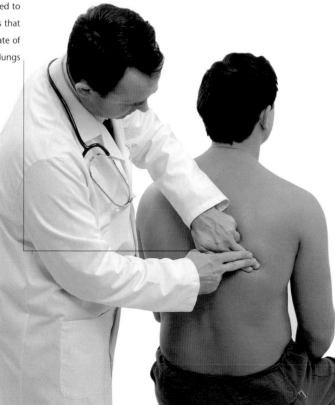

CHECKING THE HEART AND BLOOD VESSELS

The heart and blood vessels can be assessed by taking the pulse, usually at the wrist, and measuring how fast the heart is beating and whether the beat is regular. Pulses at the groin, behind the knee, behind the ankle bone and on top of the foot can be used to check the circulation in the legs. Blood pressure is measured, and the doctor will listen to the heart with a stethoscope to assess the noises made as the valves open and close (the heart sounds), and to see if there is any irregular blood flow through the heart, heard as a 'murmur'.

EXAMINING THE LUNGS

Lung function is tested by listening to several deep breaths through the stethoscope, and by determining if there is any fluid around the lungs by a test called percussion. This involves splaying one hand across the chest wall and tapping an outstretched finger with a finger from the other hand. If the sound is hollow, there is no fluid present.

NERVOUS SYSTEM

The nervous system is examined by assessing the reactions of the pupils, and by checking that the eye movements are full. The muscles of the face are tested to make sure that the movement is the same on both sides. Muscle power and tone in the arms and legs are assessed, and the reflexes in the wrist, around the elbow, the knees and ankles are tested by tapping with a tendon hammer.

ABDOMEN

Finally, the abdomen is examined to check for enlargement of its internal organs – the liver, spleen, kidneys and, in women, the pelvic organs. The activity of the digestive system is assessed by listening to the rumbling sounds produced through the stethoscope. Sometimes other tests may be included, such as a pelvic or rectal examination, or a breast check.

MEDICAL HISTORY

Medical students are taught that 80 per cent of the information needed to make a diagnosis comes from talking to the patient. The other 20 per cent comes from examination and tests. This verbal interchange is called 'taking a history'.

Doctors obtain the history by asking some direct questions requiring a yes or no answer, or more often by picking up on what the patient has said and asking questions that allow the patient to

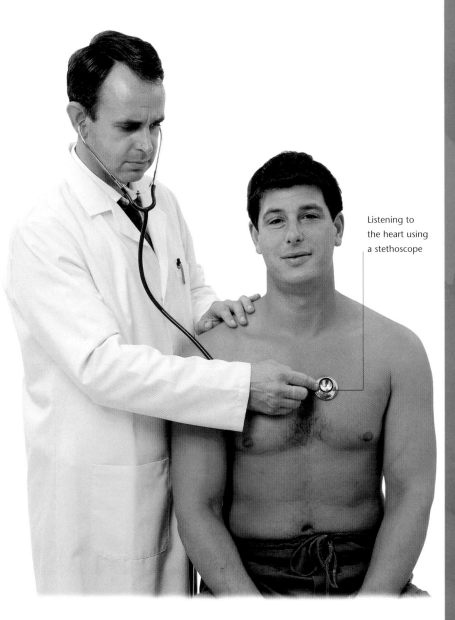

Listening to the heart using a stethoscope

provide more information in her own time. Never be worried about telling your doctor something that you feel may be irrelevant because sometimes a small detail in the history gives a vital clue to the diagnosis. Doctors are trained to trawl through all the bits of information and extract the important parts, so for that reason, it is essential that you try to answer any questions as fully as you can.

Although communication between doctors and patients is much better nowadays, it may sometimes feel as if

ABOVE *A doctor listens to sounds within the chest such as those made by the heart valves as they open and close. The doctor interprets the sounds to assess whether they are normal.*

you are both talking different languages. If there is something you do not understand, ask your doctor to repeat it or explain in a more basic fashion. Finally, remember that anything you say to your doctor is in the strictest confidence, and that this right to confidentiality will be wholeheartedly respected.

GENETIC TESTING

The normal human cell contains 23 pairs of chromosomes, each comprising thousands of genes that determine who we are and how the body works. Genetic material on a chromosome is composed of a single strand of deoxyribonucleic acid (DNA), coiled and folded to produce a compact structure. The complete complement of human genes, known as the genome, has now been discovered and mapped out. Sometimes genetic material is faulty, leading to a disorder or an increased risk of a particular illness. The development of sophisticated tests has meant that a wide range of genetic abnormalities can be identified.

WHY GENETIC TESTING IS DONE

Genetic testing examines the genetic information contained inside a person's cells to determine if that person has or will develop a certain disease or could pass a disease to his offspring. As each person has a unique set of DNA (except for identical twins), genetic tests are also used for individual identification – so-called DNA fingerprinting. This is used in forensic medicine, and for legal reasons in cases of establishing paternity.

HOW GENETIC TESTING IS DONE

Genetic testing involves examining a person's DNA, which, in the majority of cases, will entail having a blood test. However, cellular material containing DNA can be obtained from other bodily fluids such as saliva and semen, as well as from structures such as hair or skin.

Genetic testing is a complex process involving a number of stages. It requires accurate laboratory tests and reliable interpretation of results by a trained geneticist. Tests can vary in their sensitivity, and in the rate of false positives (people the test predicts will

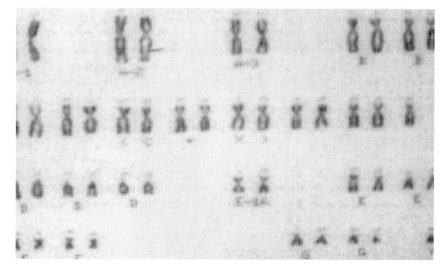

have the disorder who will be free of it) and false negatives (those given the all-clear who actually have the condition). Sometimes, close family members may also need to have the test carried out.

REASONS FOR TESTING

Individuals may decide to submit to genetic testing in a number of given situations.

Firstly, a person may be concerned that, although personally healthy, he or she might carry the genetic defect for a condition that runs in the family,

ABOVE *There are 23 pairs of thread-like chromosomes in the nucleus of every body cell, except sex cells. They contain the information that controls growth and functioning.*

for example cystic fibrosis, or a blood condition such as sickle-cell anaemia (see page 394). This is known as carrier identification.

Secondly, if an unborn child is suspected of harbouring a genetic defect, either because of family history, or because of the age of the mother, then prenatal testing is possible. Cells are obtained from the foetus early in the

The structure of DNA

Genes determine how the body works and who we are. Every cell in the body apart from the red blood cells contains a set of genes made of DNA (deoxyribonucleic acid). Two chains of DNA are shaped like a twisted ladder to form a double helix shape, with rungs of units called nucleotide bases linked together in pairs. The arrangement of nucleotides gives the cells instructions on building proteins, needed for growth and development.

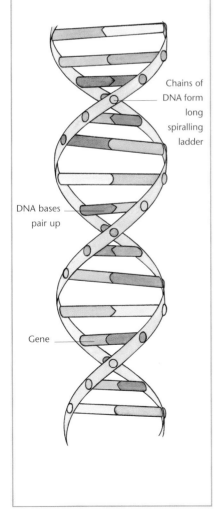

Chains of DNA form long spiralling ladder

DNA bases pair up

Gene

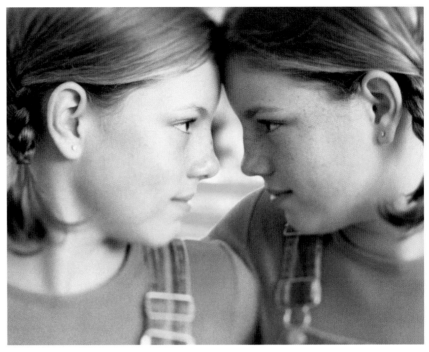

ABOVE *A third of all twins are identical. This happens when an egg divides in half after fertilisation. They are of the same sex and genetically exactly the same.*

pregnancy (either from foetal cells in the placenta or from skin cells taken from the amniotic fluid), allowing a diagnosis to be made and a decision over whether or not to continue with the pregnancy. The most common condition tested for in this way is Down's syndrome.

Thirdly, if a child is born with physical abnormalities, or learning difficulties that are not immediately identifiable, genetic testing is used to clarify the condition and allow appropriate treatment.

Fourthly, there is a number of medical conditions caused by a single gene defect that only appear later in life, with the sufferer seemingly well until the onset of symptoms. A good example is Huntington's disease, a devastatingly severe illness arising in middle age, leading to dementia and premature death. The gene defect responsible can be detected at any age.

Finally, as research progresses, a number of gene mutations (altered DNA fragments) have been identified that could be linked to an inherited tendency to certain cancers. Genetic

mutations may be responsible for 5–10 per cent of all cancers, and it is thought that around one in 300 women carry the altered genes that make them more likely to develop breast cancer.

CONSIDERATIONS BEFORE TESTING

While advances are made in this field, and genetic testing becomes more widespread, there is a number of issues that must be addressed. Anybody considering genetic testing should be thoroughly counselled with regard to the accuracy of the test, the likelihood the disease will develop if the test is positive, and the effect the result will have on that person's life and family. Employment and insurance issues should also be thought through. If testing does take place, it should only be with the written, informed consent of all parties involved.

EYE AND HEARING TESTS

You should have a vision test every two years, particularly if you are over the age of forty, to assess the sharpness of your vision and your ability to focus on near objects. If you wish to undergo a comprehensive eye test, you will need to make an appointment with an optician or an optometrist. Hearing disorders are common, and in severe cases may interfere with communication and social interaction. Sometimes the cause will be obvious, for example a build-up of wax in the ear canal, or the result of a heavy cold. If no cause is found, you will probably be referred for a hearing test, or audiogram.

EYE TESTS

Depending upon your reasons for having an eye test, whether it is because your vision has changed, or just a routine check-up, a complete eye examination will take up to 30 minutes. If abnormalities are discovered, then additional tests may be required.

HISTORY

The standard eye tests are split into a number of elements. Firstly, the optician will take a history of your eye problems, even if you have no symptoms but are attending for a routine review. If you are experiencing problems with your eyes or vision, your optician will need to know what symptoms you have, for how long you have had them and whether any changes have happened suddenly, or over a period of time.

Additionally, information about your general health, medication you may be taking, whether you have symptoms such as headaches, and what spectacles or contact lenses you wear (if any) is essential for your optician to make an accurate assessment of your eyes. Finally,

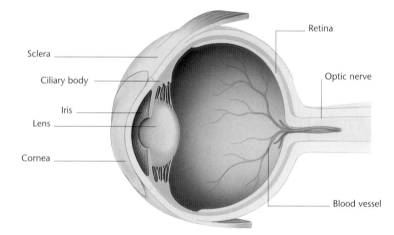

ABOVE *The structure of the eye. We have vision when light reflects from an object and enters the eye through the cornea. Light focuses on the retina where rays are turned into electrical impulses, which travel to the brain via the optic nerve.*

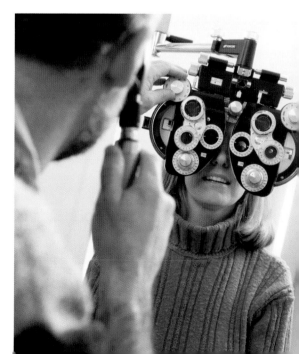

RIGHT *Eye tests are carried out by an optician to check for vision problems such as shortsightedness, longsightedness and distorted vision. A device known as a phoropter holds different lenses in front of each eye, allowing the eyes to be tested separately. Lenses are changed until you can read the letters near the bottom of the Snellen chart.*

details of any close relatives with eye or general health problems, such as glaucoma (raised pressure in the eyes), diabetes (raised blood sugar) or hypertension (high blood pressure) will complete the optician's questioning.

EXAMINATION

The second part of the eye test is the examination of the eyes, both externally and internally. Usually, the sharpness of your eyesight, known as visual acuity (VA), is checked using a Snellen chart, comprising of random letters in a variety of sizes. Normal VA, or 20/20 vision, is the ability to read letters ½ cm (⅜ in) high at a distance of 20 feet. If the vision is less than 20/20, then a refraction test takes place, where lenses of differing strengths are placed in front of the eyes to improve vision.

Following a light through the field of vision tests the external movements of the eyes. The reactions of the pupils are checked by noting the change in size in response to a bright light. The internal structures of the eye such as the lens and the retina (the light-sensitive layer inside the back of the eye) are checked using an ophthalmoscope, a device with a bright light and magnifier. Cataracts, or early changes due to diabetes or high blood pressure, are identified in this way.

Finally, if glaucoma is suspected, a device called a tonometer that fires a puff of air against the eye can measure the pressure in the eyeball. Along with pressure measurements, the field of vision in each eye is mapped out by observing randomly flashing lights, designed to distinguish early blind spots.

HEARING TESTS

A hearing test might be carried out at hospital, or at a hearing aid dispensary.

Ear tests

The ear canal and ear-drum can be examined by using an otoscope, which magnifies the inside of the ear. The ear is pulled up and back to straighten the ear canal, then the otoscope is inserted. This procedure is used to identify a ruptured ear-drum or glue ear.

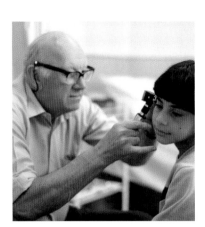

The structure of the ear

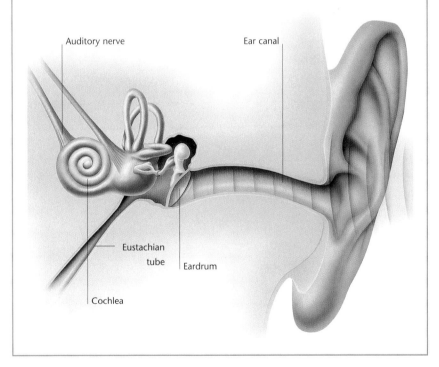

Auditory nerve

Ear canal

Eustachian tube

Eardrum

Cochlea

In an audiogram, you will be fitted with headphones, and asked to signal when you can hear bleeps at different pitches. The bleeps are gradually made quieter until they are not heard. If the audiogram suggests a hearing loss, then a bone conduction audiogram will be performed, with a special headband that conducts sounds through the bones of the skull. This helps differentiate conductive deafness, caused by an outer or middle ear disorder, from nerve deafness, caused by a disorder of the inner ear or the nerves that transmit hearing to the brain.

Sometimes, speech recognition tests are carried out if some degree of distortion of sound is suspected. In children, a special additional test, called tympanometry, is performed to see if the ear-drum is moving normally. Glue ear (fluid in the middle ear) reduces normal movement.

BREAST SCREENING

Mammography is an X-ray technique (see pages 454–55) that uses low levels of radiation to produce images of the female breast in order to detect abnormalities in the breast tissue. The radiographic film used to record the images is designed to generate high-definition pictures from minimal levels of exposure to X-rays.

HOW A MAMMOGRAM IS CARRIED OUT

The X-ray is performed by positioning each breast in turn between two see-through plates, so that the breast tissue is flattened. X-rays are then directed through the breast in two different directions to produce two images. The test is generally over very quickly, and although the procedure may involve some discomfort as the breast tissue is compressed between the plates, there are usually no after-effects.

Although in theory there may be a risk of causing changes in the breast tissue with repeated mammography, because of the low levels of radiation used, this risk is far outweighed by the benefits of early detection of breast cancer. If tumours are detected early they usually respond well to treatment. Studies have shown that the number of deaths from breast cancer in the age group 50 to 64 are reduced by 40 per cent in those who attend for breast screening.

SCREENING

Generally, there are two reasons for the use of mammography. The first of these is for screening purposes, to try to detect cases of breast cancer before the woman has developed any symptoms. The risk of developing breast cancer increases with age and the disease is most commonly diagnosed in women over the age of 50. In the UK, when a woman reaches the age of 50, she is invited to attend for mammography. If the initial examination is normal, then she will be offered a mammogram every three years until she reaches the age of 65. Continuation of screening after the age of 65 is possible if the breast screening unit considers it necessary for a particular woman.

The aim of breast screening by mammography is to pick up cancers in their very earliest form, before they could be detected by self-examination. Small cancers are less likely to have spread outside the breast to other parts of the body and may, therefore, be more responsive to early treatment.

Routine screening is not offered to women below 50 for a variety of reasons. The first of these is that breast cancer is less common in younger women. Secondly, because younger women have breast tissue that is much denser, detection of breast cancer at normal doses of radiation is much more difficult. Finally, screening in the under-50 age group has not been found to be cost-effective.

Mammography has a high sensitivity, which means that very few patients over the age of 50 who have a cancerous lump will go undetected when screened. However, there is a high false positive rate (see *Genetic Testing*, page 442), which can cause unnecessary worry. For every 10,000 women screened, 500 will be recalled for a second mammogram because something has shown up, or there has been a technical problem with the films. Of these women, about 60 will have breast cancer, meaning that around one in ten patients recalled will have a tumour.

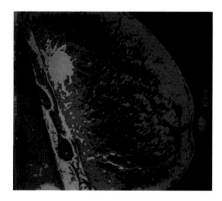

ABOVE *Lower dose X-rays are used to examine soft tissues such as the breast and they are widely used to screen for breast cancer. The image here shows a healthy breast.*

ABOVE *This CT scan uses X-rays with a computer to produce a highly detailed cross-sectional image of a breast with cancerous cells. The purple tissue is denser than normal tissue.*

INVESTIGATION

The second reason for mammography is to investigate women who have breast-related symptoms such as pain, lumps, discharge or bleeding from the nipple. In this instance, mammography can be performed at any age, although there may be a reluctance to subject women under 35 to breast X-rays.

FURTHER TESTS

Although mammography is an excellent method of detecting breast abnormalities, it is often not possible to determine whether the abnormality is benign or malignant. Further tests may be required to arrive at a final diagnosis. The most common extra

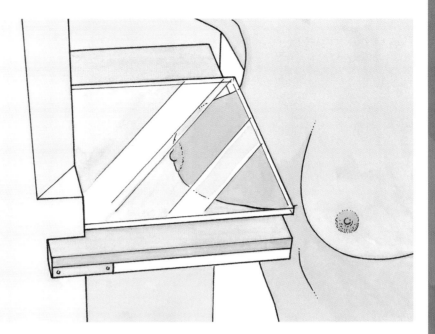

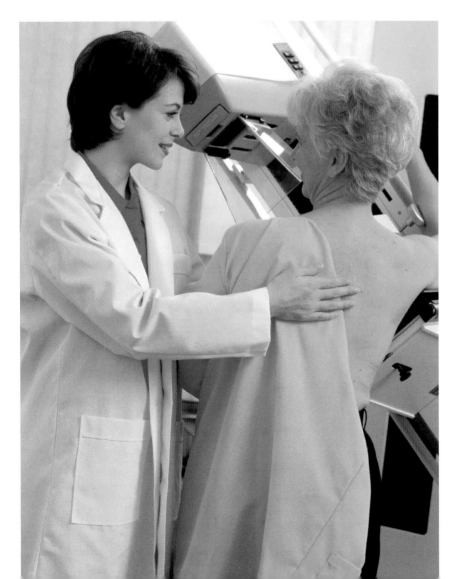

ABOVE *A mammogram is an X-ray of the breast taken to screen for indications of breast cancer and to investigate breast-related symptoms including pain, lumps and discharge or bleeding from the nipple. Each breast in turn is placed between two plates to flatten the tissue. X-rays are then directed through the breasts to produce an image.*

LEFT *Screening programmes for women over 50 are essential because the risk of breast cancer increases with age. If regular screening is not carried out, tumours may spread to other parts of the body, such as the lungs, before being detected. Small tumours are likely still to be contained within the breast and are much easier to treat.*

test is ultrasound (see page 455), which is particularly useful at distinguishing whether a lump is solid or fluid-filled (cystic). Inserting a thin needle into the lump is the most accurate way of assessing the nature of a lump, and also allows a tiny fragment of tissue to be removed for examination in the laboratory. Finally, in many cases, the only method that will give a completely accurate diagnosis of whether or not a lump is cancerous is to perform a biopsy of the lump, that is, to remove it surgically.

CERVICAL SMEAR AND PELVIC EXAMINATION

Cancer of the cervix (neck of the womb) is usually preceded by a period of time when the cells in the cervix have undergone pre-cancerous changes. These pre-cancerous changes, also known as CIN (cervical intra-epithelial neoplasia), can occur in women of all ages, and usually cause no symptoms whatsoever. For these reasons, cervical cancer screening, in the form of the cervical smear test, is offered to all women from the age of 20. The aim of the test is to detect these changes in their earliest stages, thus allowing for assessment, intervention and, if appropriate, treatment to prevent cancer developing.

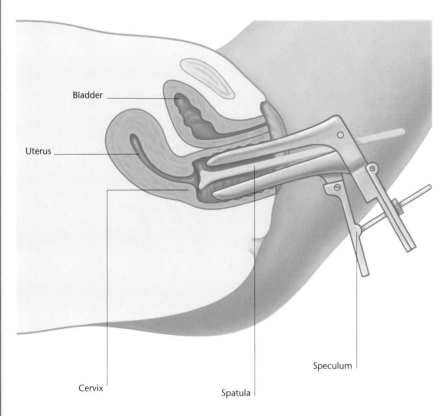

Bladder

Uterus

Cervix

Spatula

Speculum

ABOVE *A cervical smear is a screening test and a woman should not wait until she has symptoms before presenting herself for a smear. In the test, a speculum is inserted into the vagina to hold it open and give access to the cervix. A sample of cells is taken from the cervix using a wooden spatula, transferred to a slide and later examined in the laboratory.*

CERVICAL SCREENING

A cervical smear can be carried out at your doctor's surgery, either by your doctor, or a trained practice nurse within a well-woman clinic. Family planning clinics also provide a smear service. The results of all smears, from whatever source, are entered into a central computerised system coordinated by the local health authority. Screening continues on a three-yearly basis until the age of 64. Offering smears at intervals of less than three years has not been shown to reduce the rates of cervical cancer.

WHAT THE TEST CONSISTS OF

A cervical smear takes only a few minutes to perform. A metal device known as a speculum is inserted into the vagina, allowing the cervix to be identified and exposed. A sample of the cells from the cervix is obtained by scraping either a wooden spatula or a small brush across the surface of the cervical tissue. These cells are then transferred to a glass slide, preserved with fixative and transported to a laboratory, where the cells are examined under a microscope.

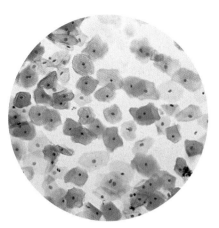

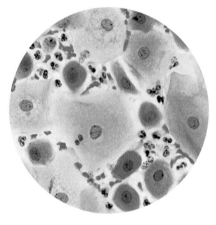

LEFT *These magnified images show a healthy smear test with cervical cells of regular shape and size (top). Cell distortion is present in the bottom picture, showing precancerous changes. Any abnormal result is followed up by further investigation in hospital, where colposcopy can allow more accurate assessment of cells in the cervix.*

Sometimes, there may be discomfort as the smear test is performed, but this is usually minimal. As the surface of the cervix has a lot of blood vessels, there can occasionally be a small amount of bleeding after the smear is carried out. This is not anything to worry about, and quickly settles.

IN THE LABORATORY

Once the smear has reached the laboratory, it is graded as normal (negative), borderline abnormal, or mild, moderate or severely abnormal. Normal smears will need repeating after three years, and borderline changes usually require a repeat examination in either three, six or twelve months.

Those smears showing the more significant changes will require further investigation. It is quite likely that some of these abnormal results, if left untreated, would progress with time to cancer of the cervix. However, it is also possible that some precancerous changes may disappear spontaneously. Unfortunately, it cannot be predicted which women might develop cancer, so all mild to severely abnormal results are followed up with a test called colposcopy.

COLPOSCOPY

Colposcopy takes place in a hospital clinic, and is performed by a gynaecologist. It involves looking at the surface of the cervix with a magnifying device known as a colposcope. Colposcopy allows a more accurate assessment of changes in the cervix, permitting samples of tissue, known as biopsies, to be taken. The tissue obtained is once again examined under the microscope.

PELVIC EXAMINATION

A pelvic examination is often carried out at the same time as a cervical smear is performed. Generally, the doctor or nurse will insert one or two fingers into the vagina while laying the palm of the other hand flat across the lower abdomen. This allows the size of the uterus (womb) and its position to be assessed. If the ovaries are enlarged, by cysts, for example, then this can be gauged. Often, the woman may be asked if she feels pain or discomfort during the pelvic examination.

A pelvic examination is a normal part of the assessment of any woman who has heavy, painful or prolonged periods, as well as lower abdominal pain. Women starting the oral contraceptive or hormone replacement therapy might also expect to have a pelvic examination.

BELOW *In a pelvic examination, a doctor or nurse may check the size of the uterus and its position, and see if cysts exist on the ovaries.*

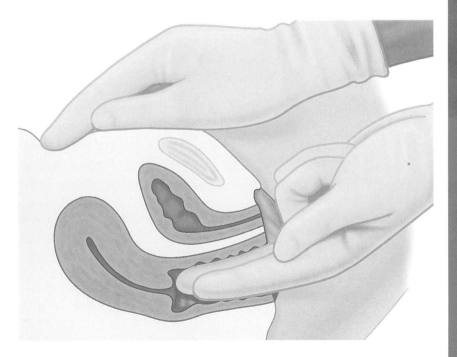

BLOOD, URINE AND STOOL TESTS

During a consultation with a doctor or nurse, a great deal of information pointing towards a diagnosis can be obtained from the symptoms and the abnormalities (if any) discovered during a physical examination. However, there are many occasions where further tests have to be carried out to help diagnosis.

BLOOD TESTS

Blood tests are widely used to help investigation of illness and to monitor long-standing conditions such as diabetes. Most blood samples are taken from veins, blood vessels that return blood to the heart. Usually, veins around the elbow are used for the test. Occasionally, a sample from an artery, a blood vessel that takes blood from the heart, is required, particularly if a person has breathing problems and monitoring of blood oxygen levels is necessary. The artery used is in the wrist. Finally, some tests are carried out on one or two drops of capillary blood (in tiny blood vessels), obtained by pricking the end of a finger and squeezing.

Blood consists of a whole range of cells, salts, minerals, proteins and hormones. For that reason, there are more than a hundred different blood tests available at hospital laboratories. However, there is no single blood test that can be used to diagnose all medical conditions. Therefore, when a blood sample is obtained, your doctor will ask for tests that are specifically related to your suspected illness.

Types of blood test

Commonly performed blood tests include a full blood count, which counts the number and size of red and white blood cells and platelets, and the level of the oxygen-carrying pigment haemoglobin in the red blood cells, to detect anaemia or deficiencies in the white blood cells involved with immunity (see page 208–9). The functioning of the kidneys, liver and thyroid gland are generally checked, especially in cases of fatigue or unexplained weight loss. Blood sugar levels to diagnose or monitor diabetes, and coagulation tests to monitor the effect of blood-thinning drugs such as warfarin (an anticoagulant drug used to treat blood clots) are frequently done.

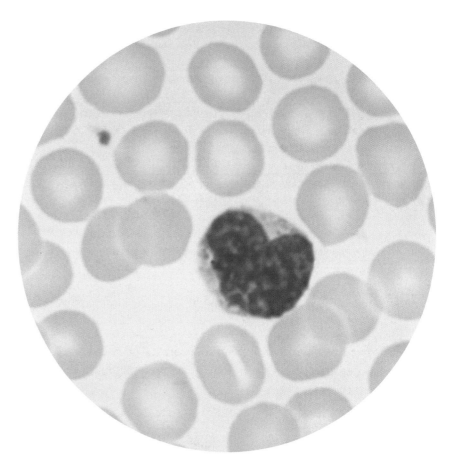

ABOVE *This highly magnified view of a drop of blood shows a normal white blood cell surrounded by red blood cells. Blood cell tests are used to investigate a number of illnesses.*

If the more general tests show an abnormality such as anaemia, then more specific blood tests, requiring further samples, might be necessary. These less commonly performed tests include measuring: vitamin levels such as vitamin B_{12} and folic acid; iron levels;

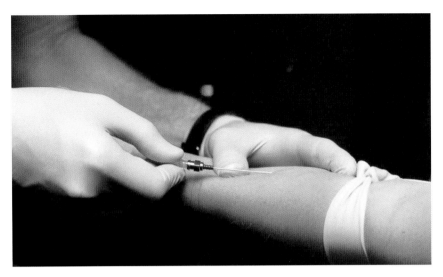

prostatic specific antigen (for prostate cancer tests); cholesterol, and levels of inflammation in the blood. Rarely, blood samples are tested for infection.

Blood tests can be intimidating for some people, particularly if they have a phobia of needles, or feel faint at the sight of blood. Pain can be minimised by smearing the area of skin over the vein with a local anaesthetic cream an hour or so before the test. Lying down while the sample is taken can reduce the risk of fainting.

URINE TESTS

Urine tests are used to detect a number of medical problems. The sample is usually obtained halfway through passing urine and collected in a sterile container. The sample is tested by dipping a special stick into the urine. Constituents of urine that are tested include sugar (for diabetes), protein and blood (for kidney disease or infection such as cystitis), white blood cells and bacteria. Squares of chemically impregnated paper along the dipstick change colour when they come into contact with one of the test substances, and these colours are compared with a chart to show the amount of substance that is present in the urine. If infection is suspected, then

ABOVE *Most blood samples are taken from a vein on the inside of the elbow. A tourniquet is applied so the vein stands out and blood is drawn up through a needle into a syringe.*

the sample is sent to the laboratory for further investigation. Measuring female hormone levels in urine is the basis of most pregnancy tests.

STOOL TESTS

Although carried out less frequently, a stool (faeces) test can be a very important diagnostic tool. In persistent diarrhoea, the stool can be examined for infection by bacteria or parasites. Samples can also be tested for hidden (occult) blood to screen for bowel cancer, or to help in the investigation of anaemia.

BELOW *In the laboratory, most chemical tests on blood or urine are analysed by machine. Several tubes, each containing a sample mixed with a chemical, are placed into the machine.*

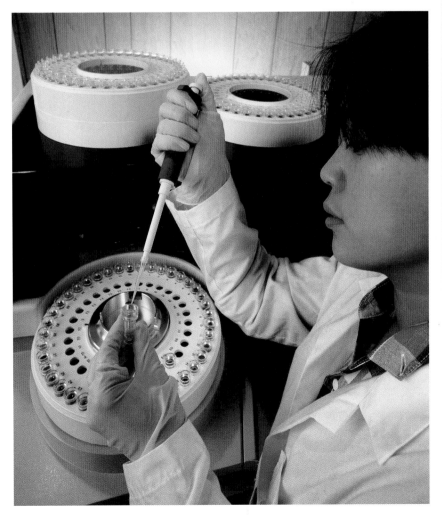

TESTING FOR HEART DISEASE

Although heart disease is very common, making a diagnosis is sometimes difficult. There are four main areas of diagnosis. The first of these is during a sudden episode of chest pain to confirm or exclude a heart attack. Secondly, people who have intermittent symptoms of chest pain or discomfort are tested to determine whether they have angina. Thirdly, some of the tests are used to see whether there is an abnormal heart rhythm if a person is complaining of palpitations. Fourthly, if the symptoms include a feeling of breathlessness, then the tests can help to establish whether the patient has heart failure.

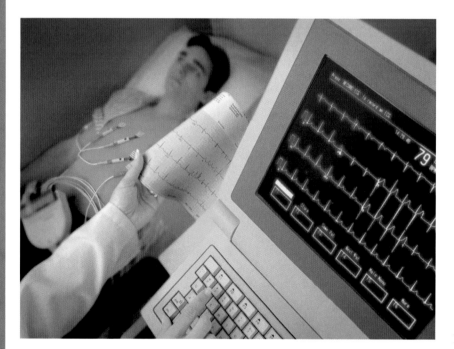

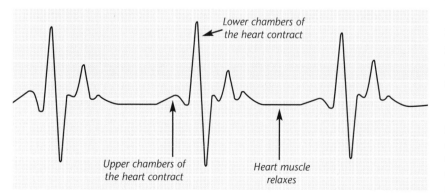

Lower chambers of the heart contract

Upper chambers of the heart contract

Heart muscle relaxes

ECG (ELECTROCARDIOGRAM)

The ECG is a test that measures the electrical activity in different areas of the heart. Small electrodes are attached to the skin to transmit the electrical activity of the heart to an ECG machine. Signals from the electrodes produce a trace, which is recorded on a strip of paper. The trace can be used to detect any abnormalities in the rate or the rhythm of the heartbeat. In addition, the ECG can demonstrate areas of damage to the heart muscle, such that might occur during a heart attack. Disease caused by narrowing of the blood vessels that supply the heart muscle (coronary heart disease) can also be identified. Most ECGs are performed with the patient lying down and inactive: a resting ECG.

Even in severe heart disease, the resting ECG can be normal, and if this is the case, the patient is asked to undergo an exercise ECG, or exercise stress test. This usually entails walking

LEFT *An ECG is used to show electrical activity in different areas of the heart. Signals from electrodes are recorded on to a piece of paper, known as a trace. Most are performed when the patient is lying down.*

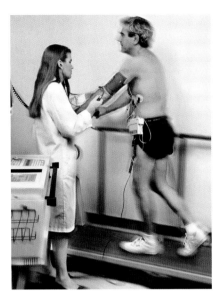

LEFT *An exercise ECG assesses the function of the heart while under stress and is used to detect severe heart disease which may go unnoticed in a resting ECG. The test involves raising your heart rate by exercising, usually on a treadmill. Small electrodes are attached to your chest, and as you exercise, the electrical activity of the heart is shown and recorded on an ECG machine.*

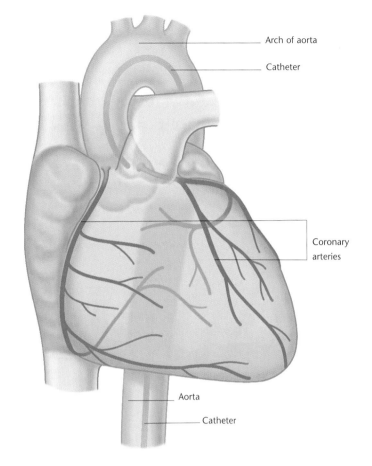

Arch of aorta

Catheter

Coronary arteries

Aorta

Catheter

ABOVE *In angiography dye is injected through a catheter into the coronary arteries so that narrowed areas can be detected on an X-ray. The catheter is inserted through the groin and positioned near the coronary arteries.*

on a treadmill until symptoms such as chest pain occur, or the pattern on the ECG changes to indicate that the blood supply to the heart muscle is inadequate during exertion.

If the patient is being investigated for palpitations, it is rare for the condition, unless very frequent, to be picked up on a resting ECG. Therefore, the patient is connected to a small machine that will monitor the ECG over a full day. This is known as a 24-hour tape, and the patient can record when symptoms are felt. Results can be compared to the corresponding part of the ECG recording.

ECHOCARDIOGRAM

This test is a form of ultrasound examination (see page 454), similar to the one used to check on the foetus during pregnancy. It is used to assess the functioning of the internal

structures of the heart, as well as indicating how efficiently the chambers of the heart are pumping blood around the body. Leaking or narrowed valves and poorly contracting heart muscle can be detected in this short test, allowing a definitive diagnosis of heart failure or heart valve disease to be made. This allows appropriate medical or surgical treatment to be planned.

CORONARY ANGIOGRAM

Angiography is the technique of producing images of the arteries in the body, in this case, the coronary arteries responsible for supplying blood to the heart muscle. A liquid dye is squirted into the coronary arteries through a soft rubber tube called a catheter. The catheter is introduced through an artery in the groin and is positioned near the entrance to the coronary arteries by following a guide wire.

Pictures of the arteries are taken in rapid succession on X-ray films (see page 454) and the whole of the procedure is monitored on a screen. Coronary angiography is the standard investigation carried out to determine the state of the coronary arteries. It is usually performed following a heart attack, or if an exercise ECG has been positive.

Angiography is mainly used to see whether the coronary arteries are narrowed and suitable for surgery, such as a bypass operation or angioplasty (where the artery is widened using a special balloon catheter).

X-RAYS AND ULTRASOUND

X-rays and ultrasound are imaging techniques that create pictures of internal organs and structures, and are often used to make a diagnosis or if the results of other tests are unclear. X-rays are the oldest form of imaging technique and are a form of electromagnetic radiation. Ultrasound scans are images of the body's internal organs produced by firing sound waves towards them and picking up the reflected sound waves with a scanner that can transmit the images formed to a monitor. The scan can be transferred to X-ray film or paper for a permanent record.

HOW X-RAYS WORK

X-rays, discovered by accident in 1895, have very high energy levels and can pass through the tissues of the human body. A specialised photographic film is used to record images produced by X-rays: the higher the energy levels reaching the film, the darker the image formed. Some parts of the body, such as the bones, which are denser than the surrounding tissue, allow less radiation through. For this reason, bones appear white on X-rays, whereas air-filled structures, such as the lungs, appear much darker. Hollow or fluid-filled structures do not show up well.

The images produced by an X-ray examination can be very informative, and allow decisions about diagnosis and therapy to be made with greater confidence than after mere examination alone. The most common use of X-rays is in the detection of broken bones (fractures). Next in line is the chest X-ray, helpful in diagnosing a range of conditions including pneumonia, asthma, bronchitis, cancer and collapsed lung (pneumothorax).

CONTRAST X-RAYS

More specialised X-ray tests can be used to look at some of the soft tissue structures and organs. In these tests, a liquid dye that prevents X-rays from passing through can be injected, swallowed or introduced into the intestines to produce a series of images of the structures to be studied.

Swallowing barium allows the oesophagus (gullet) and the stomach to be inspected for ulcers and cancerous growths and narrowings. Introducing barium in the form of an enema into

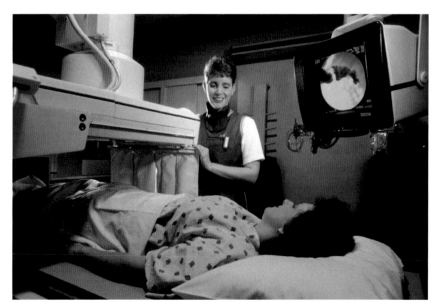

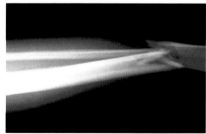

ABOVE *An X-ray produces a two-dimensional image and is particularly suitable for examining bones. This X-ray shows a clear image of a broken bone.*

LEFT *During an X-ray, the source of the X-rays is positioned directly above the area being examined. You are photographed for a fraction of a second.*

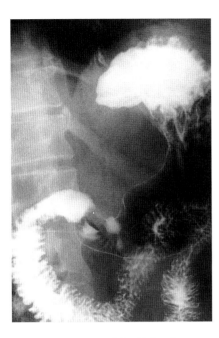

ABOVE *Barium is a thick liquid that does not allow X-rays to pass through it. Swallowing a barium solution (seen at the top) makes the stomach visible on an X-ray machine.*

BELOW *During an ultrasound examination, a device called a transducer emits high-frequency sound waves and receives their echoes to produce images on a monitor.*

the large intestine can highlight cancer, or the typical changes of inflammation present in disorders such as ulcerative colitis (see page 402) or Crohn's disease (see page 403).

Dye injected into arteries can accurately demonstrate the condition of the coronary arteries, or the blood vessels supplying the legs or other vital organs, such as the brain. In a similar fashion, the structure and function of the kidneys and bladder can be studied using a dye that is concentrated in the urine.

RISK FACTORS

Although the amount of radiation used to produce an X-ray picture is small, and there is no risk to the individual in a single test, repeated examination over a period of time might be harmful in a tiny minority of people. However, X-rays can damage the foetus, and for that reason, tests will be performed during pregnancy only if considered absolutely essential.

ULTRASOUND

Ultrasound scanning is safe, and for that reason is extensively used in pregnancy to monitor the progress of the unborn baby. Ultrasound scans are used for diagnostic purposes in numerous situations, because they can quickly and easily produce good quality images of the urinary tract, the pelvic organs, the liver and spleen, the heart and any swellings located close to the body surface. Mostly, the scanner is moved directly over the skin, using a special gel to conduct the sound waves. Sometimes the scan is performed through one of the body's openings, such as the vagina or rectum, using a small probe.

In pregnancy, scans are used in the early stages to confirm that the foetus is alive and to determine whether it is a single, twin or multiple pregnancy. The length of the foetus is measured to assess the age and calculate the due date. Later on, more detailed scans are possible to make sure the baby is developing normally. The position and health of the placenta are also assessed.

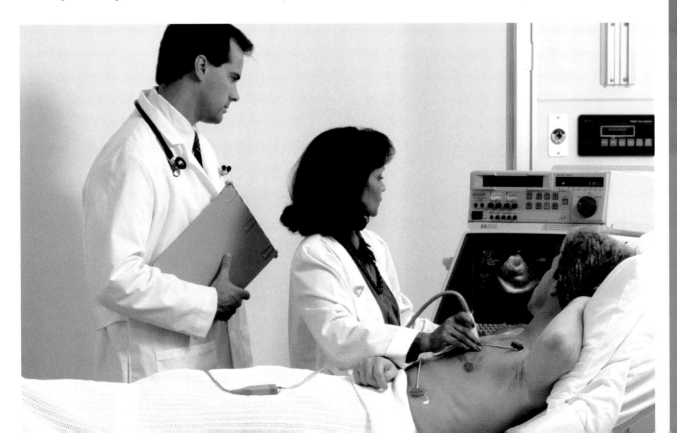

MAGNETIC RESONANCE IMAGING AND CT SCANS

Magnetic resonance imaging (MRI) is a relatively new technique, first used in the early 1980s to obtain highly detailed views of the body's internal organs. Magnets and radio waves are used to create images on a computer and, because MRI is radiation-free, it is considered to be one of the safest imaging techniques available. CT (computerised tomography) is another method of generating images of the internal organs and tissues. Using X-rays fired from a number of different angles at the same time, a computer builds up a detailed cross-sectional picture of any part of the body.

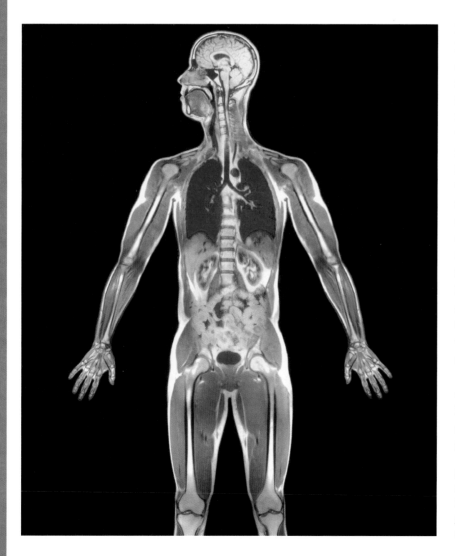

HOW MRI WORKS

MRI involves the patient lying within a strong cylindrical magnet while magnetic signals, up to 30,000 times more powerful than the Earth's own magnetic field, are directed through the parts of the body to be tested. The majority of the tissues in the human body are composed largely of water, and water contains hydrogen atoms. As the magnetic field is activated, hydrogen atoms, which usually point in random directions, are forced to line up in the same direction. When the magnetic field is switched off, the atoms move back into place, sending out radio waves of their own that are picked up by the scanner. The pattern of these radio waves is interpreted by a computer and transformed into an image.

MRI scans are performed as an outpatient procedure and, because X-rays are not used, they are safe to use repeatedly. Because the patient is lying in a powerful magnetic field it is

LEFT *MRI scans produce highly detailed images of internal organs and structures. Magnets and radio waves are used to generate a computer image, and because it is radiation-free it is a very safe technique.*

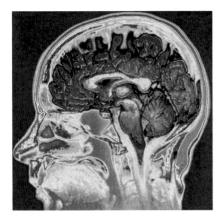

ABOVE *CT scans are often performed on the head because they clearly show the different structures and cavities within the skull.*

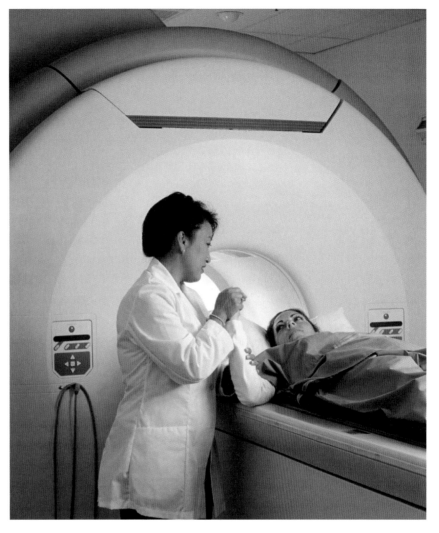

RIGHT *CT scanning uses a series of X-rays to produce pictures of many different parts of the body. You will be positioned on a motorised bed which moves you forward into the scanner. You may be given a sedative if the procedure makes you feel anxious.*

important not to wear jewellery or other metal objects, as these can interfere with the results of the scan. Medical staff should be told if a patient has a hearing aid or pacemaker, or has any metal clips within the body. Generally, metalwork relating to orthopaedic problems, such as artificial hips, are not a problem.

ADVANTAGES OF MRI SCANS

Pictures in great detail can be produced from MRI scanning, and in particular, it is the definitive diagnostic test in a number of conditions such as back pain and spinal problems, knee and shoulder pain. Initially designed to look at the brain, it is particularly useful for detecting tumours, swollen arteries (aneurysms) and bleeding within the skull. The scans can also show the early stages of some central nervous system diseases, including multiple sclerosis (see page 346). Rather like some X-ray tests, it is possible to inject or swallow dye to make some of the internal organs stand out better.

DISADVANTAGES OF MRI SCANS

The patient has to remain absolutely still during the test, and may have to lie within the scanner for up to an hour; very young children may have to be anaesthetised. Some patients can feel claustrophobic and may require sedation. The scanners make a loud banging noise during the test, which may be disturbing, although it is possible to mask this to a degree with background music.

CT SCANS

A CT scanner looks rather like a large doughnut, and the patient lies on a bed that can move, so that the part of the body to be examined lies within the ring. Once again, some people might feel claustrophobic in the machine. The machine also makes quite a loud whirring noise that may be unnerving for a few patients.

Although the main function of CT scanning is to aid diagnosis, it is also used to help guide medical staff when carrying out procedures such as tissue biopsies (removing a small part of tissue for closer examination) and planning radiotherapy for cancer treatment. Because the level of X-ray radiation is significantly higher than that used in ordinary X-ray tests, patients will not usually undergo repeated examinations.

SURGERY

With advances in medical science and the development of more effective drugs, there are many medical conditions that can be cured or controlled with medication alone. However, much of what goes wrong with the human body is not going to respond to drugs alone, and so, every day in the UK, thousands of people undergo surgical procedures, or operations.

SPECIALIST REFERRAL

If your doctor is concerned that your medical condition might require surgery, you will be referred to a specialist in a hospital. Consultant surgeons are highly qualified doctors who often deal only with a specific area of the body, such as the heart or the ear, nose and throat.

BEFORE SURGERY TAKES PLACE

After seeing the surgeon, and perhaps undergoing tests to confirm the diagnosis, the plans for a surgical procedure are discussed fully so that the patient understands what operation is necessary and the success rate, the risks and possible complications, the

time to be spent in hospital and the recuperation period. Only then can the patient make a decision about whether to proceed. This is known as giving informed consent.

Before the operation takes place, you might be invited for a preoperative check, where blood pressure is measured, and allergies and current medication are discussed. Sometimes, if you have other illnesses, such as diabetes or lung disease, an anaesthetist might need to do a more detailed physical examination and arrange blood tests or X-rays.

SURGICAL ADVANCES

Nowadays, many surgical procedures are carried out as day cases, meaning that the patient is admitted and discharged from the hospital on the same day. Some examples of day-case surgery are hernia repairs, varicose vein operations, cataract surgery and removal of the tonsils.

A great advance in the surgical world was the development of minimally invasive operations, known as keyhole surgery. A tube-like viewing instrument

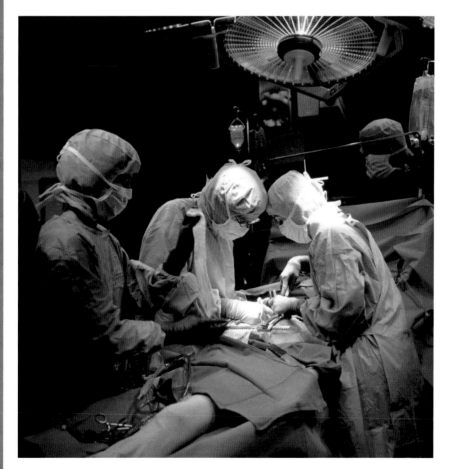

LEFT *Operating theatres are specially designed to enable the operating team to perform surgery effectively. All instruments are sterile. Lights and machinery run from an independent electricity supply in case of a power failure.*

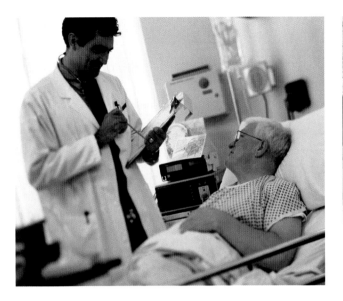

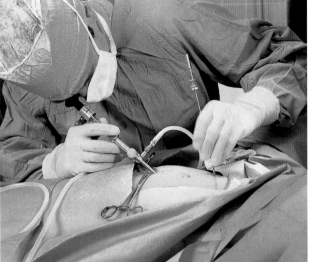

ABOVE *Before you undergo major surgery a doctor will discuss the procedure to make sure you understand why surgery is necessary, what is involved and what the risks are.*

TOP RIGHT *A viewing instrument called a laparoscope is inserted into an abdominal incision to investigate abdominal and female reproductive system disorders.*

called an endoscope is inserted through a small incision made in the body or through a natural body opening such as the rectum. This type of surgery has been used to sort out joint problems such as knee cartilage injuries for many years and is now used for a variety of other conditions, including gall-bladder removal, hernia repairs and blood vessel problems. Recovery time from such operations is shorter and there is less damage to the body.

AFTER SURGERY

After the operation, the surgeon will often discuss the findings and results of the surgery with you as you come round from the anaesthetic. If you have had day-case surgery, it is wise to have somebody with you for the discussion if possible, as the effect of the anaesthetic may make you sleepy and confused.

Anaesthesia

This is a procedure that is designed to take away the sensation of pain or feeling using specific drugs, thus allowing a surgical operation to take place. General anaesthesia is total unconsciousness; local anaesthesia abolishes pain in a limited area of the body.

Local anaesthetics involve numbing the part of the body to be treated using an injection. Usually, this means an injection directly into the skin or near the main nerve supplying the relevant area (known as nerve blocks). Sometimes a more extensive nerve block is performed, called a spinal, or epidural, anaesthetic. This is commonly used in labour, but might be used in combination with a sedative to make the patient sleepy in cases where the patient's general health is so poor that a general anaesthetic cannot be used.

General anaesthetics are used for most major operations, and involve inducing a state of unconsciousness in the patient using a combination of inhaled gases and drugs injected into the bloodstream. Although described as a form of sleep, the state of the body during a general anaesthetic is completely different from natural sleep. An anaesthetist constantly monitors the patient during the procedure, and drugs are administered to relieve pain and maintain the level of unconsciousness.

Before a general anaesthetic, patients are often given premedication, a combination of sedative drugs to induce drowsiness. Patients rarely remember anything about what happened under the anaesthetic, and improvements in the drugs used and the monitoring equipment means that deaths directly related to an anaesthetic occur only about once in every 250,000 procedures.

COSMETIC SURGERY

Cosmetic surgery, also known as plastic or aesthetic surgery, is among the fastest growing branches of medicine, as new treatments and techniques are constantly being developed. Undergoing cosmetic surgery is no longer seen as the province of the rich and famous, making it more acceptable to the general population.

WHAT IS COSMETIC SURGERY?

Cosmetic surgery can be defined as the moulding of the surface and sometimes the deeper structures of the human body to improve the appearance of the person undergoing the treatment. Many of the procedures used have been developed from reconstructive surgery, where disfigurements due to serious injury, destructive surgery (for example, the removal of malignant tumours), severe deformity present from birth, or burns, are corrected.

WHY PEOPLE HAVE COSMETIC SURGERY

Generally, patients pursue treatment for three main reasons. Firstly, they might require corrective surgery for some part of their anatomy that they are unhappy with, and about which they can do nothing themselves. This includes operations to correct bat ears (ears that stick out significantly), breast reduction, particularly if there is associated back pain, and operations to change the shape of the nose. Secondly,

treatment is sought to reverse the processes of ageing. This incorporates procedures such as face-lifts, removal of wrinkles and hair transplants. Finally, there is treatment to improve a person's attractiveness to the opposite sex, such as breast enhancement, removal of cellulite and excess fat by liposuction, and removal of tattoos.

Technological advances in other branches of surgery are being used to broaden the range of cosmetic surgery procedures. Improvements in lasers

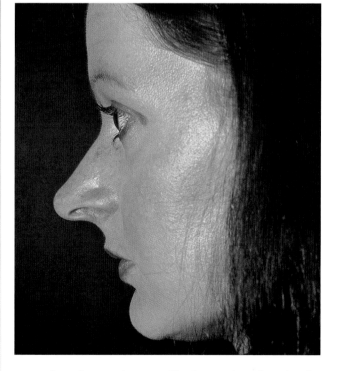

ABOVE *Cosmetic surgery known as rhinoplasty can be performed to alter the shape of the nose. This picture shows a woman before having corrective surgery on her nose to improve her appearance.*

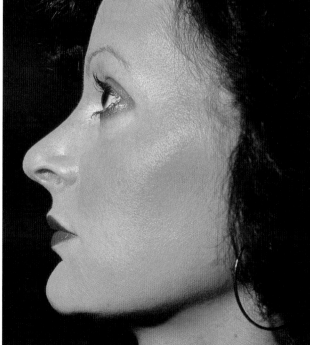

ABOVE *The same woman has been photographed after having undergone cosmetic surgery. The tip of the nose has been pared down to create a more aesthetically acceptable shape.*

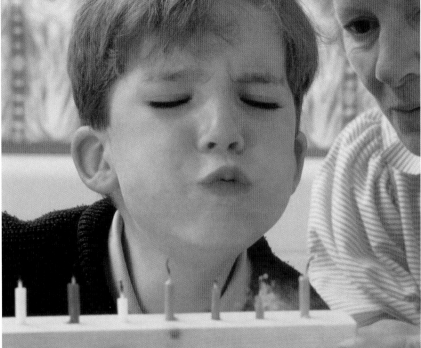

WHAT TO DO NEXT

If the idea of cosmetic surgery appeals, then the best place to start the quest for advice is your family doctor. Avoid advertisements in the back pages of magazines. Allow your doctor to refer you to somebody she knows locally who provides a reputable service. If you are too embarrassed to see your own doctor, most cosmetic surgeons will be members of the British Association of Aesthetic Plastic Surgeons (BAAPS), and it is possible to obtain a list of suitably qualified doctors and reputable clinics in your locality by contacting BAAPS by phone, or by visiting their website.

Ultimately, as almost all cosmetic surgery is unavailable on the NHS, the cost, the pitfalls and the risk of surgery must be balanced against the benefits of an enhanced appearance that could potentially be life-changing.

allow not just the removal of skin blemishes such as birthmarks with little or no visible scarring, but also permit their use in procedures to make the skin look younger. Smaller tubes used for liposuction lead to less surface scarring, and development of better breast implants means a safer long-term outlook for patients undergoing this type of operation.

Although cosmetic surgery may not win you the partner, the job or the lifestyle of your dreams, it is still a branch of medicine where most customers are delighted with the results of going under the knife. However, the final aesthetic result of any cosmetic surgery depends on the skill of the surgeon performing the operation, and this is where the pitfalls may lie. Check that the surgeon is well qualified and experienced in the techniques to be used.

ABOVE *Congenital conditions, such as cleft lip and palate, can be corrected by cosmetic surgery. Corrective surgery usually produces good results and allows speech to develop normally.*

DISADVANTAGES OF COSMETIC SURGERY

Two problems beset the world of cosmetic surgery in the UK. The first of these is the fact that a doctor does not have to hold any specific qualification in cosmetic surgery, or to have undergone training, to call himself a plastic surgeon. The second drawback is that cosmetic surgery clinics can advertise to the general public, and can make claims about treatment that are difficult to prove. Allied with the confusing array of letters after the surgeon's name, some patients are misled into having treatment that is either inappropriate or is beyond the level of expertise of the operator.

BELOW *Laser treatment is often used on the skin to destroy the cluster of blood vessels under the skin that form a birthmark. A course of treatment may be needed before it disappears.*

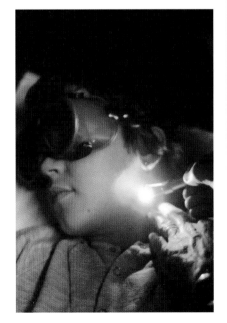

THE MEDICINE CABINET: STORING AND USING MEDICATION

Ignoring the medical products that are available over the counter from pharmacists, there are several thousand different preparations that your doctor could prescribe for you. Each of these drugs will have had millions of pounds spent on it during development, and then will have been subjected to rigorous examination by the Medicines Control Agency (MCA) to determine its safety and effectiveness.

STORING DRUGS

Most drugs can be stored at room temperature, but there are a few that should be placed in a refrigerator. Drugs in this category include some eye and ear drops and insulin (used to treat diabetes). All other drugs should be locked away out of the reach of children. If several members of the household are taking medication on a regular basis, then each person should store his drugs separately.

TAKING MEDICATION

It is vital that the instructions advising how a drug should be taken are read before the first dose is consumed. Although some medication still comes in small, child-proof, brown bottles with a label advising dosage and special instructions or precautions, many now come as a standard manufacturer's pack. This pack will, by law, contain a leaflet advising on the dose to be taken as well as all aspects of special instructions, side-effects and guidance on dealing with accidental overdose. If the instructions are still not clear, then seek advice from the pharmacist or doctor.

COMPLETING THE COURSE

There is a number of instructions that are common to several groups of drugs. In the case of antibiotics, short courses of steroids for asthma and drugs used to cure stomach ulcers, it is essential that the the full course of the medication is taken. This is to ensure that the complete effect of the drug is experienced, as symptoms will often go half-way through treatment. If medication is stopped early, partially treated conditions are likely to recur.

Similarly, many drugs for the treatment of long-standing conditions, including diabetes, raised blood pressure, heart disease, high cholesterol or asthma should not be stopped by a patient unless he has been instructed to do so by a doctor. Some of these medical problems, in particular, raised blood pressure and high cholesterol, have no symptoms, but are being treated to reduce the risk of future heart attacks and strokes.

Therefore, a patient who stops taking prescribed drugs in these conditions will not be fully aware of the potential dangers he is facing as he will feel well.

TAKING DIFFERENT MEDICATION

Many people find that they have to take a number of different drugs every day. Generally, it is safe to take a variety of tablets and medicines at the same time, but there are some groups that should be kept apart if possible as they might interfere with the way the drugs are absorbed from the stomach. If in doubt, ask your pharmacist for help. Always tell the doctor or pharmacist if you are taking any over-the-counter or complementary therapies.

DRIVING

There are several classes of medication that may cause drowsiness or sedation, and it is important that a person taking these types of drugs should not drive. Among the remedies that can have this effect are some antihistamines (for allergy), stronger painkillers and tablets for depression. The sedative effect of these drugs can be made worse by alcohol, which should be avoided.

RIGHT *When storing medicines at home it is best to keep them all in one place, ideally in a lockable wall cabinet. It should be in a dry, cool place, out of the reach of children.*

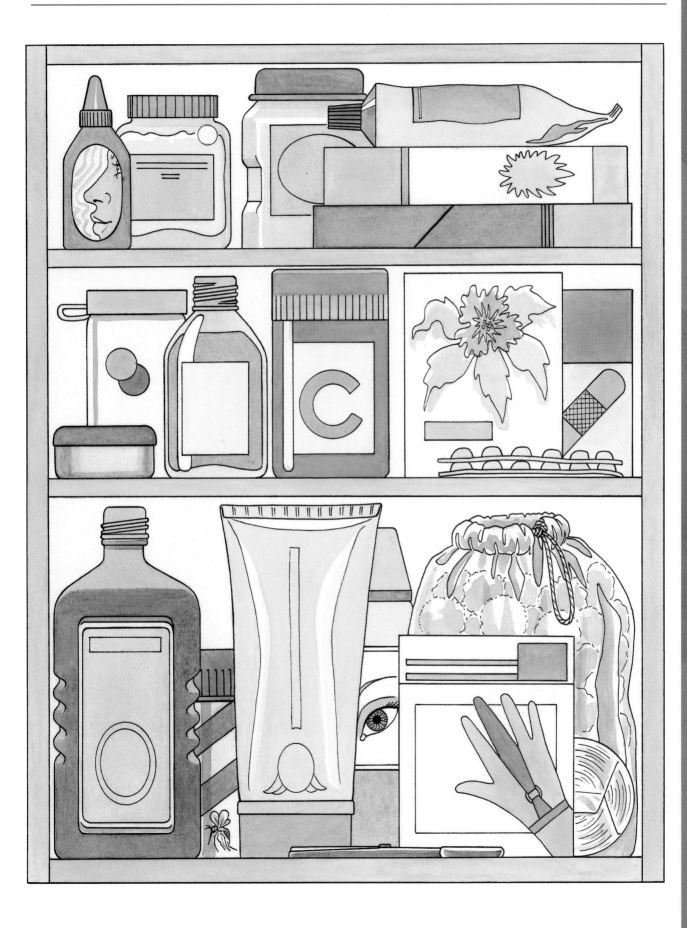

COMMONLY PRESCRIBED DRUGS: WHAT THEY DO AND SIDE-EFFECTS

Every day in the UK, medication costing millions of pounds is prescribed to hundreds of thousands of people. There are thousands of different drugs used to treat hundreds of illnesses. What follows is a general guide to some of the broad categories of medication, how they work and the common side-effects.

PAINKILLERS (ANALGESICS)

Paracetamol and aspirin are the mildest analgesics, used for headaches, joint pains, period pain and toothache. They are equally effective, but aspirin also reduces inflammation. Paracetamol can be used in children under the age of twelve. Side-effects from paracetamol are rare, but it is potentially fatal even in minor overdose because of toxic effects on the liver.

Side-effects of aspirin and other anti-inflammatories (e.g. ibuprofen) include stomach irritation and bleeding. Asthma sufferers can be sensitive to aspirin, leading to increased wheezing, and some deaths have occurred. Stronger painkillers work on the brain to reduce the perception of pain. These drugs comprise opioid analgesics, such as codeine, pethidine and morphine. Side-effects include drowsiness, constipation, nausea and vomiting.

HEART DISEASE

There are around ten different classes of drugs used to treat a variety of heart and blood vessel conditions, including raised blood pressure, blood clots, angina and palpitations. The best known of the drugs are water tablets (diuretics). They remove excess fluid from the circulatory system, lowering blood pressure and improving breathing in heart failure. Side-effects include stomach upsets, gout and rashes.

Beta-blockers reduce heart rate and lower blood pressure, but can cause tiredness, cold hands and feet and sleep disturbances. They should not be taken by asthmatics because they may trigger a fatal attack of wheezing. Digoxin is used to treat irregular heart rate and may induce nausea, vomiting and loss of appetite if the dosage is too high. Some drugs used for treating raised blood pressure can cause impotence (reversible on stopping medication).

ASTHMA

There are two types of asthma therapy. Treatment of wheezing attacks is by inhaled drugs, including salbutamol and terbutaline (known as relievers),

---

The effect of painkillers

Strong painkillers known as opioids, derived from opium, are used to relieve severe pain. Pain is transmitted in signals along nerves from the source of pain to the brain, where it passes from one brain cell to another until it reaches the part of the brain that interprets the signal as pain. Opioid painkillers block the transmission of the nerve impulses in the brain, reducing the sensation of pain.

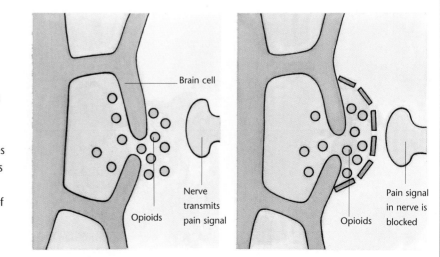

Brain cell

Nerve transmits pain signal

Opioids

Pain signal in nerve is blocked

Opioids

which open up the airways by relaxing the muscle in the walls of breathing tubes. Preventatives, such as inhaled steroids, improve breathing by reducing the amount of sticky mucus blocking the airways. Inhaled drugs have few side-effects, although steroids can cause an overgrowth of thrush (see page 425) at the back of the throat.

DEPRESSION

All drugs for depression work by affecting neurotransmitters, chemicals in the brain that pass signals between nerves. These neurotransmitters are low in depressed individuals. Older drugs called tricyclics work mainly on noradrenalin. Side-effects include drowsiness, agitation, dry mouth, constipation, blurred vision and retention of urine.

Newer drugs, such as Prozac, raise the levels of serotonin to improve symptoms. They may cause nausea, agitation, loss of appetite and sweating. Antidepressants take two to four weeks to have an effect, and should always be withdrawn slowly.

STOMACH PROBLEMS

Many stomach problems, including ulcers, heartburn and indigestion, are caused by excess acid in the stomach. The simplest drugs used to treat symptoms are antacids, which neutralise stomach acid. These drugs can form a raft on top of the stomach contents, preventing backflow from the stomach into the oesophagus.

More advanced drugs reduce acid production by blocking the action of nerves supplying acid-producing glands in the lining of the stomach (H_2 blockers), or by acting on the acid pump within the cells of these glands (proton pump inhibitors). These drugs have few side-effects, and work so well that it is difficult to persuade patients to stop taking them.

How bronchodilators work

Bronchodilators widen the airways of the lungs to ease breathing difficulties caused by conditions such as asthma. Before inhaling the drug, the airways become abnormally narrowed as the muscles in their walls contract.

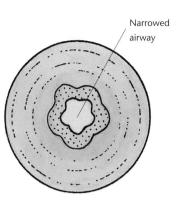

Narrowed airway

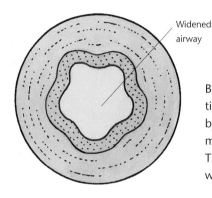

Widened airway

Bronchodilators relieve wheezing, tight chest and shortness of breath by acting on nerve endings in the muscles in the walls of the airways. The muscles relax and the airways widen, increasing airflow.

How antacids work

Acid in digestive juices may inflame the lining of the stomach and irritate the stomach walls. Antacids are used to relieve indigestion or help stomach ulcers to heal. They are mild alkaline substances taken orally that neutralise acidity in the digestive juices, allowing eroded areas in the mucous membrane lining the stomach to recover.

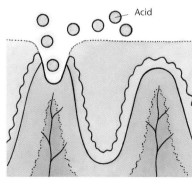

Acid

Digestive juices in the stomach contain acid, which may eat away at the mucous layer and inflame the stomach lining.

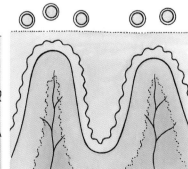

The antacid combines with stomach acid and neutralises it, reducing irritation and giving the mucous membrane time to heal.

DRUG INTERACTIONS

Drug interactions take place when a person takes two or more drugs at the same time. The drugs might be given for the same condition, for example raised blood pressure, or the person may have more than one illness requiring treatment. The effect of the interaction can vary from increased side-effects from one of the drugs to loss of effectiveness of any of the medicines involved in the interaction.

HOW DRUGS WORK

To understand how these interactions occur, it is essential to know what happens to a drug after it is swallowed, the most common way of taking medication. Generally, the drug reaches the stomach and is absorbed through the stomach wall into the bloodstream. Once in the blood, most molecules of the drug are carried along, loosely connected to proteins, until they reach their target tissues. Many drugs work by linking up to specific proteins called receptors on the surface of cells.

When the drug has performed its function, it has to be removed from the body. Most drugs are broken down in the liver and then eliminated from the bloodstream by the kidneys, which filter the remnants of the drug into the urine.

Interactions can occur in a number of ways, with the end result that either too high a level of medication is found in the blood, leading to increased side-effects, or too little of the drug is present and it will not work effectively.

TYPES OF INTERACTION

Sometimes, two drugs are taken at the same time that affect the same receptor site on the cell surface. The medication that has the strongest attraction to the receptor will prevent the other drug from having an effect. Alternatively, one drug may interfere with the effectiveness of another, either delaying or reducing it. Delayed absorption rarely has serious consequences, but reduced absorption makes a drug less effective.

Many drugs can increase the levels of the enzymes in the liver responsible for breaking down other drugs taken at the same time. This leads to lower concentrations of the affected medication in the blood, reducing its potency. This action is known as enzyme induction. When the drug causing the induction is withdrawn, levels of the second drug can increase dramatically, causing harmful effects.

SERIOUS INTERACTIONS

Many drug interactions are harmless, and even those that are potentially more serious will only occur in a small minority of patients. However, there is a number of more serious interactions, involving commonly prescribed drugs, which are important. Some of the most significant follow. The effectiveness of the oral contraceptive pill can be reduced by antibiotics and some drugs for epilepsy. Warfarin, a drug commonly used for thinning the blood, can be affected by some antibiotics, painkillers, drugs used to treat cholesterol, and epilepsy drugs. Antidepressants and tranquillisers are among the drugs acting on the central nervous system. They can have their sedative effects increased by some of the stronger painkillers available.

These are just a few of the hundreds of possible interactions that can take place. It would be very difficult for individual doctors to know all potential interactions, but almost all doctors use computers to generate prescriptions, and many of these interactions are highlighted by the computer system.

Interactions can also take place between prescription medicines and those bought over the counter from a pharmacist. This also applies to herbal medicines and homeopathic preparations. It is important to inform your doctor if you are taking any such medicines as it may influence her prescribing decision.

Drug routes into the body

There is a number of ways of introducing drugs into the body. Most drugs are taken orally in the form of pills, capsules or liquids. Intravenous injection enables a drug to take effect very quickly because it enters the bloodstream and is circulated to the part of the body where it is needed. Drugs act in a variety of ways. Some simply kill off invading organisms such as bacteria, viruses and fungi. Others alter the effects of body chemicals. Some may affect a part of the nervous system that controls a particular process.

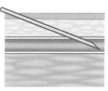

Transdermal route

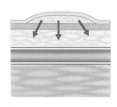

Intravenous route

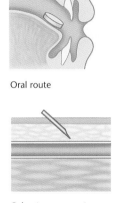

Oral route

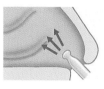

Nasal route

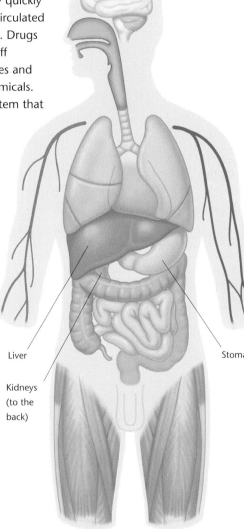

Liver

Kidneys
(to the
back)

Stomach

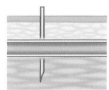

Subcutaneous route

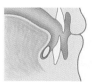

Sublingual route

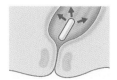

Rectal route

Intramuscular route

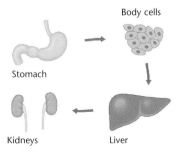

Body cells

Stomach

Kidneys

Liver

How a drug works

A drug taken orally reaches the stomach and is absorbed through the stomach walls into the bloodstream and carried to target tissues. It then has to be removed from the body, and is broken down in the liver and eliminated by the kidneys.

THE COMPLEMENTARY MEDICINE CHEST

A growing number of people use complementary remedies to treat everyday illnesses and minor accidents. These can also be used at home to speed recovery after first aid treatment, to relieve pain and calm the mind. This section gives an overview of some popular therapies, discusses what conditions they may be suitable for, and describes some remedies likely to be found in the home.

A BALANCED APPROACH

Most complementary practitioners look at the patient as a whole rather than just treating the physical symptoms of an illness. Emotional and spiritual health are considered to be just as important as physical health, and all need to be in a state of balance for a person to be truly well. The aim of treatment is to encourage the patient's powers of self-healing.

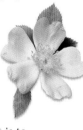

A first consultation is likely to take at least an hour as the practitioner builds up a complete picture to determine your condition and the appropriate remedy. You will be asked questions concerning medical history, diet, lifestyle and perhaps your moods, likes and dislikes. The number of sessions usually depends on the nature of the condition. Always inform your doctor if you are having this treatment because some medicines may interact with complementary remedies.

Complementary remedies are readily available from health food shops and pharmacies, but like their prescription counterparts should always be kept out of the reach of children because they may contain harmful ingredients.

AROMATHERAPY

Aromatherapy is a type of herbal medicine that uses concentrated plant essences known as essential oils to improve physical and emotional health. Essential oils are massaged into the skin or inhaled through the nose, and molecules within them enter the bloodstream. Scents released by the oils act on certain parts of the brain and in theory an aroma might affect stress levels, mood, metabolism and libido.

Most essential oils are extracted by steam distillation. Plant material is heated until it vaporises. The essential oil floats on top and is skimmed off and bottled. The most common form of aromatherapy is to massage diluted oils (combined with carrier oils such as almond or sunflower) into the skin. Inhalations are thought to be highly effective because smell receptors in the nose have direct links with the brain. Vaporisers and scented baths are also popular.

Aromatherapy is mainly used to treat stress-related conditions such as headache, anxiety, depression and sleeplessness. Various

RIGHT *A well-stocked complementary medicine chest might include: herbal remedies such as echinacea, comfrey, St John's wort, arnica; essential oils such as lavender, tea tree and eucalyptus; Bach's Rescue Remedy and various homeopathic preparations.*

oils may also be beneficial for digestive complaints (including indigestion, flatulence and diarrhoea), muscular aches and pains, skin problems such as acne, burns, stings and eczema, problems such as cystitis and thrush, and respiratory disorders (including coughs, colds, sinusitis and catarrh). Useful oils to have in stock include lavender, tea tree, eucalyptus, peppermint, rosemary, sandalwood and clary sage.

Essential oils should be stored in clear glass bottles away from light and heat in order to maintain their potency. Pay attention to instructions for dilution, and note that many oils are unsuitable for use on children. Some oils are safe to use during pregnancy or if you suffer from high blood pressure, and use inhalations with care if you have asthma or are prone to nosebleeds.

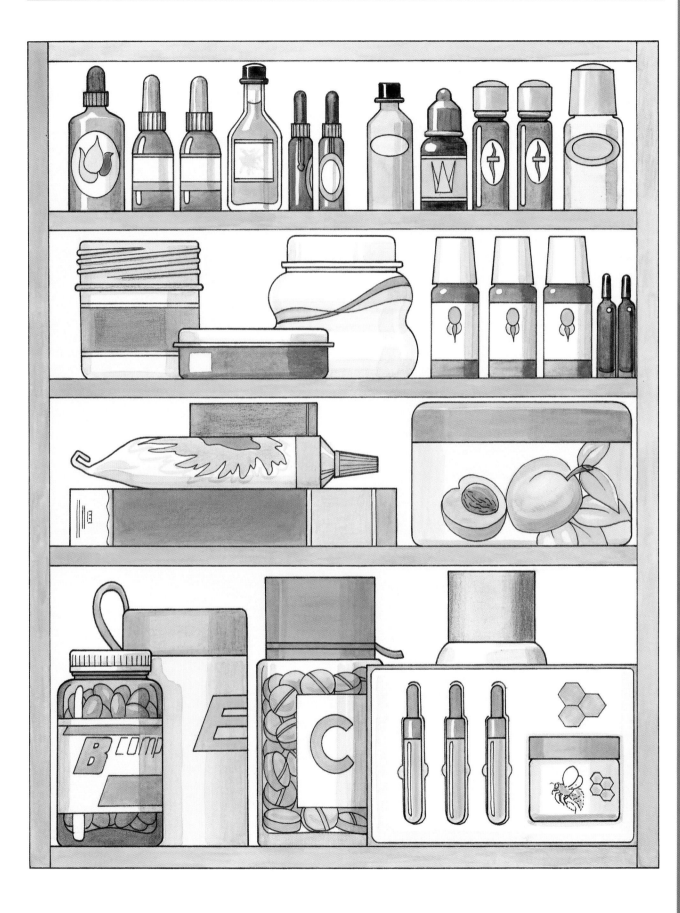

THE COMPLEMENTARY MEDICINE CHEST

BACH FLOWER REMEDIES

These remedies were developed in the 1930s by Dr Edward Bach, who believed that flowers possessed healing properties which could be used to treat emotional problems and restore physical and mental well-being. Dr Bach identified seven emotional categories (fearfulness, uncertainty, lack of interest in present circumstances, loneliness, over-sensitivity, despair and despondency, and over-concern for others' well-being), under which he grouped 38 remedies, which were developed primarily for self-help use.

Flower remedies are made by infusing or boiling plant material in spring water then preserving in alcohol, and are now available from all over the world. They are mainly used for dealing with emotional problems and stress. The compound Rescue Remedy is taken for shock, panic and hysteria, and is often found in the home.

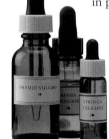

HERBALISM

Herbal remedies have been used for thousands of years throughout the world to treat disease and promote well-being. Many pharmaceutical drugs, such as aspirin and digoxin, are derived from isolated plant extracts, but herbalists believe that the therapeutic effects of plants are greater when the whole plant is used.

Wild herbs are dried and processed under strict conditions to form a variety of tablets, syrups, infusions, creams and ointments. Many of these preparations are now available from health food shops and pharmacies. Often, herbal medicines contain a number of herbs, each effective at relieving one particular symptom of an illness.

Herbal remedies are used for a variety of conditions including stress, fatigue, sleep disturbance, coughs and colds, skin complaints and menopausal symptoms. They should be avoided in pregnancy and during breastfeeding unless specific advice regarding safety has been obtained from a trained herbalist. Care should be taken if suffering from high blood pressure, diabetes, epilepsy, heart disease, or glaucoma. Useful herbal preparations for the home include comfrey, marigold, echinacea, St John's wort, feverfew, slippery elm, dong quai (for women), oil of evening primrose, ginseng, valerian and chamomile. Herbal treatments are not free from side-effects, and may interact with conventional medication. It is essential that you inform your herbalist and your doctor of any preparations being taken.

HOMEOPATHY

This is a popular system of medicine based on the principle of 'like cures like', meaning that the treatment is similar in substance to the illness it is relieving. The theory is that many symptoms experienced during an illness are a consequence of the body's own defence mechanisms attempting to cure the disease. By giving a substance that mimics the illness, the body's ability to fight off the condition is boosted. Homeopathic remedies are derived from many sources – vegetable, plant and mineral – and are prepared by making a solution of the original substance and diluting it, a process known as potentisation. The remedy is shaken rapidly after each dilution. One drop of the original solution is added to 99 drops of water and this solution has a potency of 1c. One drop of a 1c solution is then diluted again with 99 drops of water to produce a solution with a 2c strength, and so on. Most remedies are 6c or 30c potency.

According to homeopathic theory, the more diluted the remedy, the more potent it is considered to be. It seems likely that by the time the most dilute solutions are made up, there will be virtually no active ingredient left, and there is a theory that the water used to dilute the substance retains an imprint of the active ingredient, allowing it to exert its therapeutic effect. This theory is still open to debate but there is mounting evidence that homeopathy is safe, and can be an effective therapy for a wide range of conditions, often used with conventional medical treatment. Many homeopathic practitioners are also medically qualified and there is a number of NHS homeopathic hospitals in the UK.

Homeopathy can be used to treat a range of physical and psychological complaints, such as coughs and colds; digestive disorders; asthma and allergies; burns, cuts and bruises; skin rashes; menstrual and menopausal problems; anxiety and mild depression. Basic remedies, in the form of tablets, ointments and tinctures, are readily available in pharmacies and health food shops and can be used for simple maladies and first aid. Long-standing conditions such as eczema are best treated by individual remedies prescribed by a qualified homeopath.

Homeopathic remedies kept at home might include arnica, aconite, apis, carbo veg., graphites, hypericum, pulsatilla, sulphur and silica. When taking tablets, do not touch them: tap them out into the container lid or on to a clean teaspoon. Symptoms may briefly worsen after you start treatment, thought to be an effect of your immune system becoming activated. Remedies should be stored in tightly sealed containers in a cool, dark place, away from essential oils and perfumes.

NATUROPATHY

Naturopathy, or natural medicine, developed in the late 19th century and was based on ancient beliefs in the ability of the body to heal itself, given the right circumstances. It is a multi-disciplinary approach that uses non-invasive therapies to improve underlying health so that the patient is

less susceptible to infection, rather than treating symptoms directly. The most commonly used therapies include nutrition (including vitamin and mineral supplementation) and fasting, hydrotherapy, massage, osteopathy, herbalism, homeopathy, relaxation therapies, yoga and counselling. The aim is to support what is termed the "triad of health", the body's musculoskeletal system, its internal biochemistry and emotional well-being.

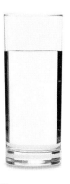

A naturopath may use a wide range of tests to build up a picture of your physical and emotional well-being. Tests may include a routine medical, X-rays, blood tests and sweat or hair analysis. Treatment is tailored to the individual's needs and will be catabolic (cleansing, to eliminate toxins) or anabolic (aiming to build up the system).

Naturopathy may be particularly beneficial for relieving stress and depression, tiredness, high blood pressure, digestive problems, skin conditions and conditions such as asthma and arthritis. Many of the principles advocated by naturopaths, such as the importance of regular exercise and a healthy diet, drinking plenty of water and deep breathing, have long been part of mainstream medical advice.

IN THE LARDER

Different foods have been used for centuries to treat illness and maintain good health. This is a part of folk medicine, the traditional beliefs, practices and materials used

in every culture to maintain well-being and fight disease in the absence of conventional medicine. Advice has been handed down from generation to generation to promote healing by supporting underlying good health, and is still used today because it works. Common conditions that respond well to home treatment include headaches, stress, anxiety and depression, respiratory disorders, skin problems, digestive problems, some forms of arthritis, premenstrual syndrome and menopause. Minor first aid conditions such as small burns, cuts, bruises, stings and sprains can also be safely treated. Serious disorders require medical attention.

Many common foodstuffs used to protect against illness are now being shown to have beneficial effects for health. Garlic, for example, may reduce levels of unhealthy cholesterol in the blood. Food can also be safely used with conventional medicine.

Traditional home remedies include onions for gastric infections, circulatory disorders, bronchitis and boils, garlic for respiratory and circulatory problems, and cabbage poultices to relieve the pain and inflammation of arthritis and to alleviate swollen, tender breasts in nursing mothers. Honey is taken to soothe sore throats or added to water to treat conjunctivitis. Lemon juice fights infection, yogurt treats thrush, cranberry juice is a urinary system bactericide and treatment for cystitis. Apply vinegar to stings to reduce swelling, add mustard powder to a footbath to treat colds and headaches, rub olive oil into the scalp to reduce flaking. For sore, irritated eyes, a slice of cucumber or a cold teabag on each eyelid will reduce swelling. To alleviate a hangover, many people swear by eating a grapefruit.

PART SIX

FIRST AID IN ACTION

CONTENTS

INTRODUCTION

This chapter covers emergency first aid: how to deal with major accidents or emergencies, should they occur. Prompt action on your part when confronted with a medical emergency can be life-saving, and everyone should know the basic first aid techniques to deal with accidents quickly, effectively and calmly. Even when a person's life is not in immediate danger, using first aid can help someone recover more quickly and avoid permanent damage.

To give first aid you need to understand and practise the techniques summarised in this section and explained in detail in Part One. You should also keep a first aid kit in your home that is easily accessible in an emergency.

The procedures in this chapter should be memorised in order to make use of them. If you have to waste time looking up relevant articles to refresh your memory, the delay in treatment could be the difference between life and death. However, to learn first aid properly you will need to complete a course of instruction and pass a professionally supervised examination.

Each spread in this section summarises a particular aspect of emergency first aid. Boxes give clear descriptions of signs and symptoms and instructions on what and what not to do. Photographic step-by-step illustrations are used throughout to clarify the procedures.

The first articles describe the most important principles of dealing with emergencies in which a person's life may be at risk. Aspects that are highlighted include checking for breathing and circulation, placing a person in the recovery position and life-saving techniques such as rescue breaths (mouth-to-mouth resuscitation) if breathing has stopped, and chest compression if both breathing and circulation have ceased. Using these techniques will ensure that vital organs such as the brain receive enough oxygen to keep the person alive until medical help is at hand.

Further articles describe how to deal with situations or injuries that could be life-threatening if not treated, such as choking, shock, burns, poisoning and severe bleeding. Asthma, heart attack, epilepsy and allergic reactions may also require emergency treatment.

Specific injuries such as head and eye injuries, broken bones and spinal injuries are also covered in this chapter. Although these may not be immediately life-threatening, first aid may help someone recover more quickly and avoid permanent damage.

First aid for children and infants sometimes requires different techniques, and this is highlighted when this is the case.

The aim of first aid is to save life, to stop the condition from getting worse and to speed recovery. However you must always remember to put your own safety first because you will not be able to help the casualty if you become a victim yourself.

ACTION IN AN EMERGENCY

DANGER

Is anyone in danger?

+ *If yes, can the danger be easily managed?*

+ *If it cannot, call for emergency help and protect the scene.*

RESPONSE

Move to the quietest victim first

+ *Gently shake the shoulders and ask her a question.*

+ *If there is a response, treat any life-threatening condition before checking the next person.*

+ *If there is no response, check the airway.*

ACT ON YOUR FINDINGS

If not breathing

+ *Give 2 rescue breaths by pinching the nose, sealing your mouth over her mouth and breathing into her.*

+ *If you are alone call for an ambulance as soon as you determine that the casualty is not breathing.*

ACT ON YOUR FINDINGS

If breathing

+ *Check for and treat any life-threatening conditions and place in the recovery position.*

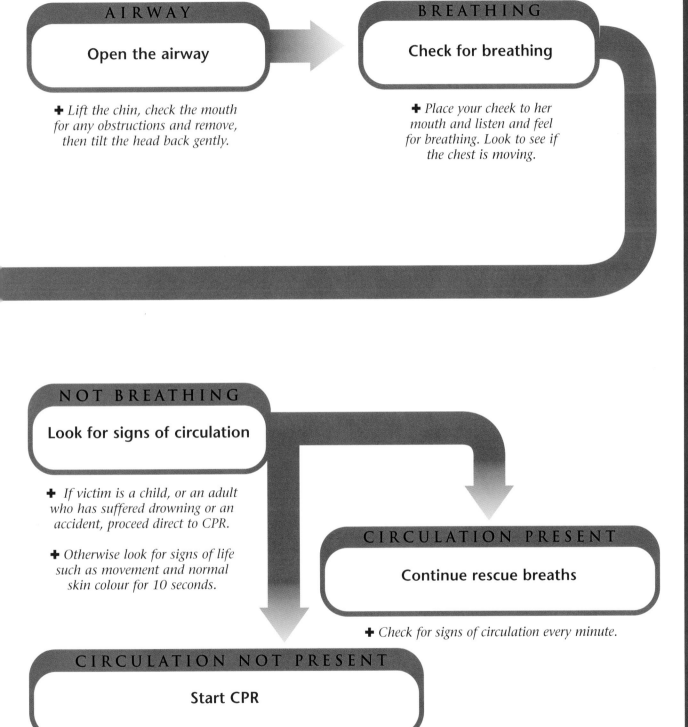

AIRWAY

Open the airway

✚ *Lift the chin, check the mouth for any obstructions and remove, then tilt the head back gently.*

BREATHING

Check for breathing

✚ *Place your cheek to her mouth and listen and feel for breathing. Look to see if the chest is moving.*

NOT BREATHING

Look for signs of circulation

✚ *If victim is a child, or an adult who has suffered drowning or an accident, proceed direct to CPR.*

✚ *Otherwise look for signs of life such as movement and normal skin colour for 10 seconds.*

CIRCULATION PRESENT

Continue rescue breaths

✚ *Check for signs of circulation every minute.*

CIRCULATION NOT PRESENT

Start CPR

✚ *Combine rescue breaths with chest compressions.*

THE RECOVERY POSITION

If faced with an unconscious person who is breathing, do a quick check for life-threatening injuries such as severe bleeding and treat if necessary. Turn the casualty into the recovery position. See also pages 22–25.

HOW TO TURN THE CASUALTY INTO THE RECOVERY POSITION

1 *Kneel beside the casualty. Remove the spectacles and any bulky objects from the pockets. Ensure that the airway is open.*

2 *Make sure both legs are straight. Place the arm nearest to you at right angles to the casualty's body, with the elbow bent and the palm facing upwards. Bring the arm furthest away from you across the chest and hold the back of the hand against the casualty's cheek nearest to you.*

3 *With your other hand, grasp the far leg just above the knee and pull it up, keeping the foot flat on the ground.*

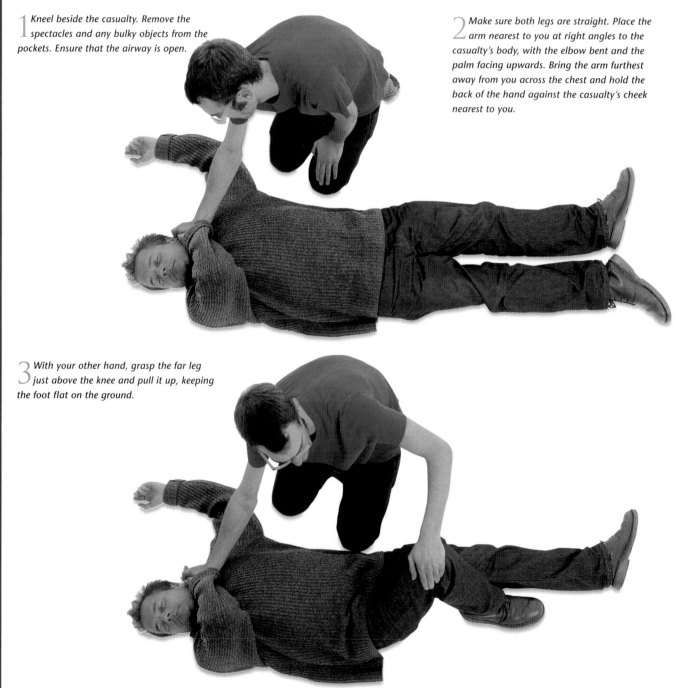

4 *Keeping the casualty's hand pressed against the cheek, pull on the far leg and roll the casualty towards you and on to his side. Adjust the upper leg so that both the hip and knee are bent at right angles.*

5 *Tilt the head back so that the airway remains open. If necessary, adjust the hand under the cheek to make sure the head remains tilted and the airway stays open.*

6 *If it has not already been done, call for emergency help.*

7 *Check the breathing regularly. Monitor the circulation in the lower arm.*

If the casualty has to be left in the recovery position for longer than 30 minutes, he should be turned on to the opposite side.

Recovery position for babies

If looking after a baby, cradle the infant in your arms on her side, maintaining an open airway by lifting the chin and tilting the baby gently to one side if vomit or mucus needs to be removed from the mouth.

The main priority is to maintain an open and clear airway.

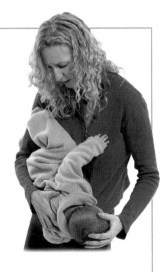

Signs and symptoms of an unconscious person

- No movement
- No, or limited, response to questioning

Managing an unconscious casualty

DO
- *Take care when turning the person over – do not rush, and consider other possible injuries by thinking about the history of the accident.*
- *Keep a careful check on the airway and breathing once the casualty is on his side.*
- *Be prepared to turn the casualty back on to his back if breathing stops.*
- *Ask for help from others.*

DO NOT
- *Waste time looking for additional injuries before turning the casualty over – do a quick check for life-threatening conditions such as serious bleeding.*

WHAT IF
- *There may be an an injury to the spine? Maintain the airway with the casualty in the position found and prepare to turn or log roll (see pages 94–95) the casualty on to his side should a problem develop with keeping the airway clear.*

RESCUE BREATHS

Vital organs such as the brain need a continuous supply of oxygen to function. If the brain is deprived of oxygen for more than three minutes, it will begin to fail. Giving rescue breaths (mouth-to-mouth resuscitation) to somebody who is not breathing could mean the difference between life and death. See also pages 26–29.

IF THE CASUALTY IS NOT BREATHING

• *Call for emergency help*
Note: if the casualty is a child or baby, give 1 minute of rescue breaths (or full CPR if required, see pages 32–33) before going for help
• *Give 2 effective rescue breaths*

Signs and symptoms

No circulation
• *No movement*
• *Loss of normal colour to the skin and blue lips*
• *Absence of normal breathing*

If there are signs of circulation
• *Continue giving rescue breaths with regular checks for circulation*
• *Do rescue breaths at a rate of 10 a minute for an adult and 20 a minute for children and babies*

If there are no signs of circulation or you are at all unsure
• *Start chest compressions*

GIVING 2 EFFECTIVE RESCUE BREATHS

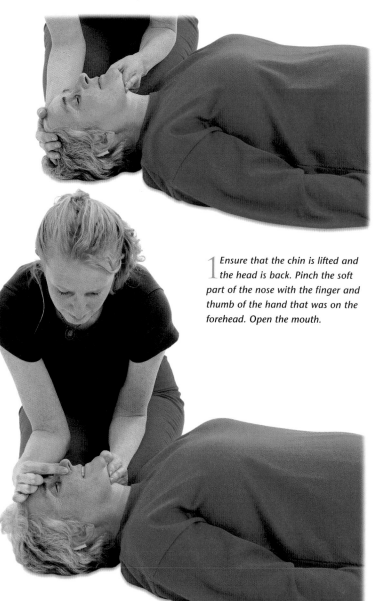

1 *Ensure that the chin is lifted and the head is back. Pinch the soft part of the nose with the finger and thumb of the hand that was on the forehead. Open the mouth.*

2 Take a deep breath to fill your lungs with air and place your lips around the casualty's mouth, making sure you have a good seal.

Keep the airway open by tilting the head back, lifting the chin and supporting with two fingers

Pinch the casualty's nose shut; take a deep breath and place your lips around mouth to form tight seal

3 Blow steadily into the mouth and watch the chest rise.

Note: for a baby, simply empty your cheeks of air rather than blowing too hard into the mouth.

4 Maintaining head tilt and chin lift, take your mouth away and watch the chest fall.

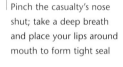

Check the casualty's chest for signs of breathing.

Giving rescue breaths and checking for circulation

DO
• *Make sure that the head is back, the mouth is open and that you have pinched the nose.*
• *Give 1 minute of rescue breaths (or rescue breaths combined with chest compressions if needed) before phoning for help if the casualty is a baby or child.*
• *Use less breath for a baby.*

DO NOT
• *Breathe too fast or forget to take a breath yourself between each rescue breath.*

WHAT IF
• *The chest does not rise? Re-open the airway, check that the nose is pinched and that you have a good seal around the mouth and try again up to a total of 5 attempts to give 2 breaths. If this is unsuccessful, move straight on to chest compressions and full CPR.*
• *There are burns or other damage to the mouth? Consider giving the breaths into the nose by closing the mouth and sealing your mouth around the nose. Come away after each breath and open the mouth to allow air to escape.*

Look for signs of circulation
Look, listen and feel for breathing, coughing, movement, normal colour or any other sign of life for not more than 10 seconds.

CPR FOR ADULTS, CHILDREN AND BABIES

These pages give emergency instructions on giving help to somebody whose heart has stopped. For more detailed information, see CPR, pages 30–33.

CHEST COMPRESSION FOR AN ADULT

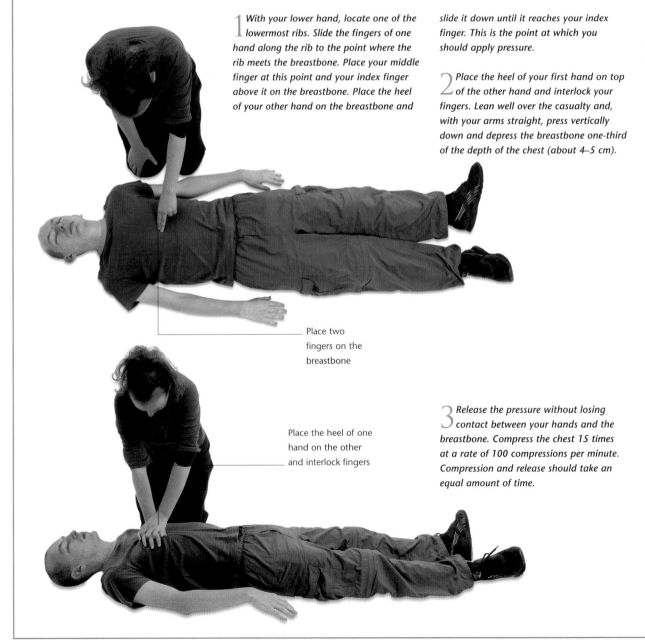

1 With your lower hand, locate one of the lowermost ribs. Slide the fingers of one hand along the rib to the point where the rib meets the breastbone. Place your middle finger at this point and your index finger above it on the breastbone. Place the heel of your other hand on the breastbone and slide it down until it reaches your index finger. This is the point at which you should apply pressure.

2 Place the heel of your first hand on top of the other hand and interlock your fingers. Lean well over the casualty and, with your arms straight, press vertically down and depress the breastbone one-third of the depth of the chest (about 4–5 cm).

Place two fingers on the breastbone

Place the heel of one hand on the other and interlock fingers

3 Release the pressure without losing contact between your hands and the breastbone. Compress the chest 15 times at a rate of 100 compressions per minute. Compression and release should take an equal amount of time.

CHEST COMPRESSION FOR A CHILD

1 *Place the heel of one hand on the lower third of the breastbone.*

2 *Compress the chest to a third of its depth.*

3 *Release the pressure without losing contact between your hands and the breastbone. Compress the chest 5 times at a rate of 100 compressions per minute.*

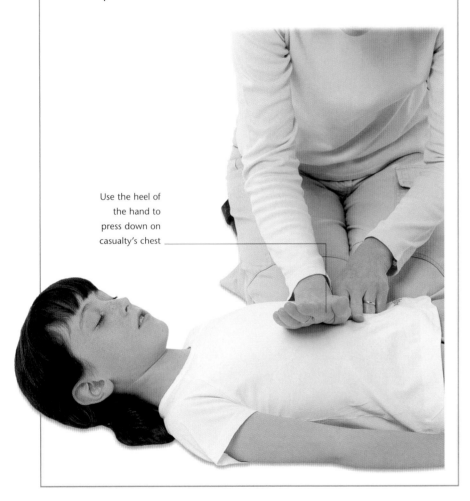

Use the heel of the hand to press down on casualty's chest

Performing CPR

DO
• *Pace yourself – CPR is tiring; swap with other rescuers if you can.*
• *Make sure that an ambulance is called as soon as possible.*

DO NOT
• *Press too hard on the chest of a child or baby.*

WHAT IF
• *The person shows signs of recovery? Stop what you are doing and return to the checks for airway, breathing and circulation. If the person is breathing for himself, place in the recovery position and monitor carefully. Be prepared to restart CPR if needed.*

CHEST COMPRESSIONS FOR A BABY

1 *Place two fingers of one hand on the lower third of the breastbone.*

2 *Compress the chest to a third of its depth.*

3 *Release the pressure without losing contact between your hands and the breastbone. Compress the chest 5 times at a rate of 100 compressions per minute.*

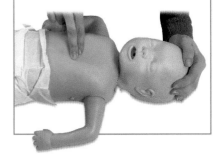

PERFORM CPR BY COMBINING RESCUE BREATHS AND COMPRESSIONS

1 *After 15 compressions (for an adult) or 5 compressions (for a baby or child), tilt the head, lift the chin and give 2 effective breaths (for an adult) or 1 breath (for a baby or child).*

2 *Do not interrupt the CPR sequence unless the casualty makes a movement or takes a breath unaided.*

3 *Continue until:*
• *Emergency help comes to take over.*
• *The casualty shows signs of life.*
• *Others offer help.*
• *You become so exhausted that you cannot carry on.*

CHOKING IN ADULTS, CHILDREN AND BABIES

Choking is due to an obstruction in the windpipe that makes it difficult to breathe. Without treatment, a person will die. See also pages 34–37.

Signs and symptoms of choking

- *Coughing at first*
- *Grasping the neck*
- *Being unable to talk, cough or breathe*
- *Red face, losing colour as breathing affected*
- *Blue lips*
- *Loss of consciousness*

Managing choking

DO
- *Encourage the victim to get the head lower than the chest – gravity helps.*

DO NOT
- *Perform abdominal thrusts on a baby.*

WHAT IF
- *The person becomes unconscious? Begin CPR (see pages 30–33). If the casualty is not breathing and the chest does not rise when rescue breaths are attempted, move straight to chest compressions without assessment of circulation. Check the mouth after every set of compressions.*

HOW TO DO BACK SLAPS

1 *Stand beside the victim. Support to bend over as far as possible.*

2 *Using the heel of one hand, hit the person between the shoulder blades.*

3 *Repeat up to 5 blows as needed to try to dislodge the object.*

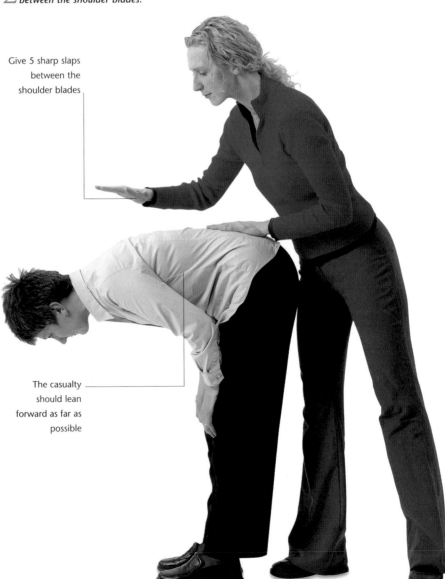

Give 5 sharp slaps between the shoulder blades

The casualty should lean forward as far as possible

HOW TO DO CHEST THRUSTS

1 *If the victim cannot clear the object, stand or kneel behind the casualty.*

2 *Make a fist and place it against the lower half of the casualty's breastbone. Grasp the fist with your other hand. Pull sharply inwards and upwards.*

3 *Perform 5 chest thrusts at a rate of 1 every 3 seconds. The aim is to relieve the obstruction with each chest thrust rather than necessarily doing all 5.*

If the chest thrusts fail, do 5 abdominal thrusts to dislodge the object.

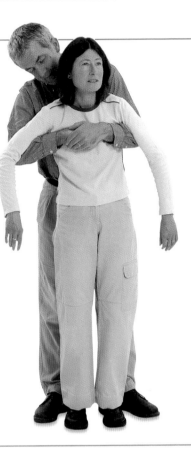

HOW TO DO ABDOMINAL THRUSTS

1 *Stand or kneel behind the casualty and put both arms around the upper abdomen. Make sure the casualty is bending well forwards.*

2 *Clench your fist and place it between the navel and the bottom of the breastbone. Grasp it with your other hand.*

3 *Pull sharply inwards and upwards 5 times. The aim is to relieve the obstruction with each abdominal thrust.*

DO NOT PERFORM ABDOMINAL THRUSTS ON A BABY.

Make a fist and position it in the middle of the abdomen, below the breastbone.

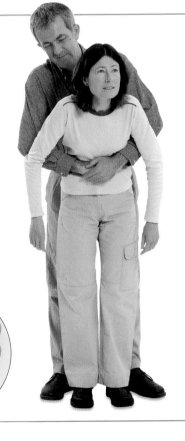

How to deal with choking

Adult
- *Encourage the victim to cough*
- *Support to bend over as far as possible*
- *Give 5 back slaps*
- *Check the mouth*
- *Give 5 abdominal thrusts*
- *Check the mouth*
- *Repeat slaps and thrusts 3 more times*
- *Go for emergency help*
- *Continue cycle*

Child
- *Encourage the victim to cough*
- *Support to bend over as far as possible or put over your lap*
- *Give 5 back slaps*
- *Check the mouth*
- *Give 5 chest thrusts*
- *Check the mouth*
- *Give 5 abdominal thrusts*
- *Check the mouth*
- *Repeat slaps and thrusts 3 more times*
- *Go for emergency help*
- *Continue cycle*

Baby (under one year)
- *Hold the baby upside down, taking care to support the back and head*
- *Give 5 back slaps*
- *Check the mouth*
- *Give 5 chest thrusts*
- *Check the mouth*
- *Repeat slaps and thrusts 3 more times*
- *Go for emergency help*
- *Continue cycle*

ASTHMA

Asthma attacks cause the muscle of the air passages to go into spasm, making it very difficult for the sufferer to breathe, particularly to breathe air out. For more information, see Asthma, pages 366–67.

TREATMENT

1 *Reassure and try to calm the person having the attack as this will have a positive effect on breathing.*

2 *Help the casualty into a sitting position leaning slightly forwards, as most asthmatics find this an easier position for breathing.*

3 *If the casualty has medication, enable her to use it – inhalers are the main form of treatment and are generally blue.*

If this is the first attack, the medication does not work within 5 minutes or the casualty is in severe distress, call an ambulance. Help the person to take medication every 5–10 minutes.

If the attack eases and the casualty find it easier to breathe she will not need immediate medical attention but should advise a doctor of the attack. The person will often be very tired so it is best to ensure that she is accompanied home.

Signs and symptoms of asthma

• *History of the condition (although some people may not realise that they are asthmatic and their first attack may be a very severe one)*
• *Difficulty in breathing, particularly breathing out*
• *Wheezing or otherwise noisy breathing*
• *Inability to speak*
• *Pale skin with potential blueness, particularly around the lips*
• *Distress, dizziness and confusion as it becomes harder to get oxygen into the body*
• *Potentially unconsciousness and then the breathing stopping*

Treatment for asthma

DO
• *Help the sufferer to take his or her own medication.*

DO NOT
• *Underestimate the seriousness of asthma. Be prepared to call for medical help if the inhaler does not ease the attack or the condition*

deteriorates. Be prepared to resuscitate if the person stops breathing.

WHAT IF
• *The casualty does not have an inhaler? Help her into the most comfortable position and call an ambulance.*

HEART ATTACK

A heart attack is caused by a blockage in the blood vessels supplying the heart with blood. A heart attack can happen at any time and can be minor, where only a small part of the heart is affected and the symptoms are minimal, or more serious, where a large part of the heart is affected and possibly even stops. For more information on heart attacks, see pages 392–93.

TREATMENT

1 *Move the casualty into a half-sitting position, with head and shoulders supported and knees bent, as this is generally the best position to breathe in.*

2 *Reassure the casualty and do not let him move, as this will place an extra strain on the heart.*

3 *Call for an ambulance as soon as possible because medical treatment for the casualty will be required.*

4 *If the casualty has angina medication, allow him or her to take this. If you have an ordinary aspirin, give him one to chew (without water).*

5 *Keep a continual check on the breathing and pulse and be prepared to resuscitate if necessary.*

Check the pulse regularly to assess circulation

Signs and symptoms of heart attack

• *Possible previous history of angina attacks or heart attacks*
• *Gripping chest pain, often described by the sufferer as 'vice-like'*
• *This pain may spread up into the jaw or down into the left arm*
• *There may be a feeling of pins and needles down the arm*
• *Shortness of breath*
• *Dizziness and confusion*
• *Anxiety*
• *Pale skin with possible blue tinges*
• *Rapid weak pulse*

Treatment for heart attack

DO
• *Check whether the person has ever suffered from angina. It may be an angina attack. Treat in the same way.*
• *Reassure the casualty – this has a very positive effect on the heart rate.*

DO NOT
• *Let the person move – this places extra pressure on the heart.*

WHAT IF
• *The heart stops? Open the airway, check breathing, call for an ambulance and give CPR.*

SHOCK

Shock occurs as a result of a loss of circulating blood from the body that can be fatal. Potential causes include severe internal or external bleeding and problems with the heart. It can also be due to loss of body fluids from burns or severe vomiting and diarrhoea. For more information, see pages 44–45.

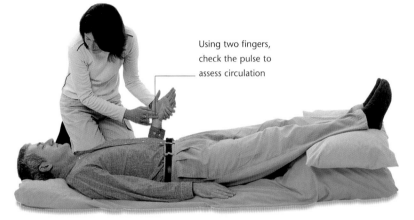

Using two fingers, check the pulse to assess circulation

WHAT HAPPENS WITH SHOCK

A severe loss of body fluid will dramatically reduce the flow of blood around the body. As blood flow slows so does the amount of oxygen reaching the brain. The casualty may appear to be confused, weak and dizzy and may eventually become unconscious. To compensate for the lack of oxygen, the heart and breathing rates both speed up. They become gradually weaker and may eventually cease.

Signs and symptoms of shock

• *Pale, cold and clammy skin*
• *Fast, weak pulse*
• *Fast, shallow breathing*
• *Dizziness and weakness*
• *Confusion*
• *Unconsciousness*
• *Breathing and heartbeat stopping*

Immediate action

WARMTH Keep the injured person warm but do not overheat. Protect from the elements.

AIR Loosen tight clothing and keep bystanders back.

REST Lie the person down with the legs raised. This reduces pressure on the heart and encourages blood flow back to the brain and other key organs.

MENTAL REST Reassure the person.

TREATMENT Treat the cause of shock.

HELP Seek appropriate medical help.

Treatment for shock

DO
• *Prevent the condition from getting worse by treating the cause, keeping the injured person at rest and reassuring him or her.*
• *Monitor and maintain airway and breathing and be prepared to resuscitate as necessary.*

DO NOT
• *Underestimate shock – it can kill. Call for an ambulance if the signs and symptoms of serious shock are present or you cannot treat the cause of the shock, for example, internal bleeding.*

WHAT IF
• *The person becomes unconscious? Open the airway, check breathing and if the casualty is breathing, turn into recovery position and call an ambulance.*
• *The casualty has the signs and symptoms of shock but no obvious cause? It is likely to be an internal injury. Treat for shock and call an ambulance.*

SEVERE BLEEDING

A large blood loss is a life-threatening occurrence leading, if left untreated, to shock and potentially death. Arterial bleeding, where the blood is pumped out under pressure, bleeding from jagged wounds (lacerations) and internal bleeding present the most danger. For more information, see Bleeding, pages 58–63.

Signs and symptoms of severe bleeding

- *Evidence of wound*
- *Blood around the site*
- *Signs and symptoms of shock: pale skin, fast breathing and heart rate, nausea, dizziness*

TREATMENT

The three main principles of the treatment of external bleeding are:

Look

Apply direct pressure

Elevate

While treating bleeding it is also vital to treat for shock and to make appropriate arrangements for secondary help.

1 *Look at the wound to check how large it is. Check that the wound has nothing in it (known as a foreign body).*

2 *Apply direct pressure to the wound. If the casualty is able to press on the wound himself, encourage her to do so. If not, apply pressure yourself, initially with your fingers and, if you have something to hand, eventually a sterile dressing or a piece of clean cloth. Applying pressure to the wound enables the blood to clot and stems the blood flow from the cut. Once applied, a sterile dressing (or whatever you have to hand) should ideally*

be held in place with a firm bandage or an improvised bandage such as a scarf or tie.

3 *Elevate the wound. If the injury is on an arm or leg, raise the wound above the level of the heart. It is harder for the blood to pump upwards and this therefore reduces the blood flow to the wound and therefore the fluid loss from the body.*

4 *Treat for shock. Keep the casualty warm. Keep the casualty at rest. Reassure the person.*

For advice on dealing with internal bleeding, see box below and pages 68–69.

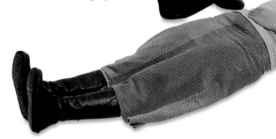

Raise injured limb above the level of the heart

Treatment for serious bleeding

DO
- *Treat for shock: keep the person warm, make her comfortable (either sitting or lying down) and reassure her.*
- *Check the injury, applying direct pressure and raising to help control the bleeding.*
- *Use a sterile dressing or clean piece of material to cover and apply further direct pressure to the wound.*

DO NOT
- *Remove anything sticking into the wound – bandage around it.*

WHAT IF
- *The bleeding is internal? Signs and symptoms of shock may be present, as well as evidence of bruising or stiffness over the site of the injury. Treat for shock and call an ambulance.*

UNCONSCIOUSNESS

Unconsciousness is an interruption of normal brain activity. It can happen suddenly or can be as a result of slow deterioration and has a number of causes. An unconscious person may still have some reactions, for example, to pain or to commands, or may have no reactions at all. For more information, see Unconsciousness, pages 54–55.

TREATMENT

Whatever the cause or degree of unconsciousness, the immediate emergency treatment remains the same:

- *Open airway*
- *Check breathing*
- *Place in the recovery position after checking for life-threatening conditions*
- *Be prepared to resuscitate if necessary*

Gently shake the shoulders and ask casualty a question

If you have time, there are some things that you can do that may provide medical staff with additional valuable information about the person's condition.

1. Monitor and record breathing and pulse rate

Take these recordings every 10 minutes and write them down if possible.

2. Assess the level of response

There is an agreed scale for assessing how responsive an injured or ill person is: the Glasgow Coma Scale. This scale focuses on measuring the person's:

Movement: for example, does the person move in response to commands or not at all?

Speech: for example, does the casualty answer coherently or does he mumble incomprehensibly?

Eyes: for example, does the person open his eyes spontaneously when you talk to him?

3. Examining the unconscious person

Check the body from head to toe looking for smaller bleeds, signs of broken bones or burns or clues as to the cause of consciousness.

Treatment for unconsciousness

DO
- *Monitor and maintain the airway, breathing and circulation throughout any check of an unconscious person.*
- *Treat any additional injuries.*
- *Hand over all information to medical staff, even if you are not sure of its value.*

DO NOT
- *Move an unconscious person unnecessarily to check him.*

WHAT IF
- *You cannot find the cause of unconsciousness? Treat any conditions and hand any clues over to medical staff.*

HEAD AND EYE INJURIES

Head injuries usually require assessment by trained medical staff. Eye injuries are potentially serious and need prompt attention to minimise the risk of impaired vision or infection. See also pages 62 and 70.

TREATING HEAD INJURIES

1 *Help the injured person to sit or lie down.*

2 *Check for any signs of head injury. Treat as appropriate.*

3 *Apply direct pressure to the wound to stop the bleeding.*

4 *Cover the wound with a sterile dressing or a clean pad. Tie this in place with a bandage.*

5 *Take or send the casualty to hospital.*

If the person becomes unconscious, monitor and maintain the airway and breathing and be prepared to resuscitate as necessary.

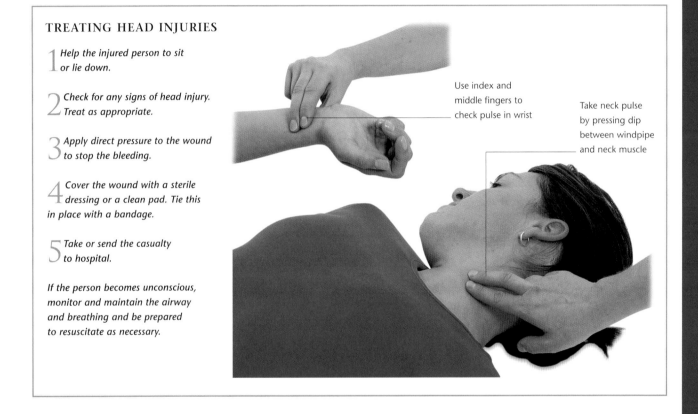

Use index and middle fingers to check pulse in wrist

Take neck pulse by pressing dip between windpipe and neck muscle

TREATING EYE WOUNDS

1 *Lay the person down, on the back if possible, and hold the head to prevent movement.*

2 *Ask the casualty to try to keep the eyes still to prevent movement of the injured eye. Ask the person to focus on something.*

3 *Ask the casualty to hold a clean pad over the eye to help prevent movement and infection. If the wait for an ambulance or other further help may take some time, you may wish to hold this pad for the*

casualty or gently bandage it in place. However, because blood loss from the eye area is not likely to be life-threatening, any bandage should be used only to hold the pad in place and not to apply pressure.

Do not attempt to remove any object embedded in the eye. If the object is very long, gently support it at its base to prevent movement. If small, ensure that the pad that you place over the eye does not push it in any further.

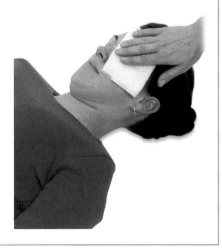

EPILEPSY

Epilepsy is a very common condition, best described as a rogue electrical discharge across the brain. As the body's functions are controlled by electrical impulses, this discharge can lead to a number of physical reactions. Many things may start a fit or seizure: tiredness, alcohol, stress or flashing lights are common triggers. For more information, see Epilepsy, pages 52–53.

Signs and symptoms

- *Potential 'aura' to warn of fit*
- *Muscle spasms followed by brief period of unconsciousness*
- *History of high temperature (for infantile convulsions)*

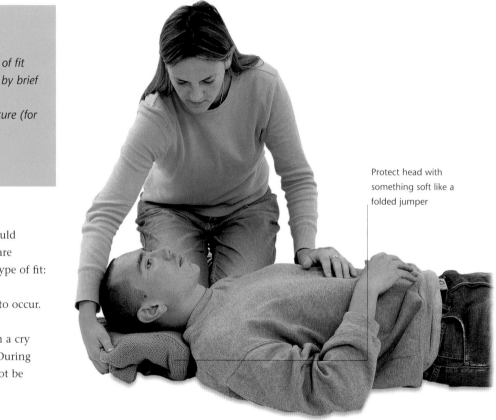

Protect head with something soft like a folded jumper

MAJOR SEIZURE

This is what most people would recognise as epilepsy. There are typically four stages to this type of fit:

1. A sense that a fit is likely to occur.

2. Falling to the ground with a cry and having muscle spasms. During this stage the casualty will not be breathing.

3. When the convulsion has finished the casualty will be in a state of unconsciousness.

4. On recovery from unconsciousness the casualty will be very sleepy.

TREATMENT FOR A MAJOR EPILEPTIC SEIZURE

1. During the fit do not try to restrain the person.

- *Do not put anything in the mouth.*

- *Do try to protect the casualty: move sharp objects out of the way, remove constrictions and, if possible, place something such as a folded coat or jumper under the head.*

2. Once the convulsion has finished, check the person's airway and breathing and be prepared to resuscitate in the unlikely event that this is necessary. Place in the recovery position while the person recovers.

3. When the casualty comes around, reassure him. He may have lost control of bladder or bowel function so cover him up and, when he is steady on his feet, help him to find somewhere to clean up. The person is likely to be very tired, so if possible find him somewhere to lie down and sleep. Most important of all, ask the person what he wants to do – most epileptics manage the condition very well and will have their own coping strategies.

INFANTILE CONVULSIONS (CAUSED BY HEAT)

Babies and young children may have
fits induced by a high temperature.
This may be the result of an infection
or because they are over-wrapped and
in a warm environment. The signs
and symptoms are similar to a major
epileptic seizure.

Treatment

1 *Make sure that the child is protected
from hitting himself on a bed or cot.
Do not attempt to restrain him.*

2 *Cool the child down by removing
bedclothes and clothing where
possible. Sponge the child's head and
under his arms with a tepid flannel or
sponge, re-soaking it regularly.*

3 *When the fit is finished, check ABC
(see pages 20–21) and take action
as appropriate.*

4 *In most cases the child will want to sleep.
Dress him in dry clothes and let him sleep.
Call a doctor for advice.*

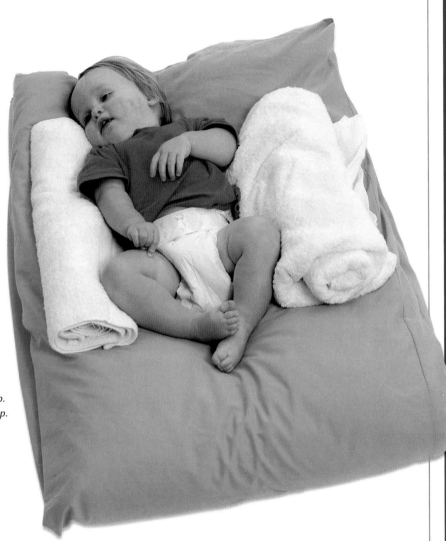

Treatment for epileptic fits and infantile convulsions

DO
- *Protect the individual during the fit.*
- *Check airway and breathing after the fit and turn into the
recovery position.*

DO NOT
- *Restrain the person during the seizure.*
- *Try to put anything in the mouth.*

WHAT IF
- *The person injures himself during the fit? Treat the injury
and call an ambulance as needed.*
- *The fit lasts for longer than three minutes or there are
repeated fits in a short period of time? Call an ambulance.*
- *The person does not regain consciousness? Open airway
and check breathing and be prepared to resuscitate. Call
an ambulance.*

HOW TO TREAT BROKEN BONES

Broken bones are known as fractures and the general rule for treating them is to keep them still, as this reduces pain and the likelihood of further injury. For more information on treating broken bones, see pages 80–91.

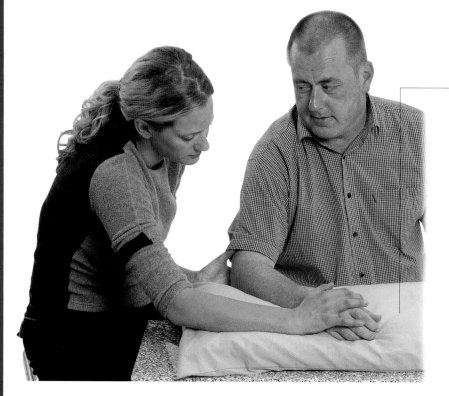

Support the injured part with padding such as a pillow

Signs and symptoms of broken bones

- *Pain*
- *Swelling*
- *Tenderness*
- *Loss of movement*
- *Loss of feeling*
- *Bruising*
- *Deformity when compared to the uninjured side*
- *Bone is visible*

Breaks or cracks in the bones can happen anywhere in in the body. Most are caused by injury such as direct impact or by twisting during a fall. There are two main types of fracture: open (compound), in which the bone pierces the skin and closed (simple) in which it does not. Treatment is a three-stage process:

1. *Help the injured person into the most comfortable position.*

2. *Steady and support the injured part to reduce pain and further damage.*

3. *Provide additional support if the wait for medical attention will be lengthy or the person needs to be moved.*

Treatment

DO

- *Listen to what the injured person tells you – he is the best judge of what is most comfortable for him.*
- *Steady and support the injured part with your hands and padding such as blankets, pillows and bandages.*
- *Seek medical advice even if you are not sure that the bone is broken.*

DO NOT

- *Move the injured part unnecessarily.*
- *Forget to check the circulation if you have bandaged the injured part.*

WHAT IF

The bone is exposed? Cover open breaks (where the bone is showing) with a sterile dressing or clean piece of material, taking care not to press on the injury.

HOW TO TREAT BACK INJURIES

Back injuries carry with them risk to the spinal cord which, if damaged, can lead to temporary or permanent paralysis or restricted movement. The treatment for a patient with suspected spinal injuries is to keep the person still, while monitoring and maintaining their airway and breathing and treating for shock. For more detailed information on treating back injuries, see pages 92–95.

Treatment

DO
• *Treat for shock.*
• *Move the head to the neutral position if you have been trained to do so (see page 95).*
• *Monitor airway and breathing.*

DO NOT
• *Move the person unnecessarily.*

WHAT IF
• *The person becomes unconscious? Check airway and breathing.*
• *If the airway is open in the position, keep him still and check breathing.*
• *If the airway is not open, get help from bystanders to move the injured person into a safer position such as the recovery position or on to his side using a log roll technique (see pages 94–95).*
• *If the person is not breathing give rescue breaths. Combine these with chest compressions if circulation is absent. If you need to turn the person over to resuscitate, do so gently but quickly.*

IF THE CASUALTY IS CONSCIOUS

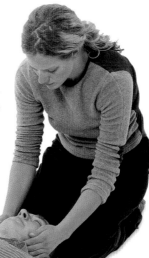

1 *If the casualty is conscious and already lying down, leave him where he is. If the person is walking around, support him down to lie on the ground. If you can, put a blanket or coat down to go underneath the person before you lay him down.*

2 *Tell the person to keep still.*

3 *Ensure that an ambulance has been called.*

4 *Hold the casualty's head still by placing your hands over the ears and laying your fingers along the line of the jaw.*

5 *Do not remove your support from the head until help arrives.*

Signs and symptoms of back injuries

BROKEN BACK
• *Dent or step in the spine which may indicate a displaced back bone (vertebra)*
• *Bruising or swelling over the spine*
• *Complaint of back pain*
• *Tenderness over the area of the break*

SPINAL CORD DAMAGE
• *Loss of movement below the site of the break*
• *Pins and needles in the fingers and*
toes or throughout the body
• *Person feels strange, possibly 'jelly-like'*
• *Numbness*

If any of these signs and symptoms are present, or if the nature of the accident indicates a potential broken bone, such as a heavy impact or fall from a height, assume that there is spinal injury. Back injury is potentially serious: seek emergency help immediately.

HOW TO TREAT BURNS

Burns are potentially very serious injuries. They carry with them three main risks: shock, infection and restriction of the airway. For more information on dealing with burns, see pages 104–105.

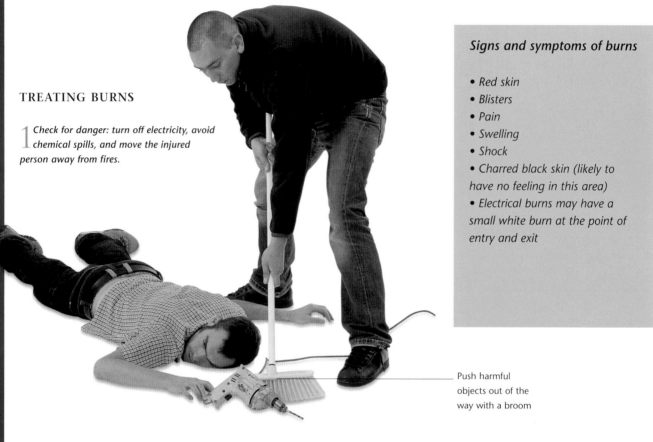

Signs and symptoms of burns

- Red skin
- Blisters
- Pain
- Swelling
- Shock
- Charred black skin (likely to have no feeling in this area)
- Electrical burns may have a small white burn at the point of entry and exit

TREATING BURNS

1 Check for danger: turn off electricity, avoid chemical spills, and move the injured person away from fires.

Push harmful objects out of the way with a broom

2 Monitor and maintain the airway and breathing and be prepared to resuscitate if necessary.

Watch to see the chest rise and fall

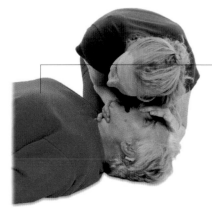

3 Cool the injured part with cool (but not very cold) water. Cool for at least 10 minutes or until the pain has stopped. Cool chemical burns for longer to ensure that all the chemicals have been flooded away.

Poor cool water over the affected part

4 *Make an appropriate decision about what help is required and call for an ambulance if necessary, for example if the injured person has any breathing difficulties, if he or she is showing signs and symptoms of shock, and if the burns are very deep or cover a large area of the body.*

Cover with a
sterile dressing
and bandage

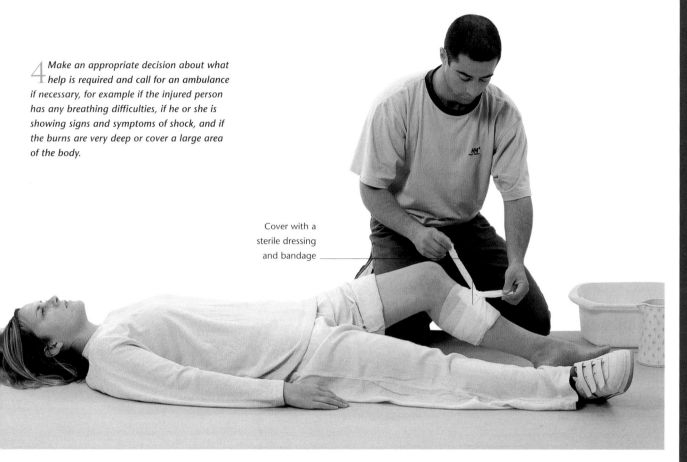

5 *Cover the injured part with a clean, non-fluffy dressing.*

6 *Treat for shock throughout your treatment of the burn.*

7 *Raise the injured part if possible.*

Treatment for burns

DO

• *Cool the injured part for as long as needed, taking care not to over-cool the rest of the injured person.*
• *Remove rings, watches or other items that may become tight around the injured part as it swells.*

DO NOT

• *Use a fluffy dressing to cover the burn. Instead, use a sterile dressing, a clean piece of non-fluffy material or a clean sandwich bag or piece of clingfilm.*
• *Apply any lotions to the burn.*
• *Remove clothing that is stuck to the burn.*
• *Burst blisters.*

WHAT IF

• *It is an electrical burn? Make sure that the source of the electricity is safe, particularly before you pour water over the burn. Electricity can affect the heart, so be prepared to resuscitate if necessary.*
• *It is a chemical burn? Take care not to contaminate yourself. Flood the injured part for at least 20 minutes, taking care that the water flows away from the injured person, any bystanders and you. Remove contaminated clothes if it safe to do so.*
• *It is a scald? A scald is a burn caused by wet heat, such as steam from a kettle. Apply cold water and cover. If possible, remove or cool clothing.*

POISONING

A poison is any substance that enters the body and causes temporary or permanent harm. In large doses many substances are poisonous, but the word is generally used to describe substances such as arsenic that are harmful in small amounts. For more information on poisoning, see pages 120–128.

Signs and symptoms of poisoning

Different poisons will have different effects on the body, and will be modified by the quantity and the time since exposure to the body.

Potential effects of poisons include:

- *Being sick*
- *The casualty becomes increasingly drowsy*
- *Difficulty in breathing*
- *Change in heart rate*
- *Erratic and confused behaviour*
- *Burns*
- *Pain*
- *Liver and kidney problems*

TREATMENT

1 *Protect yourself and any bystanders from the source of the poison.*

2 *Monitor and maintain the casualty's airway and breathing and be prepared to resuscitate if necessary.*

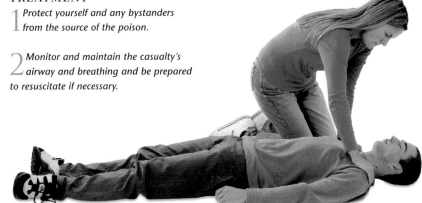

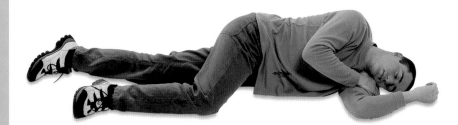

3 *Seek appropriate medical help and assistance from the emergency services to deal with dangerous substances.*

4 *Monitor the victim's level of consciousness and be prepared to turn into the recovery position if necessary.*

5 *Support the victim if he or she is sick and keep the airway clear.*

6 *Treat any burns caused by corrosive poisons if you can do so safely.*

7 *Try to identify the source of the poison and inform medical staff of your findings.*

DO
- *Protect yourself: some poisons only need to come into contact with the skin or be breathed in to cause serious problems. Wear protective clothing and a face mask if these are available.*
- *Look for clues as to the source of the poison to hand over to medical staff – but do not make assumptions.*

DO NOT
- *Try and make the person sick.*
- *Give an antidote unless you have been trained to do so.*

WHAT IF
- *The person stops breathing? Give rescue breaths; check circulation. If the person has swallowed a corrosive poison, use a face mask.*

ALLERGIC REACTIONS: ANAPHYLACTIC SHOCK

Anaphylactic shock is an extreme allergic reaction that has an intense effect on the body. Anaphylaxis can happen very quickly, within seconds, and if not dealt with promptly, it can lead to death. For further information, see Anaphylactic Shock, pages 46–47.

Signs and symptoms of anaphylactic shock

- Difficulty breathing
- Pale skin and cyanosis
- Blotches on the skin
- Rapid pulse
- Breathing or heartbeat stops
- History of contact with allergen, the thing that triggers the attack

DO
- Make an early call for emergency help.
- Help the affected person to find her own medication.

DO NOT
- Move the casualty around as this will place extra pressure on the heart and lungs.

WHAT IF
- After the person administers the injection her condition improves? Ask her what she would like to do next. Advise her to seek swift medical attention.

TREATING ANAPHYLACTIC SHOCK

1 Call an ambulance immediately. The casualty needs adrenalin to counteract the reaction.

2 If the casualty is a known sufferer, he or she may have an adrenaline injection. Help the person to take this. If the casualty is unable to do this, you may give the injection if you have been trained to do so.

3 Sit the casualty in the most comfortable position and reassure her.

If the casualty becomes unconscious, turn her into the recovery position. Monitor the casualty's breathing and circulation and be prepared to resuscitate if necessary.

RESOURCES

Many organisations throughout the UK provide information and support for specific medical conditions, including charities, self-help groups and government agencies. Only a limited number of organisations can be included in this list – You will find further useful links on the Internet.

GENERAL INFORMATION
British Medical Association
BMA House
Tavistock Square
London WC1H 9JP
Tel: 020 7387 4499
www.bma.org.uk

Department of Health
Richmond House
79 Whitehall
London SW1A 2NS
Tel: 020 7210 4850
www.doh.gov.uk

NHS Direct Online
www.nhsdirect.nhs.uk

AGEING
Age Concern
1268 London Road
London SW16 4ER
Tel: 020 8765 7200
www.ace.org.uk

ALLERGY AND ASTHMA
Anaphylaxis Campaign
PO Box 149
Fleet
Hampshire GU13 9ZU
Tel: 01252 542029
www.anaphylaxis.org.uk

British Allergy Foundation
30 Bellegrove Road
Welling
Kent DA16 3PY
Tel: 020 8303 8525
www.allergyfoundation.com

National Asthma Campaign
Providence House
Providence Place
London N1 0NT
Tel: 020 7226 2260
www.asthma.org.uk

ALZHEIMER'S DISEASE
Alzheimer's Disease Society
10 Greencoat Place
London SW1P 1PH
Tel: 020 7306 0606
www.alzheimers.org.uk

ARTHRITIS
Arthritis Care
18 Stephenson Way
London NW1 2HD
Tel: 020 7916 1500
www.arthritiscare.org.uk

Arthritis Research Campaign
Copeman House
St Mary's Gate
Chesterfield
Derbyshire S41 7TD
Tel: 01246 558033
www.arc.org.uk

BLOOD DISORDERS
Leukaemia Research Fund
43 Great Ormond Street
London WC1N 3JJ
Tel: 020 7405 0101
www.leukaemia.demon.co.uk

Sickle Cell Society
54 Station Road
Harlesden
London NW10 4UA
Tel: 020 8961 4006
www.sicklecellsociety.org

CANCER
Breast Cancer Campaign
29–33 Scrutton Street
London EC2A 4HU
Tel: 020 7749 3700

Imperial Cancer Research Fund
PO Box 123
Lincoln's Inn Fields
London WC2 3PX
Tel: 020 7242 0200
www.icnet.uk

Macmillan Cancer Relief
15–19 Britten Street
London SW3 3TZ
Tel: 020 7351 7811
www.macmillan.org.uk

CHILD HEALTH
Cancer and Leukaemia in
Childhood
12–13 King Square
Bristol BS2 8JH
Tel: 0117 924 8844
www.clic.uk.com

Children with AIDS Charity
9 Denbigh Street
London SW1V 2HF
Tel: 020 7233 5966
www.cwac.org

Great Ormond Street Hospital
for Children NHS Trust
Great Ormond Street
London WC1N 3JH
Tel: 020 7405 9200
www.gosh.org

Institute of Child Health
30 Guildford Street
London WC1N 1EH
Tel: 020 7242 9789
www.ich.ucl.ac.uk

National Children's Bureau
8 Wakely Street
London EC1V 1NG
Tel: 020 7843 2299
www.ncb.org.uk

COMPLEMENTARY THERAPIES
British Medical Acupuncture
Society
Newton House
Newton Lane
Whitley
Warrington
Cheshire WA4 4JA
Tel: 01925 730727
www.medical-acupuncture.co.uk

British Homeopathic Association
15 Clerkenwell Close
London EC1R 0AA
Tel: 020 7566 7800
www.trusthomeopathy.org

National Institute of Medical
Herbalists
56 Longbrook Street
Exeter
Devon EX4 6AH
Tel: 01392 426022
www.nimh.org

COUNSELLING
Alcoholics Anonymous
PO Box 1
Stonebow House
Stonebow Road
York YO1 2NJ
Tel: 01904 644026
www.alcoholics-
anonymous.org.uk

British Association for
Counselling
1 Regent Place
Rugby
Warwickshire CV21 2PJ
Tel: 01788 550899
www.counselling.co.uk

RELATE
Herbert Gray College
Little Church Street
Rugby CV21 3AP
Tel: 01788 573241
www.relate.org.uk

DIABETES
British Diabetic Association
10 Queen Anne Street
London W1M 0BD
Tel: 020 7323 1531
www.diabetes.org.uk

DIGESTIVE DISORDERS
British Colostomy Association
15 Station Road
Reading
Berkshire RG1 1LG
Tel: 0800 328 4257
www.bcass.org.uk

Digestive Disorders Foundation
3 St Andrew's Place
London NW1 4LB
Tel: 020 7486 0341
www.digestivedisorders.org.uk

National Association for Colitis
and Crohn's Disease
4 Beamont House
Sutton Road
St Albans
Herts AL1 5HH
Tel: 01727 844296
www.nacc.org.uk

EATING DISORDERS
Eating Disorders Association
103 Prince of Wales Road
Norwich NR1 1DW
Tel: 0845 634 1414
www.edauk.com

EPILEPSY
British Epilepsy Association
New Anstey House
Gateway Drive
Leeds LS19 7XY
Tel: 0113 210 8800
www.epilepsy.org.uk

EYE DISORDERS
International Glaucoma
Association
King's College Hospital
Denmark Hill
London SE5 9RA
Tel: 020 7737 3265
www.iga.org.uk

Royal National Institute for
the Blind
224 Great Portland Street
London W1N 6AA
Te: 020 7388 1266
www.rnib.org.uk

FAMILY PLANNING
British Pregnancy Advisory
Service
Austy Manor
Wootton Warren
Solihull
West Midlands B95 6BX
Tel: 01564 793225
www.bpas.demon.co.uk

Family Planning Association
2–12 Pentonville Road
London N1 9FP
Tel: 020 7837 5432
www.fpa.org.uk

FIRST AID
British Red Cross Society
9 Grosvenor Crescent
London SW1X 7EJ
Tel: 020 7235 5454
www.redcross.org.uk

St John Ambulance
63 York Street
London W1H 1PS
Tel: 020 7258 3456
www.st-john-ambulance.org.uk

HEADACHE
Migraine Trust
45 Great Ormond Street
London WC1N 3HZ
Tel: 020 7831 4818
www.migrainetrust.org

HEAD INJURY
British Brain and Spine
Foundation
7 Winchester House
Kennington Park
Cranmer Road
London SW9 6EJ
Tel: 020 7793 5900
www.bbsf.org.uk

HEARING DISORDERS
British Deaf Association
1–3 Worship Street
London EC2A 2AB
Tel: 020 7588 3520
www.bda.org.uk

British Tinnitus Association
4th Floor
White Building
Fitzalan Square
Sheffield S1 2AZ
www.tinnitus.org.uk

HEART AND CIRCULATORY DISORDERS
British Heart Foundation
14 Fitzhardinge Street
London W1H 4DH
Tel: 020 7935
www.bhf.org.uk

High Blood Pressure Foundation
Department of Medical Sciences
Western General Hospital
Edinburgh EH4 2XU
Tel: 0131 332 9211
www.hgpf.org.uk

The Stroke Association
Stroke House
Whitecross Street
London EC1Y 8JJ
Tel: 020 7566 0300
www.stroke.org.uk

HORMONAL AND METABOLIC DISORDERS
British Thyroid Association
PO Box 97
Clifford
Wetherby
West Yorkshire LS23 6XD
www.british-thyroid-association.org

Child Growth Foundation
2 Mayfield Avenue
Chiswick
London W4 1PW
Tel: 020 8994 7625
www.cgf.org.uk

Climb (Reserach Trust for
Metabolic Diseases in Children)
The Quadrangle
Crewe Hall
Weston Road
Crewe
Cheshire CW1 6UR
Tel: 01270 250221

Thyroid UK
32 Darcy Road
St Osyth
Clacton-on-Sea
Essex CO16 8QF
www.thyroiduk.org

INFERTILITY
Human Fertilisation and
Embryology Authority
Paxton House
30 Artillery Lane
London E1 7LS
Tel: 020 7377 5077
www.hfea.org.uk

National Fertility Association
114 Lichfield Street
Walsall
West Midlands WS1 1SZ
Tel: 01922 722888
www.issue.co.uk

LEARNING DISORDERS
British Dyslexia Association
98 London Road
Reading RG1 5AU
Tel: 0118 966 2677
www.bda-dyslexia.org.uk

Down's Syndrome Association
155 Mitcham Road
London SW17 9PG
Tel: 020 8682 4001
www.downs-syndrome.org.uk

Dyspraxia Foundation
8 West Alley
Hitchin
Hertfordshire SG5 1EG
Tel: 01462 454986
www.dyspraxiafoundation.org.uk

MENCAP
Royal Society for Mentally
Handicapped Children and Adults
MENCAP National Centre
123 Golden Lane
London EC1Y 0RT
Tel: 020 7454 0454
www.mencap.org.uk

National Autistic Society
393 City Road
London EC1V 1NG
Tel: 020 7833 2299
www.nas.org.uk

MEN'S HEALTH
Everyman, Action Against Male
Cancer
Institute of Cancer Research
Freepost LON 922
London SW7 3YY
Tel: 0800 731 9468
www.icr.ac.uk/everyman

Orchid Cancer Appeal
9 Grace Close
Hainault
Essex IG6 3DW
www.orchid-cancer.org.uk

Prostate Cancer Charity
Du Cane Road
London W12 0NN
Tel: 020 8383 8124
www.prostate-cancer.org.uk

MENTAL HEALTH
Depression Alliance
35 Westminster Bridge Road
London SE1 7JB
Tel: 020 7633 0557
www.depressionalliance.og

Mental Health Foundation
UK Office
20–21 Cornwall Terrace
London NW1 4QL
Tel: 020 7535 7400
www.mentalhealth.org.uk

MIND
15–19 Broadway
London E15 4BQ
Tel: 020 8522 1728
www.mind.org.uk

National Schizophrenia
Fellowship
30 Tabernacle Street
London EC2A 4DD
Tel: 020 7330 9100
www.nsf.org.uk

International Stress Management
Association
Division of Psychology
South Bank University
103 Borough Road
London SE1 0AA
Tel: 0700 780430
www.isma.org

MUSCULOSKELETAL DISORDERS
Arthritis Research Campaign
Copeman House
St Mary's Gate
Chesterfield
Derbyshire S41 7TD
Tel: 01246 558033
www.arc.org.uk

British Society for Rheumatology
41 Eagle Street
London WC1R 4AR
Tel: 020 7242 3313
www.rheumatology.org.uk

National Osteoporosis Society
PO Box 10
Radstock
Bath BA3 3YB
Tel: 01761 471771
www.nos.org.uk

NEUROLOGICAL DISORDERS
Motor Neurone Disease
Association
PO Box 246
Northampton NN1 2PR
Tel: 01604 250505
www.mndassociation.org

Multiple Sclerosis Society
25 Effie Road
London SW6 1EE
Tel: 020 7610 7171
www.mssociety.org.uk

Muscular Dystrophy Campaign
7–11 Prescott Place
London SW4 6BS
Tel: 020 7720 8055
www.muscular-dystrophy.org

Parkinson's Disease Society
215 Vauxhall Bridge Road
London SW1V 1EJ
Tel: 020 7931 8080
www.parkinsons.org.uk

NUTRITION
British Nutrition Foundation
52–54 High Holborn
London WC1V 6RQ
Tel: 020 7404 6505
www.nutrition.org.uk

PREGNANCY AND CHILDBIRTH
Miscarriage Association
Clayton Hospital
Northgate
Wakefield WF1 3JS
Tel: 01924 200795
www.the-ma.org.uk

National Childbirth Trust
Alexandra House
Oldham Terrace
London W3 6NH
Tel: 020 8992 8637
www.nct.online.org

TAMBA (Twins and Multiple
Births Association)
309 Chester Road
Little Sutton
South Wirral L66 1TH
Tel: 0870 121 4000

REHABILITATION
emPOWER
Rehabilitaton Centre
Roehampton Lane
London SW15 5PR
Tel: 020 8788 1777
www.empowernet.org

RADAR
12 City Forum
250 City Road
London EC1V 8AF
Tel: 020 7250 3222
www.radar.org.uk

SAFETY AND HEALTH
Health and Safety Executive
Health and Safety Laboratory
Broad Lane
Sheffield S3 7HQ
Tel: 0114 289 2333
www.open.gov.uk/hse

Royal Society for the Prevention
of Accidents
353 Bristol Road
Edgbaston
Birmingham B5 7ST
Tel: 0121 248 200

SEXUALLY TRANSMITTED DISEASES
Health Development Agency
Holborn Gate
330 High Holborn
London WC1V 7BA
Tel: 020 7430 0850
www.hda-online.org.uk

Society of Health Advisers in
Sexually Transmitted Diseases
MSF Centre
33–37 Moreland Street
London EC1V 8HA
www.shastd.org.uk

Terrence Higgins Trust
(HIV and AIDS)
52–54 Grays Inn Road
London WC1X 8JU
Tel: 020 7831 0330
www.tht.org.uk

SKIN PROBLEMS
National Eczema Society
163 Eversholt Street
London NW1 1BU
Tel: 7388 4097
www.eczema.org

Psoriasis Association
7 Milton Street
Northampton NN2 7JG
Tel: 020 7388 0266
www.psoriasis-association.org.uk

SLEEP DISORDERS
British Snoring and Sleep Apnoea
Association
1 Duncroft Close
Reigate
Surrey RH2 9DE
Tel: 01249 701010
www.britishsnoring.demon.co.uk

Narcolepsy Association UK
Craven House
1st Floor
121 Kingsway
London WC2B 6PA
Tel: 020 7721 8904
www.narcolepsy.org.uk

SMOKING
Action on Smoking and Health
102 Clifton Street
London EC2A 4HW
Tel: 020 7739 5902
www.ash.org.uk

SPEECH AND LANGUAGE DISORDERS
Association for All Speech-
Impaired Children
69–85 Old Street
London EC1V 9HX
Tel: 020 7841 8900
www.afasic.org.uk

British Stammering Association
15 Old Ford Road
London E2 9PJ
Tel: 020 8983 1003
www.stammer.demon.do.uk

TRAVEL HEALTH
Department of Health
Richmond House
79 Whitehall
London SW1A 2NS
Tel: 020 7210 4850
www.doh.gov.uk

URINARY SYSTEM DISORDERS
Continence Foundation
307 Hatton Square
16 Baldwins Gardens
London EC1N 7RJ
Tel: 020 7404 6875
www.vois.org.uk

Interstitial Cystitis Support
Group
76 High Street
Stony Stratford
Buckinghamshire MK11 1AH
Tel: 01908 569 0169
www.interstitialcystitis.co.uk

National Kidney Research Fund
3 Archers Court
Stukeley Road
Huntingdon PE18 6XG
Tel: 01480 454828
www.nkrf.org.uk

WOMEN'S HEALTH
Action Against Breast Cancer
C2
Culham Science Centre
Oxfordshire OX14 3DB
Tel: 01865 407384
www.aabc.org.uk

Breast Cancer Campaign
29–33 Scrutton Street
London EC2A 4HU
Tel: 020 7749 3700
www.bcc-uk.org

National Association for
Premenstrual Syndrome
41 Old Road
East Peckham
Kent TN12 5AP
Tel: 0870 777 2177
www.pms.org.uk

National Endometriosis Society
50 Westminster Palace Gardens
Artillery Row
London SW1P 1RL
Tel: 020 7222 2781
www.endo.org.uk

Women's National Cancer
Control Campaign
128–130 Curtain Road
London EC2A 3AR
Tel: 020 7729 4688
www.wncc.org.uk

GLOSSARY

Abdomen Part of the body below the chest (from which it is separated by the diaphragm) which contains the organs of digestion and also in women the ovaries and uterus.

Acupuncture Ancient Chinese system of healing in which thin metal needles are inserted into selected points in the skin to relieve symptoms.

Acute Disorder or symptom that comes on suddenly and is usually short-lived.

Adrenal glands Two glands on top of the kidneys producing hormones, chemical messengers that have widespread effects on the body.

Adrenaline Hormone released by the adrenal glands that increases the heart rate in response to stress, exercise and emotions such as excitement and fear.

Aeorobic Designed to increase oxygen intake and benefit the heart and lungs (when used in the context of exercise).

Allergen Substance such as pollen, dust and mould that causes an allergic reaction in a hypersensitive person.

Allergy Abnormal response by the body to a food or foreign substance, having either local or general effects, varying from asthma and hay fever to rashes and in extreme cases anaphylactic shock, whereby airway constriction, swelling, heart failure and circulatory collapse can rapidly lead to death.

Amino acid Organic substance needed to form proteins. Essential amino acids have to be obtained from food as the body cannot make them itself.

Anaesthesia Technique by which an individual's sensation of pain is reduced or abolished to enable surgery to be performed, usually effected by administering drugs, although it can also be achieved through hypnosis or acupuncture.

Analgesic Drug that relieves pain; mild analgesics such as aspirin also reduce fever and inflammation.

Angiography Technique using contrast dye and X-rays to produce images of the arteries.

Antacid Drug or remedy that neutralizes the secretion of hydrochloric acid in the stomach.

Antibiotic Substance that destroys or prevents the growth of bacteria and is used to treated infections. May alter the body's microbial balance, causing infections such as thrush.

Antibody Blood protein responsible for destroying invading antigens such as a virus, bacterium or allergen.

Anticoagulant Agent that stops blood clotting, used to prevent the formation of blood clots or break up existing ones.

Antidepressant Drug that alleviates the symptoms of depression, but may cause side-effects such as drowsiness.

Antidote Drug that counteracts the effects of overdose by another drug or poison.

Antifungal Substance used to treat fungal infections that inactivates or kills fungi.

Antigen Substance the body considers foreign and possibly dangerous, triggering an immune response and production of an antibody.

Antihistamine Substance that prevents or treats a histamine reaction and often make the person drowsy as a side-effect.

Antioxidant Agent that neutralises free radicals, naturally occurring particles that can cause cell degeneration and decay, and hence health problems.

Antipyretic Drug that lowers body temperature, thus reducing fever. Painkillers such as aspirin and paracetamol are also antipyretics.

Aromatherapy Therapeutic use of essential oils, concentrated plant essences.

Autoimmune disease Disorder, such as rheumatoid arthritis, caused by a defect in the immune system, which produces antibodies by mistake to destroy the body's own healthy tissues.

Autonomic nervous system Part of the nervous system concerned with functions such as heart-rate and breathing which do not require conscious thought. It is divided into the sympathetic and parasympathetic nervous systems, which balance each other and work by reflex action.

Bacteria Single-celled micro-organisms, some of which cause disease.

Beta blocker Drug that helps regulate heart rate, used to treat angina and reduce high blood pressure.

Biopsy Removal of a small piece of tissue for examination in a laboratory.

Biphosphonates Drugs that prevent bone loss and increase bone density, used to treat osteoporosis.

Botulism Serious form of food poisoning that affects the nervous system and can be fatal.

Bronchodilator Agent that relaxes muscles in the airways used to relieve asthma and bronchitis.

Carbohydrate Starches and sugars present in food and the body's main source of energy.

Carbon dioxide Colourless gas formed in the tissues during metabolism and transported in the blood to the lungs, where it is breathed out.

Cardiovascular Relating to the heart and all blood vessels (veins, venules, arteries and capillaries).

Cartilage Dense, protective connective tissue found in adults in the ear, spine, respiratory system and covering the surface of bones at joints.

Central nervous system Brain and spinal cord, which receive and analyse sensory data then initiate an appropriate response.

Chiropractic System of treating disease by manipulating the spine, joints and muscles.

Cholesterol Fat-like material present in blood and tissues, high levels of which can damage arteries.

Chronic Disorder or condition of long duration, but does not imply anything about the severity of the disease. Compare with **acute**.

Cognitive Behavioural Therapy Popular psychotherapy used in treating disorders such as stress-related illnesses, alcohol dependency, phobias and eating problems, that aims to teach new ways of thinking and behaving.

Complementary Alternative forms of treatment that support conventional medicine.

Compress Pad soaked in hot or cold substance and applied to the affected part of the body to relieve swelling and pain.

Concussion Condition characterised by headache, confusion and memory loss caused by head injury.

Convulsion Involuntary muscle contraction that is a feature of epilepsy; febrile convulsions are caused by fever in otherwise healthy infants.

Corticosteroids Hormones produced by the adrenal glands involved in metabolism that also help to control blood pressure and the body's salt and water balance.

CPR (cardiopulmonary resuscitation) Set of procedures applied when a person is not breathing and his or her heart may have stopped to keep the person alive until help arrives.

Crush syndrome Condition arising when toxins that have built up around the site of an injury by being trapped by an object are suddenly released into the bloodstream, flooding the kidneys. The syndrome can be fatal.

Cryotherapy The use of extreme cold to freeze and destroy unwanted tissues, such as verrucas.

CT scan (computerised tomography) Technique using X-rays and computers to produce a cross section of the part of the body being examined.

Cyanosis Bluish tinge to the skin resulting from lack of oxygen in the blood.

Defibrillation Brief electric shock given to the heart when it has stopped beating.

Diastolic blood pressure Recording that measures the relaxation of the heart between beats.

Diuretic Drug that increases the amount of urine produced, used to reduce water retention.

DNA (deoxyribonucleic acid) Molecule carrying genetic information in nearly every cell of the body.

Down's syndrome Condition arising from a genetic abnormality in which an extra chromosome is present.

Dressing Piece of material that covers a wound to staunch bleeding or protect it from infection.

ECG (electrocardiogram) Recording of electrical activity in different areas of the heart.

Echocardiogram Use of ultrasound to show the action of the heart as it beats.

ECT (electroconvulsive therapy) Treatment for severe depression and psychosis involving the passage of an electric current through the brain.

Ectopic Pregnancy that occurs outside the uterus, generally in the Fallopian tube.

EEG (Electroencephalogram) Recording of electrical activity in different parts of the brain.

Endocrine gland Gland that manufactures and releases hormones.

Endorphins Morphine-like chemicals produced by the brain to relieve pain and are also responsible for the sensation of pleasure.

Endoscope Instrument used to examine the interior of the body.

Enzyme Protein that acts as a catalyst to speed up a biological reation; essential for body function.

Epidural Term given to method of pain relief commonly used during labour, whereby anaesthetic is injected into the epidural space in the spinal cord.

Episiotomy Incision made in the area between the anus and the vagina (the perineum) to facilitate the delivery of a baby.

Essential fatty acid One of a group of unsaturated fats essential for growth.

Fat One of the three main constituents of food, needed for the absorption of vitamins and to provide an adequate supply of essential fatty acids.

Fight-or-flight response The way in which the body responds to perceived or actual danger through a series of biochemical actions, making it more efficient in fighting or fleeing.

Free radicals Natural by-products of metabolism, these particles can damage DNA and cause a range of problems from high cholesterol levels to depleted immune system.

Gas exchange Process that takes place within the alveoli in the lungs of the exchange of waste product carbon dioxide from the body cells for fresh oxygen.

Glucagon Hormone produced by the pancreas that causes blood sugar level to rise.

Glycogen Main form in which carbohydrate is stored in the body, in the liver and muscles.

H_2 blocker Drug that reduces production of stomach acid, used to treat ulcers.

Haemoglobin Oxygen-carrying substance contained within red blood cells, responsible for their colour.

Hepatitis Inflammation of the liver caused by infection, toxins or immune system problems.

Homeopathy Therapy based on the principle of 'like cures like', meaning that what causes a disease can, when given in minute amounts, cure it.

Hormone Chemical messenger produced in one part of the body that travels in the bloodstream to affect the structure or function of another part.

Hormone replacement therapy (HRT) Use of a natural or synthetic hormone to treat a hormone deficiency; normally refers to the use of oestrogen to treat symptoms of the menopause.

Hyperglycaemia Excess glucose (sugar) in the bloodstream which may lead to coma if untreated.

Hypertension High blood pressure, elevated above the normal range expected.

Hyperventilation Occurs when rapid breathing reduces levels of carbon dioxide in the blood.

Hypoglycaemia Deficiency of glucose (sugar) in the blood which may lead to coma if untreated.

Hypothalamus Part of the brain that controls the endocrine system and regulates sleep, body temperature, water content and sexual function.

Hypothermia Reduction of body temperature below the normal range.

Immune system Organs responsible for immunity, the ability to resist infection.

Immunoglobin Type of protein that acts as an antibody, destroying invading foreign substances.

Induction The starting of labour by artificial means, with drugs that stimulate uterine contractions or by rupturing the amniotic membranes surrounding the baby inside the uterus.

In-vitro fertilization Whereby an egg is fertilised in a laboratory and then implanted inside the uterus.

Infection Invasion of the body by disease-causing organisms, which multiply and cause illness.

Inflammation The body's response to injury, whether caused by chemicals, physical agents or infection. Inflammation involves pain, heat, redness, swelling and loss of function of the affected part.

Infusion Water-based preparation in which the flowers, leaves or stems of a plant are brewed in a similar way to tea.

Jaundice Yellowing of the skin or whites of the eyes caused by an excess of bilirubin (a bile pigment) in the blood, a symptom of hepatitis.

Keratin Type of protein that is the main constituent of hair, nails and skin.

Keyhole surgery Also known as minimally invasive surgery, such as that performed using an endoscope passed through a tiny incision, to enable the patient to make a faster recovery.

Lymph Fluid derived from blood that bathes tissues before being circulated into the bloodstream, and plays an important part in the immune system.

Lymphatic system Vessels and nodes throughout the body that filter and carry lymph and prevent foreign bodies from entering the bloodstream.

Mammography X-ray technique used in the diagnosis of breast cancer.

Melanin Dark pigment in the hair, eyes and skin, the production of which in the skin is increased by the action of sunlight.

Melatonin Hormone produced by the pineal gland that helps regulate the body's sleep cycle.

Menopause Time in a woman's life when the ovaries cease to produce egg cells and she is no longer able to bear children.

Metabolism Chemical processes that take place in the body, and the means by which food is converted into energy for use in the body.

MRI (Magnetic Resonance Imaging) Diagnostic technique that uses high-frequency radio waves to examine tissues, particularly those of the nervous system.

Mucous membranes Moist, mucus-producing membranes lining many structures and cavities.

Neurotransmitter Chemical released from nerve endings to transmit impulses to other nerves and the muscles or glands they supply.

Noradrenaline Hormone secreted by the adrenal glands, related to adrenaline and with similar actions. It also acts as a neurotransmitter.

NSAIDs (non-steroidal anti-inflammatory drugs) Painkillers used to relieve pain and inflammation, particularly in the muscles, ligaments and joints. They work by blocking the production of prostaglandins (released when tissue is damaged), thus reducing inflammation.

Oestrogen Hormone produced mainly in the ovaries, responsible for the growth and function of the female sex organs and the development of female secondary sexual characteristics such as breast development.

Organ Part of the body comprised of tissues that forms a structure such as the heart, responsible for a particular function.

Osteopathy System of manipulating the bones, muscles and joints to restore health.

Oxygen Colourless gas breathed into the lungs from air and essential for life because it is needed for metabolism.

Palpitations Awareness of the heartbeat when it seems to beat irregularly or more forcefully, often due to emotional causes, rapid breathing or vigorous exercise.

Parasympathetic nervous system One of the two divisions of the autonomic nervous system, which is dominant when the body is at rest.

Peripheral nervous system Parts of the nervous system lying outside the brain and spinal cord, such as the cranial nerves and the spinal nerves.

Peristalsis Involuntary wave-like muscular action; usally refers to the movement of the intestines that propels food along the digestive tract.

Pessary Solid medinical preparation designed for insertion into the vagina.

Pituitary gland Gland responsible for controlling the release of hormones into the blood from other types of endocrine gland.

Plasma Straw-coloured fluid in which the blood cells are suspended.

Pneumothorax Condition arising when air enters the pleural cavity (the space between the lung surface and the chest wall), causing the lung to collapse, often as a result of chest injury.

Progesterone Sex hormone that prepares the uterus for a fertilized ovum and maintains the uterus throughout pregnancy.

Prostaglandins Naturally occurring hormone-like substances that have many actions, such as causing muscle contractions and dilation of blood vessels.

Protein The basic material of all living cells, it is obtained from the digestion of amino acids present in food and synthesised in the body.

Proteinuria The presence of protein in the urine, which may be a sign of kidney damage.

Proton pump inhibitor Drug that reduces stomach acid, used to heal ulcers.

Radiotherapy Treatment of diseases such as cancer with radioactive waves.

Rescue breaths Method of maintaining a flow of air into and out of a patient's lungs when his own breathing reflexes are absent or insufficient.

Salmonella Type of bacterium often present in eggs or poultry that causes food poisoning.

Saturated fat Highly concentrated fat containing fatty acids and cholesterol, usually derived from animal products.

Sebum Oily substance secreted by the sebaceous glands that forms a thin film of fat over the skin, keeping skin lubricated by preventing water evaporation, and forming a barrier against bacteria.

Serotonin Substance present mainly in the blood, intestines and central nervous system. It acts mainly as a neurotransmitter, relaying information across nerve endings, and is thought to have an important effect on mood.

Shock State of collapse, which can be life-threatening, characterised by pale, cold, clammy skin, faintness, fast, weak pulse, shallow breathing, confusion and eventual deterioration into unconsciousness.

SSRI (selective serotonin reuptake inhibitor) Drug used to treat depression that blocks the reabsorption of the neurotransmitter serotonin, resulting in higher levels of serotonin in the brain.

STD (sexually transmitted disease) Disease transmitted by sexual intercourse.

Steroid drugs Artificial drugs that mimic the actions of naturally occurring hormones such as the sex hormones and corticosteroids produced by the adrenal glands.

Stoma Artificial opening of a tube such as the colon that has been brought to the surface of the abdomen in order to drain it.

Suppository Medicinal preparation suitable for insertion into the vagina or rectum.

Sympathetic nervous system The part of the autonomic nervous system that prepares the body for action.

Systolic blood pressure Measurement of pressure of blood against the walls of the main arteries when the heart muscle is contracting.

Testosterone Main male sex hormone, which stimulates the development of secondary sexual characteristics such as facial hair and the development of male sex organs.

Tetanus Infectious disease affecting the nervous system caused by bacteria.

Thrombosis Condition in which blood in a vessel becomes solid and forms a blood clot. Thrombosis in an artery obstructs the flow of blood and oxygen to the tissue it supplies, and can cause stroke and heart attack.

Tissues Collections of specialised cells that perform certain functions in the body.

Tourniquet Cord or rubber tube used to press upon an artery to prevent flow of blood through it, generally used when taking blood pressure. No longer recommended as a first-aid technique to stop bleeding because of the danger of reducing oxygen supply to other tissues.

Toxaemia Blood poisoning caused by bacteria growing in a site of infection.

Toxins Poisons and waste products produced by the body.

Ultrasound High frequency sound waves used to produce images of the interior of the body and to break up kidney stones.

Unsaturated (and polyunsaturated) fat Fat that contains fatty acids but no cholesterol.

Vaccination Means of producing immunity to a disease by using a material to stimulate the formation of appropriate antibodies.

Vasodilator Drug used to reduce blood pressure because it widens blood vessels and increases blood flow.

Vertebra One of the 33 bones which make up the backbone, through which passes the spinal cord.

Virus Minute agent capable of multiplying within living cells and responsible for many diseases.

Vitamins and minerals Essential substances needed for healthy growth and development that, apart from vitamin K and vitamin D, cannot be made in the body and have to be obtained from the diet instead.

Whiplash Damage to the soft tissues in the neck casued by sudden jerking back of the head and neck, often in car crash victims hit from behind.

X-ray Diagnostic technique using electromagnetic radiation to produce images of the body.

INDEX

Page numbers in bold indicate main references to subjects.

ACKNOWLEDGEMENTS

The publishers would like to thank the following for the use of pictures:

Corbis:
pp:145L, 156R, 157L, 208, 266, 269T, 273T, 288, 290CR, 306, 311C, 336, 364, 369BL, 372, 374T, 375T, 378C, 381T, 393, 412, 416, 418T, 442, 443T, 444B, 445T, 446, 447, 450, 451, 452, 453, 454, 455TR&B, 456, 457, 458.

GettyOneStone:
pp:12, 146T, 147B, 148, 169, 188, 198, 203, 204, 206, 228, 236, 239, 253, 259T, 277B, 283T, 295, 297, 317T, 319B, 320BR, 324, 325B, 327B, 341, 356, 368, 379T, 420, 436L, 459TL.

Image Bank:
pp:220, 229B, 246, 257B, 259B, 271LC, 279T, 29LT, 296, 300, 343, 349, 350, 353, 397T.

Science Photo Library:
pp:210, 268, 284, 290BR, 312, 326BR, 338, 346, 347, 365, 369T&R, 376, 377B, 378T, 397B, 398, 402B, 403, 407, 411, 417, 421R, 422T, 424, 428, 430B, 449, 456TL, 459TR, 460, 461.

Telegraph Colour Library:
pp:109B, 195, 207B, 227, 248, 255, 273B, 275, 276, 303B, 342, 370, 385.

Special thanks are also due to:

All models who participated in the studio photography; Anita Kerwin-Nye and Gloria Moss of The Red Cross UK, Sussex Branch for the provision of a first aid trainer and first aid equipment; Paul Clayton of J. S. Clayton Ltd for the loan of first aid boxes; *The Outdoor Centre*, Lewes, East Sussex for the loan of outdoor and camping equipment.